THE SUPREME ART AND SCIENCE OF

RĀJA & KRIYĀ YOGA

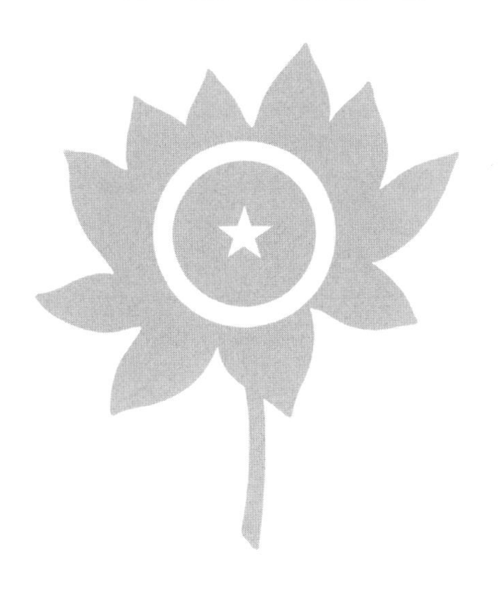

of related interest

The Four Dignities
The Spiritual Practice of Walking, Standing, Sitting and Lying Down
Cain Carroll
ISBN 978 1 84819 216 4
eISBN 978 0 85701 166 4

Mudras of India
A Comprehensive Guide to the Hand Gestures of Yoga and Indian Dance
Cain Carroll and Revital Carroll
Foreword by Dr. David Frawley
ISBN 978 1 84819 084 9 (hardback)
ISBN 978 1 84819 109 9 (paperback)
eISBN 978 0 85701 067 4

The Healing Power of Mudras
The Yoga of the Hands
Rajendar Menen
ISBN 978 1 84819 043 6
eISBN 978 0 85701 024 7

Ayurvedic Healing
Contemporary Maharishi Āyurveda Medicine and Science
2nd edition
Hari Sharma, MD and Christopher Clark, MD
ISBN 978 1 84819 069 6
eISBN 978 0 85701 063 6

Ayurvedic Medicine
The Principles of Traditional Practice
Sebastian Pole
ISBN 978 1 84819 113 6
eISBN 978 0 85701 091 9

THE SUPREME ART AND SCIENCE OF

RĀJA & KRIYĀ YOGA

The Ultimate Path to Self-Realisation

Stephen Sturgess

Foreword by Dr David Frawley

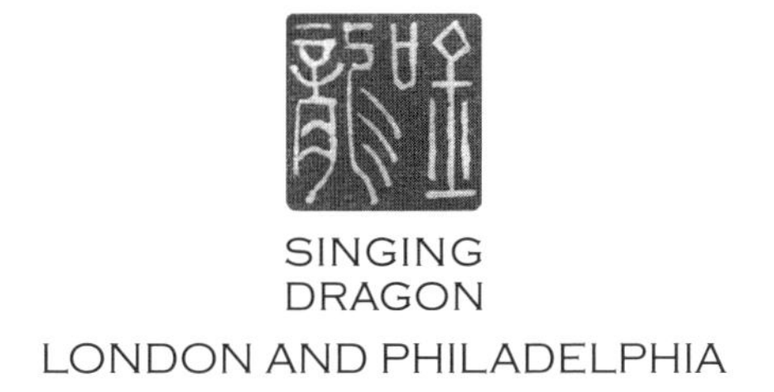

SINGING DRAGON
LONDON AND PHILADELPHIA

First published in 2015
by Singing Dragon
an imprint of Jessica Kingsley Publishers
73 Collier Street
London N1 9BE, UK
and
400 Market Street, Suite 400
Philadelphia, PA 19106, USA

www.singingdragon.com

Library of Congress Cataloging in Publication Data
Sturgess, Stephen, 1951-
The supreme art and science of Raja and Kriya yoga : the ultimate path to self-realisation / Stephen Sturgess.
pages cm
Includes bibliographical references and index.
ISBN 978-1-84819-261-4 (alk. paper)
1. Yoga, Raja. 2. Yoga, Kriya. 3. Self-realization. I. Title.
BL1238.56.R35S78 2015
204'.36--dc23
2014047510

British Library Cataloguing in Publication Data
A CIP catalogue record for this book is available from the British Library

ISBN 978 1 84819 261 4
eISBN 978 0 85701 209 8

Printed and bound in the United States

DEDICATION

I dedicate this book with love and gratitude to Swāmi Pragyamurti, my very first Yoga teacher back in 1970, who set me with my feet firmly on the authentic Yoga path. And to those four great souls whom I was personally taught by, who were direct disciples of Swāmi Sivananda of Rishikesh (1883–1963):

Swāmi Satyananda Saraswati (1926–2009)

Swāmi Vishnudevananda (1927–1993)

Swāmi Ventakesananda (1921–1982)

Swāmi Satchidananda (1914–2002)

They taught me all about Patañjali's Eight Limbs of Yoga and more.

To Swāmi Atmananda Saraswati (1939–2003), who was the first teacher to give me the Ashram experience of discipline and austerity with love.

To His Divine Grace, A. C. Bhaktivedanta Swāmi Pabhupada (1896–1977), who gave to me blessed food (*prasadam*) from his very own hand in the Krishna temple in Māyāpur, West Bengal, in India. And who initiated me with the Sanskrit name *Vratabrighu* in a dream a year after he passed away.

To Dr Swāmi Gitananda (1906–1993) of Pondicherry, Tamil Nadu, India, who taught me all about *prāṇāyāma*.

To J. Krishnamurti (1895–1986), whom I personally met in 1981, who opened my mind to a deeper understanding of living in awareness.

To Derek Ireland (1949–1998) and Radha Ireland, who taught me the rejuvenating *Aṣṭāṅga Yoga Primary Series One*, a dynamic flow of Yoga postures, in an intensive two weeks on the Greek island of Skyros in 1986.

To Swāmi Kriyananda (1926–2013), who first initiated me into *Kriyā Yoga* and who spiritually guided me for 30 years. And to Roy Eugene Davis, who in 2011 ordained me as a *Kriyācarya (Kriyā* teacher) to teach and initiate others into *Kriyā Yoga*.

To my line of great spiritual Masters: Babaji, Lahiri Mahasaya, Swāmi Sri Yukteswar, and Paramhansa Yogananda, at whose feet I lovingly and humbly bow.

To all my spiritual brothers and sisters (*gurubhais*) at Ananda.

DISCLAIMER

CONTENTS

FOREWORD

Yoga contains much depth and many dimensions that go far beyond the common Yoga classes that have now spread throughout the world. Many Yoga teachers know this, but few have mastered the deeper teachings of Yoga and can teach these in a comprehensive manner. *The Supreme Art and Science of Kriyā and Rāja Yoga* is by a modern Yoga teacher from the West, who has articulated the deeper art and science of Yoga in detail and shared it in a practical and lucid manner.

There are many branches and traditions of Yoga and many styles of *āsana* practice. Often Yoga is divided into its higher meditational practices, *Rāja Yoga*, and its foundational practices of *āsana* and *prāṇāyama*, *Haṭha Yoga*. There is considerable overlap between these two sides of Yoga and both are part of Yoga as a whole, but we must remember that the outer practices are preliminary to the inner, not an end in themselves. More accurately, we can speak of the outer Yoga of *āsana* and physical practices, and the inner Yoga of meditation or psychological practices, with meditation being the essence of Yoga.

One of the most important modern Yoga traditions in India and worldwide is the *Kriyā Yoga* tradition that goes back to Mahavatar Babaji and Lahiri Mahasaya in the nineteenth century. The *Kriyā Yoga* line is reflected in millions of followers today, particularly through the teachings of Paramahansa Yogananda, the veritable father of Yoga in the West, who lived and taught in America in the twentieth century for over 30 years. Ancient aspects of this *Kriyā Yoga* tradition may spread back through such great yogic figures as Gorakhnath, Shankara, Patañjali and Lord Krishna. This book explores and explains the greater tradition of *Kriyā Yoga*, particularly in the modern context.

The Supreme Art and Science of Rāja and Kriyā Yoga is formulated almost like a textbook or course manual for students of Yoga, specifically *Kriyā Yoga*, and covers a number of topics in a detailed manner. The book begins by awakening the reader to our inner search for immortality and union with the Divine that forms the deepest wish of our soul. This soul orientation is the foundation for true Yoga practices, not merely wanting to feel better or become fitter, which have value but are only preliminary to the real yogic quest.

The book takes a systematic approach to the many sides of Yoga, starting with an interesting discussion on the history of Yoga from the esoteric point of view of the great Yogis. It reveals the importance of Yoga in world history and the evolution of our human species overall.

It follows with an examination of Yoga and its related spiritual philosophies. We need to understand the worldview, psychology and cosmology of Yoga in order to truly practice Yoga, not only with our bodies but also with our minds. This requires study, thinking, introspection and contemplation. The yogic vision is a cosmic vision that embraces and transcends our human culture and directs us to the eternal truth.

The book explains Yoga more through the subtle body than through the physical body, linking up to the ancient Yoga traditions of *chakras*, *nāḍīs* and energy fields, which afford access to higher states of awareness. Yoga shows us the nature of the universe relative to body, energy, information, intelligence and consciousness, moving from a physical to a spiritual science that opens up the inner worlds for our experience. In this way it embraces and transcends the findings of modern physics, showing us how the entire universe dwells within our own minds and hearts.

The book, at its title indicates, explains modern *Kriyā Yoga* at some length, including the full range of its primary practices seldom taught outside of guru-disciple relationships. It follows from several recent books that have unveiled previous secret methods of *Kriyā Yoga* not shared at a public level. These are powerful practices that must be done in the right manner and sequence, and with the right concentration. *Kriyā Yoga* forms a well-structured and scientific system of inner development that can energise the Yoga practice of any sincere awakened aspirant. The book notes the need for a guru and the fact that techniques cannot work on their own, without the proper guidance, initiation, empowerment and preparation.

We must not forget that Yoga, in the true sense of the term, is a way of giving up the ego and moving beyond body consciousness to a universal Self-awareness that is not bound by time, space and karma. This inner Yoga practice is a monumental endeavour and one that requires tremendous dedication, perseverance, patience and inspiration. It can only be achieved by grace, surrender, and opening to the higher Self, not by anything we ourselves can personally do by our own energy and motivation. It is not another activity for our ordinary mind or willpower but requires that we move into the unknown and go beyond the mind. We must approach it with humility and consistency, as a way of Self-transcendence.

It is heartening to see such new books on Yoga coming out today, written by seasoned Western teachers, who know both the outer and the inner Yoga, and are carrying on older India-based Yoga traditions in an authentic and accessible manner in their own countries. The approach of the book indicates a growing maturity in the Western Yoga community.

Certainly, Yoga has its diversity of teachings and branches. The *Kriyā Yoga* tradition, like a great Banyan tree itself, has a number of important lines and representatives and several angles of approach. The current volume provides another important angle on this tradition that shows its living power, capacity for adaptation and continued relevance for all humanity.

Stephen Sturgess reflects a wide experience of Yoga and contact with many important Yoga gurus East and West. He shares this life-long yogic quest throughout the book, giving life and a personal touch to the teachings.

The author has produced other important books on Yoga and is making a notable contribution to the field of yogic studies that the greater Yoga community can certainly benefit from. *The Supreme Art and Science of Rāja and Kriyā Yoga* will provide not only extensive information about hidden aspects of Yoga, but also an opening to the deeper wisdom of Yoga within ourselves.

Dr David Frawley (Pandit Vamadeva Shastri) D.Litt.
Padma Bhushan, Vedic Education (Government of India)
Director, American Institute of Vedic Studies (www.vedanet.com)

ACKNOWLEDGEMENTS

I would like to express my thanks and gratitude to all the Singing Dragon production team, who did a wonderful job in publishing this book, and particularly to Bethany Gower and Victoria Peters, who edited this book very professionally. A big thank you to my lovely niece, Heidi Smith, who modelled for the Energisation Exercises, and to my dear Lithuanian friend, who is also a *Kriyā* initiate following Paramhansa Yogananda, Lina Kurlinkus, who kindly modelled for the Yoga and meditation poses. And a very special thank you with gratitude and great respect to Dr David Frawley (Pandit Vamadeva Shastri), Director of the American Institute of Vedic Studies, who very kindly wrote the wisdom for the foreword for my book.

PREFACE

The Supreme Art and Science of Rāja and Kriyā Yoga provides the Truth-seeker with a comprehensive and complete overview of the supreme spiritual path of Yoga, while simultaneously creating a context that inspires and guides you to place yourself consciously on the spiritual path towards Self- and God-realisation, so that you may understand and realise through your own *direct* experience the deeper meaning and purpose of your existence in your relatively brief sojourn in this world, and thereby attain your divine inheritance of inner freedom, ineffable peace, and true joy or bliss.

In its completeness, this book gives you both the sound philosophy and the practical Yoga disciplines, techniques and methods of authentic spiritual Yoga that can help and guide you on the spiritual path.

For a spiritual seeker on the quest for Truth, who wants to have that transcendent experience of Reality, it is not enough to merely practise Yoga disciplines; one also needs to have a philosophical understanding of what Truth or the Ultimate Reality is: What is the nature of Reality and our relationship to that Reality? What is the nature of mind and consciousness? Who or what is God or the Self? A seeker needs to know why he or she exists, and how to end suffering and find true joy in life. To understand the philosophy of Yoga, it is helpful to have an understanding of the Indian philosophical tradition that has its roots in the ancient Vedic culture and illustrious Sanskrit literature.

Indian philosophical literature such as the *Kātha Upaniṣad* (2.3.12) guides seekers with practical purpose by profoundly stating: 'First, accept that the Self exists, and accept that it can be known. Then its real nature is open to experience.' This should be the starting point for all sincere seekers who want to know the meaning of their existence, who want to find freedom from sorrow and suffering, and who want to attain the supreme spiritual goal of life: total freedom in Ever-New Bliss – the true nature of the Self.

You need to look within yourself and realise your own power, your own Self. You need to discover the inner reality of who you are by unfolding the Self-knowledge that is lying dormant within you. In order to realise and enjoy your totality you have to expand your limited awareness into pure, infinite Consciousness. First you will need to control your body, mind and senses, which starts from a disciplined and moral routine.

The Supreme Art and Science of Rāja and Kriyā Yoga discusses the various systems of Indian philosophy that arose as a product of the meditative insights and *direct* inner experience of various spiritually elevated seers, sages and yogis. To give a complete picture of Yoga and its spiritual dimensions, the history of Yoga and its origins are also covered in this book, and is to be read as a background knowledge to *Rāja Yoga* (the supreme or royal path of Yoga) and *Kriyā Yoga*, of which this book is primarily concerned as the supreme spiritual path to spiritual awakening or Self-realisation – to become established in our own blissful divine nature.

This book is divided into seven main parts, each part having a number of chapters:

Part 1: The Light Within. This begins with your search for Truth, discussing topics on realising your true nature, and understanding what God is, so that you may understand the deeper purpose of your existence.

Part 2: Origin and History of Yoga Philosophy. To set Yoga as an authentic spiritual path and in a wider context, Part 2 discusses the origin and history of Yoga philosophy, from the early beginnings and the Pre-Vedic period (6500–4500 BCE) to the Post-Classical period and Tantra (500–900 CE).

Part 3: Yoga in Indian Philosophy. Part 3 covers the six main philosophies (*Ṣad Darśanas*) of India: *Nyāya*, *Vaiśeṣika*, *Sāṃkhya*, *Yoga*, *Mīmaṃsā* and *Vedānta*. In relation to practising *Rāja* and *Kriyā Yoga*, this book is primarily concerned with *Sāṃkhya*, *Yoga* and *Vedānta*.

Part 4: The Subtle Bodies and the Chakras. The topics discussed in Part 4 cover the subtle anatomy: *chakras*, subtle bodies, *nāḍīs* and *kuṇḍalinī*, which all aspiring yogis should be familiar with.

Part 5: Mantras. One of the most powerful ways of focusing the mind is using a *mantra*. The Sanskrit word *mantra* means 'that which protects or liberates (*trana*) the mind (*manas*)' and is a spiritual formula or sacred sound (letter, syllable, word or phrase) which is inherently connected with the reality it represents. Part 5 gives a comprehensive view of *mantras*, their effects and how to use them. It includes the significance of *Aum* (*Oṁ*), *bīja* (seed) *mantras*, healing *mantras*, and useful *mantras* for repetition (*japa*).

Part 6: Rāja Yoga. The longest of the seven parts, *Rāja Yoga*, covers the disciplines and practices of Yoga. The relevance of Yoga to the ultimate spiritual goal is explained through such topics as Patañjali's *Yoga Sūtras*, a definitive work of *Rāja Yoga*, the Eight Limbs of Yoga: *yamas* and *niyamas*, *āsanas*, *prāṇāyāma*, *pratyāhāra*, *dhāraṇā*, *dhyāna* and *samādhi*.

Part 7: Kriyā Yoga. *Kriyā Yoga* is the essence and synthesis of all Yogas and religions, which includes the highest Yoga and meditation techniques from *Haṭha Yoga*, *Rāja Yoga*, *Laya Yoga* and *Mantra Yoga*. It became known in the West through Paramhansa Yogananda (1893–1952). Part 7 covers the teachings and techniques of *Kriyā Yoga* that Paramhansa Yogananda taught, and short biographies of the great *Kriyā* Masters.

PART 1

THE LIGHT WITHIN

1.1

OUR SEARCH FOR TRUE JOY

There comes a time in everyone's life when they begin to feel a sense of loneliness and inner emptiness; a feeling that something is missing. We may have all the material comforts that life can give us – a house, a car, the latest fashions in clothes, the latest digital technology, a good marriage or relationship, sex, family and friends, a successful career, wealth and health – all the things that are believed by most people to bring them happiness and security. But even when we attain the acquisition of wealth, power and prestige, happiness can still elude us. You may be very successful in the external world, but what good is that success if you have not found contentment, inner peace and happiness within?

From morning to night millions of people are working hard to attain some happiness. A happiness that is fleeting – sometimes we experience happiness, other times we experience sadness, sorrow or discontent. This duality causes us to continually seek something without knowing what it is.

Through not understanding the distinction between pleasure (an attribute of the senses) and happiness (an attribute of the mind), we become restless seeking the delusory charms, pleasures, thrills and temptations of the world. In trying to give meaning and purpose to our lives we fill it with events, activities, things, people, and we create circumstances that will fill our emptiness and remove our discontent.

Some people gain success in the world and become rich and prosperous, and gain distinction and celebrity status. But as we know from reading or hearing from the media, their successes in the world have not always brought them true happiness, peace and contentment. At some point in their lives they may have wondered what else there is to be achieved, and perhaps they would have come to a turning point where they questioned the meaning of their own existence.

That turning point in one's life may come through a crisis – health issues, broken relationships, economic condition, for example – or it may come in a less dramatic way in moments of quiet reflection.

Knowingly or unknowingly we are all seeking a lasting happiness: true joy of total fulfilment, and freedom from suffering, pain and sorrow. Most people in the world believe that they can attain happiness through material goals – wealth, power, position, name, fame, ownership of possessions and property. They also believe that they will find perfect happiness in another person – within a loving relationship, and with security in a marriage that brings a family, a house, a car and a career. The Lonely Hearts columns in newspapers and magazines, and online dating websites, are full of such people who believe that if they find their perfect partner they will be happy for the rest of their lives.

We are conditioned to believe that happiness comes from having a good relationship, becoming successful, or accumulating wealth. This conditioning starts from birth and continues throughout our life until we die, that is unless we have an awakening in deeper awareness to see clearly the delusion that we have been living. For most people this is not an easy task, and even the most sincere seekers struggle with it constantly. One of the most difficult things in life is to see clearly, to see things as they are.

We live in a world of ego – the separate personal self – that equates happiness with all that we long for in the external world. We have a strong desire, a wanting for something or someone; for objects outside of our own selves. The mind and the senses become excited with anticipation and intense longing for the beautiful dress, the new car, the beautiful woman or the tall, dark, handsome man. The image in our mind excites us, but also distorts our perception of reality, for we imagine that the object of our mind and senses will fulfil our happiness.

Once we have attained the object or person of our desire, there is a sense of fulfilment and happiness. But it is only a temporary fulfilment, perhaps a fleeting moment of joy, then we usually experience a process of gradual or even immediate disillusionment.

The transitory moments of happiness were equated with the thrill of wanting to acquire or possess the object or person for oneself, and the moment of attaining the object or person of desire. This wanting of instant gratification goes back to our childhood. As our ego-personality developed so did the wanting and desiring. We experienced pleasure and happiness from the gratification of our senses – the toys, the sweet lollipop and the ice-cream. Our happiness was equated with the objects of our senses. But, because it was a momentary pleasure of happiness the wanting is not pleasure, but pain. Sometimes a child may ask their mother for an ice-cream, and be refused. The wanting is so great in the child that they throw a tantrum. They cry and scream so much that sometimes it causes the mother to give in to the child by buying them an ice-cream. And for a while, the child's tension ceases as they enjoy the pleasure of their senses. They equate happiness with an ice-cream. But at this young age the child does not understand the duality of pleasure and pain.

As we continue in life through childhood, youth and into adulthood we become more conditioned. Our desires continue to grow and our wanting happiness never seems to be truly fulfilled. It's an endless tension that creates restlessness in the mind. There is a restlessness of unfulfilled desires, and the world around us does not help. We are constantly bombarded by the power of advertising, with its seductive promises of perfection that play on our fears and insecurity. Its subtle powers of persuasion entice us to find our happiness in what we think will make us happy. It creates endless desires in us and conditions us to believe that happiness and fulfilment are inherent in what they are promoting and selling.

Advertising creates the illusion of a fulfilled happiness, and many people buy into this distracting illusion only to find that this kind of happiness is elusive.

And so, knowingly or unknowingly, we continue searching for happiness in the external world, while not realising that happiness is a state of consciousness that already exists within us.

There is a beautiful story that illustrates the search for true happiness.

THE STORY OF THE MUSK DEER

Once upon a time, there lived a musk deer who was foraging for food in a dense forest. It was the time of the mating season and at this time the deer naturally secreted a powerful fragrance from a gland hidden in a pouch between its sex organs and navel.

One early morning as the musk deer was ruminating on grasses and herbaceous plants, while being inconspicuous to avoid predators (snow leopard, lynx, yellow-throated marten), he became aware of an exquisite and beautiful scent. Intrigued by the tantalising fragrance, the deer raised his head and sniffed the air. The enticing scent stirred the deer's soul so much that he became determined to find its source.

The musk deer searched everywhere. He reached up into trees and sniffed the bark, the mosses and the lichens. He looked in the rhododendron bushes and in the grass, but wherever he went the source of the beautiful scent eluded him. The undaunted deer became more and more agitated and restless in his search as he desperately looked everywhere for it. Night and day he relentlessly searched, and moved higher and higher up the steep slopes covered with coniferous trees, where there were loose rocks.

In a final desperate bid to find the source of the scent the deer precariously climbed up to a higher precipice, but lost his foothold on the loose rocks and fell into the valley below. The deer lay at the bottom of the cliff with his limbs broken and his body torn. His underside was ripped apart. The torn pouch holding the musk gland fell out and released the sweet fragrance that he had been so eagerly searching for. He sniffed the scent and, as he was dying, he finally discovered and realised that the sweet fragrance he had made great efforts to search for was within his own navel.

In the deer's last moments he expired his last breath with a joyful and serene smile. He was at last content and at peace with himself. It was the happiest moment of his life, for he had found the joy he had been searching for.

So, like the musk deer, we are in a similar predicament. We are searching outside for that which is inherent within us. We must discover the true source of happiness and joy. We need to realise that the true source of happiness, which is joy, does not lie outside of us in any thing, object or person in the world. No one can give us happiness, because it is a state of consciousness that exists within us. Joy is an inner state of consciousness, that is our true nature; we *are* that joy! Joy is another name for the Self, for God – the one and only Reality of our being. The ultimate goal of life and the true nature of God is *Sat-chit-ānanda* (Ever-Existing, Ever-Conscious, Ever-New Bliss).

> 'All things are born out of bliss, are maintained by bliss, and ultimately merge into bliss.'
>
> *Tattirīya Upaniṣad 3:6*

We seek joy in everything, because the very nature of the Self is *ānanda* (joy or bliss). Our spiritual quest is to seek that joy and realise it within ourselves. Then, having found and realised that eternal Self, the source of light and joy within, we can share it with others. For joy is the light of God, our eternal Being that is ever-present within us.

> 'True happiness is never to be found outside the Self. Those who seek it there are as if chasing rainbows among the clouds!'
>
> *Yogananda 2006, p.15*

> 'Remember that he who seeks only material pleasures will lose the divine joys hidden behind them. He that finds the cosmic joy of meditation loses the attachment to the pleasures of material life.'
>
> *Yogananda 2006, p.117*

OUR TRUE NATURE IS DIVINE

The aim of human life is to realise our Divine nature. To realise and become established in the awareness of our true Divine Self. Until we come to this realisation, no matter how many of our desires are fulfilled, we will never be happy. We will remain discontented and continue to suffer in ignorance of not understanding the mystery of our own existence. There is a feeling of being disconnected, separated, a feeling of something missing from our life, an emptiness that cannot be filled by endless desires and their promises of fulfilment. The happiness that originates outside of ourself, that we invest in things, objects and people is always elusive and transitory. Our pursuit in a futile search for happiness is a poor investment; there is no security or fulfilment in it. Our greatest investment is to regain our awareness of our Divine nature and discover the reservoir of power within us. When our life is an expression of the inner state of joy, we discover and experience true happiness and regain our freedom.

REALISING YOUR TRUE NATURE

> 'Enter eagerly into the treasure house that is within you and you will see the things that are in heaven.'
>
> *St Isaac the Syrian, in Laird 2006, p.47*

If the aim of life is to realise our divine nature, the Self, then first we need to understand the mystery of our own nature. Through our own experience we need to discover who and what we are. The realisation has to come from ourselves – no spiritual organisation, religion, teachers or books can do that for us; they can only make us aware and guide us towards Self-knowledge. We have to light our own lamp.

First know yourself. You need to regain awareness of your real nature, to awaken and transcend the illusions and limitations in which you are involved.

To regain awareness of our real nature we need to reverse the direction of the mind. The mind of the ordinary person living a worldly life is turned outwards towards the objects of the senses, and is not only concerned with things and people in the external world but is engrossed in them so completely that it is not even aware of this fact.

So the first step in becoming aware of the integrated state of consciousness and regaining the reality of our Divine Self is to direct the mind within, towards its central source of consciousness (*cit*), the light of the Self, our innermost nature which is joy (*ānanda*).

The second step is to raise the mind upwards from the lower centres (*chakras*) of consciousness to the higher centres.

This is what Jesus meant when he said, 'The kingdom of God is within you.' God can be experienced as our own Self. Turn your mind and senses inward and absorb yourself in the reality of the Divine Self within, and meditate with the awareness that you are the witness of the mind. Allow the thinking mind to become still, then when the thoughts are still, the light of the Self will shine from within.

Through meditation we can become aware of our own true nature and have a direct experience and realisation of Self, the indwelling God. Direct experience is perceiving things and beings as they really are and not as we think they are. Direct experience is intuitive and immediate. One cannot attain the Self by just doing good actions, acts of charity, or by performing rituals. Self-realisation, God-realisation, can only be attained through inner awakening of consciousness and direct knowledge. No amount of intellectual reasoning, discussing philosophy or studying of the scriptures can give us that inner awakening.

Religion, the Highest Truth, can only be known by realisation. It is beyond mere intellectual understanding. Without inner realisation of the essential truth of who we are, religious dogma, creed and doctrine will never offer freedom and joy in enlightenment. A true religious person is one who actually *feels* the presence of God within; it is an inner spiritual realisation, not a blind adherence to theology, doctrine and dogma, with its rules, laws, injunctions and morality.

The precepts of any religion, or any of the spiritual exercises – worship, prayer and meditation – have little meaning unless this realisation becomes part of day-to-day life.

A religious person's highest aspiration is not faith, but Self-knowledge. The highest purpose of religion is not to offer a reward for faith in doctrine and dogma, or to forgive punishment in return for obedience, but to lead us to that infinite freedom and joy that is God, the Ultimate Reality. God is truth, eternal and immutable, and is not limited by time, space or causation.

All religions are like different rivers flowing from different sources, winding through different regions, flowing into the same sea – the sea of Bliss and Tranquillity. The true aim and essence of all true religions is the same – God-realisation. In this sense, all true religions are One.

The word 'religion' from the Latin root, *religare*, means to reconnect or re-tie. It has the same meaning as the word 'Yoga'; the Sanskrit root for Yoga is *yuj*, which means to connect or join together. So both these words, religion and Yoga, mean in their true sense to reunite our souls to our divine Source – Supreme Being – who is our true and lasting Self. It is the awakening and realisation of our oneness with God. We are made in the image of God; when we realise the image of God-Self within us we will have true freedom and ever-new joy.

The essence of true religion is the personal discovery of the meaning of life; the Truth of life. It is an inner journey that moves us from the superficial layers of life from the unreal to the real, to the essence of our being. It is a Self-discovery – a discovery that does not need the authority, dogma or ideology of an organised religion or religious sect to indoctrinate us in what is truth. Until we understand our whole being, our divinity, we can never know truth or freedom, which is the substance of the Ultimate Reality.

Whatever we call God – *Īśvara*, Allah, Jehovah, Krishna, Supreme Being, Absolute Truth, Supreme Intelligence, Ultimate Reality, Cosmic Consciousness, Spirit, Supreme Self – the Reality that we call God is Perfect. God is infinite and so are His names. All these different names – personal or impersonal, with form or without form – refer to the undivided One God. Words fail to describe that which is beyond our limited mind. When we try to express God in language, God becomes limited and imperfect. Our limited mind cannot grasp That which is unlimited. It cannot comprehend the incomprehensible. The truest and closest definition that best describes the nature of God is the Sanskrit word *Sat-chit-ānanda*, which means Ever-Existing, Ever-Conscious, Ever-New Bliss. God exists equally in all beings at all times and in all places. As Universal Consciousness, God is Cosmic Intelligence or Knowledge. God is Bliss itself. We are all seeking that bliss or joy, because that is the very nature of the Self.

> 'True (spiritual) religion is a science. It shows how to find permanent freedom from all sorrow in the attainment of Conscious Bliss.'
>
> *Kriyananda 2003b, p.198*

The great sage, Patañjali, instructs us through his *Yoga Sūtras*, an authoritative scripture on realising the Self, that when the mind is calm and still and turns within, we perceive the Self in its true nature.

> *'Yogas citta-vṛtti nirodhaḥ.'*
> 'Yoga (the experience of Unity) results from the neutralisation of ego-feelings (*vṛttis* that produce desires, attachments, likes and dislikes).'
>
> *Yoga Sūtras 1:2*

> *'Tada drashtuh svarupe-vasthanam.'*
> 'Then the Self abides in its own (eternal) true nature.'
>
> *Yoga Sūtras 1:3*

> *'vṛtti-sārūpyam-itaratra.'*
> 'At other times when the Self is not abiding in its own true nature, there arises false identification with the ego-feeling (*citta*).'
>
> *Yoga Sūtras 1:4*

These three *sūtra*s define the essential concept of Yoga (Unity). The Reality that is attained through the practice of Yoga is accomplished by removing the obstacles that obscure one's true eternal nature, the Self.

And how do we remove the obstacles?

'Abhyāsa-vairāgyabhyām tannirodhaḥ.'
'The *vṛttis* (vortices) are controlled by practice (*abhyāsa*) and dispassion (*vairāgya*).'

Yoga Sūtras 1:12

The Sanskrit word *vṛtti* means literally a 'whirlpool' or 'vortex'. The vortices of feeling – desires, attachments, likes and dislikes – in the *citta* (centred in the heart) revolve around the ego (*ahaṁkāra*), so any movement in the *citta* is called *vṛtti*; this includes all thought processes, cognition, emotion, feeling and memory. The nature of *vṛttis* is movement; they are the cause of the restlessness of the mind. Yoga is the stilling of this movement.

Vṛttis arise from the *citta* because of the *saṁskāras* (latent impressions of past actions) and *vāsanas* (desires, latent impressions of past action). When you eliminate all *vāsanas* or desires, all the *vṛttis* will subside by themselves – then the mind becomes still.

When the *vṛtti* subsides, it leaves a definite impression in the subconscious mind (*saṁskāra*). A *saṁskāra* of an experience is formed in the *citta* at the very moment that the mind is experiencing something. All actions and experiences leave subtle impressions in the subconscious mind.

The ego-feelings (*vṛttis*) that produce the desires, attachments, likes and dislikes in the *citta* are stilled by persistent practice (*abhyāsa)* and dispassion/non-attachment (*vairāgya)*. Yoga requires enthusiastic effort, and persistent, uninterrupted practice for a long time with earnest devotion to bring the mind to a stable state in meditation. Then, when the mind is made stable, it flows unobstructed towards the object of concentration, and becomes still.

For the spiritual aspirant, the first stage of dispassion (*vairāgya)* comes with the awakening of spiritual awareness and with the redirecting of the mind from the distractions of objects of desire, both gross and subtle.

WHO ARE YOU?

When you were born, and your gender was established, your parents gave you a name, an identity to recognise you from others. They identified with your body either as a male or a female.

As you began to grow into childhood, your sense of ego-self, your sense of 'I', began to develop. 'I want an ice-cream' (and I want it now! Or I will cry and scream till I get one). The ego began to assert itself.

You began to play a particular role in your family, with your incessant questions. Your mind/memory began to absorb many facts, rules of must and must not – layer upon layer of conditioning – from your parents, grandparents, aunts, uncles, school teachers, friends and strangers.

By the time you were a teenager, and a student at college, your image of the ego-self, the 'I'-personality, had developed and become firmly established in your consciousness. You became an 'individual'. You saw and felt yourself as being different and separate from others. You identified with your mind, body and senses. A mind that produced an innumerable flow of incessant thoughts, that in turn caused a broad spectrum of feelings and emotions to arise in you – good feelings, bad feelings, likes and dislikes, fears, anger, resentment, jealousy, envy, irritation, and so on.

And because you felt yourself to be an individual personality, different and separate from others, it infused in you the concept of threat. As a consequence of your conditioning you were made to understand that the concern of your life was not only to protect yourself from whatever may threaten it physically, but to protect it from everything that would diminish any aspect of it and make it appear less than it wished to be.

The ego-self demands protection from all mental and emotional pain, and adversity. Simultaneously, the ego wants to increase the sense of Self. The ego wants to build and develop it, inflate and aggrandise it; make it feel real and permanent, and provide it with security. The ego, the 'I thought', exclaims: 'I am somebody' with more beauty, more power, more success, more money, more pleasure, more attainment. The ego arrogantly asserts: 'I am better than him or her', 'I am right and you are wrong'. The ego blocks intelligence from perceiving the truth and instead imposes its own opinions as truth. The ego-self-aggrandisement sees itself as the centre and the world as its circumference.

Through your conditioning of identifying with your ego or self-image, you cannot discriminate between the real and the unreal, between the essential true Self of your original state of being, and those attributes of body, mind, senses and emotions which you call 'myself' or 'me'. When this happens you become under the spell or power of *Māyā* (literally meaning: it is and it is not; illusion). The Sanskrit word *Māyā* is another name for God's divine power of manifestation, which remains eternally with Him, whether there is a manifestation or not. The Divine Creative Power of God makes the Absolute, formless God appear as the diverse Creation. *Māyā* is both the cause and the effect. *Māyā* creates the illusion and the duality in the world.

Take some time now to inquire who you really are. If I were to ask, 'Who are you?', your initial and conditioned response would probably be something along these lines: 'My name is John. I'm British. I'm 36 years of age. I graduated with a Business degree at university, and now I'm the business managing director of so-and-so company.'

But who are you really? You have defined yourself in terms of identification with your self-image – your name, your age, a place, and your circumstances.

How do you know that is who you are? You are assuming that you are somebody, but who is this 'I', this sense of self, behind the mind that is assuming the identification?

If you think you are the body or the mind or the senses, then who is it that says, '*my* body', '*my* mind', '*my* senses', '*my* thoughts?' Who or what is this awareness-consciousness identifying with these things we think we are? When you say '*my* body' it suggests that you possess or own a body, just as you would say '*my* car, or *my* house'. But your physical body, just like the car or house, is a temporary material structure that is subject to change and decay. It is not eternal. The physical body is born and then eventually dies.

> 'You are immortals, endowed with eternal joy. Never forget this during your play with changeable mortal life.'
>
> *Yogananda 2006, p.139*

Your physical body is not actually solid at all – it is composed of atoms, which in turn are made up of even finer particles that rotate at incredible speed around vast empty spaces. In reality it is not matter, but energy, that is emanating from the one-hundred trillion cells in your body. Even the physical body you have today is not the same body you had a few years ago, or even a few months ago. Your body loses 30,000 skin cells every minute, and by this time next month, all the skin cells on your body will have been replaced. The body is constantly changing, it is transient, it cannot be who you are. Look at your family photo album, see the photos of yourself. You will see definite changes to your body through childhood, youth and adulthood.

I may convince you that you are not the body, but then you might assume that you are your mind and thoughts:

> Are you some image thought that appears in your mind?
>
> Are you some emotion or feeling or sensation that passes through your mind-body?
>
> Are you the thinker that thinks the thoughts?

Thought is the projected vibration of the mind and intellect. It is like a ripple on the surface of a lake. When the mind is quiet it reflects, like still waters, the Reality beneath.

Thoughts come and go. In order to be perpetuated a thought needs to be thought about. It requires a thinker. Thought expresses itself through images, concepts, ideas and symbols. The forms of thought are infinite. The tendency of the mind is to be captivated and entertained by the expressions of thought. As we think we identify with our thoughts, and become immersed in and act according to the content of our thoughts. The expressions, I think and I am thinking, both mean 'I am conscious of something objective'. They cannot mean that I am the thinker, for the thinker is the object of consciousness and not the self, otherwise you could not remember having thought.

The reality of who you are cannot be thought, because thought is an instrument of knowing, which requires a subject to operate it. Therefore you are a principle transcending all that is objective to you.

It is when the non-dual witnessing principle of consciousness becomes identified with the body that the false notion of being the thinker, the ego or the I-thought, arises (I am the thinker, doer, or the enjoyer).

Thoughts and feelings are transitory, non-permanent. They are not who you are. You are the Self-awareness that is the witnessing principle, conscious of the thoughts and feelings. Thought is always a movement away from *what is*; from conscious awareness. In the state of awareness the mind is undivided, non-dual, and alive, expressing a total energy.

Each feeling is accompanied by a thought, or a constellation of thoughts, and a physical sensation. The sensation becomes a feeling at the point when the thought arises to label the sensation. Through labelling, a division arises between the thought and the experience. Labelling a sensation as desirable automatically makes its opposite undesirable. Pleasure creates pain.

Suffering begins when we identify with our body, mind, thoughts and feelings. In this world everything is subject to change – thoughts, feelings, emotions, circumstances, all objects including the human body – nothing is permanent. That which is subject to change cannot be your true nature or reality.

The delusion of the identification with the body-mind idea is the root cause of our suffering, yet it does not affect the true nature of the Self.

THE STORY OF THE LION WHO THOUGHT HE WAS A SHEEP

There is a story that illustrates this point: Once upon a time a lioness was roaming in search of prey. As she stealthily moved through the long grass, she noticed a flock of sheep grazing in a meadow across a brook. With alertness and stealth, she crept down to the brook and then quietly and eagerly watched the sheep on the other side. As she observed the sheep, she noticed that a lamb had strayed from the flock to the water's edge. So, immediately, the lioness leapt over the brook and descended upon the lamb, but at that moment the lioness gave birth to a cub and died.

From a distance a shepherd had witnessed what had happened. He cautiously proceeded towards the spot, and checked to make sure that the lioness was dead. He saw the new-born lion cub and, feeling pity for it, carried it in his arms to the sheep fold. There the lion cub was nurtured among the sheep.

As time passed, the cub grew up into a fine young lion, but never recognised itself as such. Living with the sheep constantly and seeing only sheep all around, the young lion thought it too was a sheep. And like the sheep, it grazed and lived on grass. It never heard a lion's roar, it only heard the bleating of sheep, so it learned to bleat as one of them. There was no recognition of itself as a lion, it behaved in every respect like a sheep. It happily identified itself as a sheep.

One day another lion ventured from the forest and happened to wander near the brook opposite the meadow where the sheep were grazing. He looked across to where the sheep were, and much to his surprise saw what seemed to be a young lion behaving timidly like a sheep, eating grass and bleating.

'Unbelievable! A lion who thinks he is a sheep!' muttered the lion to himself. Slowly he proceeded to the brook, sprang to the other side and quietly and inconspicuously crouched under a bush, awaiting an opportunity to catch hold of the sheep-lion.

After some time had passed, he found his moment, and pounced on the sheep-lion, who was unsuspectingly grazing. The sheep-lion was shocked with fear as it saw the attacker's deadly face and finding himself in the strong grip of the lion's paws.

'Wake up! You are not a sheep, you are a lion; you have a face and body similar to mine.'

But the sheep-lion did not believe him. So the lion dragged the young sheep-lion down to the brook and, holding him by the scruff of the neck, pointed to the reflection of their faces in the water.

'You see, your face is exactly like mine. You are not a sheep. You are a lion! You can roar. You should not be eating grass and bleating like a sheep. Come away from here and live in the forest as I do.'

With these words, he opened his mouth wide and gave out one almighty roar. As soon as the roar entered into the ears of the sheep-lion, it remembered its true identity and began to roar like the lion. The lion consciousness had awakened in the lion-sheep and with a proud roar it jumped over the brook and followed the other lion into the forest.

THE INNER SELF

'Find your Self; discovering who you are really means to find God, for there is nothing outside of Him.'

Anandamayi Ma, in Ganguli 1995, p.143

The Self is the Witness, the Consciousness which is one with the Absolute that watches the mind. When we are consciously aware and attentive in witnessing our thoughts, we discover that it is not the mind that is watching them but something else, an 'I' that is completely free and separate from the thinking process and movements of the mind. That knower who witnesses the thoughts and feelings is our true inner Self, which we can directly experience in meditation as pure awareness of 'I am' without any other self-identification.

It is because of the true Self – of the nature of Pure Consciousness – that every individual knows directly that he exists. He is aware of his own existence and the existence of all else that comes into his awareness. He is Self-aware. This Self-awareness distinguishes all sentient creatures and beings from material things. It is Self-evident and it requires no proof. We are conscious of our individual existence and therefore we transcend it. That which transcends individual existence is the changeless, impersonal Self. Since the Self transcends the mind-body, it also transcends change, including birth and death.

'The Self is never born nor dies; nor having come into existence will it again cease to be. For it is birthless, eternal, changeless, ever itself. It is not slain when the body is killed.'

Bhāgavad Gītā 2:20

TRUTH CAN ONLY BE FOUND IN ONE PLACE

'First, accept that the Self exists, and accept that it can be known. Then its real nature is open to experience.'

Kātha Upaniṣad 2.3.12

Truth can only be found in one place. It is the only thing that can be taken as a certainty, and it is the one thing that everyone shares in common. That is the fact of their own existence as awareness. Each person knows that they are, that they exist, and have always known that they are. Each person's experience of themselves as existing has remained constant for as long as they can remember. Certainly over the years, ideas they hold, the goals they strive for, and even the complexity of their thoughts, have changed, but the fact of their very existence is a constant that is never questioned.

It is the questioning of this existence that must take place. It is the only thing we can be sure of, and it must be investigated continuously. One needs to investigate as to what is this 'I'. Prior to everything is the simple sense of existing as 'I'. But what is it? Where is it? When and where does it begin and end? Remember here, you are not seeking your ideas and thoughts, but that 'I-ness' which witnesses all thoughts. The 'I Am' – the simple, pure awareness which witnesses and perceives all. Inquire into this and you will find the only true path which means anything – your Self.

SELF-KNOWLEDGE

> 'When the unreal ceases to exist, this very individual soul is definitely realised as the eternal Self. Therefore one must make a point to completely remove things like egoism from the eternal Self.'
>
> *Sankaracarya 1978, p.79*

Self-knowledge is the Self as knowledge. It is not the goal, not the Self as the knower, nor as knowledge which is the object of the Self (e.g. 'I know this') but Self as knowledge.

There is a misunderstanding that language has created. Knowledge has come to mean the object of our comprehension. When you say 'the object of my comprehension', the 'my' gets swallowed and therefore it looks as though it is an absolutely correct statement of truth. But when you also emphasise the 'my' in it, there is a problem. 'The object of *my* comprehension is knowledge' means that 'I' is here, and there is some kind of relationship or connection between me and that knowledge, so the knowledge becomes an object. And therefore, based on this misunderstanding, one tends even to create an image of self – 'I know my Self.' What is meant by that?

The expression 'I know myself' can be confusing. The knower is the Self – not knower in the sense of 'I am the knower and you are known', but knowledge. That knowledge itself is the Self – not a certain idea or ideal or image comprehended by me, but the knowledge itself.

Therefore, that is not the goal. Only if it is looked upon that way does Self-knowledge not become a goal, but an existential fact.

In that statement 'I know myself', only the middle part is truth – the other two are images. The 'I' and the 'myself' being the same, only the middle part – knowledge – is the truth. That knowledge is Self, and that knowledge is Self-knowledge. Self-knowledge is not objective, it is not a goal to go in search of. So it is incorrect to say 'I have Self-knowledge', or 'I know Self-knowledge', or 'I have acquired Self-knowledge', or 'I have obtained Self-knowledge', or 'I have reached Self-knowledge' – all of these expressions form unnecessary objects.

The Self cannot be a future goal for it is present here and now, it has never ceased to be, it is Self-existent. The Self *is* knowledge and therefore it is not a goal at all.

Yoga as Self-knowledge is Yoga as knowledge, or Yoga as Self.

Self-knowledge being natural is uncreated – it *is* – and that is the only Reality. Therefore it is not an achievement nor a goal, nor something to be created nor brought into being. That is the state of Yoga. However, if we are not in the state of Yoga, there is a confusion and a doubt, and if we formulate any questions at all, we always preface it by 'if'. 'If there were a Reality… If there were a God… which means we have a doubt. It is the doubt that is the obstruction to realisation. Doubt is a synonym for ignorance (*avidyā*). From that *avidyā*, even what you call knowledge, theory or doctrines are born, whether they are accepted as right knowledge or wrong knowledge. A kind of confusion of all this is what is called imagination.

The statement that God exists has been accepted by millions of people all over the world, and the statement that God does not exist has been accepted by millions of people all over the world. But just because these statements are widely accepted and held, they do not constitute the truth. The truth is inexpressible. These statements are either looked upon as right knowledge or wrong knowledge. Both of them are knowledge as object, and therefore there is a movement away from the centre, from Self-knowledge, or knowledge as the Self, or Self as knowledge.

Yoga as a practice (not Yoga as an unconditional existence) is merely meant to remove these obstacles.

Why should you practise Yoga? Why should you meditate?

We practise Yoga and meditate to remove the obstructions. You are not going to create the Self, you are not going to create God – It is here already. Self-God is eternally present. There is an obstruction between you and That. Become aware of the obstruction and remove it. You might discover that this obstruction that stands between you and God is the 'you'. If you put together these two statements: 'God is omnipresent' and 'I want to realise God', what stands between me and God? Wipe that 'me' out – God is omnipresent. For instance, if there is a big blackboard and you write the word 'me' in the middle, what seems to interfere with the homogeneity of the blackboard? The chalked word 'me'. Wipe it out. When it is wiped from the board there is a revelation that even behind that was the same blackboard. If God is omnipresent and I want to realise God, the obstacle here is 'me'. This 'me' has been accepted to be real. It appears to be real because I have invested it with reality. When the 'me' or 'I', the dividing factor, is dropped, that is completeness or Yoga (Unity).

You are the eternal Self, the Source and Witness of your thoughts. That is your essential nature. But because you are not aware of it, you identify yourself with the mental fluctuations of the mind and the transient forms and objects of the world, and forget your true identity as Self. Through this false identification you are unable to abide in your true essential nature. The animals and birds eat, drink, sleep, mate and multiply like us; but there is a difference: we can realise our true essential nature – the Blissful Self (*ātman*). Having been born as a human being, you must not waste this valuable opportunity in this life to realise your true nature. Life is too short to waste.

Since time immemorial, seers, sages and yogis have devoted their lives to the realisation of Ultimate Truth. The knowledge they received from their deepest states of realisation was not through sense perception or the mind, but through their inner spiritual vision of intuition during the deepest and highest states of meditation. This transcendent direct knowledge is the highest of all knowledge; it is Self-evident and experienced from the Ultimate Source of Pure Consciousness. Indirect knowledge is perceived from the external world through the intellect, the senses and the mind. Indirect knowledge is conditioned by time, space and causation, and so it cannot be the Ultimate Truth. Direct knowledge can only be attained inwardly through deep meditation.

Spiritual knowledge is not the memorisation of words in religious scripture books. It is not the study of theology, for knowledge of the Ultimate Reality is free from all dogma and doctrines. Nor is it the knowledge that is followed by blind faith and sectarian beliefs that have caused wars and separation, dividing the human race.

1.2

KNOWING WHAT GOD IS

'The light of the Self is present everywhere and in all. Whether you worship Christ, Krishna, Kali or Allah, you actually worship the one Light that is also in you, since it pervades all things. Everything originates from Light, everything in essence is Light.'

Anandamayi Ma, in Ganguli 1995, p.161

'When one finds one's Self, one has found God; and finding God, one has found one's Self.'

Anandamayi Ma, in Ganguli 1995, p.162

The dogma of religion promises the vision of God, but they do not clarify and define the concept of God. To believe in God without understanding what God is, limits our knowledge and realisation of the Ultimate Reality.

For a person to believe in God is meaningless. We cannot believe in a God unless we *know* God. Our belief in God only grows in our knowledge of God. If we merely read and hear discussions about what God is, and yet know nothing from personal experience, we cannot say that we know what God, Truth or the Ultimate Reality is. Without personal experience and practical application of actually proving God's existence to yourself, religious doctrine is of little value. Belief in God based on hypothesis, and experiencing the presence of God in every moment, are two different things. True belief, which is faith, comes after *direct* experience.

There is more to religion than mere belief. In the Christian Bible it is said: 'Faith is the substance of things hoped for, the evidence of things not seen' (Hebrews 11:1). Faith is not the same as belief. Faith springs from Self-understanding, it is the intuitive conviction of truth. Knowledge arises from experience, but first we must act on faith. The firm foundation for faith in God is faith in Self. If we cannot find our own inner strength, how will we recognise divine power? When you have no faith in the wave, how can you have faith in the ocean? Faith in Self is the basis for faith in God, for it is the divinity within that enables us to recognise the divinity in the world.

GOD – WITH FORM OR WITHOUT FORM?

Once, a disciple of Sri Anandamayi Ma asked her the question: 'Is the formless nearer to Truth than God with form?'

Ma answered: 'Is ice anything but water? Form is just as much He as the Formless. To say that there is only one formless Self and all the forms are illusion would imply that the formless was nearer to Truth than God with form. But according to this body form and the formless are He and He alone.'

God the Absolute, the Unmanifest beyond all forms, also has the power to manifest in any form. God is both transcendent and projected universe. God is like the wind – sometimes it can be awe-inspiring as it takes the form of a tornado or hurricane, and at other times it can be as gentle as a formless breeze. In the Himalayas gusts of wind blow icy cold and terrifyingly hard. On tropical shores, the gentle breeze is pleasant and warm. The wind has no form, but we know it according to its place and time. The warmth or coldness of the wind is dependent on the quality of its moving air. Its form is dependent on moisture, sunlight and the dust that it picks up. Similarly, God is ultimately formless, but we know God through His creation. He manifests to us by His appearance in the world of form. God needs form to manifest and express Himself. God is ultimately without form, but we perceive Him first through form. The form and formless are inseparably linked. Everything in the universe – from a speck of dust to enormous galaxies, from a microbe to a human being – is composed of the subtly vibrating energy of God; the Infinite Presence of Ultimate Reality. This Reality is One, the Creator is revealed in His creation. God, the All-pervading, Omniscient Ultimate Reality *is* the creation. Like the waves in the Ocean, the universe with its manifold manifestations, with varying names and forms, originates, exists and dissolves in it.

This whole universe and everything in it is God Himself. We do not have to go somewhere to seek God, because He is present here and now. God is present before you in the forms you see around you. God is in everyone and everything. Where you are, God is. You have only to be still and to look within. You cannot comprehend and realise God, who is infinite, unless you become infinite yourself by giving your whole being to God. By inner awakening to the consciousness in God as the Infinite, you will become aware of the infinite presence of God. And when you realise Self as a wave on the ocean, not different from others or from the ocean of God, the delusion of separateness, which arises from attachment, ceases to be.

God is the formless that projects all forms in the universe – gross, subtle and supreme. God is both personal and impersonal. God can be thought of and known as an impersonal Truth – as infinite Reality, infinite Consciousness and infinite Bliss. He can also be meditated upon personally with form, such as Divine Mother, or the Avatar incarnation as Christ and Krishna, or Śiva. God has also come to us in the form of *Sabda-Brāhman* (*Brāhman* symbolised through the primordial vibratory sound *Aum*).

Whichever aspect of God or Reality appeals to you, it is important to experience God directly within yourself. Feel God's presence within; your true Self shares the nature of God. Direct experience of God or Reality transcends the realms of thought and language, and it is the only valid confirmation which intellect, however rational, cannot comprehend. The knowledge gained from direct experience is complete and self-evident.

DUALITY AND NON-DUALITY

Life as we experience it is in contrast. We live in a world of duality, of contrasting opposites – light and dark, hot and cold, pleasure and pain, youth and old age, health and disease, joy and sorrow, good and evil – in which the contraries are inseparable.

In the relative universe good and evil are interrelated, one does not exist without the other. But without these contrasting opposites life would become unbearably dull and meaningless. If there were no contrast of opposites, there would be no experience. How can you know hot if you have never experienced cold? How can you know joy if you have not experienced its contrast of sorrow? We have to know both; one without its opposite is meaningless and cannot be experienced. It is like a woman who is born blind, who grows through youth and adulthood, and into old age without ever seeing and experiencing light. Behind her closed eyes all she has known is darkness.

So if life was all the same without any contrasts we would not be able to experience and grow. There would be no possibilities.

The mind desperately seeks the one to the exclusion of the other. This is the delusion of the dualities that keeps us in bondage to the vain search for security in the insecure. Everyone avoids pain and wants only happiness. Both are transient because they are bound by time. As long as there exists a sense of duality, time, space and causation will also exist. You, the pure eternal Self, are consciousness itself expressing these contrasting states, such as happiness and sorrow. These changing states are not who you are. Your true nature is pure consciousness. You are eternal, you are immortal, you are ever pure, you are full of knowledge, full of strength and full of blessedness.

> 'Pain and pleasure are transitory; endure all dualities with calmness, trying at the same time to remove yourself beyond their power.'
>
> *Swāmi Sri Yukteswar, in Yogananda 1946, p.120*

The world then is made up of dualities – a whole universe created as a means to give one some standing in what would otherwise be empty space. Because if you subtract all your beliefs, all your ideas of good and bad, all of your dualities, everything you hold on to as what you think you are and what the world is, what are you left with? Nothing. You, the person who you thought you were is dead. If you are no longer a man or a woman, an architect, a teacher, a Christian, an intellectual, a father, a mother, a human, an angel, or any other definition you can apply to yourself, then what is left? Only 'I', without definition, without location, without any parameters or limits.

When you abandon the body-mind, what is left? When you give up all identification, what remains? It is only 'I Am', without any identification attached to it. It is the 'I Am' that becomes identified. So first revert to the 'I Am' without identification. Dwell in that and see where the 'I Am' arises from. Even the 'I Am' has no location, it is not located in time and space. You cannot find its beginning or end, for it is only consciousness without objects. It is the infinite subjective state without a sense of other. Infinite Consciousness is revealed through every one of us; it is nameless and formless.

When you realise this there is nothing to strive for, nothing to fear. Then you recognise that this is your True Self. This is your changeless, eternal, spiritual Self that is outside of all concepts bound by time and space. This is who you actually are, always have been, and always will be.

THREE DIFFERENT APPROACHES TO GOD

There are three main ways in which the seeker of Truth relates to God or Reality:

1. **The Dualist (*Dvaita*):** God has *created* the universe.
2. **The Qualified Dualist (*Viśistādvaita*):** God has *become* the universe.
3. **The Non-Dualist (*Viśistādvaita*):** God appears *as* the universe.

The Dualist views God as a personal God. In this concept of duality there must be a *subject* (devotee) and an *object of devotion* (God). The God we are devoted to is both personal and external, and is worshipped through sacred symbols such as *Oṁ*, and images, and Divine Incarnations (*Avataras*) such as Jesus or Krishna, manifest in history. The major deities (both feminine and masculine) of the Indian tradition – Vishnu, Krishna, Rama, Śiva, Ganesha, Durga, Parvati, Lakshmi, Kali – are different faces of the one Divine Reality. The Divine is not only transcendent and formless but is capable of taking personal forms. The divine deities (*devas*) named above contain the full power of the Absolute in a particular aspect.

The Qualified Dualist takes the concept of God to be the cause (who has become the universe) and the universe to be the effect. The devotee is not separated from God for he is part of the whole.

The Non-Dualist has the concept of God as absolute Pure Consciousness. In this stage the meditator, the object of meditation, and the act of meditation merge into One.

In the *Rāmāyana* (meaning 'Rama's Travels', a 4000-year-old Hindu epic) Lord Hanuman, the greatest devotee of Sri Rama, beautifully describes the three kinds of relationship to Truth or God:

> 'O Lord, at moments when I am steeped in my body consciousness, I am Your slave. When I identify myself with my mind and intellect, I am part of You. And when I am one with my own nature, as the spirit, I am Yourself.'

These three different ways of relating to Reality: Dualism (Sri Madhvacharya's view of Reality); Qualified Dualism (Sri Ramanuja's view of Reality); and Non-Dualism (Sri Shankaracarya's view of Reality), are not contradicting theories but are more like progressive stages of the spiritual evolution of the spiritual seeker. All spiritual experiences of God as personal or Impersonal, with form or Formless, manifest or Unmanifest, are equally true because they are experiences of one and the same Ultimate Reality.

Everything is contained in the being of God. There is no contradiction in the One Reality being both the subject and the object. A wave is distinguishable from and identical with the ocean.

All dualism culminates in non-dualism through the intuitive direct experience of becoming one with Reality or Ultimate Truth. Direct experience of Truth removes all doubts and becomes an inseparable part of one's being.

> 'The entire universe, appearing as names and forms, is *Brāhman* (Absolute Pure Consciousness). The ingredients are *Sat*, *Chit* and *Ānanda*. In this Unconditional

Reality, the world of names and forms is just like a little foam on the edge of the ocean.'

Shankaracharya, in Clarissa 2009, p.82

GOD IS INFINITE AND UNLIMITED

In the *Purānas* – Hindu, Jain and Buddhist religious texts consisting of narratives of the history of the universe – there is a mythological story that tells us that before the beginning of creation, Brāhma, the creator, and Vishnu, the preserver, saw the Pillar of Light (*jyotir-linga*).

When Brāhma and Vishnu saw this pillar of light, they decided together to go in search of its beginning and end. So one of them went downward and the other upward along the column of light, to try and find its beginning and its end. Their search went on and on and on, from aeon to aeon. They had been gone for so long that many cycles of creation and dissolution had elapsed, and they had not found an end to the column of light After a very, very long time of searching they decided to give up and return to the original place from where they had started their search.

Brāhma looks at Vishnu and says, 'Did you find the end of the *jyotir-linga*?'

'No, did you?' replied Vishnu, looking puzzled.

'No,' replied Brāhma, who was looking equally puzzled.

God is Infinite, He exists outside of and is not limited by time, space or causation. **God is Omniscient**, He has unlimited knowledge. **God is Omnipotent**, He has unlimited power. **God is Omnipresent**, He is always present. God's infinite presence is significant because it establishes that God is eternal. God has always existed and will always exist. Before time began, God was. Before the universe was created or even matter itself was created, God was. And like in the story for the search for the beginning and end of the Pillar of Light (*jyotir-linga*), God has no beginning or end, and there was never a time that God did not exist, nor will there be a time when God ceases to exist.

'I, the (eternally) Unmanifested, pervade the whole universe. All creatures abide in Me, but I do not abide in them.

Behold My Divine Mystery! All beings seem not to exist in Me, nor I in them: Yet I am their sole Creator and Preserver!

Think of it thus: As air (which is born of ether) moves through space (*ākāśha*), but is not space, so do all creatures have their being in Me, but are not I.'

Yogananda 2006, p.378

The Bible also reveals the omnipresent aspect of God's nature to us:

'Where can I go from Thy Spirit? Where can I flee from Thy presence? If I ascend to heaven, Thou are there; If I make my bed in the depths, behold, Thou art there. If I rise on the wings of dawn, if I settle on the far side of the sea; Even there Thy hand will lead me, and Thy right hand shall hold me.'

Psalm 139:7–10

Behind every wave in the ocean there is the same boundless mass of water; similarly, behind every finite centre of consciousness there is Infinite Consciousness. And just as an apparent form differentiates a wave from the ocean without separating it, similarly the finite self is differentiated from the all-pervading Self by the veil of *ajñāna* (ignorance, the cause of all illusions; also known as *avidyā*) that creates seeming separation.

Because God is infinite, there are infinite varieties of conception of God and of paths leading to God.

GOD, LIKE INFINITY, DOES NOT CHANGE

Inside an empty glass jar is space. I can screw a top on the glass jar and say that I have captured and sealed the space inside. Outside the glass jar there is also space. The space inside the glass jar is a part of the space in the room around it, which is also a part of the space within the building that I stand in. The space within the building is a part of the space of the town, city, country, planet and universe. If I break the glass jar does the space inside change? Is the space inside the jar or the room different to the space outside the room? Space does not change, and nor does God ever change. God is Infinite, Changeless, and All-pervading.

> 'You (the Self) pervade this universe and this universe exists in you (just as a clay pot exists in clay). You are really Pure Consciousness by nature. Do not be small-minded.'
>
> *Ashtavakra Samhita 1:16, in Nityaswarupananda 1996, p.13*

> 'Just as the same all-pervading space is inside and outside a jar, so the eternal, all-pervading *Brāhman* (Pure Consciousness) exists in all things.'
>
> *Ashtavakra Samhita 1:20, in Nityaswarupananda 1996, p.16*

SAT-CHIT-ĀNANDA

> 'That beyond which there is no higher bliss, which is of the nature of existence-knowledge, which is defined as truth and is perfect – that is the supreme Self.'
>
> *Vakya-Vṛtti Verse 30, in Shastri 2012, p.36*

As said previously in this chapter, the best definition that describes the nature of Self, God or the Absolute is the Sanskrit word *Sacchidānanda*, pronounced *Sat-chit-ānanda*, which means Ever-Existing, Ever-Conscious, Ever-New Bliss. We who are manifestations of that *Sat-chit-ānanda* are non-different from it. Our physical existence is That, the one, undivided Reality. We can know it as Consciousness, which is our Self-awareness, the silent observer within that witnesses all our states of mind.

Sat – God is *Sat*, the Ever-Existing Infinite Reality. God is ever-existing in everything, in every part of creation – in humans, animals, nature, and in inanimate objects, including everything in the universe. Even if objects are broken into minute particles – into atoms, and still further broken down into finer or subtler particles –

each particle still exists. Not a single molecule, atom, proton, or even finer or subtle particle is without the presence of God as *Sat*, Ever-Existing.

Chit – God is *Chit*, Ever-Conscious in all existence. God is All-Knowing. All that we experience comes to us as something that exists in knowledge. That which *knows* is Consciousness and all it ever knows is itself. It does not need a mind or body to know itself. Consciousness knows itself directly. It is not possible for Consciousness to know or experience anything other than itself. The mind, the body, the world, and the universe are projected within Consciousness and made only out of Consciousness. Like the candlelight that makes things visible in the dark, Consciousness (*Chit*) reveals whether or not an object exists. It shines through all objects. It is the light of all lights.

Consciousness is the ever-present or ever-existing knowing of itself to be Consciousness. It is Self-luminous, Self-knowing, Self-evident and Self-existent.

The essential nature of our Self, 'I', Knowing-Being, Absolute Awareness, is Consciousness and Presence. In order for Knowing or Consciousness to be present, there must be Being. And so to experience the presence of our Being, Consciousness must be present.

Ānanda – God is Ever-New Bliss or Joy. In the *Tattirīya Upaniṣad* (3:6) it says that *Brāhman* (Ultimate Reality/the Absolute) is bliss. All things are born out of bliss, are maintained by bliss, and merge into bliss.

We seek joy in everything because the very nature of the Self is *ānanda*, bliss or joy. That joy is inherent in everything in existence.

It is only due to our own ignorance that we do not experience it as such. We have become selective and limited in our experience of joy. We do not find joy in everything, only in certain persons, places, circumstances or events.

All that we see and experience is God – *Sat-chit-ānanda*. You are made in the image of God, your nature is identical to the Absolute Reality, to God, just as the nature of a wave and the ocean are to water. You are pure existence, awareness and bliss. This is the state which you actually are, always have been and always will be, and cannot be improved upon. The Self is already perfect – there is nothing that we need to add to it. You, the light of Consciousness, are the bliss of non-being, the spontaneous arising of 'That' to experience 'Itself'. Just as the ocean raises up countless waves from itself, so the ocean of Existence-Consciousness-Bliss (*Sacchidānanda*) raises up from Itself countless individual forms of life.

The more you are in attunement with your inner Self, the more you are in attunement with *ānanda*, your own natural blissful or joyful state.

Sat-chit-ānanda or Existence-Awareness-Bliss are non-dual expressions of a singularity. Just as heat and light are non-dual aspects of fire – you cannot separate heat and light from fire – so existence, awareness and bliss cannot be separated from the Absolute. They are three aspects of the same singularity. They are not linear or causal in any way, but a simultaneous expression. For the Absolute is existence eternal. It is Being-ness or That which Is, for awareness is a symptom of existence. But awareness alone is pure subjectivity only and must by its nature be aware of an object, so expresses Itself as multiplicity in order to experience *ānanda* or Bliss.

So what Is, all that is, for no other reason than the necessity to Be and expand, is Bliss (*ānanda*). It is Awareness. It is Bliss. Every moment, every day, every thing is the Bliss of the Absolute, expressing Itself infinitely as you, me, and in everything in the universe.

Separation arises when you create an ego-personality – when you create a being separate from the Source of one Beingness, conjure up a someone to try and experience that bliss, you separate yourself from the very Bliss that you already are. Like a spark leaving the fire to experience the heat of the flames, you lose your innate bliss in a vain journey away from the true Self – *Sat-chit-ānanda* – of who you are.

ALL IS GOD

When scientists explored the atoms' nucleus, they discovered smaller particles such as electrons, protons and neutrons. They also found that protons and neutrons consist of even smaller particles called quarks. Quarks are considered elementary particles that build up matter. They are diminutive and powerful strings because of their mass and precision. The string theory postulates that everything, not only matter but energy as well, is made up of infinitesimal strings vibrating at different frequencies to give us our reality. In science it has been recognised that atoms are vast universes of empty space, and that the only tangible parts, the electrons, protons and neutrons, are really nothing but vibrational nodes in an ocean of similar material. Solid objects may appear solid to our sense perception, but they are not solid at all, nor are they separate from one another in space and time. Our senses are limited, we cannot see the subtle particles that give us the appearance of matter in the various forms and objects around us. These infinitesimal vibratory particles are fluctuations of energy existing in the vastness of space, constantly emerging from the void into creation, colliding and rebounding, and then disappearing back into empty space. The atoms and infinitesimal vibratory particles that are dancing around the universe are sharing atomic particles with each other, so that the boundaries of one to another, and thus with each individual thing in the universe, becomes extremely blurred – blurred to the point of extinction. So what the universe tells us through scientists and physicists, and through Vedic sages, is that there is only One Reality.

That One Reality is doing it all. It is the background, the foreground, and the dance itself. That One Reality can be called God.

In *Vedānta* (*advaita*, non-dualistic) philosophy, that single eternal principle essence or Ultimate Reality is called *Brāhman*. *Vedānta*, the final teaching of the *Vedās*, is based on a set of scientific, verifiable principles that are universal – they apply to all people of all time.

Brāhman is the impersonal Universal Spirit, non-dual, infinite, Pure Consciousness. The nature of *Brāhman* is *Sat-chit-ānanda* – Absolute, the basis of all awareness and the source of all bliss. *Brāhman* is both transcendent and immanent.

Brāhman is infinite. It has no beginning, no end, no change, no form. It cannot be perceived by the senses nor the mind. It has no past, no future and no dimensions. These conceptions are all in the context of time and space. *Brāhman* is beyond both. Though *Brāhman* is unseen and impersonal, it is all-pervasive. *Brāhman* is only one – the One.

Brāhman creates the universe out of itself by itself, which means that the material for creation comes from *Brāhman* alone and not from anywhere outside and that *Brāhman* is also the Creator. An example of this is a piece of fabric. Has the fabric got an existence other than the yarn it is made from? Anything created from a material is not going to be independent of that material. If you were to remove the cotton fabric from your shirt, where would the shirt be? The shirt is made of fabric, there cannot be a shirt apart from fabric. The fabric was woven to form a shirt. And what is the fabric? The fabric is yarn, a fine cord of twisted fibres. And what is the yarn made of? Is the yarn itself self-created and eternal? Does it exist by itself and in itself? What is the cause for the yarn fibres? From the point of view of the shirt fabric, the yarn is the cause. But is the yarn in itself self-sufficient to be the cause for itself? The cause for the yarn has to be cotton, silk, wool, and so on that is used to weave the fabric into the form of a shirt. We can go on still further – there is no yarn without cotton, and there is no cotton without molecules, nor are there molecules without atoms, and so on to quarks. The point is, anything created is not separate from the material it is made from.

From this example we can come to understand that we always endeavour only to have an objective understanding and not a subjective realisation of Truth. When we look at the shirt that someone is wearing we only see it as an objective form and label it 'shirt', but if we observe it more closely we can see the 'yarn' or 'thread'. Then next, we may also understand that the thread is of the substance of cotton or silk. With this realisation we know that there is in fact no difference between different kinds of cloths. Cotton is always cotton – it is only the forms (shirt, dress, sheet, curtain, etc.) of the fabric that change. The cotton is the essence. God is the fundamental fibre from which the entire fabric of the universe arises. God is everything. God is Reality itself.

THE HUMAN MIND LIMITS GOD

The human mind is limited in time, space and causation. And because it is limited we limit God to a concept. Without personal knowledge and direct experience we cannot truly know what God is.

Even the word God does not give us a direct experience of what God is. If you repeat the word 'God' over and over again expecting to experience and know God, then you need no sugar in your coffee or tea, for by repeating only the word 'sugar', you should be able to taste sweetness on your tongue. In the experience of God there are no names, no words. The Absolute, the Supreme Reality, is nameless, formless, without words, indescribable. *Brāhman* can never be defined or described for it has no attributes, but we can say that *Brāhman* is of the nature of *Sat-chit-ānanda* (Ever-Existing, Ever-Conscious, Ever-New Bliss).

The difficulty with names is that they are immediately inaccurate. The moment you name something, you have taken away any reality it had and put a label upon it which makes it a concept. We allow ourselves to define the entire universe with names, and thus lose our ability to directly experience it. This is especially true with all of the experiences which we have within ourselves. We have stopped feeling anything that arises, and have instead replaced the initial signs of something with a name that allows us to stop it in its tracks. Emotions are a perfect example of this. The moment any particular energy arises within us, we have a box that we put that feeling into that has a label – anger, fear, guilt, happiness, sorrow, and so on. Almost no one stops to actually experience the physical feelings, the thought patterns, energetic pulses, and other signs that arise throughout the day. The moment they arise they go into a box called anger, fear, guilt, happiness, pain and sorrow. The mind compartmentalises everything, putting it into boxes. In the end all we get is a box called 'I'm fine.'

We need to let go of our concepts that hold us to our own ideal of what Reality is. As long as we have concepts, ideas, belief systems, we are boxed into our own existence. We have allowed our beliefs to create who we are, and our words and language to define us. The mind separates Reality into pieces, and then decides which are right and wrong, good and bad. The mind is constantly evaluating and judging, accepting and rejecting. And when the mind of another person seems to have developed different beliefs and concepts to yours, they become wrong. They become your enemy. Wars have been and still are fought over such differences. Yet if we are to understand and know God, each of us must fully experience that we are a spiritual being having a human experience. That God's spirit is within each of us, expressing as us. You *are* life itself, and life is God. You are the Awareness which sees all equally without making any judgement. It is the mind that makes judgement, not who you are – the inner Self.

1.3

SANĀTANA DHARMA

Human beings and animals have the same instinctual sense urges – they eat, sleep and have sex to procreate, and they fight to defend themselves and their territory. They also both experience the feelings of fear – fear of danger and death. But the difference that distinguishes them from each other is the adherence by the human being to *dharma*. The Sanskrit word *dharma* is derived from '*dhr*' – to uphold, support, sustain or nourish. *Dharma* supports the existence of every living creature and thing. Its meaning is 'Natural Law', 'Universal Law', 'duty', 'that which one cannot give up' and 'that which is inseparable from itself'. The warmth of fire is inseparable from fire, therefore warmth is the *dharma*, or nature, of fire. *Dharma* is also used with the word *satya,* meaning 'truth'. *Satya* means speaking the exact true perception and realisation of truth as perceived by the mind, and *dharma* is the way of life that translates the perceived truth into action. The two words *satya* and *dharma* are synonymous, and their goal is to realise the highest Truth – the Kingdom of God within you. For one who follows *satya* and *dharma*, there is no higher path than that of practising truth in thought, word and action. This is *dharma* – the path of righteousness, equilibrium, harmony, and Truth. It can be explained in this way: to awaken spiritually, to know your true essential Divine nature, you should live in harmony with the Universal Law (*dharma*) that governs the whole Cosmos, for this is what constitutes your duty (*svadharma* – 'one's own duty') in life. Therefore, you should acquire the knowledge of this eternal science called *dharma* to understand and know yourself.

The Sanskrit word *Sanātana* means that which is eternal and everlasting. It has no beginning or end – it exists eternally, and did so before any wise teachers or gurus or religions existed. It is inclusive of all, there is no dogma, or customs or rituals as in religions. It is applicable to all people of all places and times. *Sanātana Dharma* can be roughly translated as 'the natural, eternal way of Truth'. It is the path that leads to the discovery of Truth.

Sanātana Dharma was first recorded in the *Rig Veda*, a sacred scripture, by ancient sages in India. These great sages learned the truth about the universe in relation to the human being's place in the universe.

Another important point in understanding the term *dharma*, the 'Eternal Way of Truth', is that over the course of time its concepts evolved to become synonymous with 'Hinduism'. The term 'Hindu' actually comes from the Persian word 'Sindhu', a sacred river in India (now known as the Indus). Although Hindus call their religion *Sanātana Dharma*, the term Hindu does not indicate a particular religion, but a nation of people who live in India. The term *Sanātana Dharma* has a much deeper and wider meaning, and it is certainly not to be followed as a blind faith. Wherever the universal Truth is manifest, there is *Sanātana Dharma*, for it has no limited sectarian dogmas or ideological divisions. It gives importance to individual spiritual experience over any formal religious doctrine. *Sanātana Dharma* is life itself. It is not something to be believed as in a religion of faith, but as a way of life; it is to be *lived* as a spiritual experience.

THE DIFFERENCE BETWEEN HUMANS AND ANIMALS

The fundamental difference between humans and animals is that human beings have the intelligence to inquire into the truth of their own existence. Humans have the ability to be introspective, and the capacity to discriminate wisely. They can find a solution to human suffering and realise the eternal Truth, whereas the animal cannot; it is controlled by Mother Nature, and has its own laws. The animal is not concerned with knowing its purpose in life and its relationship to Truth. This is what sets us apart from the animal, but you are no better than an animal if you do not use your human form in this lifetime to find the meaning and truth of who you are and your purpose in life. To remain in ignorance – in pursuit of sense-pleasure, money, power and fame, and being preoccupied with eating, sleeping, mating, defending, and living in fear – is to waste the opportunity to realise your true spiritual nature and achieve that true happiness and bliss, the Kingdom of God within you.

There is a universal law governing the behaviour and action of everything in the universe, from the subtle particles to the minutest material particles – from atoms and microorganisms, to the mineral and plant kingdoms, the animal kingdom and human beings. If there were not the world would not be able to function properly, there would be total chaos and destruction. It is Divine Will that all that has been created should live in happiness. It is for this reason that the law of *dharma* has been ordained for all of them. Compliance with this *dharma* ensures complete harmony. The fundamental tenet of *Sanātana Dharma* is 'All is God.' This creates a recognition that everything is a manifestation of God, and an understanding of unity with all human beings, all nations, all creatures and everything in creation.

Om Pūrṇamadah Pūrṇamidam Pūrṇāt-Purṇam-Udacyate
Pūrṇasya Pūrṇamādāya Pūrṇamévāvaśiśyate
Om Śāntiḥ Śāntiḥ Śāntiḥ.
That (God) is Infinite; this (world) is whole;
from the Infinite the becomes manifest.
From the Infinite, even if the world is taken away,
what remains again is the Infinite.

SVADHARMA

Every living being in this world has their own individual *dharma* (*svadharma*) to fulfill in this lifetime, according to their past actions (*karma*). *Svadharma* means 'one's own *dharma*'. By fulfilling your own *svadharma,* the inner law of your own being, and by living the experiences born of *karma*, you can burn the effects of *karma* and return to your original state of pure being. To follow your *dharma* is the true law of your spiritual development and unfoldment that ultimately leads to your liberation. The Divine power and presence within you will free you and release you from all *dharmas* when you live and act from your inner Divine nature and devote your whole self to the Divine.

THE FOUR PURUṢĀRTHAS – THE FOUR AIMS OF LIFE THAT LEAD TO HAPPINESS

The Sanskrit word *puruśārtha* is composed of two words: *puruśa* (human being, soul or Self) and *artha* (purpose, meaning, object of desire). These *arthas* are meant for the *puruśa,* the human beings. *Puruśārtha* means 'aim or purpose of human life' or 'object of life'. Human life without purpose would be meaningless, therefore we need a purpose, an aim towards which our actions can be directed.

Puruśārtha can be defined as an aim that is consciously sought to be accomplished either for its own sake or for the sake of utilising it as a means to the accomplishment of a goal.

Dharma, *artha*, *kāma* and *mokśa* are the four primary aims or goals of human life that cater to the spiritual and material aspirations of human beings and lead them in the right direction on the path to spiritual liberation.

Of these four aims, *dharma* and *mokśa* are the higher spiritual aims. *Artha* and *kāma* are the worldly aims that most people seek, not knowing the true aim of their life they seek happiness through sense indulgence. *Dharma*, *artha* and *kāma* all have to be attained by individual effort. *Dharma* regulates the life of a human being keeping him or her on the righteous path. To live in *dharma* is to live with our individual nature in accord and harmony with the natural law and flow of Truth, or the Divine. *Artha* and *kāma* enrich one's experience and impart valuable lessons, and *mokśa* is the transcendental aim that liberates one from delusion and suffering.

The Vedas have classified all pursuits or objectives of a human being into four categories called *puruśārthas*:

1. ***Dharma*** (righteousness)
2. ***Artha*** (securities)
3. ***Kāma*** (pleasures)
4. ***Mokśa*** (liberation)

Dharma is eternal, but neither happiness nor sorrow is eternal.

The *ātman* (soul) is eternal but that which embodies it is not; from *dharma*, *artha* and *kāma* (the way of activity) arise, which are shared by all living creatures. Of these four *puruśārthas, mokśa* (liberation) is the ultimate objective, the others are instrumental and preparatory to the knowledge of Truth, which alone gives complete freedom.

Dharma and *mokśa* are unique only to human beings, because they have the intelligence to inquire into the truth of their own existence, and the ability to be introspective. Self-realisation can only be attained by humans. Those who do not uphold the values of *dharma* (righteousness, self-discipline, discrimination, and moral and ethical values), to regulate, order and discipline their life in a harmonious and balanced way, are like animals or worse.

Dharma is the first *puruśārtha* and the primary objective in life, because the struggle for security and the search for pleasure must be governed by ethical and moral standards and virtues. *Dharma* is the Divine constitution that defines our roles and responsibilities, social and moral order, and our purpose and goals. *Dharma* is responsible for the order, regularity, harmony and control that exists in all planes and in all aspects and levels of creation. If *dharma* is violated in achieving security and spiritual standards the fabric of society would be destroyed. Spiritual unfoldment is not possible without *dharma.* Both material and spiritual progress in life must be based on living a moral and ethical life. All three aims of life – *dharma, artha* and *kāma* – have to be regulated to lead an individual to self-fulfillment in his or her search for the highest Truth.

Artha is seeking security and material wellbeing in life, which is not contrary to spiritual life. We all need a stable foundation in life. As long as we live in the world, in a physical body, we need some measure of material wealth to look after it. If life does not provide us with the basic needs of food, money, clothing and shelter, and the wealth to maintain a comfortable existence, raise a family and fulfill a higher education and successful career, we feel insecure. Insecurity, lack and limitation are not comfortable feelings, as they distract from progressing to higher goals. Therefore, acquisition of means for the material wellbeing is a legitimate social and moral purpose. However, if the desire for wealth, possessions, power or fame is motivated by greed, self-indulgence, selfishness and attachment it becomes an obstacle to spiritual realisation and liberation (*mokśa*). Worldly success cannot fulfill you completely, and its achievements are transient and subject to change. Wealth, fame and power do not survive death.

Artha helps in the attainment of *kāma*. Most people feel that money or wealth is an important factor in fulfilling their desires to attain the pleasures and comforts of life.

Wealth is not an obstacle to Self-realisation. It can be used beneficially without greed or selfishness if it is seen as a form of Divine energy to be used in the service of the Divine, for God and Nature are abundant. The path of spiritual growth and material wealth or abundance and prosperity can work mutually together.

To one who abides in the Self, he or she sees abundance or wealth as a form of the Divine, and uses it in the service of the Divine for the needs of his or her Self, family and society without any greed or attachment to it.

Kāma is concerned with the fulfilment of desires in the world. Without deep, latent desires (*saṁskāras*) that are embedded in the subconscious mind or activated desires (*vāsanās*) that take place in the present, there would be no incarnation.

Within a broader sense, *kāma* means desire for pleasure in its various forms, such as wealth, power, sexual needs, recognition and service. In a narrow sense it can refer to sexual desire. *Kāma* is enjoyment and pleasure of that which gives comfort and satisfaction in life to the mind and body. *Kāma* is the enjoyment of the appropriate objects by the five senses, assisted by the mind together with the soul. The human being can never attain permanent happiness by fulfilling the never-ending desires; it is an impossible task. Desires should be acknowledged and reasonably fulfilled in such a way that one does not become a slave to them – either by fulfilling the desires, or by sublimating them (and transforming them into a higher form of spiritual energy) or transcending them. Suppressing your desires is unhealthy and will only cause problems. Sex can be either a means to liberation and happiness in life or a great hindrance and cause of suffering, depending on how you approach it and use it. Sexual desire is the ultimate of all desires; if it is misused it can lead to attachment and the fall into delusion and suffering. Unless it is overcome, one is not free. As long as sex is not in conflict with the principles of *dharma*, and is used only for procreation and perpetuation of family, or to bring two people together in a true loving and caring relationship, it is natural. Sexual desire is a legitimate aspect of human obligations; it was created by nature to perpetuate life. Creation itself is a continuation of the union between *puruṣa* and *prakṛiti*, the male and female aspects of the manifest universe, which is symbolically represented in the form of a *Śiva lingam.*

Mokśa is liberation, the direct experience of the Absolute Truth or Reality. It is freedom from all limitations, and freedom from the life-rebirth cycle of suffering (*saṃsāra*). It is a state of non-action and Self-realisation, the direct experience of our true nature as pure consciousness. Its nature is of eternal happiness and total fulfillment. It is liberation from all desires through the realisation of your infinite blissful Self. The attainment of *mokśa* is impossible without first fulfilling the obligations of the other three *puruśārthas. Dharma* is the means to *mokśa.* One who has attained *mokśa*, enjoying the bliss of the Self is called a *jīvanmukta* (liberated living soul).

Of the six major systems of Hindu philosophy, *Sāṃkhya*, *Yoga* and *Vedānta* conclude that *mokśa* can be attained in this lifetime, although there are some differences within the sub-schools of Vedanta (*Advaita*, *Viśiṣṭādvaita* and *Dvaita*).

1.4

SIX QUALITIES OF A DEVOTEE ON THE SPIRITUAL PATH

SINCERE DESIRE TO ATTAIN SPIRITUAL TRUTH

When you decide to walk the spiritual path of Truth and live the divine life, the first requirement is to have an honest determination to be persevering and faithful towards the divine goal of discovering your spiritual nature and God, the Infinite Consciousness.

You have to awaken from the *maya*-illusion that you are your physical body, material mind and personality. You have to discover your divine spiritual nature as your Self, the principle of pure Consciousness within the temporary and transient material body that is subject to disappointment, pain and sorrow.

Living the spiritual life requires a way of living in which there is a steady and continual process of awareness and awakening. It requires a revolution in your thinking, and an opening of your heart's love and devotion for a higher spiritual ideal, above worldly pursuits. It is renouncing the negative values of material life and accepting the positive values that support you in your quest for the Divine.

In the beginning, for the sincere truth-seeker or devotee, questions will arise such as: 'Who am I?', 'Why am I here?', 'What is the meaning of life?', 'Why do I have to struggle and suffer?', 'What is my purpose in the divine plan of this life?' The answers to these deep and profound questions will only become clear to you when you discover yourself as pure Spirit, pure Consciousness.

The mind is usually in its ignorant (*avidyā*) state of being restless and agitated, and so it is continually being distracted and pulled by the senses to their objects outside in the world, and agitated by restless desires and attachments inside. So, above all other desires the spiritually awakened devotee has the greatest desire of all: a sincere desire for the Divine, God. The more you approach God through love and devotion the weaker lesser desires and attachments become.

FAITH, DETERMINATION, PERSEVERANCE AND ENTHUSIASM

Once the desire for Truth is awakened in you, then you need to re-establish mastery over your life and pursue your spiritual goal with steadfastness, faith, determination, perseverance and enthusiasm until you attain it, no matter how long that takes. Never despair or fault or doubt. To yearn and strive for the supreme Truth is the highest of all human conscious efforts and endeavours. In the struggle and urgency to satisfy lesser worldly desires you are never totally satisfied; your determination, perseverance and enthusiasm soon falls flat when you are not successful in achieving them, which brings frustration, disappointment, sorrow and unhappiness. However, if you turn that determination, perseverance and enthusiasm towards one desire of attaining the spiritual goal, the reward of fulfilment, contentment and success is far greater.

LOYALTY AND DEDICATION

On the spiritual path, the devotee seeks to reduce the ego and merge with the Divine principle. Those devotees who successfully attain that divine goal are those who have remained continuously loyal to God and Guru, and who have remained steadfast, and dedicated their life to disciplined spiritual practice of deep meditation and prayer. It is only through your devoted loyalty of keeping the presence of God and Guru ever in your heart that you can establish Oneness with the Divine. Even when the Guru is no longer physically present the loyal and faithful devotee keeps inwardly and devotionally attuned with him, for the God-realised Guru is ever present in Spirit to those who are loyal and sincere in their attunement with him. The Guru reciprocates with unconditional love for his devoted and loyal disciple. Once that bond or relationship between Guru and disciple is formed, that loyalty remains not only in this life, but for many lifetimes until the disciple attains ultimate liberation in God.

RIGHT CONDUCT AND RIGHT ATTITUDE

The practices of Yoga and meditation cannot yield spiritual realisation of your divine nature without first developing basic moral virtues and ethical values. The devotee who adheres to basic standards of right conduct and attitudes makes spiritual progress.

We do not need another person to show us right conduct, for right conduct is a function of our conscience, the inner voice, of the true Self within. You know when you are doing wrong, because your conscience tells you, and you feel it. The pursuit of a moral life is an unfolding journey, which takes us towards the Divine within. The devotee adheres to truth, love, spiritual duty (*dharma*), peace, non-violence and goodness (*sattvic* qualities), and shows respect and consideration for others in thought, word and deed. It is the observance of these noble qualities that makes us truly human and potentially Self-realised.

The great sage, Patañjali, in his *Yoga Sūtras*, has given us the five *yamas* (self-restraints) and five *niyamas* (fixed observances) for regulating and harmonising one's life. These are the foundation stones of Yoga and without them one's spiritual life would be meaningless.

Spiritual development and the higher practices of meditation are possible only for a totally integrated inner personality. This includes our attitudes towards our relationship with life and others. We have to cultivate right and positive attitudes. Actions done with the right attitude increase our vitality, whereas actions done with the wrong attitude dissipate our energy. The action itself is neither good nor bad. It is the attitude with which we do an action, the intention behind it, that matters. The devotee who has progressed spiritually has the right attitude to life and towards others. Remaining calmly centred within his true inner Self, he remains cheerful, optimistic, positive and enthusiastic. He does not give in to negative moods, brooding or sulking. He does not gossip, or judge others harshly, and is not provoked to become irritated, angry or resentful. He is not proud nor egotistic. He loves everybody and has willingness to help all.

HUMILITY

Humility, not fanaticism, is the character of the devotee who has realised the Truth. One who has humility is free from self-importance and pride, and has an understanding heart. The devotee realises that it is not he that is the Doer, but that it is God who is working through him. The devotee thinks: 'Thy Will is my will.'

DISCIPLINE

The habit of daily meditation is very important for the devotee. To meditate regularly every day you need to have self-discipline. Meditation is the highest spiritual discipline. Through meditation you come to experience inner calm and peace within yourself. You become conscious of your true essential nature: *Sat-chit-ānanda* (Ever-Existing, Ever-Conscious, Ever-New Bliss). When you become established in pure Consciousness through regular daily meditation the mind becomes one-pointed and focused on the Divine, and it is not disturbed by the transient joys and sorrows of the ephemeral world.

The devotee brings discipline into his life not only in sustaining awareness and in meditation, but also in his daily activities such as eating, sleeping, working, studying, and service to others. For without discipline of the body, mind and senses, you cannot attain spiritual transformation of awareness and experience and inner freedom. The joys of the senses are ephemeral, but the joy you attain through discipline is lasting and fulfilling. A spiritual life requires a conscious choice to live a disciplined life; it allows you to go beyond limitations, it brings transformation, success and total freedom. Self-discipline conserves energy of the mind and body so that it can be directed and focused in the right ways.

PART 2

ORIGIN AND HISTORY OF YOGA PHILOSOPHY

2.1

THE BEGINNINGS

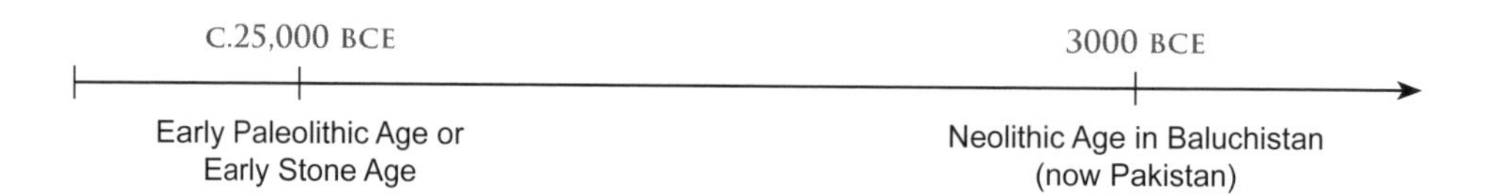

According to the *Viṣṇu-Purāna*, ancient India was originally known as Bhārat-varsa, named after King Bhārata, the son of Rsabhadeva. Much later, another Bhārata, the son of Dusyanta, became emperor, and his dynasty is also known as Bhārata. The remainder of their empire is still officially named Bhārata.

Bhārata is better known as India. In 325 BCE Alexander the Great with his great army of soldiers reached the Sindhu river, which they called 'Indus'. The word India is derived by the Greeks from the Persian form of the Sanskrit term *sindhu* (the river). The story goes that the Persians could not pronounce 'S' and so they said *Hindu* instead. From Persia, the word Hindu spread to the rest of the world, and further gave rise to such words as Indu, Indus, Industhan, and Hindusthan ('Land of the Hindus'). More recently, the religions and cultures of Bhārata (India) as a whole have been named 'Hinduism'.

The earliest date scholars can record the beginnings of India is c.25,000 BCE. The time of the early Paleolithic Age or Early Stone Age is dated c.25,000 BCE and before.

Anthropologists believe that the terrain now known as Siwaliks (a later phase of the Himalayan elevation) might have been the home of early man in India. Stone tools that were discovered in this area indicate perhaps 150,000 years ago. Geologically it is believed that during the Mesozoic era (about 230 million years ago) a great part of the present Himalayan region was beneath the sea (called the Tethys Sea). The gradual uplift of of the Himalayas is supposed to have occurred about 30 to 40 million years ago.

The middle Paleolithic Age in India corresponds to 25,000 BCE and the Mesolithic Age or Late Stone Age to 5000 BCE. Then around 3000 BCE came the Neolithic Age in Baluchistan (now Pakistan).

2.2

THE PRE-VEDIC PERIOD

6500–4500 BCE – The Treta Yuga

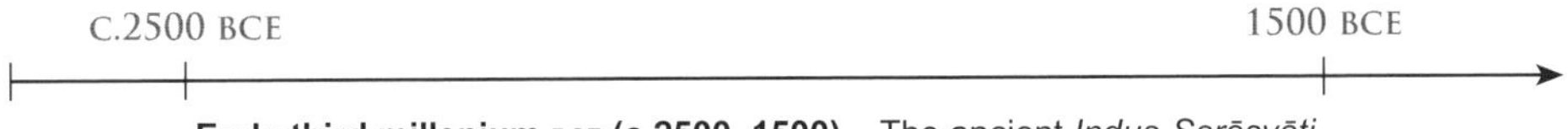

Early third millenium BCE (c.2500–1500) – The ancient *Indus-Sarāsvāti* civilisation developed on the banks of the Indus and Sarāsvāti rivers in Sindh, at **Harappa**, **Mohenjo-Daro**, and **Chanhu-Daro**.

Archaeological findings discovered from possibly one of the oldest civilisations on Earth – the Indus-Sarāsvāti civilisation, which developed around the early third millennium BCE (c.2500–1500) on the banks of the Indus and Sarāsvāti rivers in Sindh – revealed many artefacts that possibly suggest traces of the beginning of Yoga practice.

In 1921, a huge area of ancient Indus settlements was discovered. This culture, known as the Indus or Harappa culture, originated in the north-western region of the Indian sub-continent and seems to have covered an area larger than those of the contemporary civilisations of Egypt and Mesopotamia. This ancient culture was spread over parts of Punjab, Haryana, Sindh, Baluchistan, Gujarat, Rajasthan and western parts of Uttar Pradesh.

Over this vast area of ancient settlements, many of which have been explored and excavated, there are three main sites:

Harappa – on the bank of the Ravi in the Montgomery district (western Punjab). This was the first site to be excavated. It unearthed a large variety of artefacts.

Mohenjo-Daro – in the Larkana district on the river Indus, the largest Harappan settlement.

Chanhu-Daro – about 130km south of Mohen-Daro in Sindh.

The most exceptional of these three sites are Harappa and Mohenjo-Daro, 350 miles south of Harappa. Both are now situated in Pakistan. These two ancient cities were quite similar, both having an enclosed citadel fortified by crenellated walls, which may have been used for religious and governmental purposes. The main streets were laid out on a grid plan, complete with a drainage system made of burnt bricks, and sewers under the main streets. The houses had bathrooms and toilets connected to the sewers. Rubbish chutes were also evident. At Mohenjo-Daro in the citadel, a great rectanglar ritual bathing bath, constructed from bricks, which could be emptied by a drain, was also uncovered in the excavations. It has been discovered that the

Harappans were hunters and gatherers, and practised agriculture, growing peas, wheat, barley and cotton. They produced oil from sesame and mustard seeds. All this indicates that it was a highly organised and civilised culture.

The Harappans were also artisans. They spun cloth of wool and cotton, and created pottery, terracotta figurines and seals.

Among the unearthed artefacts found was the 'Paśupati Seal', a terracotta seal depicting an image of a mythological figure or a male deity, wearing bangles, necklaces and a strange head-dress consisting of a pair of horns. He is surrounded by four wild animals – on the left, an elephant and a tiger, and on the right, a rhinoceros and a buffalo. The male deity is portrayed sitting naked on a low seat. Beneath the seat are two deer. He is seated in the Yoga *āsana* called *bhadrāsana* or *kāmadahana*. His heels are locked together with the toes pointing downward, with his generative organ pointing upwards. It is believed that this figure seated in a Yoga posture was a prototype of the *Mahāyogī* or the great yogi, Śiva, the 'Lord of the Beasts' (*Paśupati*) or 'Protector of the Animals' (*Paśupatināthа*) making it probably the earliest known image of a yogi.

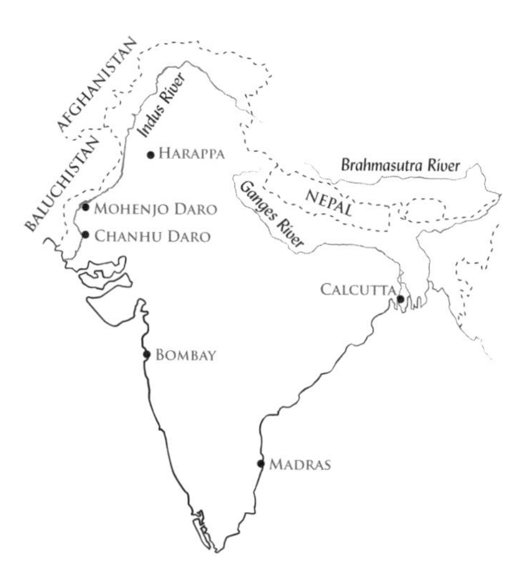

There is some speculation around the evidence of the Paśupati Seal as to whether it actually depicts a yogi or not, and anthropologists may conjecture whether the figure is truly representative of the *kāmadahana* Yoga posture, but it is evident that the feet are in the right area, the heels are under the scrotum, and the spine is upright with the hands on the knees as in meditation.

The Yoga *āsana kāmadahana* is performed by sitting with the two ankles everted under the scrotum with the toes turned backwards. There is another *āsana* that is similar, called *Bhadrāsana*, in which the yogi performs with the knees out to the sides while sitting on the heels that are pressed against each other under the perineum. The hands are crossed behind the back with them holding the big toes, and *Jālandhara bandha* (chin lock) is applied. Then with the eyes closed the yogi keeps his concentration at the midpoint between the eyebrows at the *ājñā chakra*. It is said that this *āsana* removes all kinds of diseases.

2.3

THE VEDIC PERIOD

4500–1500 BCE – During the Descending Treta/Dwapara Yugas (The Dwapara Yuga started in 3100 BCE)

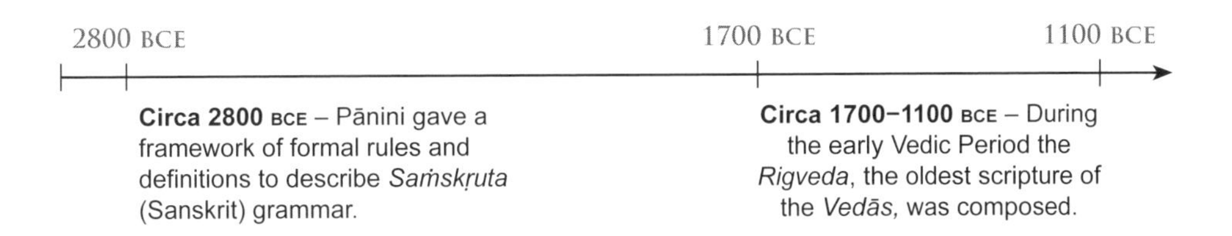

2800 BCE
1700 BCE
1100 BCE
Circa 2800 BCE – Pānini gave a framework of formal rules and definitions to describe *Saṁskṛuta* (Sanskrit) grammar.
Circa 1700–1100 BCE – During the early Vedic Period the *Rigveda*, the oldest scripture of the *Vedās,* was composed.

The period of *Vedas*, *Brāhmanas*, *Āranyakas* and early *Upaniṣads.*

Early Indian cultural history began to develop during this period. A new people, referred to as the Indo-Aryans, emerged who are believed to have settled first in North-Western India and later gradually extended their settlements over the whole of Northern India.

The Aryans ('noble ones') are generally thought to have been invading tribes of nomads from outside India, but there is now evidence, found by both Western and Indian scholars, that has determined the view that the Aryans were an indigenous population of India. It is now thought that the population of Harappa and Mohenjo-Daro, and that whole area of the Indus and Sarāsvāti River settlements, were one and the same people as the Vedic Aryans.

This view is brought to light by the authors Georg Feuerstein, Subash Kak and David Frawley in their book *In Search of the Cradle of Civilisation.* In their Chapter 9, 'Why the Aryan Invasion Never Happened', 17 arguments are given. In the fifth argument it is said:

> 'Archaeologists have argued that their digs in the Indus Valley, home of the great civilisation that was allegedly destroyed by the invading Aryans, brought no typically Vedic artefacts to light. Many of them have emphasised the marked difference between the nomadic culture they believe to have discovered in the *Rig-Veda* and the urban culture so vividly preserved in the ruins of Mohenjo-Daro, Harapa, and other sites along the mighty Indus River. However, the archaeological site of Mehrgarh, which has been dated to 6500 BCE, brought to light evidence for the use of copper, barley, and cattle at a very earlier time – all items that resemble the culture of the

> Vedic people. Additionally, many Harappan sites have yielded fire altars constructed in the same manner as those of the Vedic people, as well as sacrificial implements corresponding to those used in the *soma* sacrifice, central to the Vedic religion. Meanwhile the literary interpretation of the Vedic people as nomadic has also been revealed as an assumption of the invasion theory that is not warranted by a more critical reading of their texts, which show cities as an integral part of the Vedic culture.'

The period of the *Vedās*, *Brāhmanas* and *Upaniṣads* is termed the Vedic Period. The *Vedās*, *Brāhmanas*, *Āranyakas* and *Upaniṣads* are known as *śruti* ('that which is heard', revelation) as distinct from *smṛiti* ('that which is remembered', such as epics and legends).

The Aryans were divided into tribes which had settled in different regions of north-western India. Tribal chiefmanship gradually became hereditary, though the chief usually operated with the help of advice from either a committee or the entire tribe. With work specialisation, the internal division of the Aryan society developed along a caste system. Their social framework was composed mainly of the *Brāhmanas* (priests), *Kshatriyas* (warriors), *Vaishyas* (agriculturists) and *Shudras* (workers). In the beginning this caste system evolved as a division of occupations that was open and flexible. Much later, caste status and the corresponding occupation came to depend on birth, and change from one caste or occupation to another became far more difficult.

During the early Vedic Period (around 1700–1100 BCE) the *Rigveda*, the oldest scripture of the *Vedās*, was composed. The word *veda* is derived from the Sanskrit root *vid* which means 'to know'. *Veda* is the generic name for the most ancient sacred literature consisting of four collections. These ancient sacred writings were collected together from Vedic sages from different parts of India and compiled and organised by the great sage Vyasa into a collection of four books – the *Samhitas* (*Samhitas* – put together, joined, attached).

The ancient Vedic literature is divided into four chronological stages – *Samhita*, *Brāhmana*, *Āranyaka* and *Upaniṣad.*

THE *SAMHITAS*

The *Samhitas* are lyrical collections of hymns, *mantras*, prayers, invocations, and sacrificial and magical formulae.

Rigveda – Hymns of God. A collection of verses (*richas*) or hymns and prayers (*mantras*) to be recited during rituals and sacrifices. It consists of 1028 hymns and 10,462 *richas* distributed over ten books.

Sāmaveda – Priests' chants. An anthology of the *Rigveda*, and also a collection of songs and verses. It is a source book of great importance for the study of the ancient history of Indian music.

Yajurveda – Sacrificial formulae in prose. A compendium of sacrificial formulae (*Yajumsi*). It includes several passages of considerable astronomical significance.

Atharvaveda – Magical chants. This consists of 731 hymns and about 6000 verses grouped under 20 books. In these verses it mentions 77 diseases with references to *Āyurveda* (an ancient system of medical science), and deals with herbs, healing, and *mantras* to cure illness and combat poisons.

THE *BRĀHMANAS*

Following the four Vedic *Samhitas* came the *Brāhmanas*, the second great division of the Vedic literature. This literature is composed of astronomical, anatomical, pathological and physiological ideas and concepts with information on plant and animal life. It details the methods of the performance of various functions such as sacrifices (*yajña*). It also gives commentary on the meaning of *mantras* found in the *Samhita* portion of Vedic writings.

THE *ĀRANYAKAS*

The third division of the *Vedās* is comprised of the forest texts *Āranyakas*. These writings are the concluding portion of the *Vedās*. They are not about rituals but to do with the philosophical aspect of the *Vedās* and were intended for those people leading ascetic lives in the quiet forests. It was at this time that the doctrine of *tapas* (austerity) or asceticism and self-control found expression in the *Āranyakas* as a fruit ripening from the *Brāhmanas* and *Samhitas*. Those forest-dwelling ascetics living a life of meditative seclusion began to gain more respect than their forerunners, the priests of the *Brāhmanas*. Vedic sacrifice became more of an internal meditation than an outward oblation, and the ceremonial piety of the earlier Vedic times became more of a mystical contemplation of creation.

The forest-dwelling ascetics had discovered that the inner sacrifice was more powerful than the external sacrifice (*yajna*) of the *Brāhmanas*.

The *rishis*, seers and sages meditated and solved the cosmic mystery of reality and attuned themselves to the Absolute and attained spiritual realisation. They had actually realised the unitive Reality through their own meditative and contemplative experience. It was their spiritual revelations that formed the *Āranyakas* that lead on to the *Upaniṣads*.

2.4

THE POST-VEDIC/ UPANIṢADIC PERIOD

1500–1000 BCE – The Descending Dwapara Yuga

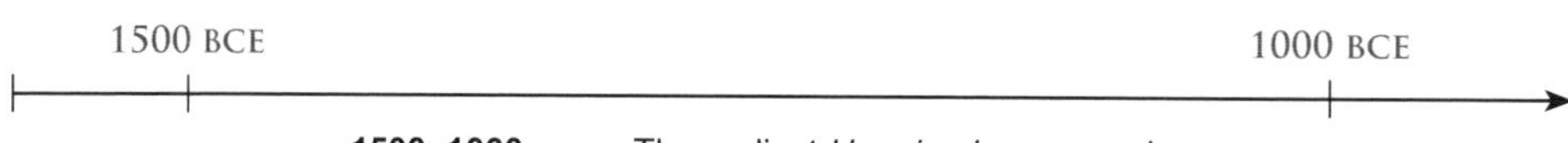
1500 BCE
1000 BCE
1500–1000 BCE – The earliest *Upaniṣads* appeared.

THE *UPANIṢADS*

The *Upaniṣads*, the fourth and last division of Vedic literature, represents the culmination of the Vedic approach. The earliest *Upaniṣads* appeared between 1500 and 1000 BCE and constituted the zenith of human thinking. They form a part of the *Āranyakas* (forest texts), because they were composed by the forest-dwelling *Brāhmanical* sages. The *Upaniṣads* are regarded as the source of the *Vedānta* and *Sāṃkhya* philosophies, and laid the foundation for the Hindu belief system of today.

The Sanskrit word *Upaniṣad* is derived from the preposition *upa* meaning 'towards', *ni* meaning 'down', and *sad* meaning 'to sit'. So *Upaniṣad* means to 'sit close beside' the sage or teacher. Many of the *Upaniṣads*, of which there are 108, and 11 that are considered important, are written in the form of a dialogue between teachers and students. In a quest for Truth, the student would sit close beside his teacher and, with attention, listen to him to learn the nature of Reality, and how to become free of worldly suffering and limitations.

There are 14 principal *Upaniṣads*: *Chāndogya*, *Brihād-āranyaka*, *Aitareya*, *Tattirīya*, *Kātha*, *Isā*, *Mundāka*, *Kausika*, *Kena*, *Praśna*, *Śvetāśvatara*, *Maṇḍūka*, *Maitrī* and *Mahānarāyana*.

The *Upaniṣads* constitute the end part of the *Vedās*, which is also termed *Vedānta*, meaning 'the end of the *Vedās*'. The basic doctrine of the *Upaniṣads* – 'the ultimate wisdom' – is that of the nature of Reality. It deals with the mystical and philosophical aspects of the *Vedās* and covers such subjects as the meaning of true knowledge, the state of oneness, the four states of consciousness, the constitution of the worlds, and the identity of the individual self (*ātman*) with the universal Self (*Brāhman*).

Vedānta is the culmination of the seeking of all knowledge and basically consist of three propositions:

1. **Man's true nature is Divine.** The soul is all-pervading Pure Consciousness individualised in a body-mind complex, and is immortal and pure. It is divine because it is non-different from God.
2. **The aim of human life is to realise this Divine nature.** The soul attains its freedom from the bondage of conditioning when it regains the knowledge of the Self.
3. Knowing that the first two propositions constitute what we understand to be 'religion', **that all true religions are essentially in agreement that the Truth, the Reality, the Eternal is one**. God as the Ultimate Reality is always one and undivided. All seekers, regardless of their religion, belief or tradition, seek the same God.

Vedānta developed and systematised certain basic doctrines that can be summarised as follows:

1. **The Ultimate Reality is described as *Brāhman***, the non-dual Pure Consciousness that is indivisible, unchanging, eternal, infinite and all-pervading. *Brāhman* is of the nature of *Sat-chit-ānanda* (Ever-Existing, Ever-Conscious, Ever-New Bliss). *Brāhman* is both transcendent and immanent. It constitutes the innermost being of a person and is the constant witness of the changing outward phenomenal world. *Vedānta* asserts that 'Truth is one; sages call it by various names' (*Rigveda* 10.114.5).
2. **The eternal Self, our permanent reality** that is distinct from the body, mind, sense-organs and intellect is called *ātman*, which is identical to *Brāhman*.
3. **The phenomenal world is not real but apparent.** *Māyā* (illusion; the very fabric of life) veils the Ultimate Reality and in its place projects various appearances. *Māyā* is God's Power of manifestation and world projection; it is both the eternal Cause and the temporal effect.

These Vedantic doctrines are central to the philosophy of *Advaita* (non-duality). Duality is merely God's illusion; there is never anything but the One. It is all God's dream-like creation. The world is neither real nor unreal for all experience of the phenomenal world is dependent on there being both a subject and an object; a seer and the seen. The one exists only so long as the other exists. Without the subject and the object, there is only the One, the Absolute. The world of experience would not exist for us without there being the duality of subject and object. It is God who has created this apparent duality of experience within Himself. He is both the subject and the object.

To go beyond this conundrum of duality we need to merge the objective and separative mind back into its Source, Pure Consciousness, God. Then we can realise truth directly, that ultimately there is only the One who has become the many. That the eternal Self, the Source and Witness of our thoughts is the only Reality.

> 'As waves, foam and bubbles are not different from water, so in the light of true knowledge, the Universe, born of the Self, is not different from the Self.'
>
> *Ashtavakra Samhita 2:4*

'The world appears as a result of ignorance of the nature of the Self, and it disappears when the nature of the Self is recognised. The illusory snake is born of the absence of knowledge of the rope, and it disappears when knowledge of the rope is attained.'

Ashtavakra Samhita 2:7

2.5

THE PRE-CLASSICAL PERIOD

1000–100 BCE – During the Descending Dwapara Yuga

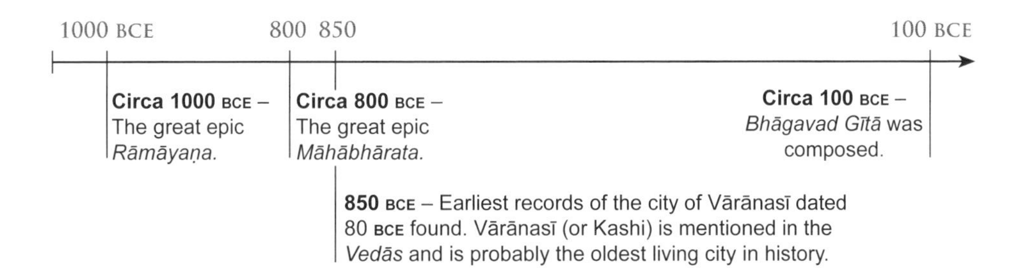

The period of the *Upaniṣads* was superseded by the period of the early great Indian heroic epics (*Mahākāvyas*) – heroic and religious tales with morals intended for popular learning and not for propounding special philosophical doctrines.

A vast body of literature was produced during this period, including the three great epics *Rāmāyana*, *Mahabharata* and *Purānas*.

The ***Rāmāyana*** (Rama's Travels) was composed by the sage-poet Valmiki and arranged into 24,000 Sanskrit verses and divided into six books. The *Rāmāyana* documents Rama's triumph over the demon-king Ravana, thereby enacting his fate as the ideal man and incarnation of the god Lord Vishnu.

The ***Mahābhārata***, composed of 220,000 lines in 18 *Parvas* plus a supplementary section on the *Harivamsa*, was written by the great sage Vyāsa. The *Mahābhārata*, like Homer's *Odyssey*, transmits the wisdom and spirit of the Vedic civilisation from where spiritual inspiration first originated and spread throughout the ancient world.

Mahābhārata means 'Great Bhārata'. *Bhārata* (with a long ā) indicates something related to King Bharata (with a short a), the son of Rsabhadeva, who is said to have ruled the whole civilised world, which was then called *Bhārata-varsa*. Much later, another Bharata, the son of Dusyanta, became emperor, and his dynasty is also known as Bhārata. Now Bhārata is better known as India.

The *Srimad Bhāgavad Gītā* (the word *Bhāgavad* refers to *Bhāgavan*, meaning 'God', and *Gītā* means 'song' – 'The Song of God') is an episode in the great epic *Mahābhārata*. The fundamental philosophical viewpoints of the *Bhāgavad Gītā* are that: all existence is a manifestation of God; God exists in all beings as their inner Self; knowledge of and union with the Self is the supreme goal of life; and ignorance of our Divinity is the cause of our suffering.

The *Bhāgavad Gītā* presents the teachings of Yoga in the form of a dialogue between Krishna and his devotee, Arjuna, on the Kurukshetra battlefield. The background story to the Yoga philosophy is an allegory: Arjuna represents the spiritual seeker and individual soul, while Sri Krishna represents the Supreme Soul, the *ātman* within each of us. Krishna instructs Arjuna on the battlefield on the nature of God, the universe and the Self, on the the four main sacred paths to Self-realisation – *Karma Yoga*, *Bhakta Yoga*, *Jñanā Yoga* and *Rāja Yoga* – and on the way to attain God.

The ***Purānas*** are supposed to have initially been compiled by the sage Vyāsa, who originally arranged and compiled the *Vedās* and were later recompiled by other sages. The *Purānas* are preserved teachings and doctrines of the sacred *Vedās* for the declining spirituality and intelligence of the human being by means of story and mythology.

The word *Purāna* is derived from *Purā* which means 'before', 'formerly', 'of old'. There are 18 known *Purānas*: *Matsya*, *Mārkendeya*, *Bhavisya*, *Bhāgavat*, *Brahmānda*, *Brāhmavaivarta*, *Brāhma*, *Vāmana*, *Varāha*, *Vishnu*, *Vāyu*, *Nārad*, *Pādma*, *Linga*, *Garura*, *Kurma*, *Skanda* and *Agni*. These sacred treatises discuss the five principal topics known as *Panchalakshana* (*pancha* means 'five' and *lakshana* means 'sign', 'characteristic' or 'quality'). The five are as follows:

1. Creation of the Universe
2. Destruction of the Universe
3. Renovation of the Universe
4. Generally gods and saints of high order or patriarchs
5. The reigns of *Manus* and the theories of the solar and lunar races.

2.6

THE CLASSICAL PERIOD

100–500 CE – During the Descending Kali Yuga

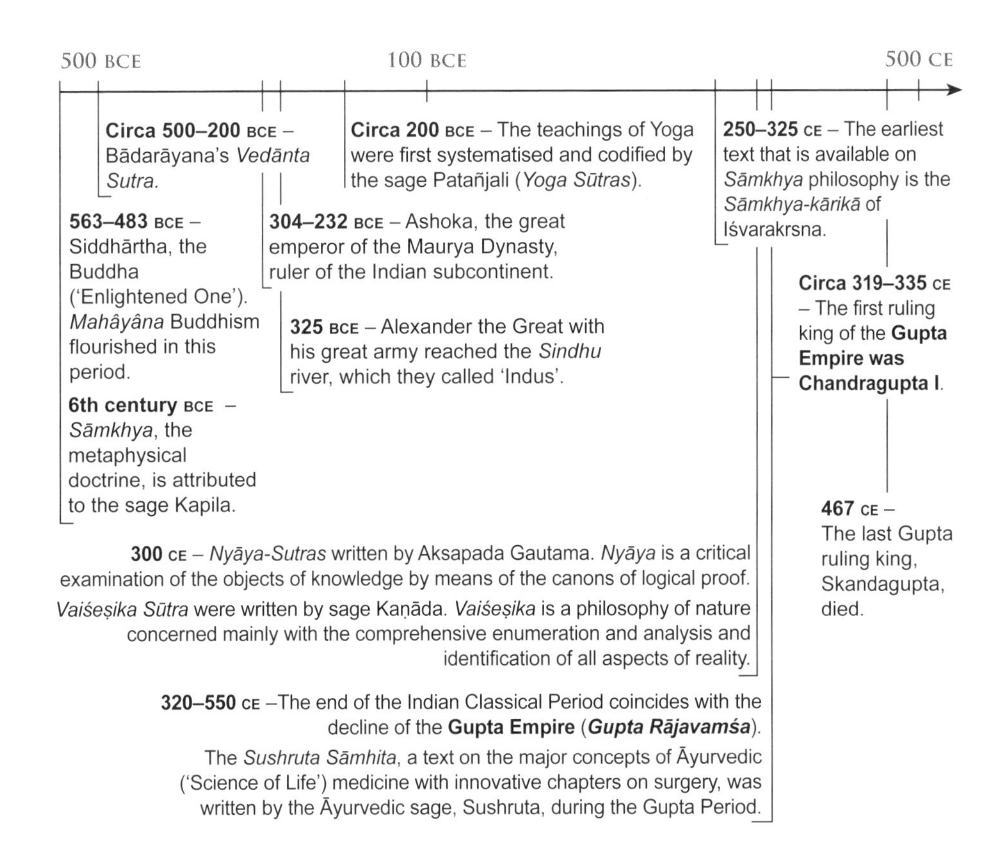

500 BCE
100 BCE
500 CE
Circa 500–200 BCE – Bādarāyana's Vedānta Sutra.
Circa 200 BCE – The teachings of Yoga were first systematised and codified by the sage Patañjali (Yoga Sūtras).
250–325 CE – The earliest text that is available on Sāmkhya philosophy is the Sāmkhya-kārikā of Iśvarakrsna.
563–483 BCE – Siddhārtha, the Buddha ('Enlightened One'). Mahâyâna Buddhism flourished in this period.
304–232 BCE – Ashoka, the great emperor of the Maurya Dynasty, ruler of the Indian subcontinent.
Circa 319–335 CE – The first ruling king of the Gupta Empire was Chandragupta I.
325 BCE – Alexander the Great with his great army reached the Sindhu river, which they called 'Indus'.
6th century BCE – Sāmkhya, the metaphysical doctrine, is attributed to the sage Kapila.
467 CE – The last Gupta ruling king, Skandagupta, died.
300 CE – Nyāya-Sutras written by Aksapada Gautama. Nyāya is a critical examination of the objects of knowledge by means of the canons of logical proof.
Vaiśeṣika Sūtra were written by sage Kaṇāda. Vaiśeṣika is a philosophy of nature concerned mainly with the comprehensive enumeration and analysis and identification of all aspects of reality.
320–550 CE –The end of the Indian Classical Period coincides with the decline of the Gupta Empire (Gupta Rājavamśa).
The Sushruta Sāmhita, a text on the major concepts of Āyurvedic ('Science of Life') medicine with innovative chapters on surgery, was written by the Āyurvedic sage, Sushruta, during the Gupta Period.

It was around 200 BCE that the teachings of Yoga were first systematised and codified by a great sage named Patañjali. In the third century BCE, Patañjali collected and systematically classified all the philosophy and practices of Yoga that were already validated by the long-existing classic tradition in practice. His work, a classical doctrine of Yoga, is known as *Yoga Sūtras*. In the form of 196 *sūtras* ('threads' – aphorisms) Patañjali gives the essential information about Yoga in order for the spiritual seeker to attain Self-realisation. Traditionally, these *sūtra*s would have been taught in Sanskrit and memorised as a chant. In this classical system of Yoga, Patañjali has established Yoga as a practical discipline. It discusses the nature and workings of the mind, its modifications, obstacles and afflictions, and the method for attaining the highest goal of life – *kaivalya* (absoluteness). In the *Yoga Sūtras* he outlines a practical discipline made up of eight limbs, known as ***Aṣṭāṅga Yoga:*** *yāma*, *niyama*, *āsana*, *prāṇāyama*, *pratyāhāra*, *dhāraṇā*, *dhyāna*, and *samādhi*.

This is also the period in which ***Mahâyâna*** **Buddhism** flourished. *Mahâyâna* means the 'Great Vehicle', and is used to distinguish itself from *Hinyaya*, or the lesser vehicle Buddhism that preceded it. The *Mahāyana* texts claim to be the teaching of the Buddha himself delivered to a special assembly of *boddhisattvas* (buddhas-to-be). These sacred texts also say that the *Mahâyâna* was concealed during several centuries until the world was ready to receive it, then it was brought forth and spread across India.

THE BUDDHA

The **Buddha**, the 'Enlightened One' or the 'Awakened One' was born around 563 BCE into the warrior tribe called the Sakyas in a village called Lumbini, in a region of India that now lies in southern Nepal.

Siddhārtha (Buddha) was born into the family of King Śuddhodāna and Queen Māyā. King Śuddhodāna ruled at Kapilavāstu, in ancient India on the border of present-day Nepal. The name given to him at birth was Siddhārtha, which means something like 'he who has attained his goals' or 'every wish fulfilled', and Gautama was his clan name.

When he was 16, Siddhārtha was married to a beautiful young princess, Yasodhāra, who bore him a son, Rahula. For a while Siddhārtha seemed to be content living the life of a prince in his father's luxurious palace. However, when he was 29 he decided to make trips outside the palace to meet his subjects in a nearby town that he had not visited before, where he saw four sights that were to change his life forever. The first sight he saw was someone who was suffering with disease. The second sight he saw was someone who was old. Then, he saw a decaying corpse. Finally, he saw a wandering ascetic, who radiated inner peace and calm, and who told him that he had renounced the world to pass beyond suffering and happiness to attain inner peace. Siddhārtha had never seen life in this way before because he had been protected from such sights by remaining in his father's palace. His mind became troubled with the thoughts of the impermanence of all life, and of the vanity and instability of all objects of desire. He was so deeply shocked by the vision of suffering that he decided to leave the palace and, following the example of the ascetic he had seen, become an ascetic himself. He shaved his head, gave away his possessions and took up the robe and begging bowl of a wandering monk, and joined a group of ascetics so that he could confront the problems of disease, old age and death.

Siddhārtha discarded his name and became the monk Gautama, or, as he is still called, Sakyamuni, the ascetic of the Sakyas, and subjected his body to great hardship and austerity. He fasted until his physical body became emaciated. But still he could not find the answer to his fundamental problem and he realised that if he kept tormenting his body with austerities he would die before finding one.

Then, one day as he lay exhausted on the bank of a river, a young village girl by the name of Sujātā came by and, seeing him exhausted, gave him a ball of rice pudding. He then withdrew from this harsh asceticism and began practising what the Buddhists call the 'Middle Path'. In other words, Gautama avoided the two extremes – self-denial and self-indulgence. Then in a place called Bodh Gaya, he sat under a great pipal tree (now known as a Bodhi tree in Bodh Gaya), and with great determination vowed to sit there in meditation until he found Truth or die trying.

After remaining in meditation for 49 days, at the age of 35, Gautama went into *samādhi* and attained Enlightenment during the night of the full moon of May. As the morning star rose, he awoke fully realised with complete insight into the cause of suffering, and the steps to eliminate it. As a fully realised being, he was Gautama no more, but the Buddha, the 'Awakened One'. It was during one of the stages of his enlightenment that he identified the **Four Noble Truths**: the universality of suffering, the cause of suffering through selfish desire, the solution to suffering, and the way to overcome suffering. This final point is called the **Noble Eightfold Path**, consisting of eight points of wisdom:

1. Right understanding leads to wisdom.
2. Right intention leads to right actions and right views.
3. Right speech leads to Truth and understanding.
4. Right action leads to self-control and self-discipline.
5. Right livelihood leads to earning one's living righteously.
6. Right effort leads to liberation of the mind, illuminated by wisdom.
7. Right mindfulness leads to serenity, insight, deep concentration and wisdom.
8. Right absorption leads to unity.

The Buddha gave his first sermon outlining the Four Noble Truths in Deer Park in Isipatana (modern Sarnath, 13 km north-east of Vārānasī, in Uttar Pradesh) and continued to teach for the remaining 45 years of his life in the Gangetic plain which encompasses most of northern and eastern India, until he passed away into full nirvana (*parinirvana*), the full deathless state, at about the age of 80 at Kushinara in 483 BCE on a full moon of May, known in the Indian calendar as Wesak. It is said that before the Buddha died, he became severely sick through some food that he had eaten, that had been offered to him by a blacksmith named Cunda. The Buddha recovered from his illness before he attained *parinirvana*.

THE GOLDEN AGE OF INDIAN CULTURE

The end of the Indian Classical Period coincides with the decline of the Gupta Empire (*Gupta Rājavamśa*), which existed from 320 to 550 CE. This period, whose first ruling king was Chandragupta I (c.319–335 CE), marks an important phase in the history of ancient India and is regarded as the Golden Age of Indian culture. During this Golden Age, many inventions and discoveries were made in science, technology, engineering, mathematics, astronomy, philosophy, art and architecture.

During this great period the *Kāma Sūtra,* by Vatsyayana, and the *Panchatantra* were written. Astronomers and philosophers postulated the theory that the earth moves around the Sun. The theory of gravity was also propounded. Aryabhatta and Varahamihira, two great mathematicians, contributed their findings to the field of Vedic mathematics; Aryabhatta estimated the value of Pi to the fourth decimal place. Algebra was developed and the concepts of zero and infinity were developed. Also, the symbols of numbers 1 to 9 were devised. These symbols came to be known as Hindu-Arabic numerals later when the Arabs adopted them. The *Sushruta Sāmhita*, a text on the major concepts of Āyurvedic ('Science of Life') medicine with innovative chapters on surgery was written by the Āyurvedic sage, Sushruta.

The ruling maharajas of the Gupta Dynasty were efficient administrators who knew how to rule with a firm hand without being despotic. Under their rulership there was relative peace, law and order. India became very rich and powerful; it was a time of peace and prosperity. Peace allowed traders to travel safely, and there was more trade between India and China.

The Golden Age was confined to the north, and the classical patterns began to spread south only after the Gupta Empire had vanished from the historical scene. The gradual decline of the Gupta Empire was brought about through substantial loss of territory and authority caused by their own feudatories and the invasion by the Hunas (the Hephthalites or 'White Huns') from Central Asia. The wars with the Hunas drained the empire's resources, which also led to the decline.

The last Gupta ruling king was Skandagupta, who died around 467 CE. Around 540 CE much of the Gupta Empire had been overrun by the Hunas, which brought an end to the Imperial Gupta Dynasty.

2.7

THE POST-CLASSICAL PERIOD – TANTRIC

500 CE–900 CE – During the Ascending Kali Yuga

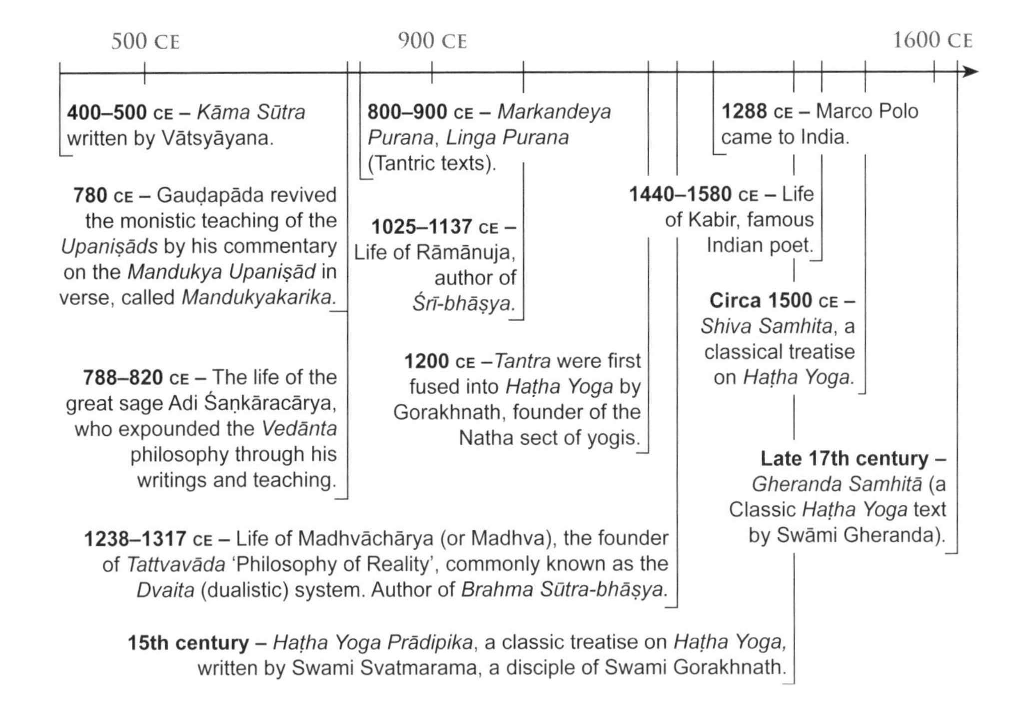

500 CE
900 CE
1600 CE
400–500 CE – *Kāma Sūtra* written by Vātsyāyana.
800–900 CE – *Markandeya Purana, Linga Purana* (Tantric texts).
1288 CE – Marco Polo came to India.
780 CE – Gauḍapāda revived the monistic teaching of the *Upaniṣāds* by his commentary on the *Mandukya Upaniṣād* in verse, called *Mandukyakarika*.
1025–1137 CE – Life of Rāmānuja, author of *Śrī-bhāṣya*.
1440–1580 CE – Life of Kabir, famous Indian poet.
Circa 1500 CE – *Shiva Samhita*, a classical treatise on *Haṭha Yoga*.
788–820 CE – The life of the great sage Adi Śaṇkārācarya, who expounded the *Vedānta* philosophy through his writings and teaching.
1200 CE –*Tantra* were first fused into *Haṭha Yoga* by Gorakhnath, founder of the Natha sect of yogis.
Late 17th century – *Gheranda Samhitā* (a Classic *Haṭha Yoga* text by Swāmi Gheranda).
1238–1317 CE – Life of Madhvāchārya (or Madhva), the founder of *Tattvavāda* 'Philosophy of Reality', commonly known as the *Dvaita* (dualistic) system. Author of *Brahma Sūtra-bhāṣya*.
15th century – *Haṭha Yoga Prādipika*, a classic treatise on *Haṭha Yoga,* written by Swami Svatmarama, a disciple of Swami Gorakhnath.

The *Tantras* are of a later origin than the ancient *Vedās*, but the essence of the Tantric rites and rituals are as old as any other form of Vedic religion. Tantric rites and rituals were prevalent among the people of India long before the *Tantras* were written. Kalluka Bhatta, the great Sanskrit scholar and commentator of the text, *Manusmṛiti*, has held the *Tantras* as a part and parcel of the *Śruti* (Vedic revelation). He says, 'There are two classes of *Śruti* – *Vedic* and *Tantric*.'

In the tenth *Mandas* of the *Rigveda* (1700–1100 BCE) there is the famous *Devi Sukta*, containing hymns to Durga, another name for Śakti (goddess Kali), the main deity of the *Tantras* and the Tantric faith. Again in the *Artharveda* (1200–900 BCE) there are many rites and rituals which are quite similar to those found in the

Tantras. These go to support the view that the underlying principles of the *Tantras* are enshrined in the *Vedās* as well.

The Tantric form of worship was also in practice at the time when the *Srimad Bhagavatam* was written. In the *Srimad Bhagavatam*, we find that the *Braja gopis* were worshipping *Yogamaya* (goddess Śakti) for obtaining Sri Krishna as their husband, and there are many references to the Tantric gods and goddesses in it. *Tantra* was also popular in the days of the *Purānas*; this is made clear from the *Markandeya Purāna*, *Linga Purāna* (800–900 CE), and many other *Purānas*. The *Purānas* are sacred texts that contain many of the ancient legends of Hinduism. There are 18 major *Purānas* or *Mahapuranas*, as they are also known. The *Purānas* are post-Vedic in nature, as the contents and style of writing clearly shows. The great sage Vyasadeva, who composed the *Mahābhārata*, is attributed to being the author of the 18 *mahāpuranas*. The name Vyasadeva was not the great sage's name, but merely a title that was conferred on him. His birth name was Krishna Dvaipayana. He was born on an island, to his parents: Satyavati and the sage Parashara.

Tantra, which originated in India, influenced Shaivism, Buddhism and Vaishnavism, and spread into Nepal, Tibet and China.

The origin of the *Tantras* and their gradual development under two categories – the *Āgamas* (literally, 'that which is received or acquired; acquisition of knowledge'; this is usually applied to non-Vedic texts that are regarded as revelation) and the *Nigāmas* – is shrouded in mystery. One school of thought subscribes to the view that the principles of *Tantra* came from China; others believe that they came from *Mahâyâna* Buddhism. Sir John Woodroffe (1865–1936), also known as Arthur Avalon (author of *The Serpent Power*), one of the greatest oriental scholars on the Tantric cult, came to the conclusion that there is no justification in favour of the argument that the *Tantras* are the offshoots of the Buddhist *mahāyana* cult.

The Sanskrit word *Tantra* literally means 'weave, loom, stretch, expand'. *Trā* means 'to protect or save'. Thus *Tantra* weaves together and expands various traditions of spiritual practices in order to protect and save us from *saṁsāra* (the cycle of birth and death).

The *Tantras* have developed a system of thought and practices by which one can reach the conclusion that the divine glories in the macrocosm are no less immanent in the microcosm, and that by purification of heart and disciplined practices one can attain a divine greatness which ultimately consumes oneself and establishes one's eternal unity with the Absolute.

TANTRA AND SĀṂKHYA

At the time of dissolution (*pralāyā*) of the universe, both *prakṛiti* (eternal principle of matter) and *puruṣa* (the Self, eternal principle of consciousness) merge into *Brāhman*, but *Sāṃkhya* philosophy has a different view on this. *Sāṃkhya* says it is *prakṛiti* that the creation merges and *prakṛiti* remains forever. According to the *Tantras*, *puruṣa* and *prakṛiti* cannot be separated from each other, while in *Sāṃkhya* it is only an instance of coexistence of close proximity. *Puruṣa* and *prakṛiti* are *Śiva* and *Śakti* of the *Tantras*, but quite different from the *puruṣa* and *prakṛiti* of the *Sāṃkhya* philosophy (which is covered in depth in Chapter 3.4, in the *Sāṃkhya* philosophy, one of the six Indian philosophies known as *Ṣad Darśanas*).

In the *Sāṃkhya* system of philosophy, *puruṣa* is not the Supreme Soul of the universe, as *Śiva* is in *Tantra*.

In *Sāṃkhya* philosophy, *puruṣa* is not indivisible, infinite and eternal, but is a multitude of souls. *Puruṣa* (or the multitude of souls) is coexistent with *prakṛiti* (primal matter), but is itself inert and inactive, and unable to produce anything. It is united with *prakṛiti* in order to contemplate her and to be distracted by her.

Sāṃkhya is a dualistic philosophy, but the *Tantras*, as we find in the *Upaniṣads*, shows *puruṣa* and *prakṛiti* to be different modes of the manifestation of Eternal and Infinite *Brāhman*. The *Sāṃkhya* philosophical account of the creation fundamentally differs from the account of the creation given in the *Tantras*. The *Tantras* do not rest on the *Sāṃkhya* system. The *Tantras* assume the existence of God as the very axiom of religion. It believes in the existence of one God and one God alone. In *Tantra*, *prakṛiti* evolves into the creation of the world as we know it, yet at the same time it always remains as *Sat-chit-ānanda* (Ever-Existing, Ever-Conscious, Ever-New Bliss). In this process of evolution, *Māyā,* 'Illusion' (the creative power of *Brāhman* that makes the absolute, formless God appear as the diverse creation), shrouds Reality and creates the duality of opposites. It is *Māyā* that binds and limits us as individual souls. According to the *Tantras*, creation is not an illusion, but real, because it is a mode of Divine manifestation. *Tantra* does not dismiss the creation totally as *Māyā*, but regards it as a Conditional Reality.

The *Tantras*' account of the creation is in essence the same as given in the *Upaniṣads*:

> 'Creation is not an act of time. It is only an emanation of God, a mode of Divine manifestation. The universe is evolved out of God. At the time of creation, Brāhma covers Himself with Māyā, as a spider covers itself with the threads of its own web. The spider weaves its thread from its own saliva. The whole creation lies merged in God; it is only when God covers Himself with His own Māyā, that He wills it and the creation emerges from it. The universe is an emergence, not a creation out of nothing.'

TANTRA AND *HAṬHA YOGA*

It was from the *Shaiva Tantra* that the *Haṭha Yoga* texts, such as *Haṭha Yoga Prādipika* (fifteenth century) and the *Gheranda Saṃhitā* (sixteenth century) originated. Traditions and body disciplines of *Tantra* were first fused into *Haṭha Yoga* by an Indian ascetic yogi known as Goraksha or Gorakhnath (c.1200 CE). Goraksha, believed to be the father of *Haṭha Yoga*, founded the *Natha* sect of *yogis* and was considered to be a revered teacher. The highest contribution of the *Tantras* towards human knowledge is the discovery and location of the centres of energy and consciousness (*chakras*) in the subtle body and their correlation to locations in the spine and brain. Along with the discovery of the *chakras* were the network of *nāḍīs* (subtle *prāṇic* energy channels) and the knowledge of *kuṇḍalinī śakti* and its awakening in the spine. All these originated from Tantric Yoga.

Rather than negate relative reality, the aim of *Tantra* is to sublimate through purification, elevation, and reaffirmation of identity on the plane of pure consciousness. The Tantric yogis celebrated the physical body, which they considered to be a sacred temple of the Divine, as a means to conquer death. To the Tantric yogi the body became the vehicle for attaining liberation.

The *Yoga Sūtras* – one of the six classical philosophies of India, that focuses on the Yoga of the mind and meditation – was formulated and systematised from the pre-existing traditions by the sage Patañjali around the turn of the Common Era (circa first to second century). There is no direct link between Patañjali's Yoga, which predates Tantric Yoga, and the discipline of *Haṭha Yoga*, whose periods of arising are distanced by over a thousand years. In fact, Patañjali makes only one reference to *āsana*, meaning 'seat' or 'posture', referring to a seated posture for sitting in meditation.

Tantra had absorbed Patañjali's eight primary practices of Yoga, known as 'The Eight Limbs of Yoga' (*Aṣṭāṅga Yoga*) early on, into the Tantric disciplines of *Haṭha Yoga*. The techniques of Patañjali's *Yoga Sūtras* were used by *Tantra*, but Patañjali's philosophy on duality was rejected. Tantric philosophy maintains that there is no division between Spirit and matter; they are inseparable. This is what is known in the *Tantras* as the union between *puruṣa* and *prakṛiti*, or between *Śiva* and *Śakti*. According to the *Upaniṣads* and *Tantra* the visible universe is a mode of Divine manifestation, hence it is inseparable from *Brāhman*. It is through the manifestation of Divine energy in the universe that we come to know the existence of God, and this energy is a mode of manifestation of *Brāhman*. The Tantrics experience this divinity in every aspect of life. There is nothing dead or inert in nature, everything is living and contains energy. God and His energy are inseparable. In *Tantra* there is no duality, there is only One.

TANTRA AND *ŚIVA* AND *ŚAKTI*

The *Tantras* emphasise the feminine aspect of the Divinity – *Śakti*, the Eternal Mother of the universe – for there is nothing more sacred and deep than a mother's love. The Tantrics worship the Divine as *Śakti*, or as She appears through the manifestation of Her Divine energy (*Mahāśakti*). *Śakti* is the personification of the Divine Energy that has brought the universe into existence, that preserves it from disintegration and dissolution. *Śiva* is the emblem of the destructive forces that lie dormant in the universe. Destruction is also an aspect of Divine Energy that coexists with the creative energy. The Supreme Lord is represented as *Śiva* and His power is represented as *Śakti*.

Like heat in fire, *Śiva* and *Śakti* are inseparable; they are ultimately one and the same, because they are two modes of the manifestation of the Eternal and Infinite *Brāhman*. In *Tantra* more prominence has been given to *Śakti*, because it is the Divine energy that has brought the universe into existence, and preserves, sustains and governs it. *Māyā* (illusion) or *prakṛiti* (the eternal principle of matter) is within the womb of *Śakti*. *Māyā* evolves into the material elements under the direction of *Śakti*.

2.8

THE MODERN PERIOD

1607–1887 – Trailanga Swāmi, famed for his spiritual yogic powers and his longevity.

1828–1895 – Shyama Charan Lahiri Mahasaya, the disciple to whom Babaji revealed the almost lost science of *Kriyā Yoga*.

1855–1936 – Swāmi Sri Yukteswar Giri, guru of Paramhansa Yogananda.

1861 – Lahiri Mahasaya's first meeting and *Kriyā* initiation with the saintly yogi, Mahavatar Babaji. The modern revival of *Kriyā Yoga* began.

1879–1950 – Ramana Maharshi, one of the greatest spiritual gurus of modern-day India.

1883 – *Kriyā* Initiation of Sri Yukteswar by Lahiri Mahasaya.

1896–1982 – Sri Anandamayi Ma ('the bliss permeated mother'), who was continuously in the highest state of *samādhi*.

1894 – Sri Yukteswar's first vision of Mahavatar Babaji.

1893–1952 – Paramhansa Yogananda, great *Kriyā* Master who brought the *Kriyā Yoga* to the West.

1906 – *Kriyā* Initiation of Mukundalal (later known as Paramhansa Yogananda).

1910–1984 – Acharya Sri Sailendra Bejoy Dasgupta (a direct disciple of Swāmi Sri Yukteswar).

1915 – Initiation into *Sannyāsa* of Mukundalal (later known as Paramhansa Yogananda).

1926–2013 – Swami Kriyananda (a direct American disciple of Paramhansa Yogananda, and founder of Ananda spiritual communities).

(1931–) Roy Eugene Davis (a direct American disciple of Paramhansa Yogananda, who was ordained by him to teach and initiate others into *Kriyā Yoga*).

1946 – Paramhansa Yogananda's classic, *Autobiography of a Yogi*, is first published.

PART 3

YOGA IN INDIAN PHILOSOPHY

3.1

THE ṢAD DARŚANAS

From the *Upanisadic* writings evolved a gradual development of the six complete systems of Indian philosophy *Ṣad Darśanas*. The Sanskrit word *sad* means 'six' and the word *darsana* is derived from the root *dris* meaning 'to see'. The term *Darsana* in Sanskrit is used for philosophy. Self-realisation, the direct experience of one's own essential nature, is the goal of all the systems of Indian philosophy; they all present a method of practice through which one can transcend suffering of the mind and body, and attain the spiritual goal of life.

Direct experience is the foundation of the six systems of Indian philosophy. The knowledge within these philosophical systems did not come from mere speculation, but were perceived by great sages (*rishis*) who had direct experience of transcendental truths through contemplative visions. In the beginning, philosophical discussions were handed down by *rishis* to their students (*chelas*) through oral traditions, who in turn became *āchāryas* (teachers). With the gradual passage of time, these realisations of truth were codified in *sūtras* (aphorisms) and written as scriptures, so that they would not be lost or forgotten. The *sūtra* style of aphorisms in literature is extremely concise and precise and avoids all unnecessary repetition. This makes the *sūtras* difficult to understand correctly in their original form without the use of commentaries (*bhāsyas*), because although they use many of the same terms, each system of the *Ṣad Darśanas* gives its own meaning to the terms used. The different expositions and commentaries given by various authors all give different viewpoints depending on their personal insights, experience, logic and reasoning. Even the Sanskrit itself, from which the *sūtras* have been translated, can give a different meaning, for a single Sanskrit word can have numerous meanings.

According to the Indian tradition, there is only one Ultimate Reality, but there are six fundamental interpretations of the Realities, called 'six insights' or *Ṣad Darśanas*. The texts of most of these six philosophical systems are considered to have been formulated in their present form sometime between 200 BCE and 450 CE.

The *Ṣad Darśanas* or the six principal philosophical systems recognised by the Hindu orthodoxy as representing valid points of view within the context of the Vedic tradition are:

1. ***Nyāya:*** founded by the sage Gautama
2. ***Vaiśeṣika:*** founded by the sage Kaṇāda
3. ***Sāṃkhya:*** founded by the sage Kapila

4. ***Yoga:*** founded by the sage Patañjali
5. ***Mīmāṁsā (purva):*** founded by the sage Jaimini
6. ***Vedānta:*** founded by the sage Vyāsa.

All other schools of thought are but variations of these six. It is of great importance when studying the Indian philosophies that one realises that the basis of all the six philosophical systems is the same. The six systems complement each other and the differences that separate them on certain points are minor. The six systems all accept the spirit as a transcendent principle, but they prove its existence and explain its essence from different viewpoints. They also accept that the involvement of the spirit (*puruṣa*) with the forces of nature (*prakṛiti*) is the cause for its bondage, but again, it is explained in different ways.

Together these philosophies form a graduated interpretation of the Ultimate Reality and are interrelated in such a way that the hypothesis and method of each is dependent upon the other. In no way are they contradictory or antagonistic to one another, because all lead to the same practical end, the liberation of the soul and the knowledge of the Absolute. The goal of each philosophical system is to transcend suffering, to make us aware of the false identification with the external objects of the world, and to inspire us to attain freedom from sorrow and suffering.

Āyurveda (Science of Life), the sister science of Yoga, is deeply related to the Indian cultural heritage. This is why it becomes difficult to explain *Āyurveda* on modern lines without having a clear knowledge of *Sāṃkhya-Yoga* and *Nyāya-Vaiśeṣika* philosophies. To understand the philosophical basis of *Āyurveda*, it is essential to have a clear idea of the *Sāṃkhya* philosophy and the concept of *panchabhuta* (also known as *panchamahābhuta*) – the basic 'Building Blocks of Existence'. In the study of *Āyurveda*, the knowledge of *Sāṃkhya-Yoga* and *Nyāya-Vaiśeṣika* is of significance in understanding the finer aspects of the subject, the basis on which it has developed; and these cannot possibly be understood by doing comparative studies with modern medical knowledge.

For those following the path of Yoga it is important to understand the underlying philosophy of *Sāṃkhya*, as it is the key to understanding the yogic concept of the mind.

The six systems of philosophy (*Ṣad Darśanas*) can be classified into three twin divisions:

Vaiśeṣika and ***Nyāya***

Sāṃkhya and ***Yoga***

Mīmaṃsā **(*purva*)** and ***Vedānta.***

Each aspect of a twin division serves as a complementary philosophy to that of the other.

For the purposes of following *Rāja Yoga*, which includes *Hātha Yoga*, Patañjali's *Aṣṭāṅga Yoga* and *Kriyā Yoga*, we really only need to be concerned with *Sāṃkhya*, *Yoga*, and *Vedānta* philosophies. So, the systems of *Mīmāṁsā (purva)*, *Vaiśeṣika* and *Nyāya* will not be covered in great depth, but only outlined here.

3.2

NYĀYA (VALID KNOWLEDGE THROUGH LOGICAL CRITICISM)

The *Nyāya* system of Indian philosophy was founded by a great sage Gautama (Gotama), who is also known as Akṣopāda, and Dīrghatapas (not to be confused with Buddha), and is said to have been born at Gautamasthāna, north-east of Darbhanga, Bihar, India. Gautama formulated the generally accepted philosophical principles of his time, and reduced the principles for the examination of Truth into their present form.

The earliest commentary on Gautama's *Nyāya-Sūtras* is by Vātsyāyana (also the author of the *Kāma Sūtra*), who is believed to have lived in the fourth century of the Common Era. He defines *Nyāya* as a 'critical examination of the objects of knowledge by means of the canons of logical proof'. The most outstanding commentary on the *Nyāya-Sūtras* is the *Tatva Chintamani* of Gangesa, which has been accepted as the final authority on the *Nyāya* system.

The term *Nyāya* signifies an analytical investigation of a subject through the process of logical reason. *Nyāya* philosophy developed out of the ancient Indian tradition of debate; its name, often translated as 'logic' (the process of reasoning), relates to its original and primary concern with the method (*nyāya*) of proof, and with the conditions of correct knowledge and the means of receiving that knowledge. *Nyāya* is also known as *Tarka Sāstra* – the science of logic and reasoning; *Pramana Sāstra* – the science of logic and epistemology; *Hetuvidya* – the science of causes; *Vadavidyā* – the science of debate; and *Anviksiki* – the science of critical study.

Nyāya is founded on the belief that only by thorough examination, through the process of obtaining valid knowledge of objects of perception, can we gain release from material bondage, and suffering. The *Nyāya* identified valid sources of knowledge and distinguished it from mere false opinions, and classified the different ways in which this knowledge is acquired.

According to *Nyāya*, there are only four sources of knowledge that are credible from a trustworthy person who knows truth and communicates it correctly:

1. **Perception** (*pratyaksha*)
2. **Inference** (*anumāna*)

3. **Comparison** (*upamāna*)
4. **Verbal testimony** (*śabda*).

This is knowledge that has been collected as the result of reasoned inquiry, made by certain extraordinary persons with divine vision or who have directly attained revelation from God. The *śrutis* such as the *Vedās* and the *Upaniṣads* remain as an external authority to tell us these revealed truths.

THE *NYĀYA* CONCEPT OF THE SELF

The soul (*atmā*) is eternal in nature because it is not limited by space and time. *Nyāya* asserts a real plurality of souls (*atmās*) – different souls in different bodies. 'I exist as an individual self.' The existence of the Self is necessary to explain the unity and coherence of my experience. One's own self (*atmā*) can be known through mental perception, whereas someone else's soul (*atmā*) can only be inferred.

Experience and cognition, thoughts, feelings and ideas are owned; they do not exist merely strung together, but as contents, objects and conditions of an individual consciousness.

The operation of the senses discloses the existence of the Self as the agent who perceives the world by means of the senses. The Self cannot be identified with the mind or intellect, with thinking, perceiving or knowing. The Self is the ultimate subject of all perception and cognition. The Self is the eternal soul. The soul is indestructible and all-pervading, though in life it perceives the world through the operation of an individual mind, which limits its ability to perceive things to those accessible to the individual body belonging to it.

Consciousness is a property of the soul, but not an essential property. Consciousness cannot exist without the soul, but the soul can exist without being conscious.

THE *NYĀYA* CONCEPT OF LIBERATION

The earliest *Nyāya* philosophers investigations led them to conclude that the essence of liberation (*mokṣa*) is absolute freedom from all pain and suffering. Liberation takes place when all effort, all activity, all consequences of activity, all tendency to incarnation, and all association with a body come to an end, and therefore all consciousness ends. *Nyāya* believes that in the final stage of liberation, the individual soul is separated from its instruments of consciousness (mind, body and senses) and abides in absolute and eternal unconsciousness. This is very different from the *Yoga* and *Vedānta* systems in which the liberated soul enters into the superconscious state.

THE *NYĀYA* CONCEPT OF GOD

According to *Nyāya*, God (*Brāhman*) is the creator, sustainer and destroyer of the universe. God is the first efficient cause of the universal forces that create the world. God creates all substances from the eternal atoms of space, time, mind and consciousness.

God causes the atoms to hold together and continue their existence in a particular order so as to maintain the physical universe.

God directs the activities of living souls. Just as an intelligent and benevolent father inspires the son to act according to his intelligence, capability and qualities, God also inspires living beings to act according to the tendencies acquired by them in the past and to win rewards appropriate to their action.

God does not take on a personal form. God is not a material cause but merely an efficient cause of creation. God is a distinct soul, and other souls are also like God. Both are eternal. However, God is distinguished from the individual souls because He is omniscient and omnipotent.

3.3

VAIŚEṢIKA (ANALYSIS OF THE ASPECTS OF REALITY)

Vaiśeṣika originates from the Sanskrit word *Viśeṣa*, meaning 'uniqueness' – the characteristics that distinguish a particular thing from all other things. *Vaiśeṣika* philosophy was founded by the sage Kaṇāda, who wrote the *Vaiśeṣika Sūtra* (third century BCE).

Vaiśeṣika is a philosophy of nature concerned mainly with the comprehensive enumeration and analysis and identification of all aspects of reality. According to *Vaiśeṣika Sūtra*, reality consists of substances that are distinct from the qualities they possess. Knowledge of reality is obtained by knowing the special qualities (*guṇas*) and essential differences which distinguish nine ultimate eternal substances (*dravyas*) or realities:

Earth (*pṛthivi*)

Water (*āpas*)

Fire (*tejas*)

Air (*vāyu*)

Ether (*ākāśha*)

Time (*kāla*)

Space (*dik*)

Soul/Self (*ātman*)

Mind (*manas*).

The first five *dravyas* (earth, water, fire, air and ether) are called *māhabhūtas*, substances that have specific qualities that can be perceived by the senses. The first seven are self-explanatory, but the last two need further clarification. The Self (*ātman*), according to this system, is omnipresent and eternal. Though present everywhere, the feelings and thoughts of a Self are confined to the physical organism it is associated with. We know directly, but the Self of others can be known only indirectly through their behaviour. Mind (*manas*) is atomic and eternal, but does not give rise to any product. Each Self has its own *manas,* which is merely an instrument of knowing like other sense organs.

It is through the mind that the relation of the Self to the sense organs and the body is established and through them the Self comes to be related to the external world.

The *dravyas* form the framework of the universe. These, together with six other categories of the system – *guṇa* (quality), *karma* (actions), *sāmānya* (generality), *viśeṣa* (uniqueness), *samavāya* (inherence) and *abhāva* (non-existence) – explain, according to the *Nyāya-Vaiśeṣika*, the whole universe.

Although the *Vaiśeṣika* system of philosophy developed independently of the *Nyāya* system, the two eventually merged because of their closely related metaphysical theories. In its classical form, however, the *Vaiśeṣika* system differed from the *Nyāya* in two crucial respects.

First, the *Nyāya* system accepted four sources of valid knowledge: perception (*pratyaksha*), inference (*anumāna*), comparison (*upamāna*) and verbal testimony (*śabda*). However, the *Vaiśeṣika* system accepted only two: perception (*pratyaksha*) and inference (*anumāna*).

Second, *Nyāya* believes that all of reality is comprehended by 16 categories (*pardārthas*). However, *Vaiśeṣika* recognises only seven categories of reality: *dravya* (substance), *guṇa* (quality), *karma* (activity), *sāmanāya* (generality), *viśeṣa* (uniqueness or specific individuality), *samavāya* (inherence) and *abhāva* (non-existence).

The 16 *Nyāya* categories (*pardārthas*) are further divided into two main categories: **that which exists** (*dravya*, *guṇa*, *karma*, *sāmanāya*, *viśeṣa* and *samavāya*) and **that which does not exist** (*abhāva*).

THE *VAIŚEṢIKA* CONCEPT OF GOD

The *Nyāya-Vaiśeṣika* philosophers maintain that the existence of God can be proved by inference without the aid of revelation, and this attitude is in keeping with the teaching of the system with its emphasis on reasoning. *Nyāya-Vaiśeṣika*, like *Yoga*, maintains that God is a distinct soul, and that other individual souls are eternal like God. However, God is distinguished from the individual souls because He is omniscient and omnipotent.

THE *VAIŚEṢIKA* ATOMIC DOCTRINE

As the *Nyāya-Vaiśeṣikas* depended solely on experience and on valid reasoning, they dismissed the *Sāṃkhya* cosmology but accepted the atomic doctrine of the four elements (*māhabhūtas*). The permanent, indivisible and eternal existence of the atoms (*paramāṇus*) of the four *māhabhūtas* **earth** (*pṛthivi*), **water** (*āpas*), **fire** (*tejas*) and **air** (*vāyu*) are not subject to change, and cannot be created or destroyed.

The fifth *māhabhūta*, **ether** (*ākāśha*), is all-pervasive and eternal but without atoms. It is regarded as the means of propagating sound; though all-pervading and thus in touch with the ears of all persons, it manifests sound only in the ear-drum, as it is only there that it shows itself as a sense-organ to manifest sounds.

According to the *Vaiśeṣika* system, there is no creation or destruction but instead an organised system of natural order of composition and decomposition of compounds.

3.4

SĀṂKHYA (ENUMERATION)

THE SEEDS OF *SĀṂKHYA* IN THE *UPANIṢADS*

In the *Upaniṣads* there is a large number of texts that describe the Ultimate Reality as the *Brāhman*, the infinite, knowledge, bliss; and speak of all else as mere changing forms and names. The word *Brāhman* in the earliest Vedic literature originally meant *mantra*, duly performed sacrifice, and also the power of sacrifice which could bring about the desired result. In many passages of the *Upaniṣads* this *Brāhman* appears as the universal and supreme principle from which all others derived their powers. Such a *Brāhman* is sought for in many passages for personal gain or welfare. But through a gradual process of development the conception of *Brāhman* reached a superior level and the One, the infinite, knowledge, the real, is regarded as the only Truth. This type of thought gradually developed into the monistic *Vedānta* as explained by Adi Shankaracharya. But there was another line of thought which was developing alongside it, which regarded the world as having a reality and as being made up of water, fire and earth. There are also passages in *Svetasvatara Upaniṣad* and particularly in *Maitrayani Upaniṣad* from which it appears that the *Sāṃkhya* line of thought had considerably developed, and many of its technical terms were already in use. But the date of *Maitrayani Upaniṣad* has not yet been definitely settled, and the details found there are also not such that we can form a distinct notion of the *Sāṃkhya* thought as it developed in the *Upaniṣads*. It is not improbable that at this stage of development it also gave some suggestions to Buddhism or Jainism, but the *Sāṃkhya-Yoga* philosophy as we now understand it is a system in which all the results of Buddhism and Jainism are found in such a manner with the doctrines of momentariness of the Buddhists and the doctrine of relativism of the Jains.

According to tradition the metaphysical doctrine of *Sāṃkhya* is attributed to the sage Kapila (sixth century BCE), of whom very little is known. Today, the sage Kapila is still venerated on the island of Sāgara in the Ganga delta region near Calcutta on the first day of the Hindu month of *Māgha* that falls in mid-January. It is believed that Kapila lived the last part of his life on the island of Sāgara.

The date of origin of *Sāṃkhya* is uncertain, like other systems of Indian philosophy. But two things are clear: that the origin of *Sāṃkhya* is due to the reaction against the performances of the Vedic sacrifices; and that it received a special sanctity in ancient scriptural literature. Pre-Classical ideas of *Sāṃkhya* are scattered in various sources. The *Śvetāsvatara*, the *Kātha*, the *Maitrāyani* and the *Chāndogya Upaniṣads* are full of *Sāṃkhya* ideas. The *Mahābhārata,* eulogising *Sāṃkhya,* speaks at one place that all kinds of supreme knowledge available in the *Vedās*, the *Purānas*, and so on, owe their origin to the *Sāṃkhya*. In the *Atharva Veda*, Pariśista speaks of the *Sāṃkhya* teachers such as Kapila, Āsuri and Pancaśikha in connection with the *tarpana* invocation. The *Sāṃkhya* teaching and its ideas form a very important part of the *Purānas*, the Āyurvedic scripture *Charaka Samhita* (*Śarirasthanam*), *Āhirbudhnya Samhita*, *Mahābhārata* (*Śāntiparva*) and Asvaghosa's *Buddha Carita*. And in the *Manu-Smṛiti* Manu is said to have learnt the knowledge of *Sāṃkhya-Yoga* first from *Brāhma*.

Sāṃkhya cosmogony is traced back to the ancient *Rigveda* (11.29) and *Arthava Veda* (10.8, 43). The earliest text that is available on *Sāṃkhya* philosophy is the *Sāṃkhya-kārikā* of Iśvarakrsna (third century CE). Later well-known commentaries are *Tattvakaumudī* (ninth century CE) by Vācaspati Miśra, and *Bhāsya* by Gaudapāda (eighth century CE).

In most of these texts the *Moksha* (liberation) Doctrine occupies the major part. Consideration of the outer world came forth only to understand what role it played in respect of bondage and liberation (absolute freedom from all pain and suffering). The *Mahābhārata* declares *Sāṃkhya* as a doctrine of liberation (*Sāṃkhya vai Moksadarśanam*), or *Sāṃkhya* and *Yoga* as the two-fold path to liberation. The purpose of *Sāṃkhya* is to provide the knowledge that will remove the cause of pain and suffering in order to liberate the soul from its bondage. According to *Sāṃkhya* the causes of pain and suffering are threefold: *adhyatmic* – causes from disorders of the mind and body; *adhibhautic* – caused by people, animals, insects and inanimate objects; and *adhidaivic* – from supernatural causes, that is, thunder, rain, cold, heat or other planets.

Yoga is often referred to as *Sankhya-Yoga*, as Yoga contains the practical methods to realise in direct experience the truths of *Sāṃkhya* philosophy. *Sāṃkhya* represents the theory and Yoga represents the application of the practical aspects.

The word *Sāṃkhya* is derived from the prefix *sām* meaning 'together' and the Sanskrit root *khya* meaning 'calculate'. Another meaning of the word *Sāṃkhya* is derived from *Samyagakhyate*, which means 'that which explains the whole'. The term *Sāṃkhya* means 'enumeration' – that which concerns number, principles of categories and hierarchical classification. *Sāṃkhya* enumerates the principles of cosmic evolution by rational analysis based on the principles of conservation, transformation and dissipation of energy. The phenomenal universe is considered as a dynamic order, an eternal process of unfolding which is infinite, that has evolved out of an uncaused Cause. In this eternal process of evolution there is an exact selection of means for the acquisition of a definite end. There is never a random combination of events and there is an order, regulation, system and division of function.

THEORY OF EXISTENCE

Sāṃkhya philosophy accepts the *Satkāryavāda* theory of causation, according to which an effect is already existent in unmanifested form in its cause. Cause and effect are seen as different temporal aspects of the same thing – the effect lies latent in the cause which in turn seeds the next effect. If the effect did not exist in the cause, then that which was non-existent would be coming into existence out of nothing. It is not possible for non-existence to become existence; nor can that which exists be entirely destroyed.

Sāṃkhya philosophy believes that there can be no production of a thing previously non-existent; causation means the appearance or manifestation of a quality due to certain changes of collocations in the causes which were already held in them in a potential form. Production of effect only means an internal change of the arrangement of atoms in the cause, and this exists in it in a potential form; and just a little loosening of the barrier which was standing in the way of the happening of such a change of arrangement will produce the desired new collocation – the effect. This doctrine is called *Satkāryavāda*, that is, that the *karya* or 'effect' is *sat* or 'existence' even before the causal operation to produce the effect was launched. The oil exists in the sesame seed, the sculptured statue in the stone, the yoghurt in the milk, the oak tree in the acorn. The causal operation (*karakaiyapara*) only renders that manifest (*avirbhuta*) which was formerly in an unmanifested condition (*tirohita*).

Advaita Vedānta philosophy differs from *Sāṃkhya*. It believes that the change of a cause into an effect is merely apparent. An example given by Vedantins is that if one mistakes a snake for a rope, it is not true that the rope is really transformed into a snake; it simply appears to be that way. *Sāṃkhya* does not accept this *vivartavāda* theory held by *Advaita Vedānta*, but holds the viewpoint of *Parināmavāda* theory, according to which there is a real transformation of the cause into the effect, as milk being transformed into curds or yoghurt; the cause being *prakṛiti* or *mūla-prakṛiti* (primordial matter).

TWENTY-FIVE *TATTVAS*

Sāṃkhya, considered to be the most ancient of all the philosophical systems, is the evolution of metaphysical doctrine. Its dualistic philosophy is primarily concerned with the evolutionary process that binds the individual soul (*puruṣa*) to matter (*prakṛiti*). *Sāṃkhya* philosophy comprehends that the universe is a sum total of 25 *Tattvas*, categories or principles (the 24 products of primordial matter, plus spirit or soul). This is no mere metaphysical speculation, but a logical account based on scientific principles of conservation, transformation and dissipation of energy.

The 25 *Tattvas* that the whole phenomenal universe evolves from are:

Puruṣa – spirit or soul

Prakṛiti – nature/matter

Māhat or ***Buddhi*** – intellect

Ahaṁkāra – ego

Manas – mind

Jñānendriyas – five cognitive senses (hearing, touch, sight, taste, smell)

Karmendriyas – five action senses (speech, hands, feet, anus, generative organs)

Tanmātras – subtle primary elements

Mahābhutas – generic gross elements.

Puruṣa and prakṛiti

> 'Without the conjunction of *prakṛiti*, there can be no conjunction of bondage in the self (*puruṣa*) who is by nature, eternal, and eternally pure, enlightened, and unconfined (unbound).'
>
> *Sāṃkhya-Pravacana Sūtra, 1.19*

Sāṃkhya philosophy is based on the theory of transformation. *Sāṃkhya* does not acknowledge a Creator or any act of creation (apart from the implied principle of continuous creation). It does not accept *Īśvara* or God, because it believes that the *puruṣa* cannot be regarded as the source of the inanimate world, because an intelligent principle cannot transform itself into the unintelligent world. The concept of *Īśvara* was incorporated into the *nirishvara* (atheistic) *Sāṃkhya* philosophy only after it became associated with the *Yoga*, the *Pasupata* and the *Bhagavata* schools of philosophy.

Sāṃkhya philosophy explains the existence of all things or substances as a mutual relationship between two basic principles: *puruṣa* and *prakṛiti* (from the Sanskrit prefix *pra*, meaning 'before or first', and the Sanskrit root *kri*, 'to make or produce'). The creation produced by *prakṛiti* has an existence of its own, independent of all connection with the particular *puruṣa* to which it is united. *Prakṛiti* has no cause but is the cause of all effects.

Sāṃkhya's twin philosophy, *Yoga*, is the practical aspect of understanding *Sāṃkhya* philosophy.

In *Sāṃkhya* philosophy the phenomenal world begins when the two principle energies, *puruṣa* (spirit) and *prakṛiti* (nature), interact with each other. Evolution cannot occur by *puruṣa* (spirit) alone because it is inactive and passive by nature; it is in itself uninvolved in the process of bondage and liberation. Nor can it be initiated only by *prakṛiti* because it is an unconscious principle. *Puruṣa* is conscious Spirit or the Universal Soul; *prakṛiti* is unconscious primordial matter. *Puruṣa* is also known as *ātman* or *jīvātma* (individual soul or self) and is considered to be conscious of its universal spirit principle, known as the *Paramātma*.

All manifestation in the universe is the interaction of these two principles, *puruṣa* and *prakṛiti*; although they co-exist together they have no independent function. They are dependent upon each other, and come into existence by their interaction with each other. In this continuous act of creation, the Spirit Principle (*puruṣa*) remains unaltered; only the Matter Principle (*prakṛiti*) undergoes transformation.

Unlike *Advaita Vedānta* philosophy and like *Purva-Mīmaṃsā* philosophy, *Sāṃkhya* believes in plurality of the *puruṣas*. The *puruṣas* (individual souls) are multiple in number and are all separate yet identical. If there were only one soul related to all bodies, then when one individual died, all individuals would simultaneously die. We know this is not true – the birth or death of one individual does not cause all other individuals to be born or to die.

These two principles, *puruṣa*, the many pure conscious intelligent individual souls who are eternal and not subject to change, and *prakṛiti*, the one all-pervading (unconscious) material cause of the universe, interact with each other to start the process of evolution. In an energy-packed state of tension, *prakṛiti*, the Matter principle, undergoes transformation, but the Spirit principle remains unaltered.

The guṇas

In *Sāṃkhya*, thought and matter are but two different modifications of certain subtle substances which are in essence three types of feeling entities. The three principal characteristics of thought and matter (sattva, rajas and tamas) are respectively the manifestations of three types of feeling substances: mental harmony, restlessness and dullness. Corresponding to these three types of manifestations as pleasure, pain and dullness, and materially as shining (*prakasa*), energy (*pravṛtti*) and obstruction (*niyama*), there are three types of feeling-substances which must be regarded as the ultimate things which make up all the diverse kinds of gross matter and thought by their varying modifications.

These three types of ultimate subtle entities are technically called the *guṇas* in *Sāṃkhya* philosophy. *Guṇa* in Sanskrit has three meanings: quality; rope; and not primary. These *guṇas*, however, are substances and not mere qualities. It may be mentioned in this connection that in *Sāṃkhya* philosophy there is no separate existence of qualities; it holds that each and every unit of quality is a unit of substance. What we call quality is a particular manifestation or appearance of a subtle entity. Things do not possess quality, but quality signifies merely the manner in which a substance reacts; any object we see seems to possess many qualities, but the *Sāṃkhya* holds that corresponding to each and every new unit of quality, however fine and subtle it may be, there is a corresponding subtle entity, the reaction of which is interpreted by us as a quality. This is true not only of qualities of external objects but also of mental qualities.

These ultimate entities were thus called *guṇas* probably to suggest that they are the entities which, by their various modifications, manifest themselves as *guṇas* or qualities. These subtle entities may also be called *guṇas* in the sense of ropes because they are like ropes by which the soul is tied down as if it were to thought and matter. The Sanskrit word *guṇa* literally means 'strand' or 'fibre' and implies that, like strands of a rope, the *guṇas* are woven together to form the universe. These may also be called *guṇas* as things of secondary importance, because though permanent and indestructible, they continually suffer modifications and changes by their mutual groupings and re-groupings, and thus are not primarily and unalterably constant like souls (*puruṣa*). Moreover, the object of the world process being enjoyment and liberation of the *puruṣas*, the matter principle could not naturally be regarded as being of primary importance. But in whatever senses we may be inclined to justify the name of *guṇa* as applied to these subtle entities, it should be borne in mind that they are substantive entities or subtle substances and not abstract qualities.

> '*Sattva*, *rajas*, and *tamas* – the (three) primary-qualities born of the Cosmos, fasten the immutable body-essence (*dehin*) to the body, O mighty-armed (Arjuna).'
>
> *Bhāgavad Gītā 14.5*

These *guṇas*, which are the foundation of reality and the essence of all things, are infinite in number, but in accordance with their three main characteristics as described above they have been arranged in three classes or types – *sattva*, *rajas* and *tamas*:

Sattva (essence, illumination) – represents the fine structure of substance and the wellspring of consciousness. *Sattva* is the power of nature that illuminates and reveals all manifestations.

Rajas (activity) – represents change, alteration and is a quality of dynamics and the basis of energy itself. *Rajas* affects and moves the other two constituents – *sattva* and *tamas* – without which they could not manifest their inherent qualities.

Tamas (inertia, darkness) – represents the quality of resistance, restraint and obstruction, and all negative and passive actions, the characteristics of which are dull, rough, coarse and heavy.

There are an infinite number of subtle substances which have characteristics of harmony, stability and illumination, and are called the c*sattva-guṇas;* those which behave as units of activity are called the *rajo-guṇas*; and those which behave as factors of obstruction, mass or materiality are called *tamo-guṇas*. These subtle *guṇa* substances are united in different proportions (e.g. a larger number of *sattva* substances with a lesser number of *rajas* or *tamas*, or a larger number of *tamas* substances with a smaller number of *rajas* and *sattva* substances, and so on in varying proportions), and as a result of this, different substances with different qualities come into being. Though attached to one another when united in different proportions, they mutually act and react upon one another, and thus by their combined results produce new characters, qualities and substances.

There is one, and only one, stage in which the *guṇas* are not compounded in varying proportions. In this state each of the *guṇa* substances is opposed by each of the other *guṇa* substances, and thus by their equal mutual opposition create an equilibrium, in which none of the characters of the *guṇas* manifest themselves. This is the state which is so absolutely devoid of all characteristics that it is absolutely incoherent, indeterminate and indefinite. It is a simple homogeneity without qualities. It is a state of being which is, as it were, non-being. This state of the mutual equilibrium of the *guṇas* is called *prakṛiti*. This is the state which cannot be said either to exist or to non-exist for it serves no purpose, but it is hypothetically the mother of all things. This is, however, the earliest stage, by the breaking of which, later on, all modifications take place.

The evolutionary process of the universe

> '*Prakṛiti* is the state of quiescence (equilibrium) of *sattva*, *rajas* and *tamas*. From *prakṛiti* evolves *mahāt* (intellect); from *mahāt*, *ahaṁkāra* (I-consciousness); from *ahaṁkāra*, the five *tanmātras* (subtle elements) and the two sets of *indriyas* (sense instruments); from the five *tanmātras*, the gross elements. Then the self. Such is the group of the twenty-five principles.'
>
> *Sāṃkhya-Pravacana Sūtra 1.16*

Sāṃkhya philosophy believes that before this world came into being there was a state of dissolution, in which the *guṇa* compounds had disintegrated into a state of disunion and had by their mutual opposition produced an equilibrium, the *prakṛiti*. Then, later on, disturbance arose in the *prakṛiti*, and as a result of that a process of unequal aggregation of the *guṇas* in varying proportions took place, which brought forth the creation of the universe.

Prakṛiti, the state of perfect homogeneity and incoherence of the *guṇas*, thus gradually evolved and became more and more determinate, differentiated, heterogeneous and coherent. The *guṇas* are always uniting, separating, and uniting again. Varying qualities of essence, energy and mass in varied groupings act on one another and through their mutual interaction and interdependence evolve from the indefinite or qualitatively indeterminate to the definite or qualitatively determinate. And through cooperating to produce the world of effects, these diverse moments with diverse tendencies never coalesce. Thus in the phenomenal product whatever energy there is, is due to the element of *rajas* and *rajas* alone; all matter, resistance, stability, is due to *tamas*, and all conscious manifestation to *sattva*.

The order of succession is neither from parts to whole nor from whole to the parts, but ever from a relatively less differentiated, less determinate, less coherent whole to a relatively more differentiated, more determinate, more coherent whole.

Evolution (*tattvantaraparinama*) in *Sāṃkhya* means the development of categories of existence and not mere changes of qualities of substances (physical, chemical, biological, or mental). Thus each of the stages of evolution remain as a permanent category of being, and offers scope to the more and more differentiated and coherent groupings of the succeeding stages. Thus it is said that the evolutionary process is regarded as a differentiation of new stages as integrated in previous stages.

Order of evolution

The relation between the two cosmic principles, *puruṣa* and *prakṛiti*, can be compared to that of a magnet and a piece of iron. *Puruṣa* itself does not come into contact with *prakṛiti*, but it influences *prakṛiti*, and as a result *prakṛiti* is prompted to produce. The radical interactions among the three *guṇas* (*sattva*, *rajas*, *tamas*) disturb the state of equilibrium in *prakṛiti*, causing a predominance of one or the other *guṇa*. The *guṇas* undergo more and more changes; *prakṛiti* goes on differentiating into numerous and various world objects, and becomes more and more determinate.

In evolution, *prakṛiti* is transformed and differentiated into a multiplicity of material objects. Evolution is followed by dissolution in which the physical existence of all phenomenal matter and worldly objects is absorbed back into *prakṛiti*, which then remains as the undifferentiated, primordial substance. This is how the cycles of evolution and dissolution follow each other.

From the combination of *puruṣa* and *prakṛiti*, evolution results in 23 different categories of objects. They comprise three elements of *antaḥkaraṇas* (internal organs) as well as the ten *bahyakaranas* (external organs).

THE FIRST THREE EVOLUTES OF *PRAKṚITI*

The first three evolutes (***māhat, ahaṁkāra, manas***) to evolve simultaneously from *prakṛiti* are termed collectively the *antaḥkaraṇa* (internal instruments). These three faculties of different functions are the outcome of the imbalance of the three causative principles or *guṇas*. *Manas*, *buddhi* and *ahaṁkāra* work together within the mind field or field of experience to create the sense of experience. *Ahaṁkāra* creates the subject–object experience that connects all the experiences of life. *Manas* and *buddhi* serve the interests of the *ahaṁkāra*.

Māhat

The first evolute to evolve is *mahāt* (the great one). The word *buddhi* (intellect) is synonymous with *mahāt*. *Mahāt*, which is predominately *sattva guṇa*, is the Cosmic Intelligence that pervades all space and permeates all manifestations, and is the state in which *prakṛiti* receives light from *puruṣa*, and sees itself.

Māhat evolves as a result of the preponderance of *sattva guṇa,* which manifests as pure light. Since it is an evolute of *prakṛiti*, it is made of matter, so it is not capable of functioning by itself. It is aware only through the pervasiveness of *puruṣa*, from which it reflects consciousness. The light of the Self reflects in the intellect (*buddhi*) just as a clear crystal appears to take on the colour of the object upon which it rests. The pure, crystal-like Self appears to take on the qualities of the *sattva-rajas-tamas guṇas*, but actually it is only *buddhi* (intellect) that takes on the condition of the *guṇas* (qualities of matter). When the crystal is removed, its own clarity becomes visible without any colouring.

Through false identification, the Self sees its reflection in the mirror of *buddhi*. It identifies with the reflected image and thinks that it is experiencing what *buddhi* is experiencing, and so forgets its true nature. The sense of 'I-ness' is transmitted to *buddhi* which starts it functioning as a conscious principle.

Māhat or intellect is a unique faculty of discrimination and intuitive wisdom that helps us in discrimination or decision-making. *Buddhi* helps us to distinguish between the subject and the object. It also helps us to discriminate between the self and the non-self, the experiencer and the experienced, as distinct entities. *Buddhi* is closest to the Self and functions for the Self. It has the predominance of *sattva*. It is radiant with the reflection of consciousness. Being identified with it the all-pervading Self becomes manifest as the individual self.

Ahaṁkāra

Closely associated with *buddhi* is the function of 'I-ness' or *ahaṁkāra*. This is the fourth principle or the next direct evolute from *mahāt* or *buddhi*. The Sanskrit word *ahaṁkāra* is derived from the personal pronoun *aham*, 'I', and the root *kri*, 'to do, make or perform'.

Ahaṁkāra refers to the sense of 'I', the ego-sense (self identified with the mind, body and senses) that creates an individual self that knows or realises that it is distinct from all other things and beings. This creates a dualistic state (subject–

object), but without a sense of individual self no further evolution is possible, for all creative activity is first formulated in a self-conscious or self-aware intelligence. The function of the ego is therefore called *abhimana* (self-assertion).

Superior to *ahaṁkāra* (ego-sense) is *buddhi* (intellect) because it is characterised by the predominance of *sattva*, while *ahaṁkāra* can have the predominance of any one of the three *guṇas* at a given time. It can transform according to the predominant proportions of *sattva*, *rajas* and *tamas*.

Manas

Manas (mind), the fifth principle, evolves from the *sattvic ahaṁkāra*.

Manas receives impressions through the senses and responds to them through the organs of action. The individual mind (*manas*) evolves from the *mahāt* (Cosmic Mind).

Manas (mind) is not a conscious entity, but is the reflection of consciousness in the mind that illuminates the mind field (*citta* – field of consciousness; field of experience). In the same way that a film projector shines light upon a screen, so does the all-pervasive consciousness reflect light on all matter and makes it appear to be conscious. It is the reflection that gives matter its individuated being or 'I-sense', which becomes self-aware, *ahaṁkāra* ('I am'). The reflection of consciousness in the mind gives us the ability to cognise. The term *manas*, which usually refers to the mind as a whole, is also used in a restricted sense. *Manas* also refers to the volitional aspect, while *buddhi* refers to the cognitive aspect of the mind. The cognitive mind (*buddhi*) is the finest of all the aspects of the mind and, being closest to the Self, reflects the radiance of consciousness.

The mind has the potency of action as well as the potency of knowledge. The potency of action becomes manifest through will and the potency of knowledge through intellect. The motive force of the organs of action in an individual is the volitional mind, and the motive force of the organs of perception is the cognitive mind.

INDRIYAS (SENSE-POWERS)

Also arising simultaneously from the *sāttvika ahaṁkāra* along with *manas* (mind), are the ten senses. These are the five cognitive senses of perception (*jñānendriyas*): hearing, touching, seeing, tasting and smelling; and the five senses of action (*karmendriyas*): verbalisation, apprehension, locomotion, excretion and procreation.

The *tāmasic ahaṁkāra* produces the five subtle elements (*tanmātras*): sound (*sabda*), touch (*sparsa*), colour/form (*rūpa*), taste (*rasa*) and smell (*gandha*). These are the subtle counterparts to the gross elements, which can be inferred but not perceived. *Rajasic ahaṁkāra* motivates the other two *guṇas* into activity.

All the *indriyas* are classified as evolutes since they are produced, and do not produce new modes of being.

THE BUILDING BLOCKS OF EXISTENCE

Tanmātras

The Sanskrit word *tanmātra* is composed of the pronoun *tad*, 'that', and the root *ma*, 'to measure'.

The *indriyas* (sense-powers) by themselves have no real existence without objects. For example, the power of seeing has no meaning without something to see, that is, colour/form (*rūpa*). So as the *indriyas* begin to manifest, their correlated subtle elements (*tanmātras*) also come into being. The objective manifestations of a being in the world are under the control of the material *tāmas guṇa*. With the increase of *tāmas*, *ahaṁkāra* (ego) produces five subtle elements of perception (*tanmātras*), which evolve in this order: sound (*śabda*), consistency or palpability (*sparsha*), colour/form (*rūpa*), flavour (*rasa*) and scent/odour (*gandha*). Each succeeding *tanmātra* retains the qualities of the preceding ones. *Shabda* has just the quality of sound. *Sparsha* has two qualities: touch and sound. *Rupa* has three qualities: form, touch and sound. *Rasa* has four qualities, and *gandha* has all five qualities. These five subtle elements are the essence of the five senses: sound, touch, sight, taste and smell.

There has been some controversy between the philosophies of *Sāṃkhya* and *Yoga* as to whether the *tanmātras* are generated from the *mahāt* or from *ahaṁkāra*. The situation becomes intelligible if we remember that evolution here does not mean coming out or emanation, but increasing differentiation in integration within the evolving whole. Thus the regroupings of *tāmas* mark the differentiation which takes place within the *mahāt* but through its stage as *bhutadi*. *Bhutadi* is absolutely homogeneous and inert, devoid of all physical and chemical characters except quantum or mass.

The difference of *tanmātras* or infra-atomic units and atoms (*paramanu*) is that the *tanmātras* have only the potential power of affecting our senses, which must be grouped and regrouped in a particular form to constitute a new existence as atoms before they can have the power of affecting our senses. It is important in this connection to point out that the classification of all gross objects is not based upon a chemical analysis, but from the point of view of the five senses through which knowledge of them could be brought home to us. Each of our senses can only apprehend a particular quality and thus five different ultimate substances are said to exist corresponding to the five qualities which may be grasped by the five senses. In accordance with the existence of these five elements, the existence of the five potential states of the *tanmātras* was also conceived to exist as the ground of the five gross forms.

Panchamahābhūtas

From the five subtle elements (*tanmātras*) come the five gross elements or the five fundamental Building Blocks of Existence, the *panchabhuta* or the *panchamahābhūta* in the same order as their corresponding *tanmātras*: ether (*ākāśha*), air (*vāyu*), fire (*tejas*), water (*āpas*) and earth (*prithvī*) – the five primordial elements or the essential states of matter from which the universe and phenomenal world evolves into being.

The three qualities (*guṇas*) of the matter principle (*prakṛiti*) produce the distinctive properties of the five Building Blocks of Existence (*panchamahābhūta*) which are as follows:

Tamas (inertia) gives rise to the element (*bhuta*) earth (*prithvī*).

Tamas (inertia) and the psyche qualities of *sattva* give rise to the element of water.

Sattva (essence) and the dynamically active fundamental quality *rajas* (dynamics) give rise to fire (*agni* or *tejas*).

Rajas (dynamics) gives rise to the element of air (*vāyu*).

Sattva (essence) gives rise to ether (*ākāsha*).

All the *guṇas*, the fundamental qualities, are in fact present in all the *bhutas* (the elements or Building Blocks of Existence), but the disturbance of the equilibrium results in the dominance of one or two qualities (*guṇas*) in each element (*bhuta*).

Ahaṁkāra produces both the subtle and the gross elements. These gross elements are produced by various combinations of subtle elements. For example *shabda* (sound), which is the first *tanmātra* to evolve that serves as a medium in which the other *bhutas* can manifest, is derived from *ākāsha* (ether), the space element. *Akāsha* is the subtlest of the *bhutas*. Spoken messages, carried by radio waves, can be heard in a satellite in space through the ether (which is full of charged particles).

Shabda (sound) is born out of the creation of space. Together with *sparśa* (touch) they produce *vāyu*, the air element, the principle of motion that can be felt and heard: for example, when a breeze blows we can feel the changes in pressure of the air flow on our skin. Without movement, there is no sense of touch.

The fire element (*tejas*) is derived from the essence of colour/form (*rūpa*). Its combined qualities of colour/form, sound and touch make it seen, felt and heard. The perceptions of fire are light and heat, which are produced from the pressure and friction inherent in movement, for example when two wooden sticks are rubbed together to start a fire. Light gives colour and form to objects and is associated with the sense of sight.

Sound, touch, colour/form and taste produce the building block water (*āpas*), the primary constituent of all living forms, perceived by the sense of taste (*rasa*). It is interesting to note that without a flow of saliva (water) on the tongue one is unable to taste anything. *Āpas* (water) embodies the principle of liquidity and cohesion – it can bind or hold together; for example, particles of earth mixed with water stick together, forming a lump of mud.

Prithvī (earth), the principle of solidity, has the function of cohesion. All structure, whether in an atom, a molecule, a leaf, a rock, a mountain or solar system is determined by *prithvī*. It is produced from the special property of smell (*gandha*) and the general qualities of sound, touch, form and taste. Thus it can be perceived by the five senses.

The five gross elements (*panchamahābhūta*) combine in different ways to form all material or gross objects. All the gross objects in the world are perceivable.

Sound (*shabda*) cannot exist without space (*ākāsha*) and lack of resistance, qualities of *ākāsha*. Touch depends on vibration or movement, aspects of *vāyu*; sight occurs because of light and heat, characteristics of *tejas*; taste cannot function without the liquid and cohesive nature of *apas*; and smell needs *prithvī*'s solidity and form.

The following shows the relation of the *panchamahābhūta* to one another:

Ether (*ākāsha*)	*shabda*
Air (*vāyu*)	*shabda + sparsha*
Fire (*tejas*)	*shabda + sparsha + rūpa*
Water (*apas*)	*shabda + sparsha + rūpa + rāsa*
Earth (*prithvī*)	*shabda + sparsha + rūpa + rāsa + gandha.*

These *panchamahābhūta* are the last evolutes of *prakṛiti*. All manifestations in the phenomenal world are said to be modifications of these principles and not the creation of anything new. The *ahaṁkāra* and the five *tanmatras* are technically called *aviseśa* or indeterminate, for further determinations or differentiations of them for the formation of newer categories of existence are possible. The 11 senses (*indriyas*) – organs of knowledge (*jñānendriyas*), the five organs of action (*karmendriyas*) and the mind (*manas*), which is an organ of knowledge and activity – and the *panchamahābhūta* are called *viseśa*, that is, determinate, for they cannot further be so determined as to form a new category of existence. It is thus that the course of evolution which started in the *prakṛiti* reaches its furthest limit in the production of the senses on the one side and atoms on the other. Changes no doubt take place in bodies having atomic constitution, but these changes are changes of quality due to spatial changes in the position of the atoms or to the introduction of new atoms and their rearrangement. But these are not such that a newer category of existence could be formed by them which was substantially different from the combined atoms.

CHART SHOWING THE EVOLUTION OF PRIMORDIAL *PRAKṚITI*

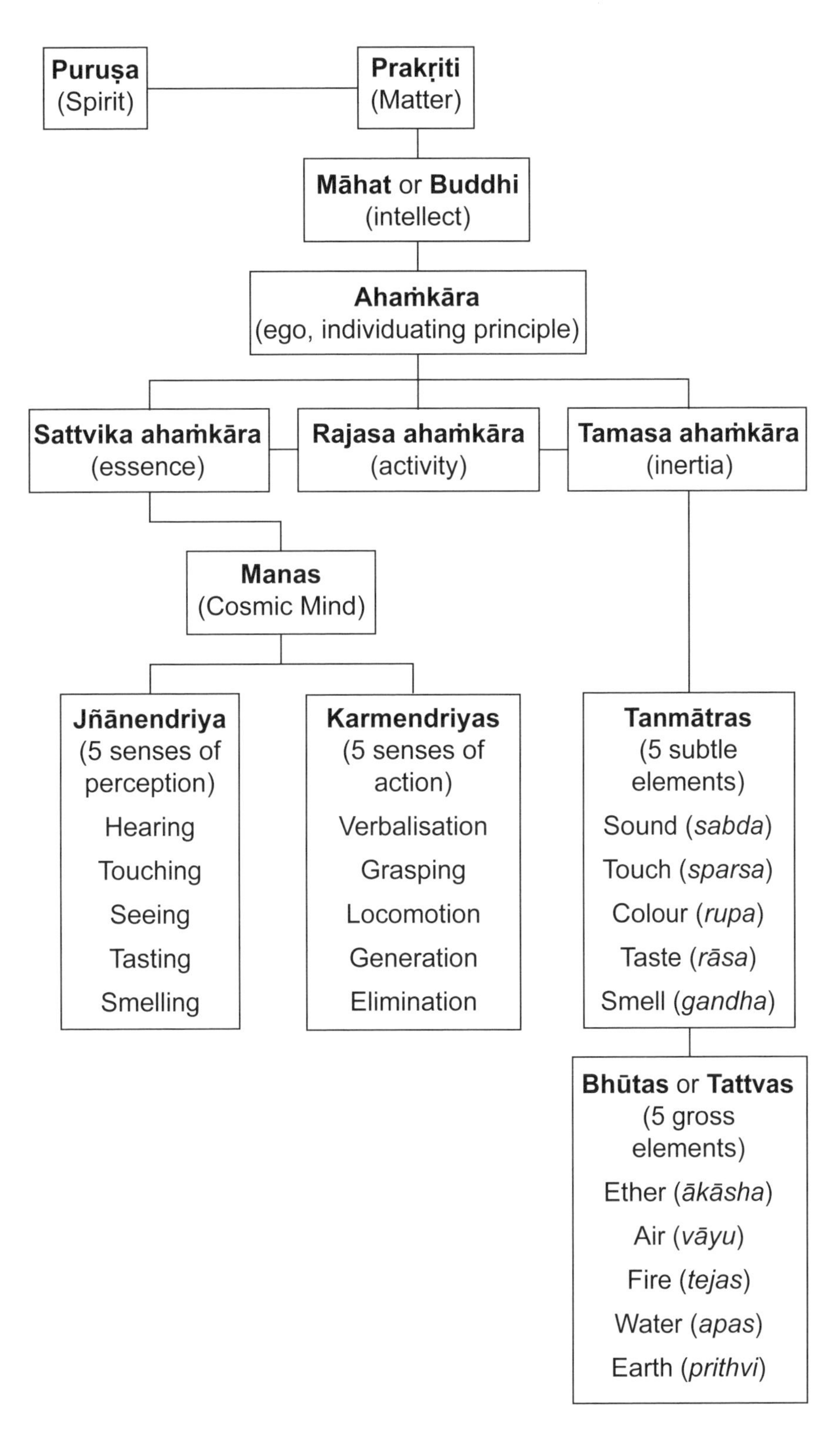

CHANGE IN MANIFESTATION

Change is constantly taking place everywhere, from the smallest and least to the highest. Atoms and *māhabhūtas* are continually vibrating and changing places in every object. At each moment the whole universe is undergoing change, and the collocation of atoms at any moment is different from what it was in the previous moment. When these changes are perceivable, they are perceived as *dhārmaparināma* or changes of a quality; but perceived or unperceived the changes are continuous.

THE EXISTENCE OF TIME

Sāṃkhya-Yoga does not admit an existence of time as does an independent entity such as the *Nyāya-Vaiśeṣika* philosophy. Time represents the order of moments in which the mind grasps the phenomenal changes. It is hence a construction of the mind (*buddhi-nirmana*). The time required by an atom to move its own measure of space is called a moment (*kṣana*) or one unit of time. One unit movement of the *guṇas* is a moment. When by true wisdom the *guṇas* are perceived as they are, both illusory notions of time and space vanish.

SĀṂKHYA AND THE CONCEPT OF GOD

The oldest text on the *Sāṃkhya* system, the *Sāmkhyākarikā* by Iśvarakrsna, does not accept the existence of *Īśvara* (God). It asserts that the existence of God can not be proved and that God does not exist. It argues that if God exists and if God is eternal and immutable, then He can not be the active cause of the world. A cause has to be active and changing. *Sāṃkhya* gives *prakṛiti*, the eternal and ever-changing unconscious manifest principle, as being the ultimate cause.

Because the body is individuated, the Intelligence inhabiting the body was looked upon as being individuated, differentiated and separated. That is how it was presented and explained by the early *Sāṃkhya* system. However, some of the later commentators of *Sāṃkhya* philosophy seem to accept the existence of God. These metaphysical philosophers explain that it is very difficult to explain the nature of the universe and of oneself without accepting *Īśvara* (God).

3.5

YOGA (THE SCIENCE OF THE SOUL)

There is a lovely story in the *Yoga Vasishta*, a mystical work of Indian philosophy that the great sage, Vasistha, imparted to Lord Rama. Someone prays to God and does some penance and eventually sees God standing in front of him. God says, 'I am pleased with you. Ask for a boon.'

He asks, 'Please give me something which is unending' – such as unending happiness, unending peace. He does not mention that, but only says, 'Give me something unending, infinite', so it is not the infinite, but must *lead* to the infinite. God replies, 'Enquire who you are.' That is the only unending thing, because even if you have happiness or peace, that also becomes boring sooner or later, and you want something else. So the practice of enquiring who I am, or who 'I' is, is unending. That enquiry can come to an end only when the enquirer has come to an end.

The seeker is absorbed in the seeking all the time, and when he finds what he is seeking, he finds he is seeking the seeker, himself. It is like a doll made of salt diving into the ocean to measure its depth and width and volume. As long as it is there it is still diving. When it dissolves, it finds the depth of the ocean, the width and volume. It has become one with it.

The individual soul (*jiva*) gets circumscribed in an individual and separative consciousness. When this veil of ignorance is removed, it realises its identity with the Supreme Consciousness. To remove this veil is the purpose of Yoga.

WHAT IS YOGA?

The Sanskrit word *Yoga* comes from the Sanskrit root *yuj*, which means to yoke, join, unite, connect, fasten, harness. The word *yuj* also has common roots with the Latin word *jungere*, which means 'to join'; this has given rise to subsequent words in other European languages – *jouge* in French, *joch* in German and *yoke* in English, which means a frame with which two working animals, such as oxen, are joined together. The ultimate meaning is the union between the individual self and the universal Self. It is establishing oneness between the finite and the Infinite, between the inner being and the Supreme Being.

Yoga signifies both the means and the end. It is the aim of human existence. Yoga, which is both a philosophy and a science, is based on direct experience, not mere theoretical philosophy. From time immemorial great sages and yogis dedicated their entire lives to discovering the deepest secrets and mysteries of life, Truth, Ultimate

Reality, God. After reaching perfection themselves they discovered the ultimate way to freedom from sorrow and the attainment of true bliss, Self-realisation/God-realisation. This ultimate way to spiritual realisation is called Yoga.

The true purpose of religion is to awaken the human mind to the Supreme Goal of life – Self- and God-realisation – and to lead the way to its attainment.

Although Yoga is *not* a religion, it shares the same goal. Yoga is the supreme science of true spiritual unfoldment that leads to the awakening and realisation of our true essential spiritual nature, that is beyond time, space and causation. Our essential nature is divine and the aim of human life is to realise this divine nature and to live life consciously in this awakened state. All human striving, knowingly or unknowingly, is directed towards this aim – the universal goal of human aspiration to attain freedom from pain, sorrow and suffering, and to attain perennial joy or bliss (*ānanda*).

Yoga is the discovery of God-consciousness on two levels:

- Discovering your true essential spiritual nature – the Self.
- Discovering and re-uniting with the Ultimate Reality or Universal Spirit – God.

In the West, Yoga has become extremely popular, but the emphasis has been mainly on the physical side. It seems that the practice of Yoga postures (*āsanas*) has become synonymous with the totality of Yoga. The Yoga postures have been taken out of the context of the particular Yoga system to which they truly belong. This incomplete view and misconstruing of the significance of the Yoga *āsanas* is due to the excessive emphasis laid upon their practice, ignoring their more important utility in the internal discipline of the whole system for a higher spiritual purpose.

The *āsana* is not an end in itself, but a means to a higher purpose; but for many Western Yoga enthusiasts, Yoga has become a physical fitness system that has been commercialised and marketed as a commodity to sell. This in turn has created a myriad array of trends, styles, attitudes and 'new' Yoga philosophies around the practice of Yoga *āsanas*, creating narcissism and competition, which is more to do with achieving outward results.

Yoga is not merely a practice, or a set of practices, but the whole science of life itself. Spiritual life is a total life. It is not fragmented, nor separated. We practise Yoga not merely to attain a healthy, fit and supple body, but to attain Self-realisation in order to discover that we are non-separated units of soul-consciousness of the Infinite, Immortal Being. The purpose of all spiritual practices is to gradually unfold our divine nature, the perceiving Consciousness.

Yoga, as union, implies perfect harmony of *body*, *mind* and *spirit*. On the physical level, it implies health and vitality. On a mental level, it implies the harmonious integration of the personality, and the corresponding elimination of psychological 'complexes'. On the soul level, Yoga implies union of the individual consciousness with its Infinite Source: God.

To be understood correctly, Yoga postures (*āsanas*) need to be seen in the context of Patañjali's *Aṣṭāṅga Yoga* (Eight Limbs of Yoga), that is, as a spiritual discipline that integrates and balances the mind and body.

For clarification of the entire theory and practice of Yoga we need to turn towards the earliest known written, comprehensive synthesis of Yoga, Patañjali's *Yoga Sūtras*, which dates back to somewhere between 500 BCE and 200 BCE.

Patañjali's own definition of Yoga is:

> *'Yogas citta-vṛtti nirodhaḥ.'*
> 'Yoga (the experience of Unity) results from the neutralisation of ego-feelings (that produce the thought-waves in the mind).'
>
> *Yoga Sūtras 1:2*

> *'Tada drashtuh svarupe-vasthanam.'*
> 'Then the Self abides in its own (eternal) true nature.'
>
> *Yoga Sūtras 1:3*

In the *Bhāgavad Gītā*, Krishna gives a number of definitions of Yoga from different viewpoints. There are some single clearly defined definitions such as:

> *'Yogah karmasu kausalam.'*
> 'Yoga is skill in action.'
>
> *Bhāgavad Gītā 2:50*

> *'Samatvam Yoga uchyate.'*
> 'Equanimity of mind is called Yoga.'
>
> *Bhāgavad Gītā 2:48*

These definitions of Patañjali and Sri Krishna are guidelines to the means of attaining the ultimate goal of Yoga: Self-realisation/God realisation. But in the *Bhāgavad Gītā* there is another definition of Yoga, which is perhaps the most comprehensive of all definitions, because it defines Yoga by the ultimate attainment of what is universally sought by us all – 'freedom from pain and suffering'.

We are all aspiring to attain eternal ever-new joy (bliss), to secure release from pain. Sri Krishna gives us this remarkable definition:

> *'Dukhasamyoga-viyogam.'*
> 'Yoga is the avoidance of contact with pain.'
>
> *Bhāgavad Gītā 6:23*

Krishna has the last word on the subject. What is Yoga? Yoga is the avoidance of contact with pain – not getting rid of pain, but avoidance of contact with pain, with sorrow. Sorrow or pain arises when 'I' is dissatisfied with the present condition and seeks another condition. The rejection of the present is sorrow, pain; and the seeking of the future, or something else other than 'what is', is again an admission of sorrow.

In his *Yoga Sūtras*, Patañjali reflects something similar to Sri Krishna. Patañjali instructs us to examine life and see that everything is tainted by misery and unhappiness, and therefore we need to overcome it. How?

> *'Heyam dukham anagatam.'*
> 'Whatever unhappiness/pain has not come to you, avoid it.'
>
> *Yoga Sūtras 2:16*

How do I do that? Practise Yoga! Yoga, union of the Seer, the individual soul (*puruṣa*) and seen, Primordial Nature (*prakṛiti*) is the cause of that avoidable pain.

> *'Drastr-drśyayoh sanyogo heya-hetuh.'*
> 'The cause of (pain and suffering) to be avoided is the union of that which sees and that which is seen.'
>
> *Yoga Sūtras 2:17*

If you are an intelligent being and you look around and examine your life, you will see that everything is tainted by misery and unhappiness. If you seem to be happy now, even that is tainted by unhappiness, because there is recognition (whether at the conscious, unconscious or subconscious level) that it is passing away. You and your partner are happy *now*, but tomorrow you may not be together – there is already unhappiness. Time is passing, everything is changing. You get bored with the same happiness repeated often, so there is unhappiness there; which means that either the external world changes, or 'I' changes – change being inevitable. Happiness also undergoes this change and therefore must come to an end.

The fundamental theme of the *Yoga Sūtras* (as also the teachings of the Buddha) seems to have been: 'Whatever unhappiness has not reached you, avoid it.' Life is full of sorrow – this is an undeniable fact – but it is possible for me to understand how sorrow reaches me; how I become unhappy. How do I become unhappy? Unhappiness can (and should) only be avoided, not got rid of. Anything that you do to get rid of the unhappiness that you have already is going to make you more unhappy. So do not try that, you have tried it long enough. The unhappy situation you are in already is passing – it is not eternal, permanent. Unhappiness came to you from somewhere for some reason, and if left to itself it will move away from you. Leave it alone. But utilise that opportunity, that situation of unhappiness you may be in, to look within, to see how it is that 'I' was caught in this.

So, Yoga is that which frees the individual from pain, suffering and sorrow for all time, giving eternal establishment in lasting perfection in that eternal joy and peace which is God. Yoga re-establishes us in our original state; it is the reintegration with this state that each individual soul – knowingly or unknowingly – seeks. The happiness and fulfilment that each self longs to experience and that motivates all of its actions is but a poor and gross projection of *Sat-chit-ānanda* (Ever-Existing, Ever-Conscious, Ever-New Bliss).

THE ORIGIN OF YOGA

The knowledge of Yoga, which is both a philosophy (*darśana* – direct vision of Truth) and a science, originated in India. Spiritual knowledge can be called timeless or eternal (*nitya*), because Truth is eternal. Yoga is the most ancient and perfected science by which a human being can attain Self- and God-realisation.

The historical antiquity of Yoga is explained in the *Bhāgavad Gītā*, 4:1–3. Krishna informs Arjuna that many ages ago he illumined the 'Deity of the Sun' – Vivasvat (symbolic of God's omnipresent light and Cosmic Energy) – with the understanding of the imperishable knowledge of Yoga (the eternal science of unifying the individual self, *jīvātma*, with the Supreme Self, *Paramātma*). Vivasvat imparted this knowledge to his son Vaivasvat Manu, the first man and progenitor of the human race. Manu in due course revealed the eternal Truth to his son, King Ikshvāku, the founder of the Solar Dynasty of the *Kshatriyas*. Then, from Ikshvāku the knowledge of Yoga was passed on to many *rajarshis* (royal *rishes* and sages), generation upon generation, in traditional succession.

After a long lapse of time, and with the coming of *Kali Yuga* (the Dark Age), recollection of the immutable knowledge of Yoga, the eternal Truth, dimmed, and the power of the teaching diminished. So, on the battlefield of Kurukshetra of the great Mahābhārata war, Krishna once again reveals to Arjuna the same eternal and immutable science of Yoga which in those ancient times he first transmitted.

In Paramhansa Yogananda's translation and commentaries of the *Bhāgavad Gītā, God Talks with Arjuna*, he explains that the first two verses in chapter four describe the symbolic aspects of the various stages of the evolution of the soul from the Infinite to the finite.

In the beginning, the soul emerges from Cosmic Consciousness and enters the vibratory state of Cosmic Light (*Vivasvat*). In the next stage, the soul becomes individualised and limited by identification with the mind (*manas*). This is termed the *Manu* state of the descending soul. In the next stage it flows down into astral life and consciousness (*Ikshvāku*). The soul then continues to descend into a sense-identified state (*Rajarishis*).

After a endured length of time, the individual self (*jīvātma*) identified with the mind, body and senses forgets its unity with the Supreme Self (*Paramātma*). It gets entangled in the web of *Māyā* (Illusion) and caught in the trammels of materialism – desire, sense enjoyments, and bad habits (*rajarishis*) – where vice (*adharma*) prevails.

Through the successful practice of the unifying science of Yoga the individual self (*jīvātma)* can be re-established in virtue (*dharma*) and once again ascend and be liberated in the Cosmic Light (*Vivasvat*).

The imperishable knowledge of Yoga is preserved through the ages by being passed on in disciplic succession from guru to disciple. If this knowledge is forgotten or even distorted, God's omniscience appears on earth as a divine incarnation (*avatar*) in a liberated soul such as Krishna, Rama, Jesus Christ, Buddha, Mahavatar Babaji.

> 'O Bharata (Arjuna)! whenever virtue (dharma) declines, and vice (adharma) is in the ascendent, I incarnate Myself on earth (as an avatar). Appearing from age to age in visible form, I come to destroy evil and to re-establish virtue.'
>
> *Bhāgavad Gītā 4:7–8, in Yogananda 2008a, p.181*

In this way the knowledge of the eternal science of Yoga can never be lost, but is preserved for all time. That is why the ancient Indian religion is called *Sanatana Dharma*. The meaning usually given for *Sanatana Dharma* is 'Eternal Religion' or 'Eternal Way'. The word *Sanatana* means 'Eternal Truth' – that which exists beyond time and space. *Dharma,* from the Sanskrit root *dhri*, means 'to uphold or support', and refers to the natural laws of righteousness that uphold or support the divine order of the universe and of mankind. *Dharma* is the foundation for Yoga to proceed in an authentic way.

Because the word 'religion' has the connotations of worship and ritual associated with it, a better translation would be 'The Way to Eternal Truth'. *Sanatana Dharma* has its basis in the eternal science of Yoga and shows the way to eternity through Yoga practice. The true spiritual religion, then, is the science of Yoga, that shows how to find permanent freedom from pain, suffering and sorrow in the attainment of conscious bliss. The supreme goal of life is liberation (*moksha*) – the realisation of the soul's identity with the absolute Reality. It is not merely the ending of suffering (*dukha*), but the positive experience of Divine Joy, Supreme Bliss.

> 'If a man is able to realise *Brāhman* (Ultimate Reality) here, before falling asunder of his body, then he is liberated; if not, he is embodied again in the created worlds.'
>
> *Kātha Upaniṣad 2.3.4*

As the *Upaniṣads* point out, Self-realisation is to be attained in this life. Why wait for a future life to become Self-realised, when you can become awakened now? Self- and God-realisation does not mean waiting to go to a far-off heaven in the next life; it is awakening now in this life. Self-knowledge is knowing that the 'Kingdom of God is within you' (Luke 17:21). It requires that we turn the mind from its normal outward course inward upon itself, and focus on our true Source, and Essence, as pure Being – *Sat-chit-ānanda* (Ever-Existing, Ever-Conscious, Ever-New Bliss). Our real Self, which is identical to the absolute Reality, to God, is already perfect. We do not need to improve it or add to it. We only need to free our Consciousness, to remove the limitations we have placed on our Self by our false ideas of who we think we are. It is only the ego, the illusion of separate Self, that keeps us from realising that we are truly divine.

THE FOUR MAJOR PATHS OF YOGA

The paths to God-realisation vary widely according to the natures of individuals. Everyone must begin their search for Truth from their own view of understanding. This understanding determined by our characteristics is revealed in the *Bhāgavad Gītā*. Krishna instructs us that there are four main paths to God, according to each person's temperament, capacity and tendency. Truth can be attained through different ways. To attain the Absolute Truth, there are various paths that lead to the same summit, but essentially Yoga is one. These paths of Yoga are not antagonistic to one another. The four paths of Yoga all lead to Self-realisation:

Karma Yoga – the path of action

Bhakti Yoga – the path of spiritual devotion and love

Rāja Yoga – the path of meditation

Jñanā Yoga – the path of discriminating wisdom.

Bhakti Yoga, *Rāja Yoga* and *Jñanā Yoga* all do the same thing. They take a particular aspect of the human being and through that enable the individual soul to realise its identity with the Supreme Self.

As human beings we are endowed with intellect, emotion and the faculty of introspection. If the intellect is predominant, the path of knowledge or *Jñanā Yoga* is resorted to by that seeker. If emotion is the predominating faculty, the approach to Reality is made through *Bhakti Yoga*, the path of spiritual devotion. And if the faculty of introspection is predominant with an inward temperament, then *Rāja Yoga* is followed. Whether you are a *Bhakti* yogi, a *Rāja* yogi or a *Jñanā* yogi, *Karma Yoga* is necessary, and is common to all. We all need to work in this world without getting attached to the results of our actions.

Each path of Yoga contains elements of the other Yogas. For example, to be fully involved in *Jñanā Yoga* does not require the elimination of the feelings and emotions of devotion (*Bhakti*) or to not practise the *āsanas* and *prāṇāyama* of *Haṭha Yoga*. These elements can certainly be included in the *Jñanā* yogi's practice. The *Jñanā* yogi, being primarily of an intellectual nature, utilises the principle of discrimination as his or her main practice towards Self-realisation.

The four paths of Yoga are closely allied, yet each path is perfect and complete in itself. The spiritual seeker of any of the four main paths of Yoga can arrive at the same goal and attain the same realised state.

Karma Yoga

Karma Yoga is the path of action that deals with the law of cause and effect. Those who perform their duties skilfully and selflessly, giving up the fruits of their actions, are called *Karma* yogis. The Sanskrit word *karma* means 'to do, to act'. Any mental or physical action is called *karma*.

On the path of action (*Karma Yoga*) Self-realisation is said to be attained by performing actions that do not create bondage, and that are performed for the Lord alone. Performing all one's actions skilfully and selflessly in daily life with enthusiasm, and offering the fruits or rewards of those actions to God and for the wellbeing of others on the path, brings freedom from the law of karma. Those who renounce both actions and their fruits also follow the path to Self-realisation.

Those yogis who renounce the desire for pleasure are called *sannyasins* or renunciants. One is the path of action and the other is the path of renunciation. These two paths are distinct and separate. It is only the rare few who have already burned their actions, desires and motivations for self-enjoyment that walk the path of renunciation, for on the path of renunciation all action is renounced. For the renunciant there is only one action: doing action for the welfare of others. There remains only one desire: the desire for Self-realisation. It is total dedication and devotion; all the renunciant's energy is directed towards Self-realisation. But for most of us, the path of action by performing our duties skilfully, selflessly and with non-attachment is the preferable and sustainable option. *Karma Yoga* is valid for everyone.

We cannot live without doing actions. When we perform actions we reap the fruits of those actions. The reaping of the fruits involves us and leads us to continue creating further actions and reaping the fruits over again and again. Thus we get caught in the bondage of *karma*. The way to attain freedom from that karmic cycle is not attained by inaction or by continuing to do actions, but by surrendering the fruits of those actions to others. It is the fruits of the *karma* and the desire to reap the fruits that create bondage.

All actions are performed by the governing nature of the universe, *prakṛiti*. The Self, unattached and unaffected, within one's being, is always established in inner calmness and stillness as the eternal Witness. It is only the ego-self, the sense of 'I', that leads one to think and feel that he is the doer, the performer of actions, and that he has the right to reap the fruits of his actions. The ego-self forgets the real Self, the inner source of consciousness and knowledge.

Bhakti Yoga

Bhakti Yoga is the path of spiritual devotion and love. The goal of *Bhakti Yoga* is the attainment of divine love through the union of the individual soul with God. The individual soul is the same nature as God: *Sat-chit-ānanda* (Ever-Existing, Ever-Conscious, Ever-New Bliss). God is the Universal Consciousness of love.

The Sanskrit root of *bhakti* is *bhaj*, 'to engage with affection'. The *Bhakti* yogi knows his beloved God to be omnipresent and sees Him in all things. Through rendering loving service and chanting devotional songs, the devotee merges his entire heart and mind, together with the intellect, ego and senses, in divine love with God.

Without love and devotion, *Jñanā Yoga* becomes intellectually dry. *Karma Yoga* becomes mere social service, and *Rāja Yoga* becomes a practice limited to one's own individual accomplishment of attaining a meditative experience, which reinforces the ego of a separative consciousness. *Bhakti Yoga* develops devotion by opening the heart. It develops faith, and destroys the hindrances to concentration and meditation.

Rāja Yoga

Another means of attaining God-realisation is through *Rāja Yoga*. The Sanskrit word *Rāja* means 'Royal'. *Rāja Yoga* is the 'Royal Path', the classical system of Yoga philosophy. It is the Yoga of meditation (which combines meditation with elements of love, wisdom and service – encompassing the teachings of all the Yoga paths).

Rāja Yoga is a practical, systematic and scientific discipline that leads one to ultimate Truth. *Rāja Yoga* steadies the mind and makes it one-pointed. By following the path of *Rāja Yoga* we can learn to control our desires, emotions, thoughts, and even the *saṁskāras* (subtle impressions dormant in the unconscious mind). Through *Rāja Yoga* we can transcend all human limitations and experience our true essential nature.

Rāja Yoga is also known as ***Aṣṭāṅga Yoga*** (Eight Limbs of Yoga), because it was organised in eight parts by the sage Patañjali who systematised and codified the teachings of Yoga into 196 *sūtras* or aphorisms (*Yoga sūtras*), around the second or third century of the Common Era.

This formalised practical system of the science of Yoga is paired with *Sāṃkhya* in the scheme of the six philosophies (*Darśanas*) of Hindu thought.

The eight limbs of *Aṣṭāṅga Yoga* comprise:

Yama – moral and ethical restraints – social discipline

Niyama – observances – individual discipline

Āsana – posture

Prānāyāma – control of the life-energy through the breath

Pratyāhāra – withdrawal of the senses from external objects

Dhāraṇā – concentration

Dhyāna – meditation

Samādhi – absorption, union with the Divine.

The first four limbs or steps – *yama*, *niyama*, *āsana* and *prānāyāma* – comprise the path of *Haṭha Yoga*. *Rāja Yoga* is used to signify the last four limbs together – *pratyāhāra*, *dhāraṇā*, *dhyāna* and *samādhi* – the royal path of meditation.

In the *Bhāgavad Gītā*, Krishna states:

> 'It is the ignorant, not the wise, who speak of the paths of wisdom (*sankhya*) and Yoga as being different from one another. One who is truly established in either receives the benefits of both.
>
> The state attained through wisdom (*Jñanā Yoga*, the path of discrimination known as *Sankhya*) is the same as that attained by action (the science of Yoga). The two paths lead to one single realisation.'
>
> *Bhāgavad Gītā 5:4–5*

Here Krishna has clearly defined that the final attainment is the same whether one follows the *Jñanā Yoga* path of wisdom, a direct approach to Self-knowledge as propounded by *Vedānta* (one of the six philosophies of Indian thought), or the path of Yoga through Patañjali's *Aṣṭāṅga Yoga* (Eight Limbs of Yoga).

In the next chapter of the *Bhāgavad Gītā*, Krishna states:

> 'The yogi is greater than those ascetics who (strive for spiritual perfection through) discipline of the body, greater even than those who follow the path of wisdom (*Jñanā Yoga*) or of action (*Karma Yoga*). Become, O Arjuna, a yogi!'
>
> *Bhāgavad Gītā 6:46*

Jñanā Yoga

Self-knowledge is another means of attaining Self/God-realisation. The *Śvetāśvataropaniṣad* says:

> *'Jnātvā devam sarvapāshāpahāniḥ.'*
>
> 'Through knowledge of God, all (mental) fetters are destroyed.'
>
> *Śvetāśvataropaniṣad 1:11*

The Sanskrit word *pāśa* means 'fetter' (restrictions), which exist in the mind as negative modifications of consciousness, keeping the mind in bondage. *Jñanā Yoga* removes the veil of ignorance and develops the power of discrimination.

Shankaracharya (sevenhth or eighth century), a Self-realised yogi who realised the nature of the Self to be absolute, transcending all phenomenal appearance, explains in his classic work *Atma-bodha* ('Self-knowledge'), that knowledge alone destroys ignorance:

> 'The Self alone is knowledge, is truth. Knowledge of the diversity is ignorance, is false knowledge. Yet ignorance is not apart from the Self, which is knowledge. Are the ornaments different from the gold which is real?'
>
> *Maharshi and Shankara 2002, p.130*

The path of *Jñanā Yoga* is for those who have a philosophical and rational temperament. The *Jñanā* yogi uses his or her discrimination to distinguish between the Real and the unreal to directly perceive the nature of Self/God, the nature of Reality.

The Self, our true essential nature, is immutable and eternal. Being pure intelligence, it is self-evident. No one doubts their own existence. One may doubt or deny the existence of everything else, including God, but not one's own existence. Even in denying oneself, one has to affirm oneself. Nothing can be denied or affirmed without presupposing the self-intelligent knower. For the *Jñanā* yogi the Self is the first thing that is real; the existence or non-existence of everything else rests on the reality of the Self.

The *Jñanā* yogi does not objectify the Self, but simply recognises the Self. Through discrimination, contemplation, ceaseless meditation on the Self, and intense longing for liberation, the yogi attains union with it. In realising the Self we realise God. The Self and God are subjective and objective views of the same Reality, which is beyond relativity and is neither the subject nor the object.

As was said before, a *Jñanā* yogi can integrate the other Yogas into his or her practice for the realisation of Self-knowledge. For example, the *Jñanā* yogi may practise *Haṭha Yoga* to make the physical body a fit and healthy vehicle for the expression of the Self. The body should not be neglected no matter what path of Yoga one is following.

YOGA AND THE CONCEPT OF GOD

According to *Sāṃkhya* philosophy, *puruṣa* and *prakṛiti* are a duality and the two remain separate. Patañjali's philosophy of Yoga agrees with this view of the separate existence of innumerable *puruṣas* (individual souls), but also includes a special *puruṣa* called *Īśvara* (God, or the Lord). This divine being is eternal, unborn, immortal and unlimited.

The purpose of nature, of matter (*prakṛiti*), is to provide an opportunity for the *puruṣa* (individual soul) to experience its own nature, its own existence and its separateness from *prakṛiti*. What is *puruṣa*, what does it do? *Puruṣa* is ever-seeing (*draṣṭā*). It is not the experiencer, only the Seer. You are not the experiencer, nor the doer. It is *prakṛiti* that is the doer and experiencer.

You – the *puruṣa*, the individual soul, the Self, the *ātman* – are only the Seer (*draṣṭā*). It does not do anything. It just is.

> *'Draṣṭā dṛśi-mātraḥ śuddho api pratyayānupaśyaḥ.'*
>
> *draṣṭā* – the Seer; *dṛśi* – the power of seeing; *matraḥ* – only; *śuddhaḥ* – pure; *api* – although; *pratyaya* – ideas or images of the mind; *ānupaśyaḥ* – witnesses
>
> 'The Seer is merely the power of seeing; (however,) although pure, he witnesses the images of the mind.'
>
> *Yoga Sūtras 2:20*

Yoga is theistic, it postulates the existence of God as *Īśvara*. *Īśvara* is derived from the verb *īśa*, which means 'to have extraordinary power and sovereignty'; capacity to rule. *Īśvara* is God, the ruler, the knower of past, present and future. This term *Īśvara* does not refer to a personal god, or a particular god; Patañjali is referring simply to the word *Īśvara* as a principle that permeates life. He does not refer to *Īśvara* as divine, he just says, 'that which permeates everything'.

Patañjali in his *Yoga Sūtras* (1.23–1.32) presents dedication and devotion to *Iśvara* as one option of how to attain the ultimate goal of Yoga.

Sūtra 1.23

> *'Īśvarapraṇidhānād vā.'*
>
> *Īśvara* (from the verb root *īśh*, 'to have power over') – the ultimate Seer, God; *praṇidhānāt* (*pra* – with, *nidhānā* – dedication to, devotion, self-offering; *vā* – or
>
> 'Through devotion, offering the ego (the sense of 'I') and the fruit of one's actions to God.'

Self-surrender to *Īśvara* (God) means to contemplate on the Supreme Being's intrinsic attributes and to resolve to cultivate those attributes in oneself.

Sūtra 1.24

> *'Kleśa-karma-vipākāśhayair aparāmṛṣṭaḥ puruṣa-viśeṣa Īśvara.'*
>
> *kleśa* (from *kliś:* to cause pain) – affliction, cause of suffering, miseries; *karma* (from *Kri:* to do) – action; *vipākā* – result, fruition of actions; *āśayaih* (*āśhaya* means 'that which lies dormant') – repository of seed impressions of latent desires, storehouse; *aparāmṛṣṭaḥ* – unaffected, untouched; *puruṣa* – the spiritual principle, soul; *viśeṣaḥ* – extraordinary, special, distinct, unique, particular; *Īśvara* – Ruler of creation, omniscient Self, God
>
> '*Īśvara* is the Supreme Self unaffected by the afflictions of life, actions (*karma*) or results of those actions, or by impressions of desires.'

Īśvara is a special Self (*puruṣa-viśeṣa*) that stands apart from creation. He is the union of *puruṣa* and *prakṛiti* before the manifestation of creation and is unaffected by afflictions (*kleśa*), actions (*karma*), fruition of actions (*vipākā*) or impressions of desires (*āśayaih*).

The individual soul (*puruṣa*), the experiencer of the fruit of actions, is rooted in *buddhi* (intellect) which has the attributes: *kleśa*, *karma*, *vipākā* and *āśaya*. But *Īśvara* (God) is untouched or unaffected by the five afflictions (*kleśa*) of life that cause pain and suffering: ignorance (*avidyā*), sense of 'I am' (*asmitā*), attachment (*rāga*), aversion (*dveṣa*), attachment to life or fear of death (*abhiniveśhā*). God also has freedom from all fruits of karma arising from the *kleśas*.

These five afflictions are the attributes of *buddhi* (intellect), which is composed of the three *guṇas* of *prakṛiti* (matter principle).

Sūtra 1.25

'Tatra niratiśāyam sarvajñatva-bījam.'

> *tatra* – there, in him (God); *niratiśāyam* – unsurpassed, unequalled, unexcelled, without limit; *sarvajñatva* – omniscience; *bījam* – origin, seed, source

'In *Īśvara* (God), the seed of omniscience is unsurpassed.'

Omniscience is knowing the totality of the dimensions of all individual things, whether past, present or future.

Īśvara (God), the special *puruṣa*, is omniscient, omnipresent and omnipotent. God is all-knowing, the source of all knowledge. He has absolute knowledge, a wisdom that transcends intellectual knowledge. It is unsurpassed.

Sūtra 1.26

'Pūrveṣām api guruḥ kālenānavacchedāt.'

> *pūrveṣām (purva* means 'preceding') – of the ancients; of those who came before; *api* – also; *guruḥ* – teacher, spiritual preceptor; *kālena* – by time; *anavacchedāt* – not limited or conditioned by time

'Unsubjected by Time, *Īśvara* is also the Supreme Teacher of the ancient teachers.'

Īśvara is the union of *puruṣa* and *prakṛiti*. *Īśvara* is the infinite, eternal principle that precedes the creation and is not limited or conditioned by time. Therefore, *Īśvara* is the Supreme Teacher of all teachers. The word *guruḥ* means both teacher and master, but in this *sūtra* the emphasis is on Teacher.

Sūtra 1.27

'Tasya vācakaḥ Praṇavaḥ.'

> *tasya* – of that; *vācakah* – speech, expression, designation; *Praṇavaḥ* – *Oṁ* (*Aum*), the inner sound current

'The expression of that (*Īśvara*, God) is *Oṁ*.'

The sacred sound syllable (*mantra*) *Oṁ* or *Aum*, the vibration of consciousness that is always in the present, eternal and infinite, signifies God. In ancient times *Oṁ* was referred to as *Praṇavaḥ* (reverberating; sounding).

Oṁ is the primal sound, the Cosmic Vibration and energy of creation that exists prior to the manifest activities of the three *guṇas* (*sattva*, *rajas*, *tamas*). The relationship between *Īśvara* and *Oṁ* is eternal; the Creator and the energy of creation cannot be separated.

Sound is an evolute of *prakṛiti*. On this level *Oṁ* remains a sound vibration and *Īśvara* remains a special and distinct transcendental Being. But on another level *Oṁ is* non-different from *Īśvara*: it is permeated by *Īśvara* and so it manifests the qualities of *Īśvara*.

The mind, which is also an evolute of *prakṛiti*, is unable to comprehend that which is more subtle than itself. The mind can only come into direct contact with *Īśvara* through the Cosmic Vibratory sound *Aum*, in which *Īśvara*'s divine presence, grace and potency is permeated and empowered. The sacred syllable *Oṁ* can be compared to fire permeating an iron ball. All the qualities of fire – heat, light and energy – are manifested.

Sūtra 1.28

'Taj-japas tad-artha-bhāvanam.'

tad – of that; *japah* – repetition; *tat* – its; *artha* – meaning; *bhāvanam* – absorbing oneself in and listening to the sound of *Aum*; deeply meditating (on *Aum*) with faith and devotion, contemplating the meaning of *Praṇava* (*Aum*)

'Its (of the cosmic vibratory sound *Aum*) repetition in deep meditation reveals its meaning.'

We can experience *Īśvara*'s (God's) presence by continually repeating (*japa*) his name, the *mantra Oṁ*. The *mahābija* (the great seed of spiritual consciousness) *mantra Oṁ* can be chanted aloud, softly or mentally, and listened to within in deep meditation. To invoke awareness of the presence of God and to go deeper in meditation, *Oṁ* should be recited with deep concentration, devotion and respect, in inner silence, while meditating on its meaning, and listening to the inner vibratory sound of *Aum*. As the mind becomes more absorbed in *Oṁ*, it becomes still in the present moment. In a state of one-pointedness the consciousness expands and experiences God's qualities of omnipotence, omnipresence and omniscience. With expansion of consciousness the yogi enters *Aum samādhi* and attains the bliss of oneness with God vibrating in the universe as Cosmic Sound.

The word *japa* is composed of *ja* and *pa*. *Ja* means 'going back to again and again, moving toward'; *pa* means 'protection, guidance'.

Japa means receiving protection and guidance by going back to the Source – *Īśvara* (the Supreme Being, God). That Supreme Reality is signified by the sacred syllable *Oṁ*, and you are That. You are That because you exist in the Supreme.

Sūtra 1.29

'Tataḥ pratyak-cetanādhigamo 'pyantarāyabhāvaś ca.'

tataḥ – from that; *pratyak* – inner, inward; *cetanā* – consciousness; *adhigamaḥ* – attainment, realisation; *api* – also; *antarāya* – obstacles, block, impediments; *abhāvaḥ* – disappearance, absence; *ca* – and, also

'From that comes the realisation of the inner consciousness (Self) and the disappearance of all obstacles.'

By the dedicated and devotional absorption (*Īśvara praṇidhāna*) in *Īśvara* as manifested in the transcendental sound *Oṁ*, by the practice of *japa* (repetition) of *Aum*, and listening to it inwardly in deep meditation, the yogi attains direct experience of his or her own essential nature (Self). By absorption in *Īśvara* (God), one realises one's own self as part of *Īśvara*.

It is by the regular practice of *japa* of *Oṁ* that the various impediments and obstacles (*antarāya*) on the path to Self-realisation are gradually removed.

Sūtra 1.30

'Vyādhi-styāna-saṁśaya-pramādālasyavirati-bhrānti-darśanālabdha-bhūmikatvānavasthitatvāni citta-vikṣepās te'ntarāyāḥ.'

vyādhi – disease, mental ailment; *styāna* – dullness, mental laziness, idleness; *saṁśaya* – doubt; *pramāda* – carelessness, negligence; *alasya* – laziness, sloth; *avirati* – non-abstention, lack of detachment, failure to maintain a dispassionate state; *bhrānti* – confusion, error, delusion; *darśana* – perceiving, seeing; *alabdha-bhūmikatva* – non-achievement of gaining (higher) ground, inability to comprehend the goal, inability to attain a higher state; *anavasthitatvāni* – inability to maintain constant awareness, inability to maintain that state that has been attained earlier; *citta* – feeling; *vikṣepāḥ* – distractions; *te* – these; *antarāyāḥ* – disturbances, impediments, distractions

'These disturbances that cause distraction to the mind are disease, idleness, doubt, carelessness, laziness, lack of detachment, delusion, inability to comprehend and reach the goal, and inability to remain grounded.'

In this Yoga *sūtra*, Patañjali cautions us that there are many obstacles on the yogic path to *kaivalya* (liberation) and offers solutions to them. He lists the nine disturbances (*antarāyāh*) that occur along with the *vṛttis*, the vortices of feeling, that cause disturbance and distraction in the faculty of feeling (*citta*). These disturbances that are produced by *rajas* and *tamas* can be overcome by the practice of *Īśvara praṇidhāna* (devotional self-surrender to God), and by practising *Oṁ japa*, which turns all the mental faculties inward towards the centre of consciousness, thus bringing freedom from all obstacles.

Sūtra 1.31

'Duḥkha-daurmanasyāṅgam-ejayatva-śvāsa-praśvāsā vikṣepa-sahabhuvaḥ.'

duḥkha – pain, suffering; *daurmanasya* – depression, frustration; *angamejayatva* – nervousness, unsteadines of the limbs; *śvāsa* – inhalation; *praśvāsāh* – exhalation; *vikṣepa* – disruptions, agitations; *sahabhuvaḥ* – accompany, occur with

'Suffering, depression, restlessness of the body, and irregular breathing accompany the mental distractions.'

The nine disturbances in the previous *sūtra* 1.30 produce these additional accompanying disruptions that disturb the mind, making it very difficult to meditate. And until these distractions are remedied, one will remain in the *vikshipta* (distracted) state of mind and will not be able to achieve *samādhi*, which requires *ekāgra* (one-pointed) state of mind.

All these disturbances or impediments (*antarayas*) that weaken concentration and distract us from realising the Self can eventually be eliminated through the practice of *Oṁ japa* (repetition of *Oṁ*), and absorption in the presence of *Īśvara* (God).

Sūtra 1.32

'Tat-pratiṣedhārtham eka-tattvābhyāsaḥ.'

tat – that; *pratiṣedha* – to prevent, to overcome; *artham* – for the purpose of; *eka* – one, single; *tattva* – principle; *abhyāsaḥ* – practice

'Practice (of fixing the mind) on one principle is the way to overcome those obstacles (physical and mental disturbances and distractions).'

In this *sūtra*, Patañjali reinforces the idea of how to gain inner stability and embrace the truth by focusing the mind at the Spiritual Eye, at the midpoint between the eyebrows, in a devotional mood on the one principle: *Īśvara* (God), through continuous, uninterrupted practice of *Oṁ japa*. This is the quick and easy method to eliminate the nine disturbances and the five conditions accompanying them.

The one-pointed (*ekāgra*) state cannot be attained in the *vikshipta* (distracted) state of mind. One-pointed concentration (*ekāgra*) is only developed when the mind is concentrated on *eka tattva* (one principle or one object of meditation), then the mind comes under control and is freed from all distractions and their accompaniments. Also, to achieve one-pointed concentration, strong, persistent practice (*abhyāsa*) and dispassion (*vairāgya*) are also needed.

'Draṣṭā dṛśi-mātraḥ śuddho 'pi pratyayānupaśyaḥ.'

draṣṭā – the seer; *dṛśi* – the power of seeing; *matraḥ* – only; *śuddhaḥ* – pure; *api* – although; *pratyaya* – ideas or images of the mind; *ānupaśyaḥ* – witnesses

'The Self (that which sees), is merely the power of seeing; (however,) although pure consciousness, the Self witnesses the images of the mind.'

Yoga Sūtras 2:20

3.6

MĪMAṂSĀ (INQUIRY; INVESTIGATION)

The Sanskrit word *mīmaṃsā* means to 'examine, investigate, inquire, critically review'. The term was applied to one of the six Indian philosophical *darsanas*, viewpoints on ritual traditions rooted in the *Vedās* and the *Brāhmanas;* as opposed to *Vedānta,* which relies mostly on the *Upaniṣads*. In this context *Mīmaṃsā* would have meant 'the investigation of the proper interpretation of the Vedic texts'.

The founder of *Mīmaṃsā* was the ancient sage, Jaimini, a former disciple of Bādarāyaṇa, founder of the *Vedānta* System. Jaimini formulated the first systematic interpretations (*Mīmaṃsā-Sūtra*) around the third century before the Common Era, a time when the priestly ritualism of Vedic sacrifice was being marginalised by Buddhism and *Vedānta. Pūrva Mīmaṃsā,* along with other groups, counteracted the challenge by demonstrating the validity of the Vedic texts by rigid formulation of rules for their interpretation.

The *Mīmaṃsā* system is better known as *Pūrva Mīmaṃsā*, meaning the prior or earlier system of investigation, because it is concerned with the earlier section of the *Vedās*. *Vedānta* is alternatively called *Uttara Mīmaṃsā* as it studies the later (*uttara*) part of the *Vedās*. *Pūrva Mīmaṃsā* is sometimes called *Dharma Mīmaṃsā* as it is an investigation into the *dharma* established by the *Vedās*.

The main purpose of *Pūrva Mīmaṃsā* is to inquire into the nature of right action (*Dharma*), understood as a set ritual, obligations and prerogatives to be performed properly. According to *Mīmaṃsā,* 'action' is the very essence of human existence, and without action human destiny cannot be fulfilled.

According to *Pūrva Mīmaṃsā*, the correct performance of the Vedic rituals is the means of salvation, which is its main concern, not liberation. An individual soul is considered to be liberated when it ascends to heaven (*svarga*). It discusses in detail the nature of ritual obligations (*karma-kānda*) and ethical and moral duties (*dharma*) based on correct interpretation of the Vedic scriptures.

Pūrva Mīmaṃsā strongly contends that the *Vedās* are not authored by anyone. Since they are 'self -revealed' (*apaurusheya*), they manifest their own validity. Thus *Pūrva Mīmaṃsā* accepts the *Vedās* as the eternal source of 'revealed truth'. The *Vedās* are eternal and uncreated. They are the expression in sacred words and sound (*shabda*) of the eternal, ritual, sacrifice (*yajna*), and moral order of the world. Hymns of the *Vedās* are the *mantras* with inherent meanings and powers to reveal the truth. To establish the truth of Vedic injunctions, *Pūrva Mīmaṃsā* tries to prove that words and their meanings and the relationship between the two are eternal. As the world is eternal, the idea of God as the ultimate cause is seen to be unnecessary. The existence of a God who decides the fruits of the *karma* (deeds) of individual souls is not recognised by *Pūrva Mīmaṃsā*. Instead, it is believed that the *karma* in an individual is the product of the fruit in one's life.

Pūrva Mīmaṃsā is a pluralistic realist. It endorses the reality of the world as well as that of the individual souls (*jivas*). The soul is accepted as an eternal (*nitya*) and infinite substance. Consciousness is an accidental attribute of the soul, which is distinct from the body, mind and senses.

In the first two *sūtra*s of the first chapter of *Mīmaṃsā-sūtra*, Jaimini states:

> 'Now is the enquiry of *dharma*.'
>
> '*Dharma* is an object distinguished by a command.'

The Sanskrit word *atha* ('now' or 'henceforth') is an auspicious word, and signifies a sequence, implying that something must have occurred prior to the study of *dharma*. What must have occurred prior to the study of *dharma*? Vedic study. After a person has completed his Vedic study, he desires to know *dharma*.

The Sanskrit word *dharma* is not translatable to any other language. It has a number of meanings, and is often translated as 'righteousness', 'virtue'or 'duty', but on their own these words seem to apply to outer behaviour, and so are not really correct for the inner meaning of *dharma*. In his book *The Holy Science*, the great *Kriyā* yogi, Sri Yukteswar, guru of Paramhansa Yogananda, expresses the meaning of *dharma* as 'the mental virtues of the internal world (inner consciousness)'.

Dharma is derived from the Sanskrit root verb *dhri*, 'to hold, support, sustain, preserve'. Its approximate meaning is 'natural law'. So *dharma* means that which holds, supports and preserves those principles of reality which are inherent in the very nature and design of the universe. On an individual level it refers to that code of conduct that sustains the soul, and enables an individual to fulfil his or her higher potential and divine destiny.

> 'It is better to fail attempting to follow one's own duty (*dharma*) than to succeed in following the dharma of another. One incurs no sin in trying to fulfil his own duty.'
>
> *Bhāgavad Gītā 18:47*

Each individual needs to correctly understand what their real nature of duty is in life, to follow their own *dharma*, to understand their place in the universal unfoldment of consciousness, and to fully express their highest potential. The highest of all duties is to realise one's own inner Self, while allowing others to do the same; for disturbing others causes disharmony in the cosmic flow and natural rhythm of life, and that is called *adharma*. One who is completely non-attached and continues to perform their duty as best they can, renouncing the fruits of their actions, is a true renunciate. That person attains the highest of perfection.

Dharma, the underlying principles that keep all things in harmony and sustain their higher growth and development, is the same for all beings. Another name for Hinduism is *Sanatana Dharma* (The Eternal Natural Law or Way), which suggests that it is eternally existing and is not limited by time, space or person. The Sanskrit word *sanatana* denotes that which is *anadi* (beginningless) and *anantha* (endless) and does not cease to be, that which is eternal. It is also *apaurusheya* (without a human founder). It is defined by the quest for Truth, just as the physical truth is defined by science. *Dharma* is that out of which our earth and humanity itself emerged.

Sanatana Dharma represents a code of conduct and a value system that has spiritual freedom as its centre. Any spiritual path that accepts the spiritual freedom of others may be considered as part of *Sanatana Dharma*. To live in alignment with, and to know the true nature of, that *Sanatana Dharma* is one of the ways of describing the spiritual aim of life. It gives reverence to individual spiritual experience over any formal religious doctrine. Wherever the Universal Truth is manifest, there is *Sanatana Dharma*. It is comprised of natural spiritual laws which govern human existence.

Yoga instructs us to follow our highest potential by following a *dharmic* approach to spiritual life to know the essence of our true nature; to lead us from the unreal to the real; from ignorance to Self-realisation. *Dharmic* actions bring peace, harmony and happiness. In contrast, *adharmic* actions limit our consciousness, causing restless desires and inharmony.

3.7

VEDĀNTA (THE ULTIMATE TRUTH)

The term *Vedānta* literally means 'the end (*anta*) of knowledge or wisdom (*veda*)'. In other words it means the concluding portion and ultimate aim of the *Vedās*. Thus *Vedānta* is that highest spiritual knowledge, knowing which there remains nothing further to be known. It is Self-knowledge (*Ātmavidyā*), and knowledge of the Absolute Truth (*Brāhmavidyā*). *Vedānta* teaches the real, essential nature of God, the universe, and the individual being (Self) and its oneness with God. The quintessence of the *Vedānta* teachings is that *Brāhmān* (God), which is Ever-Existing, Ever-Conscious, Ever-New Bliss (*Sat-chit-ānanda*), is the only Reality and that the universe is an illusory appearance; it is not the ultimate Reality. Oneness of the Self (*ātman*) and God (*Brāhmān*) is the goal of *Vedānta*.

The teaching of *Vedānta* can be summed up in four great revelations (*mahāvākyas*) that were revealed through direct knowledge:

'Pure consciousness is *Brāhman*' – *prajñānam brahma.*

Aitareyopaniṣad 3.1.3

'This Self is *Brāhman*' – *ayam ātmā brahma.*

Bṛhadāranyakopaniṣad 2.5.19

'You are That' – *tat tvam asi.*

Chandogyopaniṣad 6.8.7

'I am *Brāhman*' – *aham brahṁāsmi.*

Bṛhadāranyakopaniṣad 1.4.10

About the period 780 CE, Gauḍapāda revived the monistic teaching of the *Upaniṣads* by his commentary on the *Mandukya Upaniṣad* in verse, called *Mandukyakarika*. This nontheistic, *Advaita* school of philosophy propounded that *Brāhman* is the sole Ultimate Reality, eternal and unchanging. Gauḍapāda's disciple Govindapāda was the teacher of Śaṇkāra (788–820 CE). Śaṇkāra's commentary on the *Brāhma-sūtras* is the root from which sprang forth a host of commentaries and studies on Vedantism of great originality, vigour and philosophic insight. Thus Anandagiri, a disciple of Śaṇkāra, wrote a commentary called *Nyayanirnaya*, and Govindanānda wrote another commentary named *Ratna-prabha*. Vacaspati Misra, who flourished about 841 CE, wrote another commentary called the *Bhamāti*. The list continues of many others who wrote commentaries.

Vedānta philosophy is the philosophy which claims to be the exposition of the philosophy taught in the *Upaniṣads* and summarised in the *Brāhma-sūtras* of Badarāyāna. The *Upaniṣads* form the last part of the Vedic literature, and its philosophy is therefore also called sometimes the *Uttara-Mīmaṃsā* or the *Mīmaṃsā* of the later part of the *Vedās* – as distinguished from the *Mīmaṃsā* of the previous part of the *Vedās* and the *Brāhmānas* as incorporated in the *Purva Mīmaṃsā sūtras* of Jaimini. Though these *Brāhma-sūtras* were differently interpreted by different exponents, the views expressed in the earliest commentary on them now available, written by Śaṇkāracārya, have attained wonderful celebrity, both on account of the subtle and deep ideas it contains, and also on account of the association of the illustrious personality of Śaṇkāra. So great is the influence of the philosophy propounded by Śaṇkāra and elaborated by his illustrious followers that whenever we speak of the *Vedānta* philosophy we mean the philosophy that was propounded by Śaṇkāra.

THE ORIGINAL SOURCE OF THE *VEDĀNTA*

The original source of the *Vedānta* is the *Upaniṣads*. The *Vedānta sūtras* are but an extremely condensed summary in a systematic form. Śaṇkāra did not claim to be the inventor or expounder of an original system, but interpreted the *Brāhma-sūtras* and *Upaniṣads* in order to show that there existed a connected and systematic philosophy in the *Upaniṣads* which was also enunciated in the *sūtras* of Bādarāyaṇa. The *Upaniṣads* were a part of the *Vedās* and were thus regarded as infallible by the Hindus. If Śaṇkāra could only show that his exposition of them was the right one, then his philosophy being founded upon the highest authority would be accepted by all Hindus. The most formidable opponents in the way of accomplishing his task were the followers of the *Mīmaṃsā* philosophy, who held that the *Vedās* did not preach any philosophy, for whatever there was in the *Vedās* was to be interpreted as issuing commands to us for performing this or that action. They held that if the *Upaniṣads* spoke of *Brāhman* and demonstrated the nature of its pure essence, these were mere exaggerations intended to put the commandment of performing some kind of worship of *Brāhman* into a more attractive form.

Śaṇkāra could not deny that the purport of the *Vedās* as found in the *Brāhmānas* was explicitly of a mandatory nature as declared by the *Mīmaṃsā*, but he sought to prove that such could not be the purport of the *Upaniṣads*, which spoke of the truest and the highest knowledge of the Absolute by which the wise could attain salvation. He said that in the *karmakanada* – the (sacrificial injunctions) *Brāhmānas* of the *Vedās* – the purport of the *Vedās* was certainly of a mandatory nature, as it was intended for ordinary people who were anxious for this or that pleasure, and were never actuated by any desire of knowing the Absolute Truth; but the *Upaniṣads*, which were intended for the wise who had controlled their senses and become disinclined to all earthly pleasures, demonstrated the one Absolute, Unchangeable, *Brāhman* as the only Truth of the universe. The two parts of the *Vedās* were intended for two classes of persons.

Śaṇkāra thus did not begin by formulating a philosophy of his own by logical and psychological analysis, induction and deduction. He tried to show by textual comparison of the different *Upaniṣads*, and by reference to the content of passages in the *Upaniṣads*, that they were concerned with demonstrating the nature of *Brāhman* (as he understood it) as their ultimate end. He had thus to show that the undisputed testimony of all the *Upaniṣads* was in favour of the view which he held. He had to explain all doubtful and apparently conflicting texts, and to show that none of the texts referred to the doctrines of *māhat* (cosmic mind) or *prākṛiti* (matter), of the *Sāṃkhya* system of philosophy. He also had to interpret the few scattered ideas about physics and cosmology that are found in the *Upaniṣads* consistently with the *Brāhman* philosophy. In order to show that the philosophy of the *Upaniṣads* as he expounded it was a complete consistent system, he had to remove all the objections that his opponents could make regarding the *Brāhman* philosophy, to criticise the philosophers of all other schools, to prove them to be self-contradictory, and to show that any interpretation of the *Upaniṣads*, other than that which he gave, was inconsistent and wrong. This he did not only in his *bhasya* on the *Brāhma-sūtras* but also in his commentaries on the *Upaniṣads*.

THE LIFE OF *ĀDI ŚAṆKĀRACĀRYA*

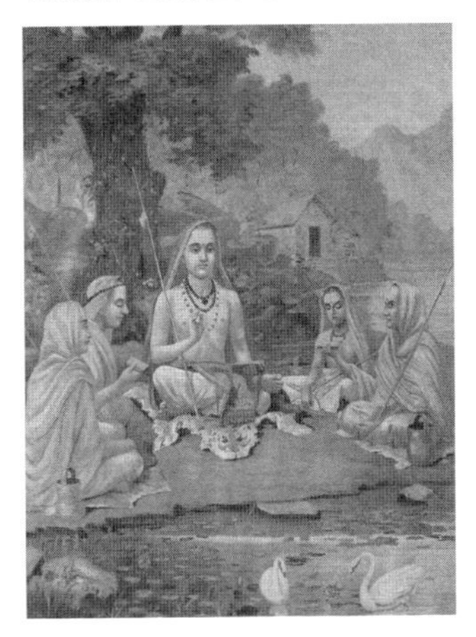

ĀDI ŚAṆKĀRACĀRYA BY RAJA RAVI VARMA (1904)

It is regarded as almost certain that Śaṇkāra (also known as Śaṇkāracārya and Ādi Śaṇkāra) was born between 700 and 800 of the Common Era in the Malabar country in the Deccan, India. His father Śivaguru was a pious *Yajurvedi* Brahmin of the *Tattirīya* branch, who was married to a woman named Aryāmba. The couple had been childless for a long time, and prayed for children at the Vrishacāla temple in nearby Trichur, in Kerala. Śiva is said to have appeared to the couple in a dream and promised them a choice of one son who would be short-lived but the most brilliant philosopher of his time, or many sons who would be mediocre at best. The couple decided to have the brilliant, but short-lived, son and so Śaṇkāra was born.

Many miracles are attributed to Śaṇkāra, and he is believed to have been the incarnation of Śiva. He turned ascetic at the very early age of eight and joined a hermitage on the bank of the river Narmadā, where he became the disciple of a renowned sage named Govindapāda (disciple of Gaudapāda, author of the *Mandukya Karikas*). Śaṇkāra was accepted as a disciple by Govindapāda, who initiated him into the *Paramhansa* order of *Saṅnyāsa*, the highest renunciation for a monk, and instructed him in the teachings of the *Brāhma-sūtras*.

It is said that Śaṇkāra wrote his illustrious *bhasya* (commentaries) on the *Brāhma-sūtras* of Vyasa when he was only 12 years old. Later on he also wrote his main commentaries on ten *Upaṇiṣāds* (*Iṣa*, *Kena*, *Kātha*, *Praśna*, *Mundāka*, *Maṇḍūka*, *Aitareya*, *Tattirīya*, *Bṛhadārānyāka* and *Chāndogya*) and the *Bhāgavad Gītā*. He also commentated on Vyasa's *bhasya* to Patañjali's *Yoga Sūtras* and wrote treatises called *Prakarana Granthis*, including the *Upadeśasahasrī*, *Mohamudgara*,

Daśaślokī, *Ātmabodha* (Self-knowledge), *Vivekacūdāmaṇi* and *Aparokṣhānubhūti*, and commentaries on *Viṣṅusahasranāma* and *Sanatsujātīya*.

By the time Śaṇkāra had reached the age of 32 (the age when he died), he had expounded the *Vedānta* philosophy through his writings; he had attracted many intelligent disciples to him, who could continue the Vedantic tradition; and he had established monastic centres (*māthas*). His life had been short, but eventful and successful. He retired to the Himalayas and disappeared inside a cave near Kedarnāth. This cave is traditionally pointed out as the site of his *mahāsamādhi*. However, other traditions place Śaṇkāra's last days at Karāvirpitham or at Mahur in Mahārāshtra, Trichur in Kerāla or Kancipuram in Tamil Nadu.

The major topics discussed in Śaṇkāra's writings are the concepts of *Brāhman* (the Supreme Consciousness), Self (*ātman*), *Māya* (cosmic illusion), the universe, God and liberation. Śaṇkāra's philosophy of non-duality *Vedānta* can be characterised by the formula from the *Brahmājñānāvalīmālā*:

God is the Reality – *brāhma satyaṁ*

The world is illusory – *jagan mithyā*

The soul (self) is, indeed, none other than God – *jivo brāhmaiva napāraḥ*.

The concept of Brāhman (God)

Śaṇkāra states that there is only one Reality, and that is *Brāhman* – the eternal, Ever-Self-existent, immanent and transcendent Supreme and Ultimate Reality. *Brāhman* is the limitless Awareness, the Universal Consciousness that is experienced in the deep meditative state. The word *Brāhman* is derived from the Sanskrit root *bṛh*, 'to grow, expand, increase', meaning that which has reached its ultimate expansion or development.

Brāhman creates, sustains, and dissolves all that is in the universe. Nothing exists separate from *Brāhman*. The phenomenal world cannot exist by itself; it is completely dependent on *Brāhman*. At the end of each world cycle (*yuga*) of dissolution (*pralaya*) the universe returns into *Brāhman*. This is the time when the infinite variety of forms are destroyed and are reabsorbed back into the eternal source from which they appeared. This is not a state of non-existence any more than there is a non-existence of clay when the various forms (pots, figure sculptures, etc.) into which it has been cast have been destroyed. The clay still exists, but there is no being or manifestation of the forms which it is capable of assuming. We can also use the analogy of electricity to represent *Brāhman*, which is unlimited, yet manifests in the limited forms of light and heat, without ever becoming exhausted.

The concept of ātman (Self)

The Self (*ātman*) is the absolute unconditional Reality. It is all-pervading, self-illumined Consciousness, beyond all time, space and causality. The Self (*ātman*) is the very source of consciousness that cannot be experienced by the mind or the sense-perceptions, for it is beyond them. The Self is the witness of the mind. If we inquire, 'Who am I? Am I the body? Am I the mind or the intellect?' in truth we will realise that we are none of these; we are the pure Consciousness that witnesses the body, mind and intellect.

Ask yourself now, who is looking out from behind the eyes reading this? Then look up from your book and ask yourself, who is witnessing all these forms and objects that I see around me? Is it only the senses? Only the mind? No. You cannot be the mind, because you are witnessing the activity of your mind. When you are sleeping and you enter the dream state, who watches the dreams and remembers them upon awaking? And when you were in deep sleep, who was it that experienced that deep blissful state of inner peace? In all three states there is an unchanging Consciousness that is uninvolved, that is only witness to them. This Witness is the true essential Self of who you are and have always been.

You are the eternal Self, the Source and witness of your mind and its thoughts. It is through the lost awareness of our true divine nature that we identify with the thoughts, feelings and emotions and transient limited forms of the manifested world. This false identification is the cause of our suffering.

The Self (*ātman*) is the ultimate Reality, the essence of consciousness and bliss. The Self is *Brāhman*, the Universal Consciousness. *Ātman* and *Brāhman* are two words for the same Reality.

The concept of Māyā

The Sanskrit term *Māyā* means illusion, the cosmic illusion of duality, appearance as opposed to Reality. *Māyā* has two functions: *āvarana* ('covering') and *vikṣepa* ('throwing out, projecting'). The first conceals the Inner Reality from us, and the second deceives us into believing that fulfilment lies without. It projects the unreal. *Māyā* pervades the universe, but its presence is inferred only from its effect. *Māyā* is an inherent power of *Brāhman*, through which it veils itself.

Śaṇkāra states that there is only one Reality, and that is *Brāhman*. The world is not the ultimate Reality, it is not real but apparent. In perceiving a world there is an apparent duality. Although there is always one eternal Reality, there is the appearance of two – there is a duality. Just as the rays of the Sun are inseparable from the Sun, so is *Māyā* inseparable and undifferentiated from *Brāhman*. The Sun and its rays appear as two things, but actually they are one. It would be untrue to say that the rays of the Sun are real or unreal, for they have no independent reality, they do not exist independent of the Sun – their source. Similarly, the world is a manifestation of God – the two are one. The difference is that God is eternal, and the world is a transient finite appearance.

Māyā covers or veils the Ultimate Reality and in its place projects various appearances. Beyond *Māyā* there is no time or space and no universal cause because only *Brāhman*, the Ultimate Reality, remains.

Māyā is an illusion of separation from the unity of *Brāhman*, whose nature is *Sat-chit-ānanda* (Ever-Existing, Ever Conscious, Ever-New Bliss) – which is also the reality of our own true Self (*ātman*).

THREE PROMINENT SCHOOLS OF *VEDĀNTA*

Over the course of centuries, several Indian philosophers have interpreted and developed the commentaries on the *Upaniṣads* and *Brāhma-sūtras* according to their own understanding and the need of the times they live in. The most prominent of the Vedantic schools that developed were Śaṇkāra's non-dualism (*Advaita*), Ramanuja's Qualified Non-dualism (*Viśiṣṭādvaita*) and Madhava's Dualism (*Dvaita*).

Non-dualism (Advaita) and Qualified Non-dualism (Viśiṣṭādvaita)

Rāmānuja, the founder of the *advaita* system, was born in 1027 CE in Śṛperumbudūr, a town located a few miles west of Madras. He studied *Vedānta* under under Yādavaprakāśa of Conjeevaram; and was initiated by Perianambi, disciple of Ālavandār.

Śaṇkāra and Rāmānuja were both outstanding philosophers of their time, but the difference between them was that Śaṇkāra was a great intellectual logician, while Rāmānuja was more intuitional and devotional in setting forth his spiritual views, stressing the theistic aspect of the *Upaniṣads*. Rāmānuja embraced all in devotional feeling, while Śaṇkāra united all in the realm of reason.

Rāmānuja's purpose was to reconcile the *Vedāntasūtras*, the *Upaniṣads* and the *Bhāgavad Gītā* with the faith and beliefs of the Vaiṣnava saints. His doctrine is salvation through devotion (*bhakti*) to God. His philosophical view is that the Ultimate Principle (*Brāhman*) is the basis of the world, and it is not an illusion, as is argued by Śaṇkāra. Rāmānuja agrees that the Ultimate Principle is real and exists, but he qualifies his position by arguing that souls are also real, though their reality is dependent on the Ultimate Principle. He believes that the world, individual self (*ātman*) and God are all real, and that the world and the individual self depend on God.

According to Rāmānuja, salvation is not the disappearance of the individual self but its release from limiting barriers. The self cannot be merged into God. One substance cannot be dissolved into another.

Rāmānuja agrees that, in the end, there is nothing but *Brāhman*, but maintains that, during the period of manifestation, the world and individual souls are separate in order to serve God.

Dualism (Dvaita)

Madhvāchārya (or Madhva), the founder of *Tattvavāda* ('Philosophy of Reality'), commonly known as the *Dvaita* (dualistic) system, was born in 1238 CE in a village near Udipi, in the district of south Kanara, north of Mangalore. At an early age he took the renunciant vow and became a *saṅnyāsin*. In the same village where he grew up he founded a Krishna temple, where he taught until his death at the age of 79 in 1317 CE.

Madhvāchārya evolved a dualistic system of philosophy from the *Prasthāna-Trāya* (the *Upaniṣads*, the *Bhāgavad Gītā* and the *Brāhma-sūtras*). It is known as Unqualified Dualism.

Madhvāchārya makes an absolute distinction between God, and animate and inanimate objects. God is the only independent Reality. The animate and inanimate objects are dependent realities. Madhva's dualistic *Vedānta* is the philosophy of distinction, the doctrine of absolute differences. He insists on five great distinctions (*pancha-bheda*): (1) between God and the individual soul, (2) between God and matter, (3) between the individual soul and matter, (4) between one soul and another, and (5) between one material thing and another.

Although these dependent realities are eternal and distinct in their own right, they only exist through the consent and sanction of God. Suffering in this world is the result of improperly understanding these differences. One who correctly understands these five differences has attained knowledge and is fit for liberation (*moksa*).

Madhva maintains that reality is composed of three basic categories (*tattvās*): God (*Īśvāra*), soul (*jiva*) and matter (*prakṛiti*). All three of these categories are real and distinct, but with one essential qualification, soul and matter are dependent on God.

THE WORLD – A REALITY DISTINCT FROM GOD

God is the efficient, but not the material, cause of the world. *Prakṛiti* is the material cause of the world. It evolves into the visible world.

According to Madhva, the world is not an illusion. It is not also a transformation of God, as curd is of milk. Madhva does not admit that the world is the body of God. The distinction between God and the world is absolute and unqualified. Hence the system of Madhva is called *Dvaita* or Unqualified Dualism. *Dvaita* means duality.

THE INDIVIDUAL SOUL

There is an infinite number of souls (*jivas*). They are all of atomic size. The entire universe is filled with individual souls. Madhva says in his *Tattvanimaya*: 'Infinite are the souls dwelling in an atom of space.' No two souls are alike in character; they are essentially different from one another.

The *jivas* (souls) are different from God, and from matter. Madhva regards the distinction between *Brāhman* and *Jiva* as real. Though the *jiva* is limited in size, it pervades the body owing to its quality of intelligence. The *jivas* are active agents, but they depend on the guidance of God. God impels the *jivas* to action in accordance with their previous conduct. They are eternal and, by nature, blissful. But the connection with material bodies due to their past karma makes them suffer pain and undergo transmigration – from birth to death, and from death to birth. When their impurities are removed, they attain salvation. The natural bliss of the soul becomes manifest at the time of salvation.

The soul does not attain equality with God, it is entitled only to serve Him. Souls attain the salvation through the grace of God. The grace of the Lord is in proportion to the intensity of devotion.

SĀṂKHYA, YOGA AND *VEDĀNTA* – SUMMARY OF DIFFERENT VIEWPOINTS REGARDING PRIMORDIAL PRINCIPLES

Both the systems of ***Sāṃkhya*** and **Yoga** regard *puruṣa* (individual spirit) and *prakṛiti* (nature) as two independent and eternal principles.

Vedānta integrates *puruṣa* and *prakṛiti* into a single non-dual principle called *Brāhman*.

Sāṃkhya and **Yoga** believe in the multiplicity of *puruṣas*. ***Vedānta*** identifies the individual soul (*ātman*) with *Brāhman*.

Sāṃkhya and **Yoga** believe *prakṛiti* to be real and eternal.

Vedānta understands *prakṛiti* to be the illusory manifestation of *Brāhman* through its *maya* power.

Sāṃkhya is a dualistic philosophy. It acknowledges two aspects of reality: *prakṛiti* (nature, the unconscious principle) and *puruṣa* (the Self or consciousness). The earliest text, the *Sāṃkhya Kārikā*, does not discuss the existence of God. The acceptance of the existence of God came in later developments of *Sāṃkhya* philosophy, when the *Sāṃkhyan* philosophers pointed out that in metaphysical discussions it is difficult to explain the nature of the universe and of oneself without accepting a Supreme Being. The *Bhāgavad Gītā* states that the unmanifested *prakṛiti* gives birth to the universe and sustains it as guided and directed by God.

> 'Such is My lower nature (*Apara-prakṛiti*). Understand now, O Mighty-armed (Arjuna)! that My other and higher nature (*para-prakṛiti*) sustains the soul (*jiva*), which is individual consciousness, and sustains also the life-principle of the universe.'
>
> *Bhāgavad Gītā 7:5*

> 'Know that all beings, (both) the pure and the impure, are born of this twofold *prakṛiti*. I (alone) beget and dissolve the (whole) universe.'
>
> *Bhāgavad Gītā 7:6*

Yoga, the practical aspect of *Sāṃkhya*, recognises the existence of God. The Yoga system agrees with *Sāṃkhya* in the separate existence of innumerable souls (*puruṣas*), but Yoga also adds a special being *puruṣa*, with godly attributes, called *Īśvara,* that is the union of *puruṣa* and *prakṛiti* before the manifestation of creation, and is thus considered the Creator.

Vedānta does not accept the existence of *Īśvara* (God). The Vedantic view is that *Īśvara* is the projection of *Brāhman* (the Ultimate Reality). *Brāhman* is without attributes.

PART 4

THE SUBTLE BODIES AND THE CHAKRAS

4.1

THE SUBTLE BODIES

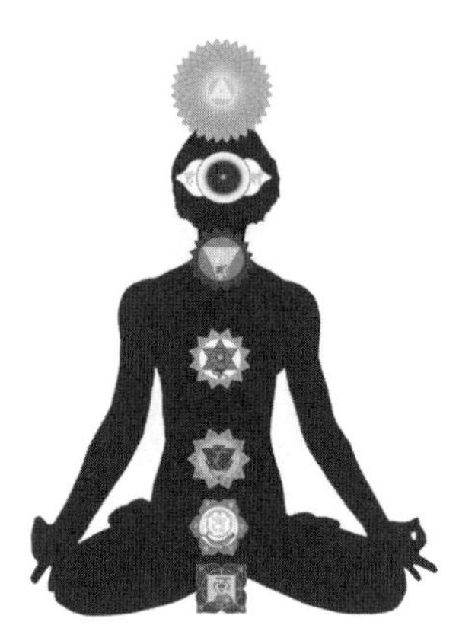

FIGURE IN MEDITATIVE POSE AND THE SEVEN CHAKRAS

Although our physical bodies appear to be dense and solid, at the most fundamental level they are composed of trillions of molecules and atoms, or energy in constant transformation. In addition to the physical body, the soul (the indwelling pure spirit – the essential reality of who we really are) has several interdependent non-material, subtle bodies or energy fields surrounding and interpenetrating the physical form, each of which is a luminous field of energy vibrating at a particular frequency level and density. These human energy fields are the manifestation of Universal Energy.

We are spiritual beings, immortal spirit-souls temporarily embodied in both material and non-material fields of energy. These non-material fields of energy or subtle bodies interpenetrate and surround each other in successive layers. Each succeeding subtle body is composed of finer substances and higher vibrations than the preceding body that it surrounds and interpenetrates. The abode of the conscious *ātman* or *puruṣa* (soul) in this body composed of material elements is likened to a castle. There are three parts of this castle: physical, astral and causal. Each of these parts, or bodies, condition the soul-consciousness to varying degrees.

The individual soul-consciousness expresses itself through five sheaths (*koshas*), which are divided between the three bodies – the *physical* body and two surrounding subtle bodies, the *astral* body and the *causal* body.

The physical, astral and causal bodies serve respectively as mediums for our daily experience in the three states of mind – waking (*jagrat*), dream (*swapna*) and dreamless deep-sleep state (*suṣhupti*). The soul is beyond these three states, being a witness to them.

The five sheaths (*koshas*) and three bodies (physical, astral, causal) are inert, modifications of matter; they have no permanent reality. They appear to be have consciousness because they reflect the consciousness of the Self (*ātman*). The entire *antaḥkaraṇa* ('internal instrument of cognition'; consisting of consciousness, intellect, ego, and mind) is the centre of energy for the soul (*jīvātman* or *puruṣa*). Although inert, *citta* (feeling) receives consciousness from its contact with the soul (*jīvātman*). Thereby it becomes active and goes on generating life every moment in the form of subtle *prāṇa*; with the help of ego it infuses life in the causal, astral and gross bodies. Essentially, this *citta* generates the energy of knowledge and action, rather like positive and negative electrical energy. The energy is generated to such an extent that it is difficult to measure it, and because it is so subtle it is very difficult to visualise it with the general light of meditation. Rising from the field of consciousness, and coming out of the orb of ego, this process appears in the form of subtle *prāṇa*. Out of these currents, the positive current of knowledge nourishes *citta* and *buddhi tattva*, and the negative current of activity continues offering energy of action to ego (*ahaṁkāra*) and mind (*manas*). The essence of the life-principle is *sūkshma prāṇa* (subtle vital air) which shines like luminous vapour outside the orb of ego; it mixes with the astral body which is seated in the brain, wrapped in the five *tanmātras* (subtle forms of the elements); it sustains, nourishes, irrigates and conducts the physical body that is constituted of five gross elements.

> 'Man as an individualised soul is essentially causal-bodied. That body is a matrix of the thirty-five ideas required by God as the basic or causal thought forces from which He later formed the subtle astral body of nineteen elements and the gross physical body of sixteen elements.
>
> The nineteen components are intelligence; ego; feeling; mind (sense consciousness); five instruments of action, the mental correspondence for the executive abilities to procreate, excrete, talk, walk, and exercise manual skill; and five instruments of life-force, those empowered to perform the crystallising, assimilating, eliminating, metabolising, and circulating functions of the body. This subtle astral encasement of nineteen elements survives the death of the physical body, which is made of sixteen gross metallic and nonmetallic elements.'
>
> *Swāmi Sri Yukteswar, in Yogananda 1946, p.408*

THE PHYSICAL BODY

The *Annamaya Kosha* (the food sheath) is the physical sheath of the gross body, which is subject to birth, growth, disease, decay and death. It is called the food sheath because of its dependence on gross *prāṇa* in the form of food, water and air. *Prāṇa* is the vital life-energy which sustains life and creation. *Prāṇa* permeates the whole of creation and exists in both the macro-Cosmos and the micro-Cosmos. Without *prāṇa* there is no life. *Prāṇa* is the essential link between the astral and physical bodies; when this link or supply is cut off, then death takes place in the physical body. Both the *prāṇa* and the astral body depart from the physical body.

Using the analogy of the castle, the physical body is the main gateway for approaching the soul. This physical body is made up of five material elements (ether, air, fire, water and earth), and is born of past actions (*karma*). It offers gross services to the individual soul or *jīvātman*, lord of the castle.

THE ASTRAL BODY

The subtle or astral body is composed of five subtle elements – *ākāśha* (ether), *vayu* (air), *tejas* (fire), *apas* (water), and *pṛithvī* (earth) – which produce the five gross elements on the physical plane.

The physical body does not have the energy to serve the soul. This energy comes from another body that pervades throughout the whole physical body. This is the subtle or astral body (*Sūkshma Sharīra*), which is the conductor of the physical body. All actions of the physical body take place by the energy and the prompting of the astral body.

The subtle or astral body has three parts: *Manomaya Kosha* (Mind Sheath), *Vijñanāmaya Kosha* (Intellect or Intelligent Sheath), and *Prānamāyā Kosha* (Vital Air Sheath).

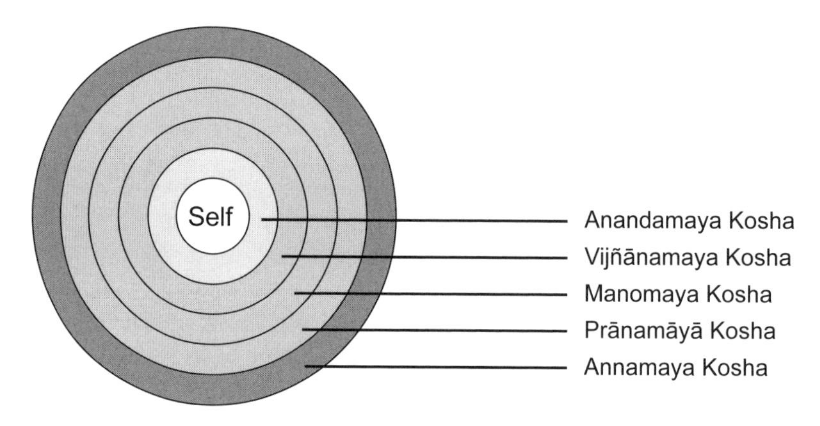

THE KOSHAS: THE FIVE LAYERS OF CONSCIOUSNESS

The Manomāya Kosha

The *Manomāya Kosha* (Mind Sheath) is more subtle than the vital *prāṇic* sheath. It holds the *Annamaya Kosha* (Food Sheath) and *Pranamaya Kosha* (Vital Air Sheath) together as an integrated whole. The Mind Sheath functions as a messenger between each body, communicating the experiences and sensations of the external world to the *Vijñanāmaya Kosha* (Intelligent Sheath), and the influences of the causal and astral bodies to the physical body.

The real Self, being identified with the Mind Sheath, experiences the world of duality. It is the mind that is the cause of bondage, but also the means to liberation. The mind is subject to change and various modifications so it cannot be the real Self.

The Vijñānamaya Kosha

The Intelligent Sheath, or discriminating faculty, functions as the knower and the doer, and being the subtlest of all the aspects of the mind, it reflects the radiance of soul consciousness or the Self. It appears conscious because it reflects the intelligence of the Self. The focus of this reflection is the ego (I-consciousness).

It is composed of the cognitive mind (*manas*), the intellect (*buddhi*) and ego (*ahaṁkāra*) conjoined with the five subtle sense organs of perception.

Both the *Manomāya Kosha* and the *Vijñānamaya Kosha* are especially important, because they are the means of individual as well as universal knowledge of all objects of creation, from gross to the most subtle.

The Intellect Sheath cannot be the real Self, since it is subject to change – the fluctuations of ideas.

The Prānamāyā Kosha

This *prāṇic* body (the Vital or Etheric Sheath) provides energy and vitalises the physical body. It is a channel for the manifestation of cosmic energy. It is approximately the same size and shape as the physical body.

The Vital Sheath is composed of five *pranas* (life-energies), which have distinct functions in the working of the physical body:

> ***Vyāna***, 'outward moving air', is the vital air that regulates the overall movements of the body, coordinating the other vital airs. It permeates the whole body.
>
> ***Udāṇa***, 'upward moving air', functions between the throat and the top of the head, activating the organs of sense: eyes, nose, ears, tongue. It has an upward movement that carries the *kuṇḍalinī shakti* (a person's potential spiritual energy or vital energy force, lying dormant at the base of the spine, in the *mulādhāra chakra* or base energy centre). When awakened, this creative, vital energy force passes through the main subtle nerve channel (*sushumna nādi*) in the centre of the spinal cord, ascending to the crown *chakra* (*sahāsāra*).
>
> At the time of death, *udāṇa* separates the astral body from the physical form. *Prāṇa* (vital life-energy) is a specific manifestation of cosmic *prāṇa* (the cosmic life-energy that pervades both the macro-cosmic universe and the micro-cosmic unit of the body). The cosmic *prāṇa* enters the body through the medulla oblongata at the base of the brain. It then descends and ascends through the astral spine, where it is modified by the *chakras* and differentiated into the vital airs (*vayus* – *prāṇic* air currents).
>
> ***Prāṇa***, 'forward moving air', functions between the throat and the top of the diaphragm, activating the respiration. It also raises the *kuṇḍalinī shakti* to *udāṇa*.
>
> ***Samāna***, 'balancing air', functions in the abdominal area between the navel and the heart, activating and controlling the digestive system, the heart and the circulatory system.
>
> ***Apāṇa***, 'air that moves away', functions from the region of the navel to the feet, activating expulsion and excretion. It has a downward movement, but carries the *kuṇḍalinī* upwards to unite with *prāṇa*.

These five airs (*vāyus*) are conjoined with the five subtle organs of action (speech, hands, legs, organs of evacuation and procreation), which have their counterparts in the physical body.

The vital energy, the modification of cosmic energy, enters the body after its conception and leaves it at the time of its dissolution.

This *prāṇic* body or Vital Sheath, which is a vehicle for the Self, is not the real Self, since it too is subject to change and has a beginning and an end.

THE CAUSAL BODY

> 'In thirty-five thought categories of the causal body, God elaborated all the complexities of man's nineteen astral and sixteen physical counterparts. By condensation of vibratory forces, first subtle, then gross. He produced man's astral body and finally his physical form.'
>
> *Swāmi Sri Yukteswar, in Yogananda 1946, p.408*

The causal body is known as the *Kāraṇa Sharīra* or the *Linga Sharīra*. It is even more subtle than the astral body. It has a finer and higher vibration and pervades the astral body, giving life to it. Although it gives energy to the astral body, its own vitality has a different abode, called the *Ānandamaya Kosha* (Bliss Sheath). This is a body of light that reflects the blissfulness of the Self. It is the cause of both the subtle and gross bodies. Like the other sheaths, it too is a product of matter and is subject to change, and therefore cannot be the real Self.

4.2

THE SOUL

> 'The soul is not inside the body. The soul projects itself as the body and the mind. It finds a location in space-time and broadcasts or telecasts itself through the body.'
>
> *Chopra 2006, p.63*

The human being is a soul wearing a physical body. The soul is extremely subtle, even subtler than ether, mind and energy. Consciousness and intelligence are attributed to the soul, not the gross body. Consciousness is evidence of the existence of the soul.

The bodies or sheaths obstruct the true spiritual knowledge about the concealed soul or the kingdom of God within. When the obstruction veils are removed, the Self is realised. The knowledge of the soul is already present within us, but because of the entanglement into the 24 categories of *prakṛiti* (material nature) due to *avidyā* (ignorance), it is forgotten. When these categories of *prakṛiti* that bind the soul are transcended through the systematic practices of Yoga, the true nature of the Self is realised and liberated from all suffering and bondage.

The individual soul or spirit (*puruṣa* or *ātman*) resides within all three bodies (physical, astral and causal), witnessing all of their activities. The soul is the ever-shining consciousness, perfect and complete, having no limits and without beginning or end. It is infinite and eternal. The light of knowledge that flows through *manas* (mind), *citta* (feeling), *buddhi* (intellect), *ahaṁkāra* (ego) and then through the *indriyas* (senses) is called consciousness.

The source of knowledge and intelligence, by which we know, exist and act, is our true Self. The realisation of God's existence is inseparable from the knowledge of our Self. From this centre of consciousness the life-force flows in varying degrees. When a lamp has many shades, the light is very dim, but after removing the shades one by one, finally you find the centre of radiant light whose radiance illumines them all. Similarly, the soul, the centre of consciousness, is covered by the three bodies (physical, astral and causal).

The individual soul (*Jīvātman*) is an image or reflection of the Supreme Soul (*Paramātman*). Just as the Sun is reflected in different bowls of water, so also the Supreme Soul is reflected in different minds of different persons. All souls (*jīvas*) are the radiance of God, the one Self. All forms are God's expressions. The one Consciousness has expanded and extended Itself from Its eternal Pure-Mind state to appear as countless individual living beings in a temporal universe of myriad forms. Each form, possessing Consciousness, relates to the world as a subject to an object; that is, 'I am the seer, and what I experience is the seen.'

These conscious soul-beings are forgetful of their true essential nature, they identify with their body, ego-mind and senses, and regard themselves as being separate entities with specific desires and goals. Through lack of memory and unawareness of our true soul-identity we suffer unhappiness and feel there is something missing or incomplete in our life. Eventually we must all awaken to our true Divine nature.

In the second chapter of the *Bhāgavad Gītā*, Krishna reminds us of our immortal and eternal true nature:

> 'As we observe life the change of a youthful body to an old one, so too after death, the soul adopts another body. Those who have understood the true nature of life are not deluded by these changes.'
>
> *Bhāgavad Gītā 2:13*

> 'The indwelling Self never takes birth and will never die. It has always existed and shall never cease to be. For it is birthless, eternal, immortal and unchangeable. It is not slain when the body is killed.'
>
> *Bhāgavad Gītā 2:20*

> 'As a person discards worn-out clothes and acquires new clothes, so also the embodied soul abandons a worn-out body and enters into another one which is new.'
>
> *Bhāgavad Gītā 2:22*

> 'The Self cannot be cut; fire cannot burn it; water cannot drown it; nor can it be dried by the winds.'
>
> *Bhāgavad Gītā 2:23*

> 'The Self is indivisible and indissoluble and cannot be transformed by fire or air. The soul is everlasting, omnipresent, unwaveringly steady and ever-existent.'
>
> *Bhāgavad Gītā 2:24*

> 'Realise that the soul, the spirit-self, is unmanifested, it is beyond the mind's ability to conceive and cannot be changed. Therefore, knowing this, transcend your unfounded anxieties and grief.'
>
> *Bhāgavad Gītā 2:25*

4.3

THE CHAKRAS

The Body's Energy System

WHAT ARE THE *CHAKRAS*?

Chakra is a Sanskrit word meaning 'wheel', 'circle' or 'revolving disc'. For those who are able to see the *chakras*, by observing the aura (a rainbow of light surrounding the body) or luminous energy field within the 'subtle' or astral spine, they are seen in cross-section as fast-moving whirlpools or vortices of energy containing colours, and taking the form of a luminous funnel-shaped structure, somewhat like a convolvulus flower. Each *chakra* has its own specific plane and direction of rotation. The first and third *chakras* rotate in a clockwise direction; all the other *chakras* rotate counterclockwise.

The Yoga and Tantric Traditions recognise seven major *chakras*, confluences of consciousness and energy, distributed along the midline of the body, located above the crown of the head, the forehead, the throat, the chest, the navel, the genital area, and at the base of the spine. In the texts of *Hātha Yoga* and *Kuṇḍalinī Yoga* the *chakras* are represented and visualised as luminous lotus flowers or *pādmas* with various numbers of petals, *bīja* (seed-syllable) *mantras* inscribed in each petal, and symbols within the centres of the lotuses. These representations of the *chakras* are images of energetic experiences in symbolic form. The petals, radiating light, are small rotating vortices whirling at very high speeds. Each vortex metabolises an energy vibration that resonates at its particular whirling frequency. The colours in each *chakra* are related to the frequency of energy being metabolised at its particular rate.

The lotus, a beautiful and captivating symbol of the *chakras*, represents to us the nature of the *chakra* as a living force. The lotus (Latin – *Nelumbo nucifera*, Sanskrit – *pādma*; *kokanada rakta-kāmāla* – reddish lotus, *pundarika* – white lotus), which can be seen growing in lakes and ponds throughout Asia in such countries as India, Sri Lanka, Thailand, China and Japan, is very beautiful to observe. The lotus flower grows from the bottom of streams, muddy ponds and lakes to rise above the water and bloom. Its roots are deeply buried in the mud far below the surface, yet its petals are not soiled by the mud, which just rolls off it. The leaves are coated with a film, upon which water forms magnificient, glittering droplets. The flower stalk rises above the leaves, ending in large, sweet-perfumed, white or pink blooms which appear one at a time. Symbolically the lotus flower can be related to the human condition, being fully grounded in earth, with its density and heaviness, yet reflecting the upward aspiration of human consciousness towards the light and the divine. And just like the lotus, the *chakra* can be closed, in bud, opening or blossoming.

'Do not go to the garden of flowers!
O friend! go not there;
In your body is the garden of flowers.
Take your seat on the thousand petals of the lotus, and there
gaze on the infinite beauty.'

Kabir (fifteenth century Indian mystic and poet)

The petals of the lotus symbolise subtle nerves (*nāḍīs*) which resonate to a specific sound vibration. If the hue of the petal is muddy or dull, the sensitivity to sound is decreased. Purity of the sounds through spiritual practice energises the petals so that they turn and point upwards. This increases the smoothness with which the *chakra* rotates. The rhythm of the rotation is perfect when the lotus petals are pointing upward and in full bloom.

Essentially, *chakras* are energy centres situated within the astral body – the subtle body that mirrors the physical body's informational and energy content. The *chakras* energetically connect the five sheaths (*koshas*) that embody the soul to the functions of the physical body, primarily through the endocrine glands and the nerve plexuses in the spine. They access all emotional, mental and spiritual states of our being.

The *chakras* act as dynamos of cosmic energy, which allow our energy bodies to plug into the universal power source. They serve as transformers and act as regulators to receive, assimilate and distribute energy (*prāṇic* life-force) to the subtle body, which then distributes the energy to the spinal nerve plexuses where it is in turn transferred to the blood circulation and organs of the physical body.

CHAKRAS AND ENERGY

'The astral body is not subject to cold or heat or other natural conditions. The (subtle) anatomy incudes an astral brain, or the thousand-petalled lotus of light, and six awakened centres in the *sushumna*, or astral cerebro-spinal axis. The heart draws cosmic energy as well as light from the astral brain, and pumps it to the astral nerves and body cells, or lifetrons.'

Yogananda 1946, p.403

Ultimately even our bodies are nothing but energy. The body is composed of cells, which are composed of atoms, which in turn are made up of particles (leptons, quarks, mesons) that spin around at incredible speeds around empty spaces. It is all a ceaselessly changing pattern of energy. Think of the body as a pattern of intelligence in a field of pure consciousness.

The subtle *prāṇic* life-force enters the body at the base of the brain (medulla oblongata) and flows to the higher brain centres. Then it filters downward through the six major *chakras* or energy centres. As this energy and light filters and spirals down through each *chakra*, it becomes increasingly more dense. At the lowest *chakra* at the base of the spine (*muladhāra chakra*), the vibrational frequency is lower and slower than those above it. The higher the *chakra*, the more subtle and finer the vibrational frequency. These higher *chakras* are closely related to the innermost sheaths and higher levels of consciousness.

The energy that filters down through the *chakras* ultimately spirals down from cosmic energy, produced from cosmic light, which is created by the will and energy of God – the Ultimate Reality.

Consciousness moving becomes energy. As consciousness descends in a spiralling movement of energy, it subdivides and stretches out, and when the movement is slowed down, it becomes matter. As it condenses into matter it forms the five elements: ether, air, fire, water and earth – first the subtle elements, then the gross elements. The difference between one element and the other is a difference in their vibratory wavelength frequencies.

As consciousness descends and moves in space, it becomes air. When air moves there is friction and therefore fire, when the gases collide and fire is generated, water is also generated; and then water condenses into solid substances (earth). These elemental stages describe the stages of the descent of soul-consciousness into matter.

The process of Yoga is a reversal of this descent into matter. Through definite stages of spiritual awakening in our awareness of our true identity as the Self, the soul-consciousness can return to the freedom and oneness in Spirit from matter.

CHAKRAS AND THE ELEMENTS

The elements associated with the *chakras* should not be confused with the chemical elements known to modern science. In their pure states the elements are not visible and are known as *mahābhūtas* (generic gross elements) which evolve in this specific order: *ākāśha* (ether), *vāyu* (air), *tejas* or *agni* (fire), *apas* (water) and *pṛithvī* (earth). These have evolved out of the five *tanmatras*, which evolve in this specific order: *śabda* (sound), *sparśa* (touch), *rūpa* (colour/form), *rasa* (taste) and *gandha* (smell). Each of the *mahābhūtas* is a compound of all the five *tanmātras*, one of them dominating in each. Sound dominates in ether (space), touch in air, form in fire, taste in water, and smell in earth.

The earth centre (*mūlādhāra chakra*) is that part of your anatomy which comes into contact with the earth. A little above there is the water element (*svādhiṣṭhāna chakra*), the next subtle element, located where water collects. At the navel centre (*maṇipūra chakra*) is the fire region – when we talk about digestion, we think of the gastric fire (*agni*) there. Above the navel is the heart region (*anāhata chakra*), which represents air – the region in which the lungs and oxygenation operate. Above the heart is the throat region (*viśuddha chakra*) – a little space (ether) in the throat. Higher still is the Spiritual Eye (*ājñā chakra*) at the midpoint between the eyebrows, which represents the mind.

CHARACTERISTICS OF THE *CHAKRAS*

The *chakras* vibrate at different frequencies as they transmit energy. Each is associated with a vibrational frequency, a characteristic colour, a petal sound, a seed-syllable (*bīja*) *mantra*, an element, a planet, a spiritual quality, a presiding deity, a symbolic animal, a sense organ and an endocrine gland.

Kuṇḍalinī Yoga, *Laya Yoga*, *Tantric Yoga* and *Kriyā Yoga* are the main branches of Yoga that specifically concentrate on the *chakras*.

Besides the *chakras* manifesting the specific sounds of the *bīja-mantras*, they also manifest the following inner astral sounds, which can be heard by meditating on the *chakras* in deep meditation:

ājñā chakra – *Aum* (*Oṁ*)

viśuddha chakra – Roar of the ocean

anāhata chakra – Long-drawn-out deep bell sound; deep gong

maṇipūra chakra – Harp

svādhiṣṭhāna chakra – Flute

mūlādhāra chakra – Humming sound, like a bumble bee.

All of these subtle sounds are manifestations of the Cosmic Vibration of *Aum*. These six subtle sounds can be heard in meditation by listening with deep concentration in the right ear. The inner *Aum* (*Oṁ*) sound is heard in meditation with the inward gaze at the Spiritual Eye (at the midpoint between the eyebrows) mentally chanting *Oṁ*, while simultaneously listening with deep concentration.

> 'As the various vital centres (*chakras*) begin to open up, different sounds are perceived inwardly and the devotee comes to feel the sounds of conches, bells, flutes, etc. all merging in the cosmic rhythm of one great voice of infinite silence. At that stage no thought or object of the outside world can distract his attention. As he advances, his being gets dissolved in the bottomless depth of that blissful music that pervades the whole universe, and he finds eternal repose.'
>
> *Sri Anandamayi Ma, in Lipski 1988, p.69*

FUNCTIONS OF THE *CHAKRAS*

Every *chakra* governs a specific kind of energy related to various human attributes. For example, the heart *chakra* is the centre of consciousness, of the mind, feeling and emotions. If the heart *chakra* is functioning in a balanced way, the person will be able to relate to others in a caring, understanding,and unselfish way. Love and ability to forgive are attributes of a balanced heart *chakra*. Conversely, those persons who tend to close themselves off from others or are dominated by emotions suggests that there are energy blockages in the heart *chakra*.

Essentially, the *chakras* relate to our individual growth and development. The first three *chakras*, the lower centres of consciousness, are primarily concerned with the primal issues of survival and self-preservation, sexuality and power, while the upper *chakras* are concerned with issues of personal expression, spiritual insight and spiritual realisation. We begin individual growth and development at the first *chakra* or 'root' *chakra* (*muladhāra*) in infancy and develop our upper *chakras* as we mature into adulthood.

The lower *chakras* or centres of consciousness give us a firm stability in life. This foundation becomes unstable when we hold fears and misconceptions in our consciousness, creating blockages in the flow of energy to and from the *chakra*. We need to understand that the *chakras* are conduits that conduct and transform subtle energy (*prāṇa*) into matter. If the channels are blocked then imbalances will occur.

Although the higher *chakras* reflect the aspiration of human consciousness towards Self-realisation, all the *chakras* remain important to a person's overall state of health and wellbeing. One should not think, for example, that development of the sixth *chakra* (*ājñā chakra*), the centre of insight and intuition, is more important than development of the second or sacral *chakra* (*swadhisthana chakra*), the centre of procreation, creative instincts and self-fulfilment. In fact, the balanced development of the second *chakra* is an important step for the development of the sixth *chakra*. For instance, in some cases, there are persons who have taken vows of celibacy on entering a spiritual community, an ashram, a convent or a monastery who have an unbalanced second *chakra* (*svādhiṣṭhāna chakra*) through suppressing their sexual energy rather than naturally transforming and redirecting it into other areas of creativity. This causes a blockage in the second *chakra*, causing the person to become unbalanced in their energy and attitude towards sexuality. A person's sexual energy is connected to their life-force; it is a source of vitality. If the energy in that *chakra* is blocked it will have the unhealthy effect of lowering physical and natural sexual vitality.

In the tradition of *Kuṇḍalinī Yoga*, *Tantric Yoga*, *Haṭha Yoga* and *Kriyā Yoga*, there are spiritual practices that involve *āsana*, *prāṇāyama*, *mantra* and meditation to transform and redirect the sexual energy through different energy channels. The energy is directed upwards through the central channel and power current of the inner spine to the higher *chakras* and brain centres, to be transformed into higher vibratory energy.

CHAKRAS AND THE ENDOCRINE SYSTEM

On the physical level each *chakra* is related to, and has a significant effect on, a ductless gland. The *chakras* function as transmuters of energy, distributing *prāṇic* energy to the physical body. The *chakras* absorb the universal or cosmic energy, break it up into component parts, and distribute it via a network of channels (*nādīs*) to the nervous system, the endocrine glands, and then the blood circulatory system to nourish the body. The endocrine system, which regulates different systems in the body, plays a vital role in the health and wellbeing of the body.

When there is a balance between the astral and the physical systems, the life-current energy becomes harmoniously connected and synchronised. However, if the flow of energy is blocked and imbalanced in the *chakras*, the corresponding endocrine gland will be affected, causing malfunction in the physical body, with mental and emotional changes.

The endocrine system is a collection of internal glands and cells that secrete hormones directly into the circulation to regulate various functions of the body. Hormones are complex chemical substances that are secreted into the bloodstream to regulate body functions such as the metabolism, growth and sexual reproduction. The control centre of hormone secretion is in a part of the brain called the hypothalamus, which secretes 'releasing factors', which in turn control the secretion of hormones from the pituitary gland.

Relationship between the *chakras* and the endocrine glands

Chakra	**Endocrine gland**
Sahasrāra (crown centre)	Pineal
Ājñā (brow centre)	Pituitary
Viśuddha (throat centre)	Thyroid/parathyroids
Anāhata (heart centre)	Thymus
Maṇipūra (navel centre)	Pancreas
Svādhiṣṭhāna (sacral centre)	Adrenals
Mūladhāra (root centre)	Testes/ovaries

CHAKRAS AND THE NERVE PLEXUSES

The *chakras* are also related to the nerve plexuses, which are located along the physical spinal cord, and appear to be attached by their 'stems' very close to the major nerve plexuses. Each nerve plexus is like a computer. It receives information from the senses and the internal organs (input), processes the information within the brain (data processing), and transmits nervous impulses and energy to the various body parts (output). This in turn causes the activation of the various organs in the body, such as muscles and glands, by the nerves leading to them.

Relationship between the *chakras* and the nerve plexuses

Chakra	**Nerve plexus**
Sahasrāra (crown centre)	None
Ājñā (brow centre)	Medullary plexus
Viśuddha (throat centre)	Cervical plexus
Anāhata (heart centre)	Cardiac plexus
Maṇipūra (navel centre)	Solar plexus
Svādhiṣṭhāna (sacral centre)	Sacral plexus
Mūladhāra (root centre)	Coccygeal plexus

The *sahasrāra chakra* is associated with the cerebral cortex and the pineal gland.

4.4

NĀḌĪS

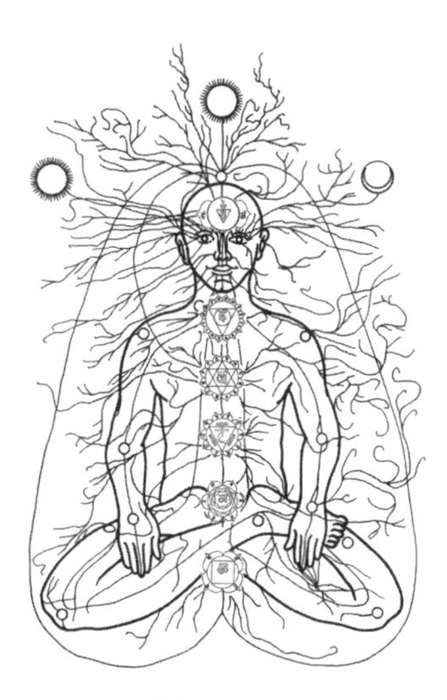

THE NĀḌĪS

The anatomy and physiology of the gross physical body is patterned from the blueprint or template of the subtler etheric body (between the astral and physical bodies) composed of a luminous matrix of web-like lines of force in constant motion, scintillating with a bluish or white light. It acts as a receiver, assimilator and transmitter of *prāṇic* energy.

The etheric body of light channels the flow of life-energy (*prāṇa*) to create and sustain the physical body through a vast network of fine subtle *prāṇic* channels called *nāḍīs* (*nāḍī* literally means 'flow' or 'motion'), astral nerve conductors of *prāṇa*. Any mental or emotional disturbances that a person experiences in life will create blocks to this flow of life-energy which are registered in the astral body, and stored in the *chakras* – the main energy centres of the astral body. This in turn will influence the energies of the physical body and will have an effect on the health and wellbeing of the individual.

The physical spine and the ganglia of the sympathetic nervous system alongside the spine correspond to the astral spine (*suṣumnā*) with its subtle channels (*nāḍīs*) of the *iḍā* on the left side, and *piṅgalā* on the right side, of the central astral channel (*suṣumnā*).

The *suṣumnā*, which corresponds with the central nervous system, consists of the *śirobrāhman* (cerebrum) contained within the cranium, the *suṣumnā śirśakam* (medulla oblongata) and the *suṣumnā kandam* (spinal cord within the vertebral canal).

The *parisariya nāḍī maṇḍalam* (peripheral nervous system) consists of a series of nerves by which the *suṣumnā* (central nervous system) is connected with the various tissues of the body. This is classified into three groups: cranial, spinal and autonomic nervous systems.

The central nervous system as a whole corresponds with the *suṣumnā.* The autonomic nervous system is called *iḍā,* corresponding with the parasympathetic nervous system, and *piṅgalā,* corresponding with the sympathetic nervous system.

The source of the *nādīs* in the astral body is an egg-shaped centre of nerves called the *kanda*, which is located between the anus and the root of the reproductive organs, just above the *mulādhāra chakra*. From this source 72,000 *nādīs* (350,000, with 14 main channels, according to the *Śiva Samhita* 2:13; the *Darśana Upaniṣad* 4:6 says there are 72,000, with 14 main channels), invisible vital *prāṇic* current channels flow out to the entire subtle circuitry of the astral body. This is the junction where the *nādī* that passes through the spinal column is connected to the *muladhara chakra* at the base of the spine. Corresponding to this centre in the physical body is the *cauda equina*, a fibrous network at the base of the spinal cord, that tapers off to a fine silk-like thread.

There are two views regarding the origin of *nādīs* – one is the *kanda sthāna* and the other is the solar plexus in the navel. The text *Jābāladarśanopaniṣad* states that the centre is nine finger breadths above the *mulādhāra* (root centre), in the navel region. But the text *Yogi Yājñavalkya-Saṃhitā* (4:16–17), which mentions only 14 *nādīs*, gives its location as being nine finger breadths above the navel, and that it is egg-shaped, four fingers in breadth, width and height. The text *Yogaśikhopaniṣad* states that the navel encircled by the *vilamba nādī* as the *nābhi chakra* is egg-shaped, and it is from here that the *nādīs* originate.

The solar plexus is the main storage battery of *prāṇa* and large amounts of *prāṇa* can be stored to give vitality to the physical body, through the practice of *prāṇāyama*. The *nādīs* can be purified by this practice particularly through *Nādī Shuddhi* or *Anuloma Viloma prāṇāyama* (alternate nostril breathing). If the *nādīs* are not purified, then the *prāṇa* cannot flow into the *suṣumnā nādī* (the main central channel in the astral spine).

The life-energy or *prāṇa* which flows through the *nādīs* is used by the soul in its expression through the physical and astral manifestations. Without light from the indwelling Self or soul, the brain, mind, body organs, senses, and even *prāṇa*, cannot function. It is the Self that sustains the body by agency of *prāṇa*.

FOURTEEN IMPORTANT *NĀDĪS*

1. ***Suṣumnā*** – carries the *kuṇḍalinī śakti*.
2. ***Iḍā*** – carries the mental energy.
3. ***Piṅgalā*** – carries the *prāṇic* energy.
4. ***Gāndhārī*** – is situated by the side of *iḍā nādī* and helps to support it. *Gāndhārī nādī* stretches from below the corner of the left eye to the big toe of the left foot. Affects the excretory system.

5. ***Hastijihvā*** – is a complementary *nāḍī* to *iḍā*. *Gāndhārī*, *iḍā* and *hastijihvā* form the left channel. The *hastijihvā nādī* stretches from below the corner of the right eye to the big toe. Affects the excretory system.
6. ***Kuhū*** – originates from the throat and terminates at the genitals. Affects the liver, and when this *nādī* is balanced, it keeps the stomach and the blood circulation functioning well.
7. ***Sarāsvāti*** – is seated on the tongue and runs parallel to *suṣumnā nādī*. Affects the spleen, and controls the temperature of the stomach.
8. ***Pūṣā*** – extends from the left big toe to the right ear. This *nādī*, along with *yaśasvinī nādī*, forms the right channel and is complementary to *piṅgalā*.
9. ***Śankhini*** – originates from the throat and passes between *sarāsvāti* and *gāndhārī nādīs* on the left side of *suṣumnā nādī*, terminating in the anus. Affects the kidneys; its main functions are purification of the blood and urinary excretion.
10. ***Payasvinī*** – flows between *pūṣā nādī* and *sarāsvāti nādī. Pūṣā* is complementary to *piṅgalā* on the right side of the *suṣumnā*, and to *sarāsvāti* on the left. Directly linked to the gallbladder, it controls the level of bile in the body and affects the digestion.
11. ***Vāruṇī*** – situated between *yaśasvinī* and *kuhū nādīs*. *Vāruṇī nādī* assists in keeping *apana vayu* free of toxins. Together they help each other in the body's process of excretion.
12. ***Alambuṣā*** – begins at the anus and terminates at the mouth. It affects the mind and the metabolic system. An important *nādī* because all feelings of the senses are conveyed to *suṣumnā* through it, which is then carried to the brain. It affects the mind and the metabolic system.
13. ***Viśvodarī*** – flows between *kuhū* and *hastijihvā nādīs* and is located in the area of the navel. *Viśvodarī nādī* is related to the adrenal glands and the pancreas. Affects the intestines, and controls the metabolism and catabolism. *Viśvodarī,* working together with *vāruṇī nādī*, improves the distribution and flow of *prāṇa* throughout the body, especially the *prāṇa* rising through the main channel (*suṣumnā*). The Yoga practices of *Uḍḍīyānabandha* and *Nauli Kriyā* energise the *viśvodarī nādī.*
14. ***Yaśasvinī*** – extends from the right big toe to the left ear. It affects the excretory system.

THREE MAIN *NĀDĪS – IḌĀ*, *PIṄGALĀ* AND *SUṢUMNĀ*

In the *BrihadĀranyaka Upaniṣad*, one of the oldest *Upaniṣads*, dating from about 800 BCE, states that the *nādīs* are as fine as a hair split into 1000. Out of the network of 72,000 *nādīs*, the subtle channels through which the *prāṇa* (life-force), consciousness and vital energy flows to sustain and maintain the organs of the body, there are ten important *nādīs*. These ten *nādīs* are the main channels of the distribution of life-energy and consciousness to the whole body. From these ten *nāḍīs*, there are three that are important, they control the complete network of the 72,000 *nāḍīs*: *iḍā*, *piṅgalā* and *suṣumnā*.

Iḍā nāḍī, the left-hand current, transits mental energy (*citta shakti*) and controls all the mental processes. *Piṅgalā*, the right-hand current, transits the vital life-force (*prāṇa śakti*) and controls all the vital and physiological processes. The central channel, *Suṣumnā*, is for the awakening of spiritual consciousness; it transits spiritual power (*atma shakti*). Both *iḍā* and *piṅgalā nāḍīs* control our normal consciousness and are constantly active, even during sleep. The *suṣumnā nāḍī* is mainly dormant in the majority of people who are not consciously and actively engaged in spiritual development through such practices as Yoga and meditation. Their consciousness is limited to the lower *chakras* on the worldly plane; they have not yet spiritually awakened.

SUṢUMNĀ – THE PATHWAY TO GOD

The *suṣumnā* ('most gracious'), the major central *nāḍī* in the astral spine corresponding to the spinal cord in the physical body, is also called *brāhma-nāḍī* ('Path to God'), *brāhma-dandu* ('God's staff'), *divya-mārga* ('Divine Path'), *meru-daṇḍa* (Mount Meru is *axis mundi*, the supporting pillar of the earth, running from the underworlds to the heavens) and *vaisnavi-nāḍī*. Most of the Vedic texts and Yoga texts consider the *mulādhāra* (root *chakra*) at the base of the spine to be its origin, and the *Brāhmarandhra* at the crown of the head to be where it terminates. *Suṣumnā* corresponds with the sacred river *Sarāsvāti*.

The *mulādhāra chakra* is located and experienced between the genital root and the anus in males, and at the cervix, or base of the uterus, in women. From the *mulādhāra chakra*, the *suṣumnā nāḍī* ascends slightly backward and upward to the second energy centre, *svadisthāna chakra*, which is located at the point in front of the coccyx where the *Suṣumnā nāḍī* enters the spinal column. From the *svādiṣṭhāna chakra* the *Suṣumnā* continues upwards through the spinal column, through the navel centre (*maṇipūra chakra*), heart centre (*anahata chakra*), throat centre (*vishuddhi chakra*), the point at the base of the brain where the spinal column ends (medulla oblongata), and passes through *ājñā chakra* (the psychic passage which runs from the eyebrow centre to the medulla oblongata at the back of the head). *Suṣumnā* terminates at *sahasrāra* ('Gate of *Brāhman'*) at the crown of the head.

Suṣumnā nāḍī is composed of three subtle currents of force, each concentric tube arranged one within the other. The innermost channel is *citriṇī* (pale like the moon), and has a *sattvic* nature. The second inner channel is the active and forceful *vajriṇī* (sunlike), and the outer channel is the *suṣumnā* itself. When *kuṇḍalinī* energy, the psycho-spiritual power, is awakened, it passes through the *brāhma nāḍī*, a very fine canal inside the *citriṇī nāḍī*. It enters through the 'Door of *Brāhman*' (*brāhma-dvāra*) at *mulādhāra chakra* (at the base of the spine) and blissfully ascends to *sahasrāra chakra*, the Thousand-petalled Lotus of supreme consciousness at the crown of the head. In a general sense the *suṣumnā nāḍī* itself is called the *brāhma nāḍī* because it is within the *suṣumnā nāḍī*.

IḌĀ AND *PIṄGALĀ*

The Sanskrit word *iḍā* means 'comfort'. The *iḍā nāḍī* is the 'comforting' channel due to its cooling effect on the body.

Iḍā is associated with feminine and lunar energy possessing cooling qualities. It corresponds with the sacred river Ganges (*Gaṅgā*), which is nourishing and purifying. *Iḍā* controls all the mental processes, and is *sattvic* in nature.

The origin of the subtle *prāṇa* and the breath lies in the astral body. When there is an upward movement of *prāṇa* in the *iḍā nāḍī* this is astral inhalation. Astral exhalation is when there is a downward movement through the *piṅgalā nāḍī*.

In *Svāra Yoga*, *iḍā* represents the breath flowing in and out of the left nostril. During the ascending moon cycle, from the new moon to the full moon, *iḍā nāḍī* is dominant for nine days in a fortnight at the time of sunrise and sunset.

There are some yogis who follow *Svāra Yoga* who create a *sattvic* balance in body and mind by keeping the flow of breath in the left nostril during the day. This balances the solar energy that is received during the daylight hours.

In Sanskrit, *piṅgalā* means 'tawny-red', which is derived from the word 'tan' symbolising the action of the Sun. The *piṅgalā nāḍī* is associated with masculine and solar energy, possessing heating qualities. *Piṅgalā* corresponds with the sacred river Yamunā, and controls all the vital processes. *Piṅgalā* represents the breath flowing in and out of the right nostril. *Piṅgalā* is more active during the descending moon cycle, from the full moon to the new moon, and operates for nine days in a fortnight at the time of sunrise and sunset.

The *Svāra Yoga* practice of keeping the right nostril open at night, when solar energy is less strong, is said to maintain a balance in a healthy body. This can be achieved in sleep by lying on the left side of the body. Keeping the left nostril (*iḍā nāḍī*) open and predominant during the day, and the right nostril (*piṅgalā nāḍī*) open and active at night, increases vitality and longevity.

The two *nāḍīs* run up either side of the spine – *iḍā* on the left side, and *piṅgalā* on the right side of the central channel in the astral spine (*suṣumnā*). *Iḍā* and *piṅgalā* correspond with the sympathetic nerve ganglion on either side of the spine, while *suṣumnā* runs between them in a position corresponding to the spinal cord. At certain locations along the spine, these three energies converge into whirling vortices – the *chakras*.

Iḍā and *piṅgalā* emerge from *mulādhāra chakra* at the coccygeal point of the base of the spine. This junction where the three *nāḍīs* meet is known as *Yukta Triveni* (*yukta*, 'combined'; *tri*, 'three'; *veni*, 'streams'), the point at which three rivers converge – Ganga, Yamuna and Sarasvāti – corresponding respectively with *piṅgalā*, *iḍā* and *suṣumnā nāḍīs*. (In India these three rivers meet at a place called Prayag.) From *mulādhāra*, the base *chakra*, *piṅgalā*, emerges from the right side of the spine in a semi-circular curve, and crosses the *suṣumnā* at *svādiṣṭhāna chakra* (sacral plexus). It then curves up on the left side, joining the *suṣumnā* at *maṇipūra chakra* (solar plexus). Continuing in a series of curves crossing back and forth over the *suṣumnā*, *piṅgalā* goes to the right and *iḍā* goes to the left. *Iḍā* and *piṅgalā* move in opposite directions, and cross each other at the *chakras*, finally meeting at the sixth *chakra*, *ājñā chakra*. This meeting point of the three streams is called *Mukti Triveni* (*mukta*, 'liberated'). *Iḍā* and *piṅgalā* end in the left and right nostrils, respectively.

The spiral patterned movement is likened to the double helix of our DNA, or a pair of intertwined serpents as seen in the symbol of the caduceus of medicine. The caduceus is a winged staff, with two serpents, and is carried by the Greek god, Hermes, who is said to be the messenger of the Gods. Together, *iḍā* and *piṅgalā* form the two serpents or snakes of the caduceus, while *suṣumnā* forms the staff. The snakes intersect at the *chakras*, as do the *nādīs*. At the *ājñā chakra*, at the midpoint between the eyebrows, there are two petals, one on either side, just as there are two wings at the top of the caduceus. Although the caduceus symbol was only adopted as a Western symbol for medicine about a century ago, we can see the representation of the entire system of *kuṇḍalinī shakti*.

RELATIONSHIP OF *IḌĀ* AND *PIṄGALĀ* WITH HEMISPHERES OF THE BRAIN

The cerebrum, the largest part of the brain, is made up of two halves, called hemispheres and known as the left and right cerebral hemispheres. These halves are interconnected by a pathway of nerve fibres along which information continuously passes. The cerebrum is divided into four lobes paired according to the skull bones next to them: frontal, parietal, temporal and occipital lobes. The grey matter of the cerebrum is located in the outer layers of the brain known as the cortex as well as in 'islands' of grey matter within the white matter.

The cortex of each hemisphere controls the opposite side of the body and contains various centres – motor centres that control the voluntary muscles, the sensory centre for receiving skin sensations, the visual centre that processes stimuli arriving from the eye, and the hearing centre.

The specific functions of the two hemispheres of the cerebrum correlate with the activities of *iḍā* and *piṅgalā nādīs*. *Iḍā* is connected with the right hemisphere, which governs the left side of the body. *Piṅgalā* is connected with the left hemisphere and governs the right side of the body.

The right hemisphere (non-dominant hemisphere), in relation to *iḍā*, contains centres for spatial orientation, extra-sensory perception, intuition, and creative, artistic and musical abilities. The right brain moves from whole to parts, holistically. It reviews the big picture first, not the details. It is also random – its tendency is to jump from one track to another.

The left hemisphere (dominant hemisphere), in relation to *piṅgalā*, is concerned with logical, rational and analytical abilities. Information is processed in a linear, sequential and logical manner. It processes from part to whole. It takes parts, lines them up, and arranges them in a logical order; then derives conclusions.

Mind and *prāṇa* are interrelated and interdependent. When the *pranas* are disturbed the mind also becomes disturbed; and vice versa, when the mind is disturbed the *prāṇas* become disturbed. The practices of *Hātha Yoga*, *Svāra Yoga* and *Rāja Yoga* help bring a balance between the alternating activities of the *iḍā* and *piṅgalā nādīs*, ensuring that they operate in rhythm with the movements of the external sun and moon. The Sanskrit word *Haṭha*, as in *Hātha Yoga*, represents the moon (*ha*) *iḍā* lunar current, and sun (*tha*) *piṅgalā* solar current.

There is one particular *Hātha Yoga* practice called *nāḍī sodhana* (alternate nostril breathing) that is the best technique to calm the mind and nervous system. *Nāḍī sodhana* purifies the *nāḍīs* or vital channels of energy. The exercise also produces optimum function to both sides of the brain, that is, optimum creativity and optimum logical verbal activity. This creates a more balanced person, since both hemispheres of the brain are functioning properly.

PRĀṆA AND THE *NĀḌĪS*

Iḍā and *piṅgalā* are related to the two nostrils in the body. *Iḍā*, the cooling lunar current, also called *chandra nāḍī*, flows through the left nostril; and *piṅgalā* (*sūrya nāḍī*), the heating solar current, flows through the right. The *nāḍīs* are channels or pathways for carrying *prāṇa* into the *chakras* situated along the spinal column in the astral spine. To consciously activate a *chakra* one can either direct *prāṇa* to the *chakra* or, using mental visualisation, concentrate on its location and form. The word *prāṇa* comes from two Sanskrit roots. *Pra* means 'first', and *na* is the 'smallest unit of energy'. *Prāṇa* is therefore the first breath, the primal or atomic beginning of the flow of energy. Out of this first unit of energy manifests all aspects and levels of the human being. It is one and the same as *kuṇḍalinī śakti*.

The *kuṇḍalinī*, manifesting as *prāṇa*, flows in certain patterns, or channels that are called *nāḍīs*. *Prāṇa* is the life-force that links the physical with the mental, and the mental with the spiritual.

4.5

KUṆḌALINĪ

Kuṇḍalinī is the primordial energy of consciousness (*caitanya śakti*) that lies dormant at the base of the spine in the causal body of all beings, and in every atom of the universe. It is the spiritual potential force of the Cosmic Power. *Kuṇḍalinī* maintains the individual soul through the subtle *prāṇa*. The subtle *prāṇa* is connected with the subtle *nāḍīs* and *chakras*, and the *nāḍīs* are connected with the mind, which is connected to all the parts of the body. When *kuṇḍalinī śakti* is dormant or is active only in the lower three *chakras*, a person has only a finite experience. When *kuṇḍalinī* is aroused and ascends upward, she withdraws into herself the moving powers of creation, and unites with pure consciousness (*Śiva*). This is the reverse process of the evolution of the mind and the five gross elements. In reality *kuṇḍalinī* has no form, but the mind and intellect require a particular form on which to concentrate initially, so the subtle, formless *kuṇḍalinī* has symbolically taken the form of a coiled serpent or snake. In the *mulādhāra chakra* there is a self-existent point, at which the *suṣumnā nāḍī* is attached to the *kanda*. The sleeping *kuṇḍalinī* serpent lies face downwards at the mouth of *suṣumnā nāḍī* on the head of this point. She is coiled like a serpent with three and a half coils around the *svayambhu* ('self-born') *lingam*. The unawakened *kuṇḍalinī śakti* remains coiled around the *lingam* with her tail in her mouth. The three coils represent the *kuṇḍalinī* energy within us, compressed like a spring, ready to change from potential static energy (dormant) into kinetic manifestation (awakening). The half coil represents the state of transcendence. There are also other meanings: the three coils also represent the three *guṇas* of *prakṛiti* – *sattva*, *rajas* and *tamas* (equilibrium, activity and inertia); the three states of consciousness (waking, sleeping, dreaming); and the three *matras* of *Oṁ* (*Aum*).

Kuṇḍalinī comes from the Sanskrit word *kundal*, which means 'coiled'. But a more correct meaning of *kuṇḍalinī* is derived from the word *kunda*, which means 'pit' or 'cavity'. *Kunda* refers to the concave cavity in which the brain, resembling a coiled, sleeping serpent, nestles. *Prāṇic* energy and consciousness (*caitanya śakti*) are the two forms of *kuṇḍalinī*. *Prāṇic* energy is the cause of action, and consciousness (*caitanya śakti*) gives rise to knowledge and wisdom. When *kuṇḍalinī* is activated these two energies, *prāṇa śakti* and *caitanya śakti*, are activated in all the brain centres.

KUṆḌALINĪ AWAKENING

> 'The *kuṇḍalinī*, in its latent form, is coiled like a serpent. One who causes that *Śakti* to move (from the *mūladhāra* upwards) will attain liberation.'
>
> *Haṭha Yoga Pradīpikā 3:108*

In *Tantra Yoga*, *kuṇḍalinī* is an aspect of *Śakti*, the divine female energy and consort of *Śiva*. The one Consciousness is polarised into static (*Śiva*) and dynamic (*Śakti*) aspects for the purpose of manifestation. The object of *Kuṇḍalinī Yoga* is to awaken the latent coiled-up cosmic energy (*Śakti*) in the spine and unite it with Pure Consciousness (*Śiva*). The consummation of the blissful union between *Śakti* and *Śiva* in the *sahasrāra chakra* is the union of the individual soul (*jīva*) with the supreme Self, or Divine Consciousness. The duality becomes one.

If the positive and negative forces of *iḍā* and *piṅgalā nāḍīs* are completely balanced, an awakening can occur which activates the latent *kuṇḍalinī* to rise from its dormant state. There are degrees of awakening; sometimes there may only be a mild awakening in which *kuṇḍalinī* rises as far as *svādhiṣṭhāna chakra* and then drops back to *mūlādhāra*, the root support. That is why it is important to purify and balance the *nāḍīs* through the *Haṭha Yoga* practice of *prāṇāyama*. The *chakras* also need to be purified and in balance.

When activated, the *kuṇḍalinī* energy, which was lying dormant and static in the *mulādhāra chakra*, becomes kinetic and dynamic. It travels up the psychic pathway in the *suṣumnā nāḍī*, the central axis, criss-crossed in a helix by the *iḍā* and *piṅgalā*. As the *kuṇḍalinī* climbs up on its spiritual ascent towards the *sahasrāra chakra*, the seat of consciousness at the crown of the head, it activates all the *chakras* in the subtle body in succession. They are stimulated into intense activity by the force of the *kuṇḍalinī* as it travels upwards. Layer after layer of the mind becomes fully opened, causing the yogi to experience visions, powers, knowledge and bliss.

Kuṇḍalinī can also be awakened in an individual *chakra*. For instance, if *kuṇḍalinī* is awakened in the second *chakra* (*svādhiṣṭhāna*) it ascends directly to *sahasrāra chakra*. Similarly, if *kuṇḍalinī* is awakened in the third *chakra* (*maṇipūra*) it ascends straight to *sahasrāra chakra*.

After having made its ascent through the six centres of consciousness to the awakening at *sahasrāra*, the *kuṇḍalinī* descends back down through the *chakras* to its root support at the *mūlādhāra chakra*. The luminous ascent through the *chakras* is a resorption (*laya*) of all the cosmic powers into *kuṇḍalinī*, culminating in a freedom that transcends the phenomenal world in which consciousness is bound and conditioned by space, time and causation. As *kuṇḍalinī* makes the return journey or descent to her root support at the base of the spine, she revivifies and illumines what she had previously absorbed.

The latent force of *kuṇḍalinī* may be activated through various means, such as birth, *mantra* (a method used in *Bhakti Yoga*), austerity (*tapasya*), meditation, *prāṇāyāma*, *Kriyā Yoga*, *Rāja Yoga*, *Śaktipāt* (the transmission of spiritual power from the guru to the disciple), *Karma Yoga*, *Bhakti Yoga* and *Jñanā Yoga*.

In some circumstances, *kuṇḍalinī* can even occur without Yoga practice, for instance due to a shock or an accident. But in these kinds of circumstances the person has no conscious control over the power, and so there is no guarantee of true spiritual awakening.

When the *kuṇḍalinī śakti* passes up along the *suṣumnā* piercing the *chakras* as it goes, the yogi experiences different kinds of knowledge, powers and bliss. But for the vast majority of people whose minds operate only in the lower levels of consciousness the *suṣumnā* is generally closed at the base of the spine.

THE THREE PSYCHIC KNOTS – OBSTACLES TO *KUṆḌALINĪ* AWAKENING

Within the *suṣumnā nāḍī* there are three psychic knots of energy, known as *granthis*. The Sanskrit word *granthi* means a knot, a tied-up force, or an obstacle to one's spiritual growth. These knots restrict human life to instinctive, emotional and intellectual levels. If lower desires become dominant in a person, the flow of *prāṇa* gets obstructed and short-circuited at the first knot or *Brāhma granthi*, diminishing the flow of energy to the higher centres. The path of the *kuṇḍalinī* is obstructed, preventing its upward movement to the crown centre (*sahasrāra chakra*).

When *kuṇḍalinī* is activated it rises upward through the *chakras*, and pierces successive veils of ignorance in the form of knots (*granthis*), which changes the perception of reality and consciousness.

The *granthis* are a protective mechanism, like safety valves or circuit breakers, that effectively prevent premature entrance of the *kuṇḍalinī* energy into the *chakras* above the second centre (*svadhisthana chakra*). The three knots are named after the presiding deities of these knots: *Brāhma granthi*, *Vishnu granthi* and *Rudra* (*Śiva*) *granthi*, which respectively are the creative, preservative and transforming forces that are involved in the presence of any object. These three forces are involved, one in the other.

For the spiritual aspirant or yogi, it is important to loosen these knots and make the *iḍā* and *piṅgalā* function smoothly so that they are in balance, with a clear flow of *prāṇa*. The *nāḍīs* need to be purified and strengthened to allow for the strong surge of energy to rise up the spine.

Brāhma granthi. The first knot is located at the root *chakra* (*mūladhāra chakra*), and is related to the physical body. This knot is connected with our entanglement in the world of names and forms. It creates instinctive drives and strong, demanding, sensual desires with attachment.

Vishnu granthi. The second knot is located at the heart *chakra* (*anāhata*), and is related to the astral body. This is associated with emotional life, attachment, and understanding ourselves through the concept of ego (*ahaṁkāra*).

Rudra granthi. The third knot is located in the *ājñā chakra* or Spiritual Eye, and is related to the causal body. This is the point where the *iḍā* and *piṅgalā nāḍīs* cross over each other. *Rudra granthi* is concerned with intellectual obsessions, and attachments to psychic phenomena and psychic powers, and our mortal insecurity. When the *kuṇḍalinī* loosens this knot, it can continue its upward journey to the crown *chakra* (*sahasrāra*), enabling the yogi to attain transcendental bliss.

4.6

THE SEVEN MAJOR CHAKRAS

'Just as you find that earth, water, fire, air and the space beyond the atmosphere, interpenetrate one another, so also these six main centres lie inside the body apparently one above the other, but functioning in mutual interdependence as one vital chain. A little reflection will convince you that the play of life goes on in the upper centres (*chakras*) of your body when your thoughts are pure and full of bliss.'

Sri Anandamayi Ma, in Lipski 1988, p.68

The *chakras* are specific life-energy centres that control the living formative forces or *tattvas*, without which our physical bodies could not be animated. The *chakras* are the link between the physical realm and the spiritual dimensions of existence. Each *chakra* facilitates the flow and interchange of energies from the subtle dimensions by stepping them down, so that they can be utilised by the physical body. The frequency of energies can also be stepped up so they can be used at the subtle realm. To become aware of the more subtle levels of our spiritual existence, meditation on the *chakras* can help us to transcend our identification with the impermanent physical body.

In the Yoga and Tantric traditions the *chakras* have been represented as diagrams and *yantras* in the form of lotuses (*pādmas*) with various symbols, colours, *mantras* and deities, representing the different energies and consciousness of each centre. In reality the *chakras* do not actually look like this; the *yantras* are visual metaphors, corresponding to inner states of human consciousness through which we can discover our inner spiritual identity. *Yantras* function as revelatory symbols of spiritual truths – they are instruments or maps for visualisation and meditation that can help the spiritual aspirant to transcend the *tattvas* (elemental nature or quality), which dominate the five basic centres from *mūlādhāra* to *viśuddhi*. The *chakras* in the form of diagramatic *yantras* helps the meditator to concentrate the mind on the spiritual reality symbolised by the form. Through the form the meditator reaches the Formless, and as a result the meditator feels the presence of the Omnipresent Being. Knowledge about the *chakras* can help an individual to develop a deep inner experience in meditation and in life. The dormant powers and energy in these *chakras* can be purified, balanced, strengthened and activated.

Each *chakra* appears as a lotus with a particular number of petals with a Sanskrit letter for each petal. The number of petals in each *chakra* is determined by the number and position of the *nādīs* around the *chakras*. The entire 50 letters of the Sanskrit alphabet are present in the 50 petals of the lotuses (*chakras*). The letter represents the sound vibration produced by each petal, and denotes the *mantra* in latent form of *kuṇḍalinī*. These *mantras* can be manifested and their vibrations experienced during meditation.

When the *kuṇḍalinī* is lying dormant at the *mūladhāra chakra*, the petals of the *chakras* hang downward. When *kuṇḍalinī śakti* is awakened, the petals turn upward towards the head.

MULADHĀRA CHAKRA (ROOT SUPPORT) – FOUR-PETALLED LOTUS

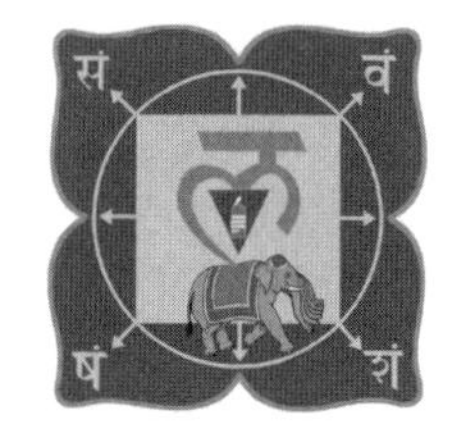

> 'Now we come to the *Ādhāra* lotus (*muladhāra chakra*). It is attached to the mouth of the suṣumnā, and is placed below the genitals and above the anus. It has four petals of crimson hue. Its head (mouth) hangs downwards. On its petals are the four letters from *va* to *sa*, of the shining colour of gold.'
>
> *Ṣaṭ-cakra-nirūpaṇa, verse 4*

(The *Ṣaṭ-cakra-nirūpaṇa* is a part of the sixth *Patala* of the *Śrī-tattva-cintāmani*, a Tantrik work composed in Sanskrit in 1577 CE by the Tantrik *sadhaka*, Pūrnaṇānda, who attained spiritual perfection.)

The upward journey of *kuṇḍalinī śakti* begins at the 'root support' centre, the foundation for the development of our personality, and the basis from which the possibility of higher realisation arises.

The *mūladhāra chakra* is also referred to as the 'base' or 'root support' centre (from the Sanskrit word *mūla,* pronounced 'moola'). *Mūladhāra chakra* is the seat or base where *kuṇḍalinī śakti* resides, and it is also the basis of our existence. It is located between the origin of the reproductive organ and the anus. It is just below the *kanda* and the junction where *iḍā*, *piṅgalā* and *suṣumnā nāḍīs* meet. In the male the seat of *mūladhāra* is situated slightly inside the perineum, midway between the scrotum and the anus. In the female, it is located on the posterior side of the cervix.

SVĀDHIṢṬHĀNA CHAKRA – SIX-PETALLED LOTUS

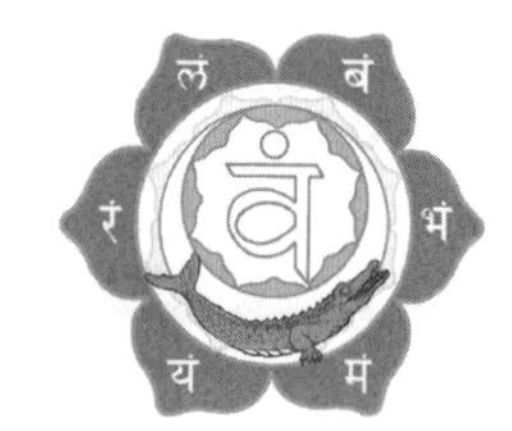

> 'There is another lotus (*svādhiṣṭhāna chakra*) placed inside the *suṣumnā* at the root of the genitals, of a beautiful vermillion colour. On its six petals are the letters from *Ba* to *Puraṁdara* (the letter *La*), with the *Bindu* superposed, of the shining colour of lightning.'
>
> *Ṣaṭ-cakra-nirūpaṇa, verse 14*

We began our journey through the *chakras* at the *mūladhāra chakra*. Now we arrive at *svādhiṣṭhāna*, where we can start to express ourselves creatively. The evolution of consciousness towards Pure Consciousness begins in *svādhiṣṭhāna chakra*.

The Sanskrit word *Svā* means 'one's own' and *ādhiṣṭhāna* means 'dwelling place', so *svādhiṣṭhāna* means 'one's own place'. It has been suggested by some yogis that this refers to a distant time when the seat of *kuṇḍalinī* lay dormant within *svādhiṣṭhāna chakra*, but for some reason there was a fall and *kuṇḍalinī* came to rest in *mūladhāra chakra*.

Svādhiṣṭhāna is the second *chakra*, located in the sacral region of the spine at the level of the coccyx (tailbone), behind the sexual organs.

MAṆIPŪRA CHAKRA – TEN-PETALLED LOTUS

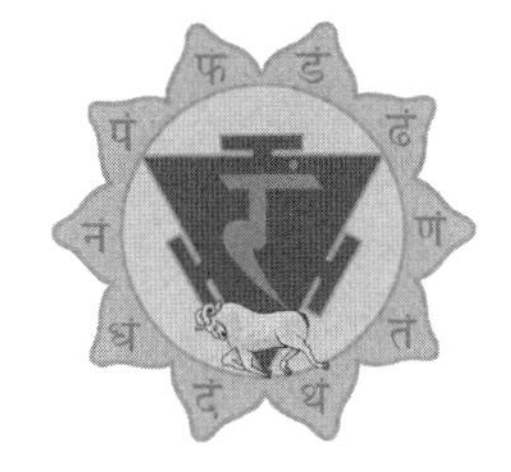

> 'Above it (*svādhiṣṭhāna*), and at the root of the navel, is the shining lotus of ten petals (*maṇipūra chakra*), of the colour of heavy-laden rain clouds. Within it are the letters *Ḍa* to *Pha*, of the colour of the blue lotus with the *Nada* and *Bindu* above them. Meditate there on the region of Fire, triangular in form and shining like the rising sun. Outside it are three *svastika* marks, and within, the *bīja* of Vahni himself.'
>
> *Ṣaṭ-cakra-nirūpaṇa, verse 19*

On our journey upwards from the inert stability of *mūladhāra chakra*, and the fluidity and adaptiveness of *svādhiṣṭhāna chakra*, we now rise to the dynamic fire of *maṇipūra chakra*. This third centre radiates its fiery energy like a bright sun. The element of this *chakra* is fire. The first two lower *chakras* are predominantly *tamasic* (lethargic and negative), but *maṇipūra*, the third lower *chakra*, is predominantly *rajasic* (active, intense). Both *svādhiṣṭhāna* and *maṇipūra* are the seat of *prāṇāyama kosha*. *Maṇipūra* is a very important centre because it is the centre of willpower, energy, vitality and achievement. It generates and distributes *prāṇic* energy throughout the whole body, and controls our energy balance, vitality and strength.

ANĀHATA CHAKRA – TWELVE-PETALLED LOTUS

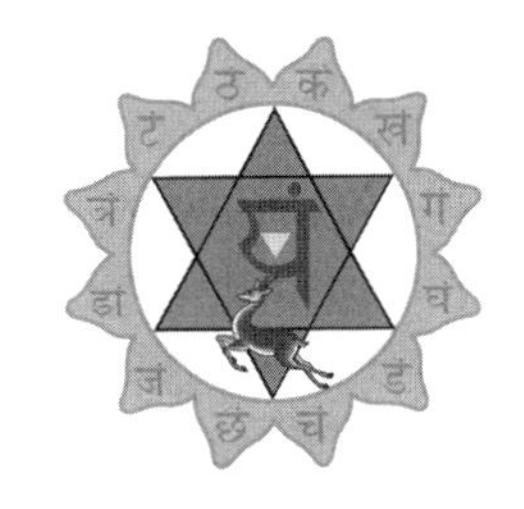

> 'Above that, in the heart, is the charming lotus (*anāhata chakra*), of the shining colour of the *Bandhūka* flower, with the twelve letters beginning with *Ka*, of the colour of vermillion, placed therein. It is known by its name of *anāhata*, and is like the celestial wishing-tree (*kalpa-taru*), bestowing even more than (the supplicant's) desire. The Region of Vāyu, beautiful and with six corners (interlacing triangles), which is like the colour of smoke.'
>
> *Ṣaṭ-cakra-nirūpaṇa, verse 22*

From the *maṇipūra chakra* we rise above the limitations of perception in the two lower centres: *mūladhāra* and *svādhiṣṭhāna*, and we ascend to the fourth centre of consciousness, *anāhata chakra*. The three lower *chakras* relate primarily to the physical body; the fourth centre (*anāhata chakra*) takes us beyond the limits of the ego-self. The heart *chakra* is the pivotal point of transition, the plane of balance between the three lower *chakras* – related to the world of body, mind and senses and associated with survival, security, sensuality, sex and power – and the *chakras* above, related to a higher and more evolved consciousness.

The Sanskrit word *anāhata* literally means 'unstruck'. It refers to the inner subtle sound vibration (*nada*) experienced in meditation. It is called 'unstruck' because it is not created by physical friction.

There are two kinds of *nada*: *ahat nada* – all external or struck sounds, such as musical instruments played; and *anāhata nada* – all sounds which do not have any external source, or 'unstruck' sound.

The *anāhata chakra* is also the seat of the subtle life-force (*prāṇa*). Within this subtle heart resides the individual soul (*jīvātman*), together with mind (*citta*) and ego-principle (*ahaṁkāra*). Various scriptures affirm that the heart is the seat of the individual soul:

> 'God is seated in the hearts of all beings. His cosmic delusion (*Māyā*) causes them to revolve as though they had been mounted on a machine.'
>
> *Bhāgavad Gītā 18:61*

> 'By meditation upon the heart the *ātman* is realised.'
>
> *Yoga Sūtras 3:34*

> 'Which is the self? This Omnipresent Being (*puruṣa*) that is identified with *buddhi* and is in the midst of the organs, the (self-effulgent) light within the heart.'
>
> *Brihadaranyaka Upaniṣad 4:3.7*

According to the *Chandogya Upaniṣad* the location of the self is in the heart. The physical body is referred to as *Brāhmapuram* (the city of *Brāhman*), because *Brāhman* resides here as the internal ruler with a retinue of attendents, such as the ten organs and the mind. His abode is the small lotus of the heart. Non-dual *Brāhman* (Pure Consciousness), who is immanent in the universe, is the all-pervading Being (*puruṣa*). But His direct manifestation in the phenomenal world is the innermost self of every individual, shining as the central principle of consciousness in the centre of the heart.

> 'In this city of *Brāhman* there is a small lotus, an abode. Inside this there is a tiny space (*ākāśha*). That which is within this one should seek and yearn.'
>
> *Chandogya Upaniṣad 8:1.1*

Paramhansa Yogananda's guru, Swāmi Sri Yukteswar said:

> 'The heart's natural love is the principal requisite to attain a holy life. When love, the heavenly gift of Nature, appears in the heart, it removes all causes of excitation from the system and cools it down to a perfectly normal state... When this love becomes developed in man it makes him able to Understand the real position of his own Self as well as of others Surrounding him... Love, the heavenly gift, is the principal requisite for the attainment of holy salvation; it is impossible for man to advance a step towards the same without it.'
>
> *Yukteswar 1990, p.37*

> 'All love in its native purity, is God's love... Love is a condition of the mind and heart which essentially transcends all relationships. We worship God above all through all these relationships.'
>
> *Yogananda 2007a, pp.130–131*

VIŚUDDHI CHAKRA – SIXTEEN-PETALLED LOTUS

'In the throat is the lotus called *Viśuddha*, which is pure and of a smoky purple hue. All the (sixteen) shining vowels on its (sixteen) petals, of a crimson hue, are distinctly visible to him whose mind is illumined. In the pericarp of this lotus there is the ethereal region, circular in shape, and white like the full moon. On the elephant white as snow is seated the *bīja* of *Aṁbara*, who is white of colour.'

Ṣaṭ-cakra-nirūpaṇa, verse 28

The word *viśuddha* means 'pure'; *viśuddhi* means 'purity'. *Viśuddha* is derived from the Sanskrit words *visha,* meaning 'impurity', and *śuddhi*, meaning 'to purify'. It is the centre of purity.

The fifth centre of consciousness, *viśuddha chakra*, is located in the cervical plexus, directly behind the base of the throat.

Viśuddha chakra is the centre for communication, creativity, self-expression, non-attachment, and learning to accept and receive. When this *chakra* is balanced and open the powers of communication and creativity become awakened. In the raising of consciousness, *viśuddha chakra* is an important bridge from the *anāhata chakra* to the higher *chakras* above, belonging to the mind principle.

The inner qualities of *viśuddha chakra* are calmness and expansion. When we quieten the mental restlessness by directing the energy inward and upward in meditation, we reach a deep level of inner calmness and an expansion of consciousness. Even-minded calmness is clarity of perception and intuition; calmness is the enjoyable experience of the Self. Until we learn to think, talk and act with calmness and even-minded attitude, we cannot make our life productive. Paramhansa Yogananda said that calmness is more dynamic and more powerful than peace, because calmness gives one the power to overcome all the obstacles in one's life.

ĀJÑĀ CHAKRA – TWO-PETALLED LOTUS

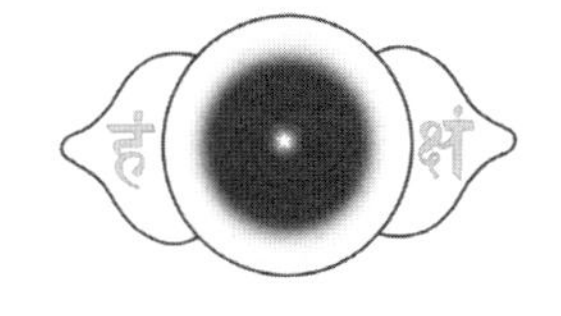

'The lotus named *Ājñā* is like the moon, (beautifully white). On its two petals are the letters *Ha* and *Kṣa*, which are also white and enhance its beauty. It shines with the glory of *Dhyāna*. Inside it is the *Śakti Hākini*, whose six faces are like so many moons. She has six arms, in one of which She holds a book; two others are lifted up in the gestures of dispelling fear and granting boons, and with the rest She holds a skull, a small drum (*ḍamaru*), and a rosary (*japa* beads). Her mind is pure (*śuddha-citta*).'

Ṣaṭ-cakra-nirūpaṇa, verse 32

The Sanskrit word *ājñā* (pronounced 'agya') literally means 'command'. It means 'to obey', and 'to know'. It is the seat of the mind-space and 'inner Master', indicating that wisdom and knowledge are realised in all actions. The *ājñā chakra* is the instruction and command centre that guides the other *chakras*.

Ājñā chakra is the *chakra* of the mind and the seat of concentration. It represents a higher level of awareness. It is the centre of extrasensory perception, intuition, clarity and wisdom, and it forms the boundary between human and Divine consciousness. This chakra is the sixth centre of consciousness. It is located in the *suṣumnā nāḍī* and its corresponding centre in the physical body is in the brain directly at the midpoint behind the two eyebrows.

> 'When the devotee reaches beyond the highest vital centre which is situated between the eyebrows, his mental powers merge in the supra-mental, his ego dissolves in *mahābhāva* (highest ecstasy, supreme love for God) and he finds his eternal refuge in *svarūpa* (His own true Self). He then goes into *samādhi*, a state of perpetual bliss.'
>
> *Sri Anandamayi Ma, in Lipski 1988, pp.68–69*

The Spiritual Eye

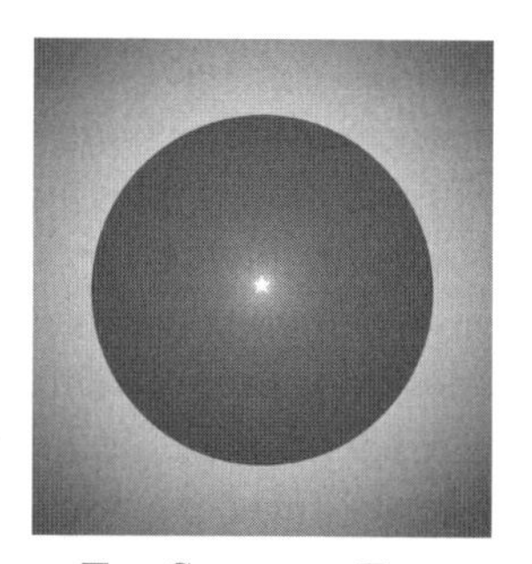

The Spiritual Eye

> 'Stop beholding only the little toy show of this world; close your physical eyes and plunge behind the screen of darkness. Lift the veil of silence, and behold the magic of soothing, rolling fires of planets, of trillions of multi-coloured dancing atoms. Behold life-force dancing in the hall of electrons. Behold one layer of light lying within another. Behold consciousness dancing in the sphere of living light. Behold the Bliss-God and His blessed angels dancing in the thought fashioned, wisdom lighted Eternal Chamber of Perpetual, ever-new Bliss. Lift all curtains of light and behold God in the glory of bliss. The Spiritual Eye is the tunnel through all veils of light, leading straight to God.'
>
> *Yogananda 2003, p.5*

Ājñā chakra has two poles: a positive and a negative. The positive pole is the 'Spiritual Eye' or 'Christ centre' as Paramhansa Yogananda referred to it, which is located at the midpoint between the eyebrows (ruled by the sun). It is associated with Divine joy. The negative pole is the medulla oblongata (ruled by the moon), located in the brain stem of the spinal cord at the base of the skull. It is the seat of the ego. The moon is a symbol of the ego. The moon has no light of its own, it only reflects the light of the sun; similarly, the ego having no reality of its own reflects the light of the Self. The mind reflects the object on which it meditates, and takes on the qualities of that object, as a mirror takes on the qualities reflected in it. In other words we see the mind's activity by the light of the Self. Neither the mind nor the intellect has the ability to illumine the Self. The source of light does not need another light to illumine it; similarly, the Self needs no other knowledge to make itself known, as its nature is Knowledge itself. The ego-mind is differentiated from the luminous Self in the same way that the physical body, sense-organs and external objects are. In respect to this, Patañjali in his *Yoga Sūtras* (4:19) states: 'The mind is not self-luminous, because of its nature as the (visible) object of inner perception.' The mind in itself is not perceivable.

Both the Spiritual Eye and the physical eye are reflections of the medulla oblongata. By concentrating on the midpoint between the eyebrows (Spiritual Eye) one can see the medulla reflected as one light. This is the meaning behind Jesus Christ saying: 'If, therefore, thine eye be single, thy whole body shall be full of light' (Luke 11:34–35). When the two physical eyes manifest the single Spiritual Eye, then one can perceive, by continuous spiritual development, the physical body as filled with the illumination of the astral body.

The medulla oblongata (the negative pole of *ājñā chakra*) is where the Conscious Cosmic Energy (life-force; *prāṇa*) primarily enters into the body, and remains concentrated in the brain as the thousand-rayed lotus. *Prāṇa* is stored in the *sahasrāra chakra* and distributed throughout the whole body through the astral nerve channels (*nādīs*). It descends into the body through the spinal cord and the sympathetic nervous system.

It is also interesting to note that images of *Śiva* are depicted with the moon symbol resting in his hair at the crown of the head (*sahasrāra chakra*), showing that his ego-consciousness is totally one with the Cosmic Consciousness.

When we are meditating with deep calm concentration at that point between the eyebrows, with a feeling of joyous aspiration, it is possible to see the spiritual eye. This inner eye of luminous light is seen as a circular sphere of blue light, haloed with a ring of gold light, and at its centre a white star with five rays of luminous scintillating light.

Suṣumnā, the major central *nādī* in the astral spine corresponding to the spinal cord in the physical body, (also called *brāhma nādī* 'Path to God') is comprised of three astral tubes or currents of life-energy. The *suṣumnā* is like an electrical wire with two or three coverings to insulate it. The outermost covering or sheath is the *suṣumnā* itself. The second inner covering or tube is the sun-like *vajrinī nādī*, which covers the third inner astral tube, the moon-like *citriṇī nādī*. Within the *citriṇī nādī* is a very fine astral current called the *brāhma nādī*. The Spiritual Eye is a cross-section of the *suṣumnā* or astral spine, showing the various sheaths or coverings for the energy in the spine. The concentric astral channels (*nādīs*) – *suṣumnā*, *vajrinī*, *citriṇī* and *brāhma* – are reflected in the Spiritual Eye. The sun-like *vajrinī nādī* is reflected in the Spiritual Eye as a halo of gold light, which the meditating yogi experiences as the Cosmic Vibration, *Aum* (the Holy Ghost). The spiritual eye elongates first into a golden tunnel, and then into a tunnel of blue as the yogi's consciousness enters into the blue sphere of light (moon-like *citriṇī nādī* – the causal world), giving the experience of Christ Consciousness or *Kūtastha Caitanya*. Finally at the end of the tunnel of blue is a silvery-white star with five rays of luminous, scintillating light (*brāhma nādī*) representing the Kingdom of God beyond all creation. Here the meditating yogi enters the light uniting his or her consciousness with Cosmic Consciousness.

SAHASRĀRA CHAKRA – THOUSAND-PETALLED LOTUS

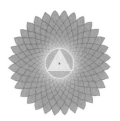

'Above all these, in the vacant space (*parama-vyoma*, the supreme Ether) wherein is *śaṅkhini nāḍī*, and below Visarga is the lotus of a thousand petals (*sahasrāra chakra*). This lotus, lustrous and whiter than the full moon, has its head turned downward. It charms. Its clustered filaments are tinged with the colour of the young Sun. Its body is luminous with the letters beginning with A, and it is the absolute bliss (*Brāhman* Bliss).'

Ṣaṭ-cakra-nirūpaṇa, verse 40

The Sanskrit word *sahasra* means one thousand; *sahasrāra* means 'thousand petalled'. The *sahasrāra chakra* is also called the crown *chakra* and is also known as *Niralambapuri* ('dwelling place without support'); and *Brāhmarandhra* ('the Door of God').

The *sahasrāra chakra*, the seventh centre, strictly speaking is not actually a *chakra*, as it does not belong to planes of consciousness of the mind and body. It is an extended field of consciousness that is experienced above the head as the highest centre of Pure Consciousness. The attainment of superconscious awareness of the Self as the Infinite at the *sahasrāra*, is symbolically shown in many religious paintings as a halo of light above the crown of the head.

The *sahasrāra* lotus has one thousand *nāḍīs* symbolised as petals emanating from it. The vibrations made by the *nāḍīs* are represented by Sanskrit letters. The thousand petals of *sahasrāra* carry the total sound-potential represented by all 50 letters of the Sanskrit alphabet. The 50 letters are repeated 20 times, 50 in each layer (20 x 50 = 1000).

Sahasrāra chakra is a shining moonlike white lotus of a thousand petals and the light of a thousand suns. It lies about three inches (8 cm) above the crown of the head with its face or petals pointing downwards. This differentiates it from the other six *chakras*.

In *ājñā chakra* there was still the experience of a Self apparently differentiated from the 'object' of God, but in *sahasrāra* the experience, the experienced and the experiencer become one and the same. They all become unified and liberated. The illusion of individual self is dissolved.

When the *kuṇḍalinī śakti* (creative energy-power) awakens, she ascends to unite in one form above the crown of the head with *Śiva* (Pure Consciousness), whose manifest energy she is through the *chakras*. *Śakti* merges with *Śiva* in *Laya Yoga* (Absorption).

Through deep meditation the yogi finally attains the goal of Yoga by uniting his or her consciousness in *nirvikalpa samādhi* (the highest level of superconsciousness, *samādhi*) at the *sahasrāra chakra*. All the *vṛttis* of the mind come to complete stillness, and the yogi attains fulfilment and liberation in the union of knowledge, the knower, and the object of knowledge. To reach this divine union in *sahasrāra chakra* we must first awaken the *ājñā chakra*, which is the gateway to it. Self-realisation takes place at the *ājñā chakra*. Here you have the first union with God in the blissful state of *savikalpa samādhi*. And finally comes the highest experience, which is identification with the Absolute in *nivikalpa samādhi*, which liberates the Self. Liberation (*kaivalya*) takes place in the *sahasrāra chakra*. First *samprājñāta-samādhi* is established, then it develops into *asamprājñāta-samādhi*, finally culminating in *kaivalya*. *Samādhi* is attained by faith, energy, memory, meditation and the awakening of wisdom.

To give you some idea of what *asamprājñāta-samādhi* is, think about the following comparisons of time that a meditator can concentrate for.

Concentration on an object for 12 seconds is called *dhāraṇā*. If the period of concentration is increased to 12 times that of *dhāraṇā*, to 144 seconds, it is called *dhyāna*. And if the concentration lasts for 12 times the period of *dhyāna*, to 1728 seconds (28 minutes 48 seconds), it is called *asamprājñāta-samādhi*.

LOCATING THE *CHAKRAS*

The seven centres of consciousness (*chakras*) are situated in the Astral Body. Here they are shown in relation to the Physical Body.

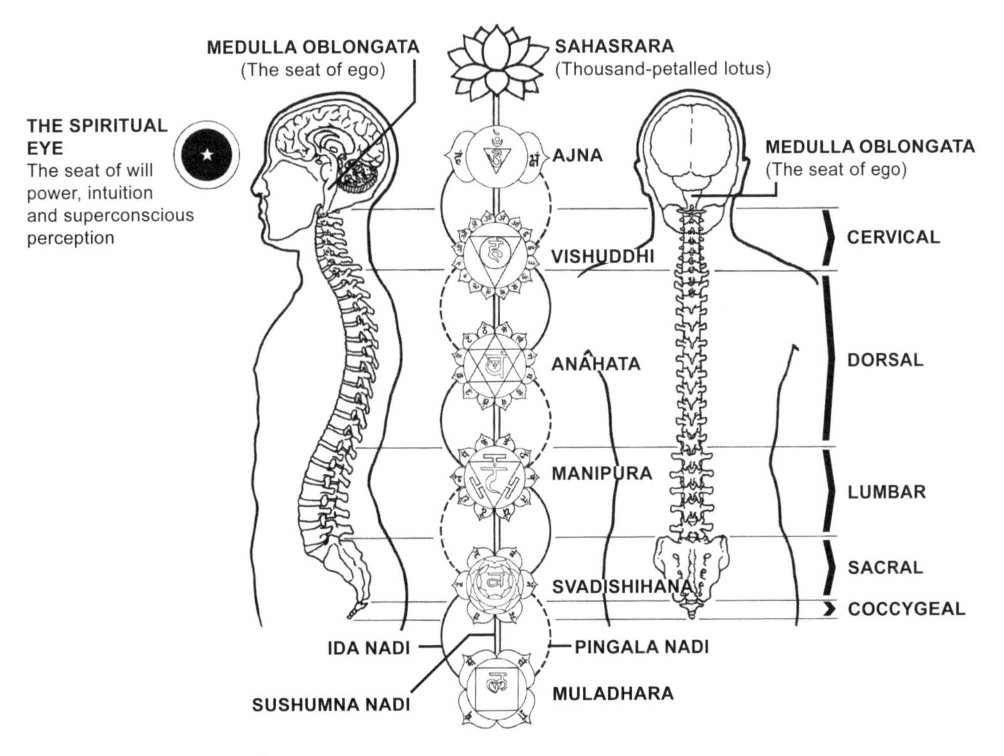

THE CHAKRAS IN RELATION TO THE PHYSICAL BODY

The following exercise is for locating the *chakras* in your spine.

Sit in a comfortable and relaxed meditation posture with your head, neck and spine aligned. If you are unable to sit with your legs crossed, then sit in an upright chair. It is important to keep your spine upright so that the energy can flow unimpeded to the higher brain centres.

First, become aware of your astral spine as a tube of light by placing your left hand at the base of your spine and your right hand at the base of your skull at the medulla oblongata (one of the three vital regions of the brain stem that regulates heart rate and breathing rate). Close your eyes and calmly look into your Spiritual Eye (at the midpoint between the eyebrows). Inhale and feel your breath rising up from the base of your spine to the medulla oblongata. Exhale and feel the breath moving down through the astral spine. Practise 12 breaths.

Now place your left hand at the Spiritual Eye while keeping your right hand at the medulla oblongata. As you inhale, feel the breath flow through the psychic passage in the brain from the medulla oblongata (negative pole of *ājñā chakra*) to the Spiritual Eye (positive pole of *ājñā chakra*). Exhale and feel your breath and energy flow from your Spiritual Eye to the medulla.

In the second part of this exercise you will contract and relax certain parts of the physical body, and visualise each *chakra* as a lotus flower.

Mūladhāra

Mūladhāra chakra is located on the posterior side of the cervix. *Mūladhāra* is the direct switch for awakening *ājñā chakra.*

For men: Contract and relax the perineum muscles located midway between the anus and the scrotum.

For women: Contract the vaginal muscles inwards and upwards so that the walls of the upper vagina contract. Try to do this without contracting the anus or the front part of the perineum (clitoris and urinary opening).

During contraction visualise a lotus with its petals closed and pointing downwards. Then visualise this lotus turning through 180 degrees so that it is pointing upwards, opening its petals. Now mentally chant the *mantra Oṁ* three times. Relax the contraction and direct the energy (the lotus rays of energy from the petals) up to the next *chakra.*

Svādhiṣṭhāna

Svādhiṣṭhāna is located at the level of the coccyx or tailbone. The trigger point for *svādhiṣṭhāna* is at the region of the pubis, at the level of the pubic bone.

For men: Bring your awareness to the urethra (urinary passage) inside the penis and try to draw it upwards. Contract the urethra as when controlling the urge to urinate, then relax. This is called *vajroli mudrā.*

For women: Contract the urethra in the same way as when trying to control the urge to urinate.

Repeat as above, visualising the lotus and mentally chanting *Oṁ* three times. Direct the energy up to the next *chakra.*

Maṇipūra

Maṇipūra is located directly behind the navel on the inner wall of the spine. The trigger point is situated at the navel. Contract and draw the navel sharply in towards the spine and hold it there, feel the pulse beat at this point.

Repeat the visualisation and mental chanting as above and move the energy to the next *chakra*.

Anāhata

Anāhata is located in the spine on the inner wall, directly behind the centre of the chest, at the level of the depression in the sternum. This is the *hridayākāśha* (the space within the heart where purity resides). Contract and pull the shoulders back, and place one hand on the centre of the chest, and concentrate on the sensation in the heart space of this *chakra*.

Repeat the lotus visualisation and mental chanting as above and direct the energy up to the next *chakra*.

Viśuddha

Viśuddha is located in the cervical plexus directly behind the throat pit. The trigger point is in the front of the neck, at the throat pit. Place three fingers of one hand on the throat pit and three fingers of the other hand on the spine directly behind. Gently press both points and feel the sensation at this *chakra*.

Repeat the visualisation and mental chanting as before and move the energy to the next *chakra*.

Ājñā

Ājñā corresponds to the pineal gland and is located inside the brain directly behind the eyebrow centre, in the midline of the brain directly above the spine.

Concentrate deeply at the point between the eyebrows by turning the eyes upwards to this point. *Ājñā chakra* is located inside the brain at a point directly behind the eyebrow centre and on top of the spinal column, where the pineal gland is situated. Try to feel a subtle pulsation within this *ājñā chakra* region and synchronise the *mantra Oṁ* (mentally) with the pulsation, so it becomes *Oṁ*, *Oṁ*, *Oṁ*, *Oṁ*, *Oṁ*...

Mūladhāra is the direct switch for awakening *ājñā chakra*, so by practising *aśvinī mudrā* (contraction and relaxation of the anal sphincter muscles) at a medium speed, you should be able to feel the *ājñā chakra*.

Sahasrāra

Sahasrāra is the supreme seat of higher expanded awareness situated at the crown of the head. It is correlated to the pituitary gland in the brain. The power of the *chakras* resides in *Sahasrāra*.

Transcendence and Self-realisation begin at the sixth centre, *ājñā chakra*, in *savikalpa samādhi*. But final enlightenment and final liberation are attained in *nirvikalpa samādhi* or transcendental Cosmic Consciousness, which occurs in *sahasrāra*, the seventh centre at the crown. So we meditate at the *ājñā chakra* until realisation or enlightenment is attained. Then when the gateway opens, and the currents of energy flow together up to *sahasrāra*, the thousand-rayed cerebral light, human consciousness is united and expanded with Cosmic Consciousness.

4.7

THE DESCENT AND THE ASCENT OF THE SOUL THROUGH THE CHAKRAS

THE DESCENT

Higher Consciousness is not something we have to find, or develop, acquire, possess, or build up, because it is always present here and now. It is not out there or up there somewhere. The kingdom of God is within you. It is here, and is available at all times, but because we are not giving any attention and awareness to it, the Truth/Reality remains hidden from us. The belief that one is the ego obscures the realisation of the reality of the Self. The constant identification with the body-mind-ego complex keeps us in bondage. The ego deals in form and definition, so it is unable to comprehend the Self, which is beyond all form.

The sun is always shining brightly until the clouds cover it, or so it seems. Moving away, the clouds do not cause the sun to shine but merely reveal that which was temporarily obscured. Similarly, the higher conscious Reality or Infinite Presence is always present. Everybody in this world has descended from the subtle causal state to the gross physical state. The majority of the nine billion souls here on Earth have no conscious awareness or true knowledge of the divine nature of the being (the eternal Self that does not exist in time and space) that dwells within their own material personality form of mind-body.

We feel finite, separate from the Divine Reality we call God, separate from one another, and mistakenly identified with this transitory and impermanent physical form.

The individual soul

God is the Supreme Being undivided and unrelated to creation, and yet the same God is also made up of an infinite number of individual shining souls. Just as there is a boundless ocean of water behind each and every wave, similarly the Supreme Consciousness is behind each and every individual consciousness. The one Supreme Consciousness has extended Itself from Its eternal pure-mind state to appear as innumerable individual souls living in a temporal universe of forms.

God is in the heart and soul of every being. And yet God remains undivided; the Supreme Being never loses Itself by becoming many. Just as water can be taken from the ocean and divided into numerous cups, without losing its quality of water, similarly, the ocean of God's presence behind the wave of your consciousness always retains its original nature.

From the *sahasrāra chakra* at the crown of the head, Divinity descends to the *ājñā chakra*, located in the centre of the brain, behind the junction of the eyebrows. Here the soul makes its entry into the physical body through the negative pole, the medulla oblongata, of the *ājñā chakra*. It is here that the individual soul has come into existence, distinct from God. The soul has not forgotten God, but there is a separation, a duality.

As the soul descends from *ājñā chakra* in the astral spine, to the fifth centre, *viśuddha chakra*, at the level of the throat, the soul is no longer in conscious union with God. The soul still feels God's presence; there is still an intensity of feeling for God but it is not very clear.

The soul continues its journey downward in the spine to the level of the heart, *anāhata chakra*. At this level of the descent, the soul has awareness of God but the intensity of feeling for God has lessened.

The soul comes to rest

God is still within the heart and soul of the individual being as it descends through the *chakras*, but as it descends further below the three highest *chakras*, the soul's awareness becomes more and more obscured. Below the level of the heart the soul enters the next centre at the navel, *maṇipūra chakra*. Here identification with the body-mind-ego is beginning to take effect, and the awareness of God is fading.

The soul then passes deeper downward in the spine through the *svādhiṣṭhāna chakra*, becoming more entangled in bondage to matter. Finally, the soul reaches the lowest centre at the base of the spine, *mūladhāra chakra*. In this last stage of the downward journey through the *chakras* the soul comes to rest. Now the soul has become more aware and identified with gross matter, with the material form of the body-mind and a separate ego-personality, making it bound, conditioned and dependent in a world of objects, names and forms; in a world of duality. Clothed in the physical form, the individual soul has forgotten its real identity and true divine nature and so has also forgotten God. The primal life-force known as *kuṇḍalinī śakti* that brought the soul down in its descent through the *chakras* now lies latent at the base of the spine.

THE ASCENT

Now if we made our home or remained at the level of these lower centres of consciousness, the soul would essentially be conscious only of eating, sleeping and procreation. A human being functioning only from these lower planes of consciousness is behaving essentially like an animal.

The soul's real nature is divine, and the aim of human existence is to realise this divine nature: that you are *Sat-chit-ānanda* (Ever-Existing, Ever-Conscious, Ever-New Bliss). It is bliss or joy that we seek, because joy is our true nature. Everybody will eventually awaken to some degree to that divine Consciousness present in their lives. As souls we may turn to God, or as the Self we may turn within to our own identity; in both we experience the one Light, the one Pure Consciousness.

Know the Truth

Eventually there comes a time when the soul becomes aware of its higher nature and spiritual ideas begin to enter the mind. The human soul begins to think, 'There must be more to life than just eating, sleeping, procreating and enjoying the senses', 'Who am I?', 'Where did I come from?', 'What happens after death?', 'What is my true purpose and what is the meaning of life?', 'Who or what is God?', 'What is the Ultimate Reality?' There is a deep desire to know and be the knowing.

As we become increasingly disillusioned with the nature of the world, we begin to understand the inherent limitations of this life. We live in a world of dualities – life and death, growth and decay, knowledge and ignorance, happiness and sorrow, health and disease, success and failure – these opposites coexist. The world cannot be made perfect, but it can be used as an instrument, as a means to perfection. Jesus Christ said: 'Know the truth and the truth will set you free.' Know the truth of your essential nature, the Divine Self, the fountain of Infinite Joy within you, then you will find true freedom.

Now there is a glimmer of light, there is some hope. The individual soul aspires to something higher than what it has experienced in the states of the lower *chakras*. The soul tries to remove the veil of ignorance by meditating in God. When the mind turns towards God, the Divinity within, the spiritual ascent begins. *Kuṇḍalinī* begins to wake up. Now the soul becomes more and more disidentified with the mental-physical form and rises above the three lower *chakras* to the subtle state. Through deep God-conscious meditation the soul ascends through the same path it descended in the astral spine, reversing the primal life-force and consciousness from matter, and retracing its steps back attains unity in Supreme Consciousness.

The world of inner Light

In its upward journey, when the soul reaches the heart level of the *anāhata chakra*, it has left the world of darkness and has entered into the world of inner Light, giving the individual soul a wonderful sense of relief and freedom as it moves towards the innermost Consciousness. But at this level of the heart something of our attachment to the world is still left. There is still the danger of falling to a lower stage.

When the soul in its journey upwards advances to the level of the *viśuddha chakra* it is secure. Here the mind is no longer limited or bound by time and space. The mind is transformed from the lower to a higher consciousness, into a finer state, transcending the seeker's negative and material vibrations. In *viśuddha* all the elements are purified and transmuted into their refined essence of *ākāśha* (ether/space). It is then that the individual soul is established in pure consciousness.

The next stage of the soul's ascent is from *viśuddha* to *ājñā chakra*, the sixth centre of consciousness at the midpoint between the eyebrows. At *ājñā chakra*, you have the first union with God in *samādhi*, in which the finite self as the meditator, the process of meditation and the object of meditation – the Supreme Self (God) –

become one. Consciousness of the body, and the sense of 'I' or ego consciousness, disappears, and knowledge of the external world is lost. In this *samādhi* state, which is called *savikalpa samādhi*, the meditator's individual consciousness merges with the Cosmic Consciousness, and experiences ever-new Bliss. Like a wave dissolving into the ocean, the individual soul is merged in an effulgent ocean of bliss.

The pinnacle of consciousness

The last stage of the soul's upward journey through the astral pathway in the spine is to the thousand-ray lotus at the *sahasrāra chakra*, the pinnacle of consciousness. Reaching this plane of inner consciousness, there is a divine awakening of the highest experience in *nirvikalpa samādhi*, which is total identification with the Absolute. The individual soul consciousness and the Supreme Consciousness become One. The finite self becomes absorbed in the Supreme Self and the identity of the two as Pure Consciousness is realised. God is experienced as the Ultimate One Reality, as undivided Pure Consciousness. The soul is resurrected from ignorance and delusion and regains its Divinity and unity. The individual soul becomes identified with the limitless Supreme Self – the two vanish, and one integral, undivided consciousness beyond subject-object relationships alone shines.

Part 5

MANTRAS

5.1

THE SPIRITUAL DISCIPLINE OF MANTRA JAPA

> 'Word, sound and *mantra* are integral parts of Indian cosmology, and cannot be separated from it. Taking cosmological principles out of the realm of theory, *japa*, or *mantra* repetition, puts them to work in a pragmatic way. It is the path from microcosm to macrocosm; it is the vehicle that carries the individual back to the Source.'
>
> *Vishnudevananda 1995, p.51*

One of the most powerful ways of focusing the mind is using a *mantra*. The Sanskrit word *mantra* means 'that which protects or liberates (*trana*) the mind (*manas*)'. It is a spiritual formula or sacred sound (letter, syllable, word or phrase) which is inherently connected with the reality it represents. Each *mantra* is unique, powerful and divine; they represent different aspects of the Infinite Creative Intelligence.

A *mantra* is a sacred sound with a radiant energy that can transform the mind. It can have a single syllable such as *Oṁ*, or a word such as *Sri Rāṁ*, or a phrase such as *Oṁ Namo Bhagavate Vasudevaya*, or a Vedic mantric prayer like the *Gāyatrī Mantra* ('May my mind be guided by Divine Light'), or the *mahā Mrityunjaya mantra* ('May the Lord lead me to freedom from fears and attachments').

> 'If one listens with undivided attention to the sounds of stringed instruments (sitar, vina, tanbura), one will, in the end, be absorbed into the ether of Consciousness and thus attain the nature of *Śiva*.'
>
> *Vijnanabhairava Dharana 18:41*

Just as a white cloth takes on the colour of the dye in which it is soaked, so does the mind absorb the qualities of the sacred sound vibration of the *mantra* that is recited. Whether recited silently inside your head, softly whispered or chanted aloud, *mantras* help to interiorise the mind and have the ability to transform the consciousness of the reciter.

The radiant energy of a *mantra* is awakened from its latent power through the power of the aspirant's spiritual practices (*sādhana*). When it is constantly repeated, the *mantra* awakens the consciousness which is latent in it. Just as a mirror acquires the power of reflection when the dirt covering it is removed, so also the mind from which the impurities have been removed acquires the capacity to reflect the pure conscious Self within.

In the Yoga tradition the spiritual and devotional discipline of repeatedly reciting a *mantra* or Name of God is called *japa* (repetition). It also reaches far back in the Christian tradition in which the desert monks and early contemplatives would give attention to a prayer word such as 'Jesus', or the ancient Aramaic formula *Maranatha* ('Our Lord, come!' or 'Come, our Lord!'; 1 Corinthians 16:22), or a phrase such as the Jesus Prayer: 'Lord Jesus Christ have mercy on me', as a contemplative discipline to focus the mind, instead of allowing its attention to be stolen by constant wandering inner chatter. In both traditions – Yoga and Christian – the aim of this practice is to open the depths within by drawing to interior stillness the restlessness and wandering of the mind, so that it becomes inwardly focused in the present here and now moment, consciously aware of its true being, the Self. St John Climacus, a seventh-century Christian monk on Mount Sinai, said, 'Let the remembrance of Jesus be with your every breath. Then indeed you will appreciate the value of stillness' (*The Ladder of Divine Ascent*, Paulist Press 1982).

When you practise *japa* correctly, with attentive awareness, it will gradually calm and integrate your mind, so that your awareness vibrates with the *mantra*. This naturally leads you into a deeper state of stillness in meditation, where you go beyond the mind to rest in your true Divine nature.

When the *mantras* are chanted aloud, the rhythmical vibrations produced by continually repeating them regulate the unsteady vibrations of the five sheaths (*koshas*). The chanting of *mantras* generates potent spiritual vibrations that penetrate the physical and astral bodies, filling the atoms and cells of the body with pure divine energy.

Japa breaks the habitual current of thought forces that are moving towards external objects. Driving away all worldly thoughts, *japa* forces the mind to interiorise and move towards the Supreme Reality within. When *japa* is practised with faith and devotion over a long period of time, it purifies and removes the impurities such as anger, greed, lust and other negative qualities from the mind, replacing them with pure thoughts and divine qualities such as love, compassion, kindness, forgiveness, cheerfulness and a sense of service to others, which strengthen the good latent impressions (*saṁskāras*) in the mind. Just as the quality of burning is natural in fire, so also the power of the *mantra* of destroying impurities in the mind, and bringing the aspirant into blissful unity with the Supreme Lord, is naturally inherent in the Name of God.

The ego imperatively requires of us some task which will satisfy its need for activity. The mind is constantly active, so to calm it, give it something to do, discipline it with *japa*: to keep the attention from chasing thoughts, let it quietly repeat a *mantra*. Let go of all other concerns, recollect yourself and gently return your attention to repeating your *mantra*. Even a little *japa* (recitation) with faith, sincere feeling, purity and one-pointed concentration on the meaning of the *mantra* removes mental impurities that veil the inner light of the Self. When there are impurities in the mind it is like a mirror covered in dust, that is ingrained with habits and attitudes that are firmly established and difficult to change. When cleaned with *mantra japa*, the mind acquires the power of reflection, the capacity to reflect higher spiritual truth, revealing the inner Light of the Self of Pure Consciousness.

SIX MAIN CATEGORIES OF *JAPA*

1. Vaikhari japa

The *mantra* is spoken or chanted aloud. This form of *japa* is particularly good for those people who are negatively emotional, dull, moody or of a restless nature. When *vaikhari japa* is practised alone or in a group of chanters the atmosphere becomes powerfully charged with energy and positive vibrations of peace and joy.

When chanting aloud, chant with love and devotion from your heart. Concentrate at the Spiritual Eye (at the midpoint between your eyebrows), drawing God's energy to you. Open your heart and listen attentively to the sound of the *mantra* that you are chanting. Sound is easy for the mind to concentrate upon. When the mind is absorbed in the mantric vibration of sound, we rise higher into a state of superconsciousness. It is then that the chanter, the chant and the process of chanting become one.

2. Upansu japa

The *mantra* is whispered. Only the one who is chanting the *mantra* can hear it. This form of *japa* is useful for those people who are practising many hours of *japa* throughout the day. It is also good for those who are practising *japa* with a special *mantra* for a specific purpose. Practise this for three months before you begin *manasika japa*.

3. Manasika japa

The *mantra* is repeated mentally. There is no movement of the lips. This is the most subtle *japa* and can be difficult for beginners in the practice of *mantra* Yoga. The mind can easily be sidetracked and wander away from the practice to other thoughts. During the practice, if you are not vigilant and attentive, sleep may overpower you. This higher practice is for those who are able to concentrate with a steady mind.

When practising mental *japa*, or any other form, the *mantra* should not be repeated mechanically or in a hurry. When mental *japa* is repeated with deep concentration, attention and awareness, it prepares the mind for meditation in stillness.

4. Likhita japa

The *mantra* is written, while being simultaneously repeated mentally. It is written down on paper hundreds or thousands of times in lines, shapes or forms (such as the shape of a lotus flower or a mandala). It is best to keep a notebook specifically for this purpose; it can be kept near your bed or the shrine where you meditate.

When you write the *mantra* use red ink, as this will help to reinforce the *mantra* in your mind. Blue and green ink can also be used. Write the letters of the *mantras* as small as possible, carefully creating a beautiful design. Practise with concentration and devotion. It is good to concentrate on the meaning of the *mantra* so that it predominates over other thoughts.

5. Akhanda japa

When a *mantra* is repeated a specific number of times without a break, or for a fixed period of time, such as from sunrise to sunset, it is known as *akhanda japa*. This may be practised as a group, each devotee taking it in turns to chant for a few hours. For example, if the group was chanting a particular *mantra* for the purpose of bringing peace and harmony to another country where there is conflict and suffering, the group could form a rota and allocate each person in the group to chant at a certain time for a certain duration. In this way many hours could be covered without the devotees becoming too tired.

6. Purascharana

In this powerful method of *japa*, one takes a spiritual vow to undertake to repeat a particular *mantra* a certain amount of times every day. For example one might take a vow to repeat the *mantra* continuously from sunrise to sunset for a specific number of days. Or one may decide to do undertake a 40-day *purascharana* of repeating a *mantra* a number of times a day. If you repeated 100,000 repetitions for each syllable of the six-syllable *mantra Oṁ Namah Śivaya* (*Oṁ-Na-Ma-Shi-Va-Ya*, the sounds that invoke conscious control over the elements which rule the *chakras*), it would actually require you to repeat 600,000 repetitions to complete a *purascharana*. One round of this *mantra* on 108 beads of the *mālā* amounts to repeating 648 syllables.

AJAPĀ JAPA

Ajapā japa is the spontaneous and automatic repetition of the *mantra* or Name of God without conscious effort.

It is best if chanting begins aloud, then gradually softens, until it fades into silent, internal chanting. The *mantra* then flows without exertion. When this happens the practice is called *ajapā japa*, or effortless repetition. The inner space of the mind becomes filled with the sound of the *mantra*, there is no mental exertion, it is more a 'listening to the *mantra*'.

Ajapā japa practice

In the practice of *ajapā japa* the awareness of the natural flow of the breath is integrated with the *mantra so'ham* (pronounced 'So-hum'). *So'ham* means 'I am He' ('He' meaning Spirit, Divine Consciousness).

You can also use the *mantra Hong Sau* (pronounced 'hong saw'), which has the same meaning as *so'ham*.

The following practice of *ajapā japa* develops awareness and concentration, and is the basis for *Kriyā Yoga*. One achieves *pratyāhāra* (sense-withdrawal) by mastering the practice of this technique:

1. Sit comfortably upright on a chair, or cross-legged on the floor with a cushion, and adjust your spine so that your pelvis, chest and head are vertically aligned.
2. Inhale deeply, and while holding your breath, simultaneously tense all the parts of your body. Then exhaling with a double breath, 'ha-haaa', release all tension and completely relax your body. Repeat tensing and relaxing your body two more times.
3. Now feel your whole body sitting comfortably and relaxed. Close your eyes and rest your attention at your Spiritual Eye (at the midpoint between the eyebrows), and become aware of your the natural flow of your breath, feeling its subtle and slow flow through the inner space of your whole body. As you breathe subtly, sense the vibration of a slow wave of breath moving in your spine. This vibration is the *mantra so'ham.*
4. Now bring your awareness to the deep inner space within your spine and as you inhale feel the rising breath from the base of the spine (*mūladhāra chakra*) to the base of your brain (medulla oblongata). As you naturally inhale, hear the mantric sound *So*. Then, exhaling down the spine from the medulla to the *mūladhāra chakra*, hear the sound *ham*.
5. Continue the technique with total concentration and awareness, listening inwardly to the sound of the *mantra* and follow the movement of *prāṇic* energy up and down the inner passage within your spine. Allow your breath to flow naturally and smoothly in an unbroken flow of inner sound – *so'ham so'ham so'ham* – so that one repetition of the *mantra* weaves smoothly into the next, and your awareness is settled in the *mantra*. As you practise, become more focused and one-pointed, gradually drawing deeper within, so that your mind rests within itself, without the support of the breath. Rest in the awareness of this calm, peace and stillness for as long as it persists. Mentally affirm: '*The quiet stillness of the Infinite permeates my being. I melt into the ocean of bliss.*'
6. To finish your practice, gently return your awareness to your natural breath, and feel the presence of your physical body by massaging your face and stretching your legs. Become aware of the environment around you, then sit quietly for a few minutes before getting up.

MĀLĀ BEADS FOR RECITING *MANTRAS*

To help you concentrate on your *mantra* and to keep count of the repetitions, it is useful to use a *mālā* (garland/necklace/rosary), a string of 108 beads. You can also use a *mālā* with only 27 or 54 beads; these are divisions of 108, which always add up to 9. In numerology, the number 9 symbolises the perfection of human life. One round of the *mālā* equals 108 repetitions of the *mantra*. Depending on your practice of *mantra japa*, your daily session might include more than one round of a *mālā*.

The number 108 is a spiritual number: 1 + 0 + 8 = 9. The number 9 cannot be destroyed, no matter how many times you multiply it or add it to its own multiple, it is the sacred number of eternity. The 1 of 108 symbolises God the Creator. The 0 added to the 1 gives it power and represents God's creation as complete. The number 8 is the symbol of eternity.

According to the *Varaha Upaniṣad* (5:119), the height of every individual is 96 finger-widths placed horizontally, as measured by his own fingers. And according to the *mahānarayana Upaniṣad* 13:7, 'The heart, which is located just at a distance of a finger span below the Adam's apple (in the throat) and 12 fingers above the navel, is the great abode of the universe (because *Paramātman*, the Soul of all, resides there).' Therefore 96 + 12 = 108, meaning that 108 signifies the union of the *jīvātman* (individual soul) with *Paramātman* (the Supreme Soul).

Each *mālā* of 108 beads has an extra bead offset from the main circle of beads. This bead is called a *sumeru* or *meru* ('mountain'), which acts as a reference point, so that the practitioner knows when he or she has completed a rotation of 108 beads. It is also said that the *meru* bead stores the power of all your recitations. *Mālās* can also come in lengths of 54 beads, as does the Catholic rosary.

The Sanskrit alphabet has 54 letters, each with a Male (*Śiva*) and Female (*Shakti*) counterpart. Therefore in total there are 108 letters in the Sanskrit alphabet. There are also said to be 108 names given to the Indian Goddesses.

Rudraksha

Traditionally, *mālā* beads are usually made from *rudraksha* seeds, *bhadrakshya* seeds, lotus seeds, beads made from the *tulasi* (tulsi) plant, the *bel* tree, or from the sandalwood tree, or from crystal beads. Each material has its own particular vibrations. Sandalwood helps to calm the mind and connects the base *chakra* with the crown *chakra*. Worshippers of Lord Śiva and the goddess Kali use sandalwood beads. For worshippers of Lord Ganesha, the *mālā* of beads prepared from the tusk of an elephant are said to be auspicious.

Rudraksha (*Rudra*, another name for *Śiva*; *aksha*, eye – literally, 'The Eye of Śiva') is considered sacred with metaphysical and healing properties by the devotees of Lord Śiva. The Eye of Śiva symbolises the *ājñā chakra*, the Spiritual Eye of intuition and direct perception.

The dried fruit of the *rudraksha* tree (*Elaeocarpus ganitus*) is grown in the foothills of the Himalayas, India, Nepal, Burma, Java and south-east Asia. This is the only fruit in which the stone and pulp cannot be separated. When the fruit is ripe, the outer pulp becomes dry, wrinkled and very hard. At this stage the seeds can be used for *malas*.

According to the *Rudraksha Jabala Upaniṣad* the root of the *rudraksha* tree is *Brāhma*, the fibre of it is *Vishnu*, and the top *Rudra*, and the fruits are all *Devas*.

Rudraksha is of many varieties. The best is that which has five or six dividing lines on the seed, or five or six faces. Each type has a corresponding deity or quality, and each *rudraksha* bead has a natural hole at the top and ridges on the sides. These ridges are known as *mukhi* (face), ranging from one (which is very rare) to 14 faces, or even more. The Hindu legend behind *Rudraksha* is that Lord Śiva opened His eyes after being absorbed in a long and deep meditation, then feeling fulfilled, He shed a single tear which grew into the *rudraksha* tree (*Rudra* means 'one who weeps', so *Rudraksha* is one who has the ability to wipe our tears and give happiness). *Rudraksha* is used in the treatment of various diseases and has a beneficial influence on the blood circulation, strengthens the heart and is recommended for those who have high blood pressure. It calms tension and gives clarity to the voice.

Tulsi

Tulsi or *Tulasi* (Indian basil) is a plant related to the herb basil (*Ocimum sanctum*). In India *tulsi* is highly venerated as a sacred plant and is worshipped by followers of Vishnu and Krishna. The branches of this plant are used for making *mālās* and the leaves have medicinal value – they are used in Āyurvedic medicine as a demulcent, diaphoretic and expectorant in bronchitis, cough, cold and fever. The leaves can be used for indigestion and poor appetite. *Tulsi* prevents and heals mosquito and other insect bites and purifies the air.

Sandalwood

There are two types of sandalwood: red (*Santalum rubrum*) and white (*Santalum album*). True sandalwood only comes from these two Indian species. *Mālā* beads made with red sandalwood help to sublimate the passions and destructive tendencies such as anger and jealousy within us. A red sandalwood *mālā* is often useful for those who are very active. They are also used for worship of the great feminine goddess energy within, when chanting *Shakti mantras*.

White sandalwood helps to induce harmonious qualities that are conducive to meditation, such as peace and calmness. It has a long-lasting, deep, sweet woody fragrance, which helps heighten the energy in the *prāṇāyāma kosha* (vital sheath, etheric body), giving one vitality and helping to bring about the inner state of meditation. Mysore sandalwood has the finest oil, which is used in perfumery and incense.

Semi-precious stones and crystals

There are many different varieties of semi-precious stones and crystals, too many to list here. Each has different qualities and can induce specific effects on the mind, body and aura.

Crystal Quartz *mālās* are used for their psychic properties. Crystal Quartz radiates all the colours of the light spectrum and so can be programmed for any use which brings light and energy into our spiritual body. It is associated with the crown *chakra* (*sahasrāra*). They are good for focusing the mind and aiding concentration for meditation. Crystal Quartz also has the powers of protection and healing.

Lapis Lazuli enhances one's awareness, insight, intuition and intellect, and is said to impart knowledge, wisdom and peace to its bearer. It assists in awakening the *ājñā chakra*, at the eyebrow centre.

In making a *mālā*, crystal beads can be strung together with *rudraksha* to add more power. Likewise, sandalwood and crystal beads make a good combination for a *mālā*.

In India, the guru traditionally blesses and purifies the *mālā* by chanting the holy *mantra* called *Sadyojāta mantra*. This *mantra* gives a new birth into spiritual life, and is therefore prayed in order to bring spiritual liberation to the reciter of the *mantra*. Then the *mālā* is worshipped by invoking creative energy into it. In the *Vārāhi Tantra*, the prayer to invoke *Devī* (Divine Goddess) is:

'O Divine Mālā, you are of the form of all wisdom.
You confer on me all joy and peace here and hereafter
and bless me to attain perfection.'

Another prayer to the *mālā* from the *Yogini Hṛdaya* is:

'O Divine Mālā, you are bringing me the blessings of
all the gods. By your Power I shall attain the Truth.
O Divine Mother, to Thee I bow.'

What to do if your mālā breaks

If the string holding the beads of your *mālā* happens to break, it is considered inauspicious. Then you need to chant the seed-syllable *mantra Hrīṃ* ('Hreem') to purify your *mālā* and chant 108 times the holy Name of God.

How to repeat your mantra using a mālā

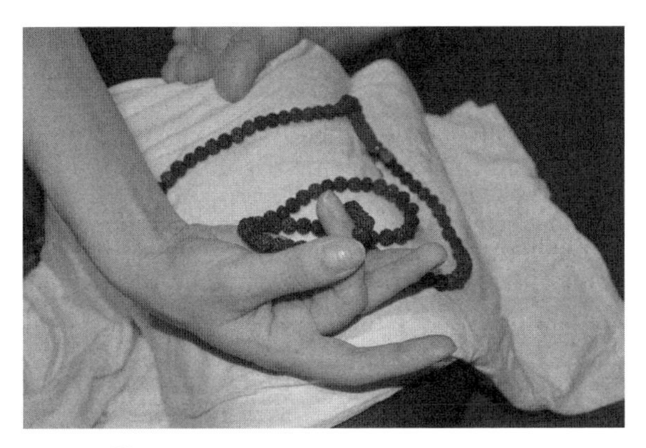

HOLDING *MĀLĀ* BEADS FOR *MANTRA JAPA*

To use a *mālā*, hold the beads in your right hand, with the beads draped over your middle finger, ring finger and little finger. Keeping your index finger free and extended, use your thumb (representing God or the divine) to rotate the beads. Do not use your index finger (representing the ego) to rotate the beads as it is considered inauspicious in *mantra* chanting. Start by repeating the *mantra* on the first bead below the *meru* bead, then rotate the next bead and so on, until you have repeated the *mantra* on all 108 beads. When you come back to the *meru* bead turn the beads and start rotating them in the other direction. You should never chant on the *meru* bead itself or cross over it. Always rotate the *mālā* towards your palm.

After your practice you can either wear your *mālā* around your neck or place it on your shrine or altar if you have one. Respect it with sacredness, and do not let other people touch it.

Using a *mālā* helps the mind to concentrate and physically releases nervous and restless energy by the movement of the hand rotating the beads.

Another way of keeping count of your rounds of *japa* is to just use your own fingers. If you look at your hand (palm upwards) you will notice that each finger has three phalanges allowing the fingers to bend. If you multiply the four fingers by three phalanges it makes a total of 12 for each hand. So, starting with your little finger and finishing with your index finger, touch with the tip of your thumb the crease of each phalange, and pronounce in your mind *Oṁ*. Do this nine times on your hand to complete *japa* of 108 *Oṁ*s.

When you repeat your chosen *mantra*, do so with the right mental attitude and *sattvic* feeling. Repeat it with devotion and faith and over time the *mantra* will free you from difficulties and obstacles, and bring you to peace and inner joy. It should be emphasised that cultivating a spiritual practice, such as using a *mantra* in *japa*, is not to reduce meditation to a technique. Techniques imply a certain control and focus on a determined outcome. Meditation is a skill, a discipline that facilitates a process that is out of one's control, but it does not have the capacity to determine the outcome. For example, a gardener uses certain techniques to cultivate the garden soil by watering, feeding, composting, weeding and pruning. But there is nothing the gardener can do to make the plants grow. The gardener's skills are necessary but by themselves insufficient. There has to be a harmonious synergy between human or self-effort and Divine grace. This is beautifully described by St Teresa of Avila in her book *The Interior Castle*, in which she describes the image of the silk worm. As the silk worm spins its own silken cocoon, from which it will one day emerge transformed into a butterfly, so the soul, who gives itself diligently to spiritual practice, is responsive enough to the promptings of grace to cooperate in its own process of transformation. Meditation practice is like the cocoon that is gradually and delicately spun and from which we will emerge transformed.

If you use a short *mantra* such as *Aum*, *Aum Guru* or *Sri Rāṁ,* your power of concentration will be much greater than if you use a longer *mantra* of many syllables.

Repeating the Divine Name such as *Aum Guru*, *Aum Jesus* or *Sri Rāṁ* with sincere love and devotion from deep within your heart is like a waterfall of pure water pouring into a glass of muddy water. After a while the mud disappears, leaving only crystal clear water in the glass. The sincere repetition of *Aum* produces sound waves that correspond to those of the Supreme Reality.

SOME USEFUL *MANTRAS* FOR *JAPA*

The following *mantras* can be used for *japa* (recitation) before meditation or at any time during the day, evening or night. By repeating such *mantras* the vibrations of the five sheaths (*koshas*) are steadied and brought into balance, and the unsteady and restless movement of thoughts of the mind are checked. The mind is usually constantly fluctuating between thoughts of the future and the past, but by practising *japa* the mind can be focused in the present now-moment, even while travelling, walking or working.

To be effective these *mantras* must be recited properly, with your mind focused, and by giving your attention to the Sanskrit syllables and rhythm.

To gain the full benefits of reciting a *mantra*, choose just one *mantra* and recite it regularly every day for at least 21 days, or for the more auspicious 40 days. The three auspicious times for reciting a *mantra* are at dawn, noon and dusk, but if this is not possible it can be done as often as you can. Use your *mālā* beads to practise a certain amount of rounds of *japa*. For example you may choose to practise three rounds of chanting your *mantra* on your *mālā* (3 x 108 = 324 repetitions of the *mantra*) once each day for 40 days. This would result in you having chanted 12,960 *mantras*. If you do *japa* of three *mālās* twice a day you would have chanted 25,920 *mantras* in 40 days.

A good *mantra* to start with is the *Ganesha Ganapathi* ('the Lord of Cosmic Consciousness') *mantra*:

> *Oṁ Gum Ganapatayei Namah*
> Salutations to the remover of obstacles.

Ganapati is another name for *Ganesha*, who is symbolised as the elephant-headed god, representing courage and strength. This very auspicious *mantra* helps one through the challenges of life and helps to remove obstacles to your true inner unity.

First set your intention for its use before doing *japa* with it. In other words affirm to yourself the obstacle you wish to overcome that will benefit your highest good.

You can also recite this *mantra* before reciting other *mantras* to clear the way of any obstacles that may be blocking your spiritual objectives. It can also be used to bless a new endeavour or project.

> *Śriṁ Hrīṁ Klīṁ*
> *Glauṁ Gum Ganapatayei*
> *Sarva Janam Me*
> *Vasha-manaya Svāhā*
> May Ganesha the great remover of energy blocks
> and obstacles that transcends this apparent
> reality bring all things that concern me under
> my control.

This longer *Ganesha Ganapathi mantra* can be used for removal of obstacles that may be blocking your way to fulfilling your spiritual objectives. It has the added power of the seed-syllable (*bīja*) shakti mantric sounds: *śriṁ* ('shreem'), *hrīṁ* ('hreem'), *klīṁ* ('kleem').

> *Oṁ namaḥ Śivāya*
> Salutations to that Pure Consciousness who abides within me.

This *mantra* is known as the *pañcākṣara mantra* and is composed of five syllables: *Na*, *Ma*, *Shi*, *Va*, *Ya*, representing the five elements that govern each *chakra*: earth, water, fire, air, and ether.

Oṁ śriṁ klīṁ namaḥ Śivāya
Salutations to Śiva, that Pure Consciousness who abides within me and in all creation.

The added seed *mantras śriṁ* and *klīṁ* help in accelerating one's spiritual progression towards Self-realisation. *Śriṁ* has the power of abundance and brings many blessings. *Klīṁ* has the power of attraction, and helps us to achieve our true wishes in life.

Oṁ śriṁ klīṁ param Īśvari svāhā
Salutations to the Divine Feminine, Shakti the power of Śiva.

This *mantra* helps in activating energy in the spine and *chakras* giving mastery over the elements of each *chakra.*

Oṁ namo Bhagavate Vāsudevāya
Salutations to the Divine indweller in me who is omnipresent and in unity with all creation.

Bhagavan means Lord (Lord Viṣṇu). *Vasudeva* means 'He who abides in all things and in whom all things abide'. This 12-syllable *mantra* is for liberating the soul with spiritual realisation. It also gives success in all undertakings. Chanting the 12 syllables of this *mantra* magnetises the energy in the spine, activating a rotation of energy around the spine, stimulating the positive and negative poles of each *chakra.*

Oṁ namo Nārāyaṇa
Salutations to Lord Viṣṇu.

Nārāyaṇa is a name for *Viṣṇu*, the Preserver or Maintainer of the universe. This is a *mantra* for liberating the soul.

Oṁ klīṁ Kṛṣṇāya namaḥ
Salutations and devotion to Lord Krishna, the bringer of love and joy.

This *mantra* with the added power of the *bīja mantra klīṁ* ('kleem') is said to give extraordinary power and spiritual development. *Klīṁ* relates to Lord K*ṛṣṇā* and so carries the power of attraction. It is also the seed *mantra* of love and devotion; it increases the love energy within the heart, and brings joy.

Oṁ śrīṁ Mahālakṣmīyei namaḥ
Salutations to the great Mother Lakshmi.

The seed *mantra śrīṁ* is the sound for the principle of abundance, of which the goddess Lakshmi is the personification. Lakshmi is the Goddess of abundance and prosperity, of both a material and spiritual nature.

Oṁ aiṁ hrīṁ sarasvatyei svāhā
Salutations to the goddess Saraswati who is the auspicious Shakti of the Lord.

Hrīṁ represents the *Śakti* (Energy) of the Lord that gives prosperity, health, clarity, growing knowledge and wisdom. *Hrīṁ* also gives the power to destroy. *Aiṁ* represents only the auspicious *Śakti* of the Lord – blessings of knowledge. *Sarasvatī* is the goddess of the power of Divine speech, knowledge and music. She empowers anything involving the mind through the *ājñā chakra* – the brow centre.

Oṁ Ram Rāmaya namaḥ
Salutations to Lord Rama.

The seed *mantra Ram* is the seed sound of the *maṇipūra chakra* at the navel centre. The two syllables *Ra* and *Ma* of *Rāma* are associated respectively with the *piṅgala* (solar channel) and *iḍā* (lunar channel) *nāḍīs* (subtle *prāṇic* channels) running along either side of the central channel (*suṣumnā nāḍī*) in the astral body. This is a powerful healing *mantra*, giving strength and helping by clearing the currents of energy in the two subtle channels *iḍā* and *piṅgala*.

Oṁ Śrī Dhanvantre namaḥ
Salutations to Dhanvantre the Celestial Healer.

To use this *mantra* set your intention for the condition you want healed and, without any expectation of how the healing will occur, chant this *mantra* 12,500 times. Dhanvantre is the Hindu god of Āyurvedic medicine and healing.

5.2

THE SIGNIFICANCE OF AUM (OṀ)

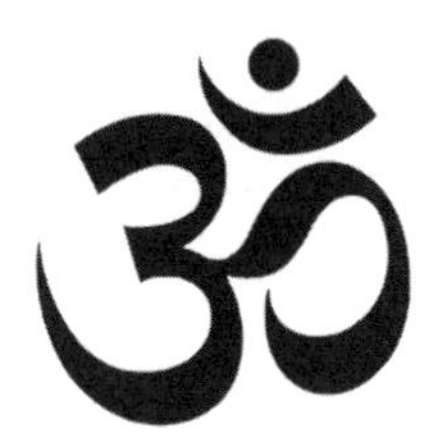

> 'Through the divine eye in the forehead (east), the yogi sails his consciousness into omnipresence, hearing the Word or *Aum*, divine sound of many waters or vibrations which is the sole reality of creation.'
>
> *Yogananda 1946, p.263*

The source of all sound vibrations is the sacred Primordial Creative Vibration and Divine Power – *Aum*.

In the *Yoga Sūtras* of Patañjali (1:27), it is stated: 'The expression of That (*Īśvara*, Supreme Lord) is *Aum* (*Praṇava*).'

The sacred sound syllable *mantra Aum* (*Oṁ*), the vibration of consciousness that is always in the present, eternal and infinite, signifies the Supreme Being. In the ancient scriptures *Ṛgvedasaṁhitā* and the *Yajurveda's Tattirīyasaṁhitā*, *Aum* (*Oṁ*) was referred to as *Praṇava* (reverberating; sounding), and refers to the vibration of consciousness itself. *Aum* is the greatest seed (*mahābīja*) among the *bīja mantras*; it is the seed of the entire creation. It is the supreme verbal symbol of *Brāhman* both as the impersonal Absolute and as *Īśvara*, the personal God.

Aum is the Primal Sound, the Cosmic Vibration and energy of creation that exists prior to the manifest activities of the three constituent aspects or *guṇas* that originate from *prakṛiti* (primordial nature): *sattva* (luminous, goodness, purity), *rajas* (activity, desire, passion) and *tamas* (darkness, inertness, ignorance).

Aum also represents the three states of human consciousness: waking, dream and dreamless sleep. *A* stands for the waking state (*jāgrat*); *u* for the dream state (*svapna*); and *m* represents deep sleep (*suṣupti*), that is dreamless. Beyond these three states of ordinary awareness and pervading them all is a fourth state called *turīya*.

The three phonemes *a*, *u* and *m* also correspond to the three levels of existence: gross, subtle and causal. When a yogi is absorbed in deep *samādhi* meditation on *Aum* the gross, subtle and causal sounds merge into the limitless ocean of consciousness until only the meaning and radiance itself remains.

The relationship between *Īśvara* and *Aum* is eternal; the Creator and the energy of creation cannot be separated.

Sound is an evolute of *prakṛiti* (Primordial Nature). On this level *Aum* remains a sound vibration and *Īśvara* remains a special and distinct transcendental Being. But on another level *Aum* is non-different from *Īśvara*; it is permeated by *Īśvara* and so it manifests the qualities of *Īśvara*.

The mind, which is also an evolute of *prakṛiti*, is unable to comprehend that which is more subtle than itself. The mind can only come into direct contact with *Īśvara* through the Cosmic Vibratory sound *Aum*, in which *Īśvara*'s Divine Presence, grace and potency is permeated and empowered.

In the next *Yoga Sūtra* (1:28), Patañjali states: 'Its (of the Cosmic Vibratory Sound *Aum*) repetition and contemplation of its meaning (is to be practised).' We can experience *Īśvara*'s Divine Presence by continually repeating (*japa*) His Name, the *mantra Aum* (*Oṁ*). To invoke awareness of the presence of the Divine and to go deeper in meditation *Aum* should be recited with deep concentration, devotion and reverence, in inner silence, while meditating on its meaning, and listening to the inner Vibratory Sound of *Aum*.

According to the *Śiva Sūtra-Vārttika*, the secret of a *mantra* lies in its psychic existence. The purpose of a *mantra* is to destroy the bondage of life and death. *Bīja-mantra* has this capacity to the maximum, and the most powerful of all is the *mantra* of all the *mantras* – *Oṁ*.

The seed (*bīja)* syllable has a mystical or magical aura around it. According to the Tantric tradition, every seed syllable must have a nasal sound which results in a divine union. Since *Śiva* and *Śakti* are considered to be two lips, their union leads to the birth of seed (*bīja*).

The nasal sound *anusvāra* is supposed to have the germ of a complete doctrine. Through *bīja-akshar* (seed syllable) a huge treatise can be compressed in a few lines. A seed syllable, by virtue of being short, is good for the repetition of a *mantra* as it creates cerebral vibrations which keep reverberating. With the help of the nasal sound (*anusvāra*), one can transfer the seed syllable to the back of the head or between the eyebrows. At a later stage the accumulated energy of a *mantra* can be projected anywhere in order to achieve the desired result.

Oṁ has a prolonged and tapering sound like the peal of a distant bell. This sound represents a movement from the gross to the subtle, from the finite to the infinite, the all-pervading Self beyond all limitations. It signifies Supreme Consciousness that is omnipotent, omnipresent and omniscient. That Supreme Self is the all-pervading Reality, the innermost essence of everything. Our power, our joy and our knowledge is limited because we do not turn to the one Source of all power, all joy and all knowledge. How can you contact that Source? By turning your thoughts towards God, by meditating on the Source with all faith and devotion.

'Oṁ (Praṇavaḥ) is the bow, the arrow is the self:
and Brāhman is its target. It must be
hit by one who is not careless:
So, like the arrow, one will become one with it.'

Mundāka Upaniṣad 2.4

Just as the bow is the cause of the arrow hitting the target, so *Oṁ* is the bow that brings about the union of the self with the supreme Self.

After hitting the mark, one should remain identified with *Brāhman* or the supreme Self.

'The entire universe is the syllable Oṁ. Everything in the past, present, and future is Oṁ. That which is beyond time, space and causation is also Oṁ.'

Māṇḍūkya Upaniṣad 1.1

The whole universe with its manifested objects and umanifested states of reality are denoted by the syllable *Oṁ*, the infinite, eternal and unmanifest power that is not subject to change. *Oṁ* represents all levels of consciousness and is also the name of the Absolute Reality (*Brāhman*). The word *Brāhman* is from the Sanskrit verb root *bṛha* or *bṛhi*, meaning expansion, knowledge, all-pervasiveness. *Brāhman* is that Absolute Reality, that Supreme Consciousness that is pure existence, pure consciousness and pure bliss. *Brāhman* is the pure being, the essence of our soul and the essence of everything. In the *Upaniṣads*, *Brāhman* is the most commonly used word for God.

'All this, whatsoever is seen here, there, and everywhere, is Brāhman. This very Self, ātman, is Brāhman, the Absolute Reality. This ātman has four aspects.'

Māṇḍūkya Upaniṣad 1.2

The essential nature of the individual Self (*ātman*) is *Brāhman*, the Universal Self (I am That). *Brāhman* is non-different from oneself.

Whether we seek to know God (*Brāhman*), or to know our Self (*ātman*), when you find the one, you will find the other as well, for they are one. *Brāhman* exists as both the subjective and the objective Reality. He may be intuited in the objective world, but He can only be directly known as the subjective Reality, from within. The subjective Reality is the perceiver, the Witness – the consciousness which we experience as our own existence.

The *Māṇḍūkya Upaniṣad* states that *ātman* (Self) is experienced on four levels of consciousness: waking (*vaiśvānara*), dreaming (*taijasa*), deep sleep (*prājñā*), and a fourth liberated state beyond the other three, called *turīya*. That fourth state, which is collectively the experience of all three realities, can be attained through deep meditation and constant contemplation.

In the waking state (*vaiśvānara*) of subject/object consciousness there is identification with the physical and *prāṇic* sheaths (*koshas*). The consciousness is constricted by time, space and causation.

In the dreaming state (*taijasa*) the mind detached from the senses is inwardly aware. It recalls the subtle impressions of previous experiences stored in the unconscious mind. Desires that are not fulfilled in the waking state are fulfilled in the dreaming state. But of course, when the dreamer awakens from the dream he realises that it was exactly that, just a dream.

The deep sleeping state (*prājñā*) is more subtle than the previous two states of consciousness, for there is neither desire nor dream. In *prājñā* the sleeper remains close to the Absolute Reality in a restful and blissful state, but is unaware of it.

The highest joy or bliss (*ānanda*) is realised only when the state of *turīya* is attained.

The *Kātha Upaniṣad* is a dialogue between a spiritual master, Yamaraja, and an ardent seeker of Truth, Nachiketa, son of Vajashrava. In this dialogue Nachiketa enquires about Truth, and the difference between *dharma* and *adharma*. Yamaraja answers his questions by saying that all the *Vedās* proclaim: that which is the goal of all spiritual disciplines, and that which seekers follow the disciplines pertaining to the knowledge of God – *Oṁ* is That.

'This eternal Oṁ is Brāhman. It is absolute. Upon
knowing this Eternal One, the seeker attains whatever he wishes.
This eternal Oṁ is the best and highest resting point.
Upon reaching this highest state of restfulness,
the seeker prospers in the realm of Brāhman.'

Kātha Upaniṣad 1.16–17

In the *Upaniṣad Amrita-Bindu* ('Immortal Point'), c.900–1200 CE, a distinction is made between the practice of intoning or sounding the mantric (*svāra*) syllable *Oṁ*, and the higher spiritual practice of listening to and meditating on the unsounded (*asvāra*) syllable of *Oṁ*: 'One should combine Yoga with the sound (*svāra*), and realise the Supreme as the Soundless (*asvāra*). Through the realisation of the Soundless, there can be no nonbeing (*abhâva*). Being is desirable.'

'That is the formless and stainless Absolute. "Knowing I am the Absolute", the Absolute is surely attained.'

'It is formless, infinite, devoid of cause or precedent, immeasurable and eternal without beginning. Knowing this the sage is liberated.'

Amritabindûpanisad 7–9

'The imperishable (*akshara*) sound (*Oṁ*) is the supreme Absolute. When that has dwindled what remains is the Imperishable. Should the knower desire Self inner peace, he should meditate on that Imperishable (*akshara*).'

Amritabindûpanisad 16

The *Upaniṣad Nâda-Bindu* (sound-point) describes the sacred syllable *mantra Oṁ* as being 'resplendent humming' (*vairâja-praṇava*). It also describes the practice of the inner sound (*nâda*), heard inwardly during meditative absorption. In deep meditation this inner sound is so prominent that it drowns out all external sounds, and manifests the inner sounds of the *chakras* (vortices of energy located in the subtle astral spine), which are vibrating at different frequencies. The *chakra* inner sounds sound like the drone of a bumblebee, a flute, a *vina* (plucked stringed instrument), a deep gong or bell, the sound of wind in the trees, and the sound of a roaring ocean.

In *Kriyā Yoga*, in the tradition of Paramhansa Yogananda, there is a technique called the *Aum* Technique, a meditation technique that does not involve the audible chanting of *Oṁ*, but listening to the subtle inner sounds. Listening to these inner sounds and concentrating on them until they recede into the background gradually helps one to become more sensitive to the more subtle astral sounds and to the sound of all sounds, the Cosmic Vibration of *Aum*.

Paramhansa Yogananda explained that *Aum* is referred to in the Holy Bible as 'the Comforter' and 'the Holy Ghost'.

> 'But the Comforter which is the Holy Ghost, whom the Father will send in my name, He shall teach you all things, and bring all things to your remembrance, whatsoever I have said to you.'
>
> *John 14:26*

According to the *Atharvaśikhopaniṣad*, the first syllable or *mātra* of *Aum* is the earth. The 'A' sound stands for the *Ṛgveda*. It has *Brāhma* as its presiding deity and the eight *Vasus* as its subsidiary deities. Its presiding metre is *Gāyatrī* and has *Gārhapatya* as its fire.

The syllable 'U' stands for the mid-ethereal region, and its area is the *Yajurveda*. *Viṣṇu* is its presiding deity. Eleven *rudras* are its subsidiary deities. Its metre is *triṣtubh* and its fire is known as *dakṣiṇa*.

The third part of the primordial sound *Oṁ* is the syllable 'M', which stands for the *Sāmveda*. *Rudra* is the presiding deity and the 12 *ādityās* are its subsidiary deities. Its metre is *jāgriti*, and has *ahavaniya* as its fire.

The half syllable or *ardhamātrā* of *Praṇava* is the fourth part, which is the lunar region. It stands for *Atharvaveda*. Its presiding deity is *Samvartakāgni* and it is in the *turīya* state. Seven *maruts* are its subsidiary deities. Its metre is known as *virāt*, and *ekarṣi* is its fire. All the systems of *Vedānta* call it *Bhāsvati*.

These parts of *Praṇava* also have different colours and form. 'A', the first *mātra*, is a mixture of red and yellow. It is presided by the great *Brāhman*.

'U', the second *mātra* is a mixture of *Kṛṣṇā* (blackish blue) and the sheen of lightning. Its presiding deity is *Viṣṇu* who is all-pervading.

The third *mātra* of the sacred word *Aum*, which is 'M', is indicative of both adversity and prosperity. Its colour is white, and its presiding deity is *Rudra*.

The final part of *Praṇava* has all the colours, shining brightly. *Puruṣa* is its presiding deity.

From the earliest times of the ancient *Vedās* it has been declared that 'the universe arises from the Word (*śabdāt prabhavati jagat*)'.

> 'Verily, *Vāk* (the Word) is the unborn one. It was from *Vāk* (the Word) that the Maker of the universe produced creatures.'
>
> *Tāṇḍya-Mahābrāhmaṇa of the Sāma Veda 20:14.2*

In the Christian tradition there is a similar view expressed by St John in the opening lines of the fourth gospel of the New Testament of the Bible, which he wrote around 85–90 CE.

> 'In the beginning was the Word and the Word was with God and the Word was God.'
>
> *John 1*

This means that before Creation, nothing existed except God the Father as pure Spirit: Ever-Existing, Ever-Conscious, Ever-New Bliss. God created the universe and everything in it through his Word, the Cosmic Sound vibration *Oṁ* (the Holy Ghost or Holy Spirit). God the Father, or Christ Intelligence, guides the Cosmic Vibration to create all finite matter.

The Cosmic Vibration *Oṁ* is used by Hindus as *Aum*, Muslims as *Amin*, and Christians as *Amen*.

Paramhansa Yogananda said that John the Baptist was baptised by the omnipresent sound *Aum* (the Holy Ghost), and that in a previous incarnation he was Jesus' guru, called Elias. (Matthew 11:13–15 and 17:9–13 demonstrate support for the doctrine of reincarnation.)

Jesus became the Christ after being baptised by his guru, John. In the Bible, John says, 'I saw the Spirit descending from heaven like a dove, and it abode upon him (Jesus).' Potentially, Jesus was a Master from birth, but it was actually at the time of his baptism or initiation by John the Baptist that he became a Master, Jesus the *Christ*. The Word (Holy Ghost or *Aum*) had descended into Jesus (symbolised in the Bible and paintings of the baptism as a pure white dove). His human consciousness had expanded with the Cosmic Sound Vibration of *Aum*. Jesus embraced the vastness of Infinite Vibration. His consciousness became identified with the Christ Consciousness, which is the only reflection in all creation of God, the Father beyond creation. 'Christ' means 'the anointed of God' or 'chosen by God'.

The conception of the Word (Sanskrit – *Vāk*, Hebrew – *Memra*, Greek – *Logos*) as the creative principle was prevalent in varying forms among the ancient Hebrews and the Greeks. The word *Vāk* is from the root *vach*, 'to speak'. Literally, it means 'voice' (Latin – *vox*). It signifies the word, uttered or written, which has a meaning, idea, thought or reason. The Sanskrit *Vāk* and the Greek *Logos* have the same etymological sense. Synonymous with *Vāk* is the Sanskrit term *śabda* (sound or word). A word is the verbal symbol of a concept, that is, *Oṁ* signifies *Īśvara* (Supreme Lord, God). *Īśvara* and His creative thought or Word are inseparable. The Divine Word signifies the Divine Ideation or the creative thought of God.

> 'By the Word of the Lord were the heavens made; and all the host of them by the breath of his mouth.'
>
> *Psalms 33.6*

The primary meaning of *Logos* (from *lego*, 'to speak') is 'meaningful word', which connotes 'active reason'.

St John, author of the Fourth Gospel, got the idea from Philo Judaeus, the Jewish philosopher of Alexandria, and adapted it to the personality of Jesus Christ as the Saviour. He sought to harmonise the speculative philosophy of Greece, particularly Stoicism and Platonism, with the tenets of Judaism and developed his doctrine of the *Logos*.

The significance of *Aum* is also given in the *Bhāgavad Gītā*:

> 'A person who is situated in yogic concentration by controlling all the (nine) gates (openings) of the body, confining the mind within the heart, and fixing the vital life-force at the crown of the head, and remaining steadfast in yogic on *Oṁ*, the monosyllable (Primordial Sound) signifying *Brāhman*, concentration

and remembers Me (Spirit) at the time of departure from the body, attains the Supreme Goal.'

Bhāgavad Gītā 8:12–13

There are some advanced Yogis who are able to control the life current in the body, by closing all the nine gates (*dvārāṇi*) of the senses of perception (two eyes, two ears, two nostrils, two organs of excretion and of procreation, and the mouth (tongue)), and confining the mind in the heart by not contemplating external objects. The *Kriyā yogis* use a meditation technique called *yoni mudrā* or *jyoti mudrā* to close off the senses of perception. In this *mudrā* the openings in the head are closed and the energy is directed inward and upward towards the Spiritual Eye at the midpoint between the eyebrows. The concentration is then held at the point between the eyebrows to open and illumine the Spiritual Eye, for the consciousness and life force to pass through into infinity. As the concentration deepens and the yogi becomes more absorbed in the meditation he hears the Divine *Aum* Sound Vibration that signifies God, and communes with it superconsciously, expanding his consciousness into the Infinite. As he expands his consciousness, he first becomes conscious of the Christ Consciousness underlying all creation (*Kūtastha Caitanya*), then his consciousness is absorbed into the Transcendental Absolute, beyond vibratory manifestation.

The higher yogis have made a conscious exit from the three bodies (physical, astral, causal) at the time of death through these advanced meditation methods and have attained the highest goal of God-realisation (*sa yāti paramāṁ gatim* – 'he goes to the highest goal').

AUM AND *OṀ* – SOUNDING THE *MANTRA*

Aum is an extension of the *Oṁ* energy. *Oṁ* extended becomes *Aum*, which has a greater power to expand, with a greater force and *prāṇic* energy to it.

The *mantra Aum* may be sounded aloud, whispered, or repeated mentally. In sounding the word *Aum* the three phonemes (*mātras*) – *a* (*akāra*), *u* (*ukāra*), and *m* (*makāra*) – are sounded equally. The '*a*' and '*u*' become blended into '*o*'.

The long vowel letter '*A*' (pronounced like 'aw' in 'dawn'), on an energetic level, represents Self-expansion and awareness of the Absolute. It starts at the back of the mouth, with the tongue lying relaxed on the lower palate, the sound resonating deeply from the lower abdomen. Repeat a long 'aaw', like opening your mouth to reveal your tonsils. This will expand and release the *prāṇic* energy.

The strongest of the three primal vowels, the short vowel letter '*u*' represents the Divine force unfolding and expanding in a creative and energising way. It is formed in the middle of the mouth with a long 'uuu' sound, and has a strong expansive power. The letter '*m*' is produced by closing the lips, following with the nasal resonance, the 'after-sound' (*anusvāra*), repesenting the fourth state of consciousness (*turīya*). As the full range of the mouth is used, it is said that *Aum* the *oṁkāra* or *Praṇava* contains all sounds.

The correct pronunciation of *Oṁ* is like the 'ong' in 'song' but drawn out and with the 'o' pronounced like its alphabet name. *Oṁ* is a pure vowel sound and the consonant 'm' is silent, because the 'o' sound is prolonged.

5.3

SO'HAM, HAṀSA AND HONG SAU

SO'HAM AND *HAṀSA*

> 'The breath of every person, in entering (inhaling), makes the sound of *so* and in coming out (exhaling), that of *ham*. These two sounds make *so'ham*.'
>
> *Gheranda Samhita 5:84*

> 'The Self is God, the Self is Consciousness, and the Self is always repeating its own *mantra, so'ham, so'ham*.'
>
> *Sundardas*

The Sanskrit word *haṁsa* is traditionally translated to mean 'swan', a symbol for the Supreme Spirit or *Brāhman*. According to the *Vedās* and *Purānas*, ancient scriptures of India, the *haṁsa* (swan) is the vehicle (*vahana*) of *Brāhma*, the Supreme Spirit. The flight of the *haṁsa* symbolises the escape from the cycle of birth and death (*saṁsāra*). Swans are also noted for their stamina, discipline, grace and beauty. The swan is unique in being able to separate milk from water once it has been mixed, which is symbolic of great spiritual discrimination. Similarly, the advanced yogi separates the real from the unreal, absorbing only the pure vibrations. And just as the swan lives on water but does not wet its feathers, a yogi lives in the world but is not tainted by its illusionary (*Māyā*) nature.

Those who have attained Self-God-realisation are sometimes called *Paramhansa*, 'the supreme swan', symbolising an advanced level of spiritual enlightenment. In recent times Paramhansa Yogananda (1893–1952), founder of the Self-Realization Fellowship in the USA, was one such God-realised *satguru*.

The *haṁsa* has the *mantra so'ham ahaṃ saḥ* ('I am He, He is I').

The Sanskrit word *ahaṃ* means 'I am, I exist'. *Saḥ* means 'That' (That, the Supreme Consciousness). *So'ham* represents the unity and oneness of the soul (*ātman*) with God (*Brāhman*).

The *so'ham mantra* (pronounced 'so hum') is said to have originated from the *Īśa Upaniṣad*. The *Upaniṣads* form the end (*anta*) of the *Veda* and are termed as *Vedānta*. These are the enlightened teachings of ancient seers and sages on the identity of the Self (*ātman*) and the Ultimate Reality (*Brāhman*).

When the Sanskrit *mantra haṁsa* ('I am He') is repeated continuously it becomes *so'ham*, which means 'He (the Absolute) am I'. Repeated either way the meaning is the same. *Sa* means 'He' and *aham* means 'I'. *So'ham* or *haṁsa* signifies the identity of the individual self (*jiva*) and *Brāhman* (Supreme Self).

In an early *Śaiva Tantra* (seventh century CE) it is stated that *ha* is the inhaling breath, representing *Śakti*, and *sa* is the exhaling breath, representing *Śiva*. The syllables *ha* and *sa* are joined by the nasal sounding *ṁ*, which represents the individual soul (*jiva*). Joined together *ha* plus *ṁ* plus *sa* form the *mantra haṁsa*.

In the *Vijñānabhairava*, an old meditation text, each complete breath is described as an automatic repetition of the *mantra haṁsa*, or *so'ham* when the exhalation is emphasised. The syllable *haṁ* vibrates with the experience 'I am', and the syllable *sa* or *so* vibrates with the expansive experience of 'That' (the Absolute). Therefore, when we repeat the *mantra haṁsa*, or *so'ham* with awareness, we affirm 'I am That'.

So'ham is a natural and well-known *mantra* similar to the universal *Praṇava mantra Aum* (*Oṁ*). In fact, *so'ham* is a modified version of *Oṁ*. If you delete the consonants *s* and *h* from *so'ham*, you are left with *Oṁ*. *So'ham* is the Life breath and *Oṁ* is the Soul of breath.

So'ham, the sound of that supreme Consciousness, is the natural sound of the breath – *so* with the inhalation, *ham* (pronounced 'hum') with the exhalation. The repetition of *so'ham* represents the Cosmic cycle of life flowing through the individual self and the Supreme Self. Throughout the 24 hours of the day the breath flows in and out 21,600 times in a continuous *mantra* of *so'ham*, not only in our wakeful hours but also during our sleep. Unknowingly, we are all repeating this inherent mantric sound created by the inhalation and exhalation of breath, in a process of automatic and continuous recitation. In Yoga, spontaneous recitation of a *mantra* is called *ajapā japa*. The *japa* becomes *ajapā* when the *mantra* gets repeated in the consciousness on its own, without conscious effort on the part of the yogi. This spontaneous recitation of *so'ham haṁsa* is called *ajapā Gāyatrī*. All you have to do is simply become aware of it. Just watch your breathing process and listen to *so'ham* – inhaling *so*, exhaling *ham* – and realise the true Self eternally present within you which always says 'I am He' or 'I am That' (your true divine Self).

If you were to be consciously aware of *so'ham* with each breath continuously throughout the day, connecting with the rhythm of *prāṇa* (Life Force), your breath would gradually become slower and subtler, and your mind very calm. You would connect with the space of stillness that comes from deep within you, and your awareness would turn towards the inner Self, deepening your awareness of Pure Consciousness. You would naturally become more conscious and spiritually awake. Through total understanding of *so'ham* or *haṁsa*, contemplating your oneness with the Supreme Consciousness, you can perceive and realise the Truth in this very moment. The power of this *mantra so'ham*, the seed of transcendence, is in the effect its vibrations has on our body, mind and inner consciousness, for every time we consciously connect *so'ham* to our breath we are closer to uniting the consciousness of our individual self to the Supreme Self, moving from separation to oneness in that infinite expanse of Consciousness: God, the Supreme Consciousness.

> 'This *mantra* (*so'ham*) which is called *ajapā Gāyatrī* will give liberation to all yogis. Just mental repetition of this *mantra*, will help one destroy all sins. There are no practices as holy as this, no *japa* which is equivalent to this, and no

wisdom equivalent to this, and in the future nothing equivalent to it. This *ajapā Gāyatrī* which rises from the *kuṇḍalinī* supports the soul. This is the greatest among the sciences of the soul. He who knows this will know the *Vedās*.'

Yoga Chudamani Upaniṣad 33–35

THE PRACTICE OF *SO'HAM*

Mantras can be intoned aloud, whispered or silently contemplated. Using the *mantra so'ham*, practise it mentally with awareness on your breath, with the deep inner consciousness of it affirming your true inner Self and oneness with God, the Supreme Self.

The following meditation *mantra* process can also be done using the *mantra haṁsa* ('I am He') which is *so'ham* ('He am I') reversed (*ham* as you inhale, *so* as you exhale). In the *Kriyā Yoga* tradition, my guru, Paramhansa Yogananda, used the *mantra Hong Sau* instead of *haṁsa,* which when reversed becomes *so'ham. Kriyā Yoga* disciples of Yogananda use *Hong Sau*, while other Yoga traditions use *haṁsa* or *so'ham*, but with these *mantras*, it is not that one is better than the other. It is a matter of choice, and if the *mantra* is practised correctly with love and devotion, it will surely bring spiritual illumination.

The *Hong Sau* technique will be covered separately in the *Kriyā Yoga* practice (section 7.6.1).

1. Begin your practice by sitting in a comfortable and relaxed meditative upright position, either on a chair or on the floor with a cushion to raise your hips and support you. Sit with your spine upright with your pelvis, chest, head and neck aligned. Rest your hands, one on the other, in your lap with your palms facing upwards. Or rest the backs of your hands on your thighs, close to your torso.

2. Spend a few moments consciously tensing and relaxing your body by inhaling deeply, and while holding your breath tensing all the muscles in your body. Then, simultaneously exhale and release all body tension with a deep exhalation through your mouth with a 'ha-haaa' sound.

3. Sitting still, close your eyes and bring your attention to rest at the midpoint between your eyebrows on the forehead, the centre of intuition and perception (Spiritual Eye). Then, turn your awareness to the natural rhythm of your breath. Become aware of where the inhalation and exhalation arise and dissolve. As your breath naturally flows in, the inhalation sounds like *so*, and as your breath naturally flows out, the exhalation sounds like *ham*. Synchronise the *mantra* with your breath; they arise and dissolve simultaneously together. Do not try to control the breath in any way – allow the process to happen naturally.

4. As you become increasingly more aware, and your focus more concentrated, notice that between the two movements of the arising inhalation and the subsiding exhalation there is a momentary pause or resting point of stillness. Focus your attention on this space or still point without trying to increase

or decrease its length, just simply observe it. Then as you begin your next inhalation follow the breath, with *so* until it naturally subsides, and focus on the space of stillness within. As your exhalation begins follow it with the *mantra ham* to the space of stillness outside. Again, become aware of that space by gently focusing your attention there. You the inner Self are just a witness, observing your breath with total attentive awareness, while simultaneously listening to the subtle mantric sounds: *so* and *ham*.

In those still point spaces between the breaths you are present as your true Self, pure Awareness and pure Consciousness. While resting in the present moment of those spaces of stillness, feel your oneness with the Infinite and affirm, 'I am He, blessed Spirit I am He.'

5. As you rest and focus on the timeless pauses between the breaths they will naturally increase, and you will go deeper into timeless, spacious stillness and expansion of consciousness. As your breath becomes more subtle and refined and slows down, you may notice it temporarily and naturally become suspended. Don't be alarmed if this happens, it is quite natural and the breath returns to its normal rhythm of breathing. Do not try to prolong this breathless state, just enjoy the calmness and freedom it brings. It is important to remain calm; there should be no tension or strain, just allow your awareness to merge in the space inside. Then when the breathing naturally returns continue synchronising it with the *mantra so'ham*.

   If your attention wanders to thoughts, memories and subconscious impressions or inner sensations during this meditation, just be calmly aware of them but detached, and immediately return your awareness and concentration to the continuous repetition of the *mantra*: *so* as you inhale, *ham* as you exhale, and attention on the still point or space between them. Understand, that as you repeat the *mantra*, the goal of the *mantra*, and the reciter of the *mantra* are one. Do not let your attention get caught up in any inner or outer phenomena, if this happens just keep returning to the practice of your attention on *so'ham*. If you feel you are becoming restless and tense and distracted, tense and relax your muscles as you did in the beginning of the practice, then relax and return your awareness and attention to *so'ham*, mentally intoning the *mantra* synchronised with your breathing.

6. To finish your *mantra* meditation return to awareness of your physical body, rub your palms together and gently massage your face, open your eyes, and then gently stretch your legs. Take a few minutes to remain quiet before getting up and leaving your meditation, then go about your day in the consciousness of peace, harmony and goodwill to all whom you meet. Throughout the day, whatever you are doing bring your awareness to *so'ham*, which you can intone mentally. By quietly watching your breath in relation to *so'ham* in this way throughout the day, the mind becomes calm effortlessly. In this way you harmoniously unite your conscious awareness with the inner Self-awareness.

5.4

BĪJA MANTRAS

In Sanskrit *bīja* means seed, denoting the benefits that grow from repeating these short syllable *mantras*. Seed-syllable *mantras* are powerful and potent letters, words or sounds which have evolved from the spiritual experiences of enlightened saints and yogis. Regular chanting and meditation of *bīja mantras* awaken spiritual energy; for example, the individual *chakras* in the astral spine can be activated by chanting its particular *bīja mantra*.

The seed syllable has a magical aura around it. Some *bīja mantras* have a subtle inner meaning. According to the Tantric tradition, every seed syllable must have a nasal sound which results in a divine union. Since *Śiva* and *Śakti* are considered to be two lips, their union leads to the birth of seed, *bīja*.

The nasal sound (*anusvāra* – the closing *ṁ* sound) is supposed to have the germ of a complete doctrine. Through *bīja-akshara* (seed syllable) a huge treatise can be compressed in a few lines. A seed syllable, by virtue of being short, is good for the repetition of a *mantra* as it creates cerebral vibrations which keep reverberating. With the help of the nasal sound, one can transfer the seed syllable to the back of the head or between the eyebrows. At a later stage the accumulated energy of a *mantra* can be projected anywhere in order to achieve the desired result.

According to the *Śiva Sūtra-Vārttika*, the secret of *mantra* lies in its psychic existence. The purpose of *mantra* is to destroy the bondage to life and death. *Bīja mantra* has this capacity to the maximum, and the most powerful of all is the *mantra* of all *mantras*, the *Praṇava* or *Aum* (*Oṁ*), the Primordial Sound that represents the Supreme Reality (*Brāhman*). *Oṁ*, the root of all sounds and letters, contains all the other *bīja-aksharas* (seed syllables) within it. *Oṁ* is the Supreme *Bīja*.

BĪJA MANTRAS OF THE *CHAKRAS* IN THE ASTRAL SPINE

The seed syllables of the 'Five Great Elements' (*Pañchamahābhūtas*) – ether, air, fire, water and earth – are respectively *Haṁ*, *Yaṁ*, *Raṁ*, *Vaṁ* and *Laṁ*.

The *bīja mantras* of the *chakras* (centres of consciousness) have the power to awaken the spiritual energy within the individual and bring it to the corresponding *chakra* as awareness.

Laṁ – *mūladhāra chakra* (first *chakra*, coccyx centre, 'earth')

Vaṁ – *svādhiṣṭhāna chakra* (second *chakra*, sacral centre, 'water')

Raṁ – *maṇipūra chakra* (third *chakra*, lumbar centre, 'fire')

Yaṁ – *anāhata chakra* (fourth *chakra*, dorsal (heart) centre, 'air')

Haṁ – *viśuddha chakra* (fifth *chakra*, cervical centre, 'ether').

PRIMARY *BĪJA MANTRAS*

Oṁ. The Primordial Vibratory Sound that is the ultimate transcendental Reality.

Aiṁ (pronounced 'aym'). The seed *mantra* of the Divine Mother in the aspect of Sarāsvāti, the goddess of knowledge, speech and communication, the consort of Lord Brāhma. *Aiṁ* can be used to invoke wisdom and understanding. It increases concentration of mind and awakens higher intelligence.

Hriṁ (pronounced 'hreem'). *Hriṁ* is a solar seed *mantra*, and a main *shakti mantra* that relates to the goddess Parvati, the consort of Śiva. *Hriṁ* energises and directs the power of *prāṇa*. It is an empowerment *mantra* when used in relation to a deity or object whose presence you wish to access at the heart (*hṛdaya* – the seat of feeling) level. It relates to the *prāṇic* function of the heart and brings joy and bliss.

Śrīṁ (pronounced 'shreem'). The lunar seed *mantra* of the Divine Mother in the aspect of Lakshmi, the consort of Lord Vishnu, and goddess of prosperity and abundance. *Śrīṁ* is a *mantra* of faith, devotion and surrender. It can be used to gain grace when used devotionally towards any deity.

Hlīṁ (pronounced 'hleem'). *Hlīṁ* is a seed *mantra* of joy and bliss when used at a soft level, but can also be used to neutralise or destroy. It helps in gaining control of one's own body, mind, senses and *prāṇa*, bringing one into inner stillness.

Krīṁ (pronounced 'kreem'). *Krīṁ* is the seed *mantra* of the Divine Mother in the aspect of the goddess Kali, the consort of Lord Śiva. It is a *mantra* of transformative energy – through it you can gain control of your *karma*. It gives greater power to concentration and meditation, and helps in awakening the *kuṇḍalinī śakti*.

Klīṁ (pronounced 'kleem'). *Klīṁ* relates to Krishna and is the seed *mantra* of love and devotion. It is also often called the *Kāma bīja*, in reference to Kāmadeva (Lord of Desire). This aspect of desire is distinct from greed and signifies legitimate desire, the fulfilment of which is a recognised goal of human life.

Strīṁ (pronounced 'streem'). *Strīṁ* is a seed *mantra* of the Hindu goddess, Tara, who is connected to goddess Durgā. *Strīṁ* brings an expansive energy, and is the seed syllable of peace. In sound qualities *Strīṁ* is similar to *Śrīṁ* but is stronger with a more stabilising effect.

Trīṁ (pronounced 'treem'). The indication of this seed *mantra* is similar to *Strīṁ*, but with a more fiery nature. This *mantra* is good for helping one to overcome difficulties and harmful forces.

Huṁ and ***Hūṁ*** (pronounced 'hoom'). There are two versions of this *mantra*: one has a short vowel sound (*Huṁ*), the other has a long vowel sound (*Hūṁ*). Both are used to raise the *kuṇḍalinī śakti*, when combining the *mantra* with the breath.

Hūṁ is the primal sound of Lord Śiva, the transformative aspect of the Divine Trinity (Brāhma, Viṣṇu, Śiva).

Huṁ with the short vowel sound is connected to the power of *prāṇa* and the breath, and can be used to give energy to other *mantras*.

Hauṁ. *Hauṁ* is a combination of the mantric sounds *Ha* and *Aum*. The *Ha* sound gives more power and *prāṇa* to the Cosmic Vibratory Sound of *Aum*. *Hauṁ* is an expansion of the seed *mantra Hūṁ*.

This powerful *mantra Hauṁ* can be used to revitalise your mind and *prāṇa*, and to expand your energy and awareness.

Sauṁ. *Sauṁ* is a combination of the mantric sounds *Ha* and *Aum*. The *Sa* sound empowers the *mantra* with strength and stability. *Sauṁ* indicates *Śakti* (Shakti) and relates to the principle of bliss.

Hsauḥ. *Hsauḥ* is a combination of the mantric sounds *Hau* and *Sau*. This is a very powerful seed *mantra* for energising the internal *prāṇa* and stimulating the *kuṇḍalinī śakti*.

Duṁ (pronounced with a short 'u' as in fl*u*te) and ***Dūṁ*** (pronounced with a long 'u'). *Duṁ* is the seed *mantra* of the Divine Mother in the aspect of the protective goddess Durgā, who saves us from all difficulties. So it can be used to overcome obstacles and eliminate sorrow.

Dūṁ (with a long vowel sound) has a more feminine quality and is used in *Śakti mantras* to neutralise negative forces.

Gaṁ. This is the *Ganesha-bīja*. *Ga* means Ganesha, the dispeller of sorrow.

Glauṁ. *Glauṁ* is a combination of the mantric sounds of *Ga*, *la* and *Aum*. *Glauṁ* deepens and expands the *Aum* vibration, and helps to remove obstacles.

Kṣrauṁ. *Kṣrauṁ* is related to Narasimha, the Man-Lion, the protective form of Lord Viṣṇu. It has the power to purify the ego and reduce lower desires within us.

CHANTING THE *BĪJA MANTRAS* IN THE *CHAKRAS*

Begin with a prayer

> Heavenly Father, transfer my consciousness from the physical body to the astral spine and from it through the seven chakras to Cosmic Consciousness, where Thy glory and Light reign in the fullness of Thy manifestation; where the Life Force reigns in all Thy power. Aum, Peace, Amen.

Chanting the chakra bīja mantras

Chanting is an effective way to activate energy throughout the body. This practice activates and tunes the *chakras* using the sound vibration of the *bīja* (seed-syllable) *mantras*. Each seed *mantra* has a unique power, which clears the *chakras* of blockages so that they can function efficiently. This prepares the way to meditation.

Sit comfortably and relaxed in a meditative posture with the head, neck and spine aligned. Close the eyes.

Bring your awareness to *mūladhāra chakra*. Inhale deeply and as you exhale, chant continuously aloud the *bīja mantra* ***Laṁ***. Feel the *bīja mantra* vibrating at *mūladhāra chakra* – ***laṁ***, ***laṁ***, ***laṁ***, ***laṁ***...

It will depend on the length of your inhalation and exhalation how many times you repeat the *bīja mantra*. If you have quite a good lung capacity you may be able to chant it 20 times in one exhalation.

Start at *mūladhāra chakra* and ascend through the *chakras* to *ājñā chakra*, chanting the *bīja mantras* in a focused meditative way, feeling the vibration at the six *chakras*:

Chakra	***Bīja mantras***
First chakra (Mūladhāra)	***Laṁ***
Second chakra (Svādhiṣṭhāna)	***Vaṁ***
Third chakra (Maṇipūra)	***Raṁ***
Fourth chakra (Anāhata)	***Yaṁ***
Fifth chakra (Viśuddha)	***Haṁ***
Sixth chakra (Ājñā)	***Oṁ***

Mentally chanting the chakra bīja mantras

Sit comfortably and deeply relax in a meditative posture with the head, neck and spine aligned. Close the eyes, and bring your awareness to your breath, and as you breathe in feel the spaciousness expanding in the spine. Change the centre of your consciousness from the body and senses to the spine... Feel the subtle astral spine by slightly and gently swaying the upper body from left to right... Then, feel your consciousness with the breath move up and down the spine several times, from the *mūladhāra chakra* at the base of the spine to the midpoint between the eyebrows... Now bring your attentive awareness to the first *chakra*, *mūladhāra*, breathe into this area and mentally repeat the seed *mantra* ***Laṁ*** once, feeling it vibrating and resonating in the *chakra*... At the end of the exhalation remain in the stillness for a short while. Then feeling the energy pulsating like a magnetic current in *mūladhāra*, expand it upwards to the second *chakra*, *svādhiṣṭhāna*, and mentally repeat the seed *mantra* ***Vaṁ***, feeling it vibrating and resonating in the *chakra*... Then again, pause in the stillness, and feel the intensity of energy resonating in the *chakra*.

In the same way, continue ascending through the other four *chakras*, mentally repeating the seed *mantra* for each and pausing in stillness after chanting in each *chakra*:

Ājñā chakra – ***Oṁ***

Viśuddha chakra – ***Haṁ***

Anāhata chakra – ***Yaṁ***

Maṇipūra chakra – ***Raṁ.***

Then descend through the spinal passage to each *chakra* in the reverse order, mentally repeating the seed *mantras* for each and pausing in stillness after chanting in each *chakra*:

Ājñā chakra – ***Oṁ***

Viśuddha chakra – ***Haṁ***

Anāhata chakra – ***Yaṁ***

Maṇipūra chakra – ***Raṁ***

Svādhiṣṭhāna chakra – ***Vaṁ***

Mūladhāra chakra – ***Laṁ.***

Practise nine to 12 rounds.

5.5

HŪM MANTRA

The Mantra that Brings Power to All the Mantras

By adding the additional powerful seed syllable *Hūm* (pronounced 'Hoom') to the *bīja mantra* of a *chakra* (each sounded with a long 'a'), you activate its energy.

To help magnetise, and raise the energy in the spine, and to purify the elements in the *chakras*, the *mantras* below can be chanted. The *bīja mantra Hūm* ('Hoom') is added at the end of the seed *mantra* for the *chakra*. *Hūm* is the Primal Sound of *Śiva* that brings a fire energy and power to all the *chakras* in which it is used, increasing its *prāṇic* energy.

Sit in a meditation posture with your eyes closed and focused at the midpoint between the eyebrows, and start by chanting aloud the *mantra Oṁ Lam Hūm* at the base of the spine in the *mūladhāra chakra*, and feel it vibrating and resonating there. Sit quietly and continue to feel the vibration of this *mantra* as you remain still for a while. Then, continue sounding the *mantras* listed below for each of the seven *chakras* up to the crown (*sahasrāra*) at the top of your head, pausing for a short silence between the soundings of each *mantra*.

Chakra	**Element**	***Mantra***
Sahasrāra		*Oṁ Oṁ Hūṁ*
Ājñā		*Oṁ Kṣaṁ Hūṁ*
Viśuddha	ether	*Oṁ Haṁ Hūṁ*
Anāhata	air	*Oṁ Yaṁ Hūṁ*
Maṇipūra	fire	*Oṁ Raṁ Hūṁ*
Svādhiṣṭhāna	water	*Oṁ Vaṁ Hūṁ*
Mūladhāra	earth	*Oṁ Laṁ Hūṁ*

5.6

THE TWO GREATEST HEALING MANTRAS

The greatest of all the healing *mantras* that are revealed in the Vedic scripture are the *Gāyatrī Mantra* and the *Mahā Mrityunjaya Mantra*. For those who want to attain perfection in healing it is suggested that they practise a vigorous *sādhana* (spiritual practice) of *japa* on these two healing *mantras*.

MAHĀ MRITYUNJAYA MANTRA

In the seventh Mandala of the *Ṛig Veda* (7.59), attributed to the sage Vasishtha, and also in the *Yajur Veda* (3.60) there occurs a *mantra* that is said to be life-giving and the most powerful that the ancient sages had evolved. Along with the *Gāyatrī Mantra* it holds the highest place among the numerous *mantras* used for meditation. The significance of this *mantra* lies in the fact that it has saved many people from death. It is the source of all protection – physical, mental and spiritual. It is considered one of the most potent healing *mantras*, bestowing health, wellbeing, longevity, peace, abundance, prosperity and protection. Since the *Mahā Mrityunjaya Mantra* has been repeated or chanted by many Hindus, saints, sages and yogis for the past 4000 years, this *mantra* has accumulated a very special power. Its power prevents accidents of all kinds, and keeps the devotee safe and protected. The great Swāmi Sivananda of Rishikesh gave great praise to this *mantra*: he said that the *Mahā Mrityunjaya* is a life-giving *mantra* that wards off death by accidents of all descriptions, and has a great curative effect, including diseases pronounced incurable by doctors, when chanted with sincerity, faith and devotion.

Mahā Mrityunjaya Mantra means 'the great *mantra* that removes diseases and liberates one from death'. This life-giving *mantra* is also known as the *Markandeya Mantra*, named after an ever-living master (like Mahavatar Babaji) whose abode is in the Himalayas. There is a story behind this *mantra* concerning a son, named Markandeya, born to pious parents. The story is as follows.

THE STORY OF MARKANDEYA

There was once a forest-dwelling sage called Mrikandu, who with his wife, Marudvati, practised severe penance to earn the favour and blessings of Lord Śiva. When Lord Śiva, their *ishtadevata* (the deity of their hearts), saw this he rewarded them with a boon, saying, 'You will either have a divine son born to you who will only live for 16 years or a bad son who will live for one hundred years. The choice is yours.'

Sage Mrikandu and his wife prayed together for the divine son, even though his life would be short. So, Śiva blessed the couple with a divine son, and when he was born they named him Markandeya. When Markandeya became eight years of age, he knew all the holy scriptures, the secret of the *Gāyatrī Mantra*, and all that is to be known for Self-realisation directly from the wise instruction of his father, Mrikandu.

Markandeya's parents never revealed the secret to him that his life would end when he reached the young age of 16. But because they were devotional and had faith in Lord Śiva they instructed and guided him to worship (*puja*) and meditate on Lord Śiva in the form of a *Śiva lingam* ('supreme emblem' or symbol denoting Śiva as Divine Consciousness). So young Markandeya worshipped Lord Śiva regularly, with devotion. Then on the last day of his sixteenth year, Yama, the god of death, appeared to him as he was sitting in worship of Lord Śiva. Suddenly, Markandeya's breath became disturbed as Yama threw his noose to pull his soul from his body. In that moment, with great devotion Markandeya embraced the holy *Śiva lingam* on his altar and with great faith chanted the great Śiva *mantra* known as the *Mahā Mrityunjaya Mantra*. As he uttered the great *mantra*, the protection of Lord Śiva appeared to him through the *Śiva lingam*. Śiva drove away Yama, the god of death, and in that moment stopped Markandeya's ageing process, and pronounced with a blessing to Markandeya that death would never claim him, that he would remain a 16-year-old eternally and that he would become an ever-living spiritual master of the Himalayas.

Mahā Mrityunjaya Mantra
(the Great Conqueror of Death)

Oṁ Tryambakam yajāmahe
Sugandhim puṣti-vardhanam;
Urvārukamiva bandhanān
Mrityor mukshīya māmritāt.

Oṁ. We worship the three-eyed one
(Lord Śiva; Pure Consciousness), who is
the fragrance of life, who nourishes all beings.
May He liberate me from bondage, for the sake
of immortality, even as the cucumber is severed
from the creeper and is freed from the bondage.

Oṁ – symbolises God; Absolute Reality; All-pervading Consciousness

Tryambakam – the prefix *tri* means 'three'. When it is joined to *ambakam*, the letter 'i' becomes 'y', resulting in the word *tryambakam*.

Ambaka means 'eye'. *Tryambakam* means 'three-eyed', which refers to Śiva's three eyes, the third being his 'third eye' or Spiritual Eye, at the midpoint between his eyebrows.

Yajāmahe – we worship, adore, revere

Sugandhim – *su* means 'good, sweet'

Gandha – fragrance

Puṣti – nourish

Vardhanam – one who nourishes, strengthens

Urvārukamiva – an Indian cucumber-like plant that grows as a creeper

Iva – like, just as

Bandhanān – stem of the gourd (that is attached to the cucumber vine by a strong woody stem)

Mrityor – from death

Mukshīya – free us, liberate us

Mā – not

Mritāt – immortality.

Recite *japa* daily on *rudraksha* beads of this great *mantra* with faith and devotion that Lord Śiva may bless you with protection against all accidents and fear associated with death; for your health and vitality; to attain freedom from all forms of misery; and to bless you with infinite consciousness. This *mantra* can also be recited when taking medicines, for it prepares the body and mind to make the best use of them.

According to the holy scriptures of India, to gain the *mantra siddhi* (power of the *mantra*) one would have do *japa* or recitation of *Mahā Mrityunjaya Mantra* 125,000 times, equivalent to 1250 rounds of a *mālā*.

As you recite *japa* of this *mantra* of 32 syllables, divided into four lines, each containing eight syllables, let your mind become absorbed in the mantric sounds and rhythm of each line, allowing the *mantra* to draw your awareness to your Spiritual Eye (eyebrow centre) and to your heart centre. After you have completed your recitations using your *mālā*, sit with your mind calm in the stillness of meditation, and know that *Mahā Mrityunjaya Mantra* is vibrating eternally at the heart of creation.

GĀYATRĪ MANTRA

'...the *Gāyatrī Mantra* is universally considered the essence of all *mantras*. The Sanskrit words contain the essential vibration of the upper luminous spheres of light, and all spiritual powers and potencies are within. The *Gāyatrī Mantra* is simply meditation on light.'

Ashley-Farrand 2000, p.191

The *Gāyatrī Mantra* is known as the 'Queen of *Mantras*'. It is said to have been realised by the sage Vishvamitra, and it first appears in the ancient *Ṛig Vedā* (3.62.10), and later in the *Yajur Vedā* (3.63) and *Sāma Veda*, and later still in the *Upaniṣads* (the culmination of the *Vedās*). Before the *Vedās*, there was a time when Brahmā, the Supreme Creator, was once in deep meditation when the subtle inner vibration of Gāyatrī revealed itself to Him. It was later revealed to the Vedic sage Vishvamitra, a preceptor of Sri Rāma, incarnation of Lord Viṣṇu. As a reward for his many years of deep meditation and penance, the Supreme Being revealed to him the *Gāyatrī Mantra*. This was to be a gift for all humanity.

The *Gāyatrī Mantra* is the most sacred prayer of the *Ṛig Vedā*; a prayer for light, for illumination. It is addressed to the Immanent and Transcendent Divine, which has been given the name *Savitur*, meaning 'that from which all is born'. It is said that the Absolute expresses itself as *Aum*, and *Aum* further expresses as the *Gāyatrī Mantra*.

The *Gāyatrī* may be considered as having three parts: praise, meditation and prayer. First, the Divine is praised, then it is meditated upon in reverence, and finally an appeal is made to the Divine to awaken and strengthen the intellect. The *Gāyatrī* possesses both the power of *mantra* and the power of prayer, and so has both an intrinsic power through its mere utterance alone, and also an instrumental power, which is derived from the understanding of its meaning and philosophical significance.

Gāyatrī is the essence of all *mantras*, and all spiritual powers and potencies are contained within it. Of all *mantras* the *Gāyatrī* is supreme. *Gāyatrī* is the 'Mother of the *Vedās*' (*Vedāmata*), the source of Divine Wisdom, because it stimulates revelation and allows one to intuitively understand the knowledge contained in the *Vedās* by awakening insight. *Gāyatrī* is the bestower of all that is beneficial to the person who chants it with faith.

The *Gāyatrī* is a universal prayer that can be recited by all humanity, for it is a sincere prayer to be guided by the transcendental Light of the One Supreme Being. The *Gāyatrī Mantra* can be repeated mentally under all conditions, in all sorts of places. Whether one is travelling, walking, standing, sitting, or even lying down, this *mantra* can be mentally recited in public places. To get great benefit from this *mantra* it is best repeated three times daily – in the morning, noon and evening. The benefits are so great that it is said that the *japa* or recitation of this *mantra* brings the same fruit as the recitation of all the four *Vedās* together with Patañjali's *Eight Limbs of Yoga*.

A STORY THAT GIVES THE INNER SIGNIFICANCE OF THE *GĀYATRĪ MANTRA*

The story begins with Manu, a young Brahmin, whose desire was to have the entire knowledge of the *Vedās* without actually reading them. His father was a great scholar, and Manu had inherited all the potentialities to become a wise man himself. But due to his lack of energy and enthusiasm he would not read the *Vedās*. Instead, he took a short-cut by worshipping Indra, the king of heavens.

After some time Indra appeared before Manu and said, 'I'm happy with your meditation and efforts. You may now request a boon, something that will be helpful and beneficial to your life.' Manu, who was eagerly awaiting such an opportunity, bowed down low at the feet of Indra and replied, 'My Lord, please grant me the favour to have the knowledge of all the *Vedās* without me having to read them.'

Indra, the king of Heaven, laughed at his desire and replied, 'I am sorry, Manu, I cannot grant such a boon, because nobody until today has been able to master the *Vedās* without reading them.' Having said that, Indra then disappeared.

Manu, however, was persistent, and again started to worship Indra, but this time he fasted only drinking water. Then, after some time had passed, Indra had to appear again to Manu. The king of Heaven said, 'I am very impressed by your continued effort of worship. Please tell me what I can do for you this time.'

Manu again repeated the same desire he had asked the first time. But Indra again expressed his inability to grant such a boon and then disappeared.

The next day when Manu was going for a bath in the sea, he saw a man throwing stones into it. Manu stayed and curiously watched him for a very long time, until it became almost impossible for him to resist any longer. He went up to the man and asked, 'Excuse me, but why do you keep throwing stones into the sea?'

The man replied, 'I don't like the sea so I'm trying to fill it up.' On hearing this, Manu burst into a fit of laughter, and said, 'Impossible, nobody can fill the sea up by throwing stones into it!' The man replied, 'Yes! If people can have the knowledge of the *Vedās* without reading them, I can also fill the sea up with stones.'

In that moment, Manu immediately understood who the man was, and with all humility bowed down to touch the feet of the man who was none other than the king of Heaven – Indra. But Manu, due to his laziness, was still not sure whether he would really be able to master the *Vedās*. So he asked Indra for the technique. Indra replied, 'If you want to have the wisdom of the *Vedās*, chant first the *mantra* called *Gāyatrī*. The *Gāyatrī Mantra* will help you to overcome your laziness by giving you energy and enthusiasm! By chanting this *mantra* you will feel positive, energetic and enthusiastic! It will also sharpen your intellect power and within a few days you will be a different man. Due to the amazing power of *Gāyatrī*, you will be able to master all the *Vedās*.' After giving this advice Indra disappeared.

The *Gāyatrī Mantra*

Oṁ bhūr bhuvaḥ svaḥ
tat savitur vareṇyaṁ
bhargo devasya dhīmahi
dhiyo yo naḥ pracodayāt

We meditate upon the splendour of the Divinity, the Spiritual Effulgence of That Adorable Supreme Divine Reality, the Source of the Physical, the Astral and the Heavenly Spheres of Existence. May That Supreme Divine Being enlighten our intellect so that we may realise the Supreme Truth.

The *Gāyatrī Mantra* contains all the important *bīja* (seed-syllable) *mantras*:

Oṁ – symbolises God; Absolute Reality

Bhūr – represents earth; physical plane. It also refers to the body made up of the *pancha bhutas* (five elements) that constitute *prakṛiti* (nature)

Bhuvaḥ – represents *Bhuva Loka*, the middle world; the subtle or astral plane. It is also the life-force (*prāṇa śakti*) that animates the body, that comes from the power of the Self (*Ātma śakti*)

Svaḥ – represents the third dimension or celestial region, known as *Svarga Loka* and all the luminous *lokas* (spheres) above

Tat – That, the essential essence

Savitur – luminous, bright, sun-like, inner power of spiritual light, which leads one to Self-realisation

Vareṇyaṁ – finest, best, fit to be sought

Bhargo – effulgence; destroyer of obstacles

Devasya – Divine, resplendent, shining

Dhīmahi – we meditate

Dhiyo – our being of intelligence, intellect, understanding

Yo – who, which

Naḥ – our

Pracodayāt – may enlighten, direct, inspire.

The *Gāyatrī* invokes the splendour and power that pervades the Sun and the Three Worlds to activate the *chakras*, and awaken and strengthen the Intelligence.

The *Gāyatrī Mantra* is chanted for the attainment of cosmic consciousness and for awakening the intuitive powers. It has the power to destroy all delusions, energise *prāṇa*, bestow health, longevity, radiance and illumination. Unless the intellect is illumined the Truth remains hidden and veiled by the forces of *tamas guṇa* (dark forces) and *rajas guṇa* (passion). The light of *Gāyatrī Mantra* removes the obstructions of *tamas* and *rajas* from the mind's mirror, and reflects the Light of Truth in it by which the mind is illumined. The Radiant Light of *Gāyatrī* burns *karma* and blesses with liberation.

Meditation on the Gāyatrī

'Among hymns, I am Brihat-Saman; among poetic meters, I am *Gāyatrī*.'

Sri Krishna, Bhāgavad Gītā 10:35

Through meditation on the *Gāyatrī*, one can become aware of the inner motivating principle of the *pancha bhutas* (five elements) that constitute *prakṛiti* (nature), the five *prāṇas* or vital airs in the body, and the five sheaths (*koshas*), which enclose the soul (*ātma*).

The best times to repeat the *Gāyatrī* are at dawn, noon, and dusk. These times are known as the three *sandhyas*. Sit facing east or north. These auspicious times are beneficial for spiritual practices. But the repeating of *Gāyatrī* is not limited only to these times. As long as the mind and heart are pure when repeating *Gāyatrī*, and it is pronounced clearly and correctly with concentration, and without haste or hurry, it can be repeated at any time of the day or night, and everywhere.

This *mantra* should not be repeated in a mechanical way with the mind wandering on other thoughts. The *Gāyatrī Mantra* is synonymous with the Divine and therefore it should be repeated with reverence, faith and love. In this way, if the *Gāyatrī Mantra* is chanted correctly the atmosphere in which you are chanting it will be illumined by the vibrations produced by the *mantra*. The *Gāyatrī Mantra* will illumine your intellect and light your spiritual path.

To realise the *Gāyatrī Mantra*'s blissful effect one needs to chant it regularly for a considerable period of time. *Gāyatrī* activates the nerve ganglia and the *nāḍīs* (subtle *prāṇic* energy channels), activating the power that yields spiritual knowledge. Repetition of the *Gāyatrī Mantra* produces notes which mingle with the vibrations already existing in nature (*prakṛiti*). This activates the centres of power in the *chakras* and the brain. Divine spiritual light and power are infused into the *chakras*, connecting them to the higher spiritual realms, aligning us with the forces of nature, both subtle and gross, and increasing our connection to the vital force of the sun. The mind becomes infused with solar spiritual energy, and our spiritual perceptions increase.

Gāyatrī Mantra Sādhanā (spiritual practice)

When you sit for meditation, chant the *Gāyatrī Mantra* for a minimum of 108 times, which will take approximately 15 minutes to recite. This is one *mālā* (a rosary of 108 meditation beads); you can use your *mālā* beads to count, using one bead for each recitation. The maximum benefit of chanting the *mantra* is said to be obtained by chanting it 108 times. However, one may chant it for three, nine or 18 times when pressed for time.

For your spiritual practice (*sādhanā*) of meditation on the *Gāyatrī Mantra*, start by practising one *mālā* every morning. If you can devote more time, then chant three to five *mālās*. If you are on a personal spiritual retreat you may wish to chant ten *mālās*, which will take about two and a half hours. You can also do a 40-Day Discipline of chanting ten *mālās* each morning for 40 days. This is called a *Gāyatrī Purascharana*. Or you can choose a number of repetitions per day, and chant that for 40 days.

An extended practice of chanting the *Gāyatrī Mantra* (*purascharana* – 125,000 repetitions of a *mantra*, equivalent to 1250 rounds of a *mālā*) is said to give the meditator a noticeable level of *mantra siddhi* (power of the *mantra*).

By chanting the *Gāyatrī Mantra* for many repetitions over a period of time, the *chakras* become tuned to the energy of each of the seven planes of light. Eventually, after long devoted practice of chanting the *Gāyatrī Mantra*, the entire subtle body becomes attuned with all the planes of spiritual light, making the aura radiant.

> 'If one practises this spiritual discipline sincerely, one realises God in a very short time. So, practise this *Gāyatrī Mantra* meditation regularly and attain illumination… Practice of *Gāyatrī* meditation destroys all *karmas* and sins. By purifying the heart and the mind, it opens the third eye of illumination.'
>
> *Keshavadas 1997, p.58*

The *Gāyatrī* is a cosmic rhythm consisting of 24 syllables arranged as a triplet of eight syllables each. The individual syllables contain an energy seed for each of the seven celestial planes of light. The syllables of the *Gāyatrī Mantra* are constructed and arranged in such a way that the major portion of *vayu* (air) inhaled during the process of chanting moves downward towards the seat of *kuṇḍalinī śakti*. The escape of *vayu* is minimised by the nature of the chest cavity's contraction caused by the systematic chanting of the *mantra*. The collected *vayu* descends to the *mūladhāra chakra* and the heated *prāṇa vayu* strikes the *kuṇḍalinī*, activating it to ascend upward through the *chakras*.

Chanting the syllables of the *Gāyatrī Mantra* positively affect all the *chakras* in the subtle body. The cyclic chanting of the *Gāyatrī Mantra* stimulates the subliminal power centres in the subtle body. The pressure of the tongue, lips, vocal cords, palate, and the connecting regions in the brain generated by continuous chanting of the 24 syllables of the *Gāyatrī Mantra* creates a resonance or a vibration in the *nāḍīs* of the subtle body. This awakens the *chakras* and a sublime magnetic force arouses in the meditator that attracts the vital currents of *Gāyatrī śakti* immanent in the Infinite realms.

The practice of Gāyatrī Mantra meditation

There are two forms of *Gāyatrī Mantra* – the short form and the long form.

Meditation on the short form of Gāyatrī Mantra

> *Oṁ bhūr bhuvaḥ svaḥ*
> *tat savitur vareṇyaṁ*
> *bhargo devasya dhīmahi*
> *dhiyo yo naḥ pracodayāt*
>
> We meditate upon the splendour of the Divinity, the Spiritual Effulgence of That Adorable Supreme Divine Reality, the Source of the Physical, the Astral and the Heavenly Spheres of Existence. May That Supreme Divine Being enlighten our intellect so that we may realise the Supreme Truth.

Sit facing east or north in a comfortable and relaxed meditation posture, with the head, neck and spine aligned. Close your eyes and bring your focused attention to the midpoint between the eyebrows at the Spiritual Eye, on the Light of Truth.

Chant the *Gāyatrī Mantra* clearly and rhythmically without strain:

Begin first by inhaling and then chant ***Oṁ***.

Pause…inhale again, and chant ***bhūr bhuvaḥ svaḥ***.

Pause…inhale, and chant ***tat savitur vareṇyaṁ***.

Pause…inhale, and chant ***bhargo devasya dhīmahi***.

Pause…inhale, and chant ***dhiyo yo naḥ pracodayāt***.

When you have chanted all the syllables of the *mantra*, meditate upon its meaning with feeling of joy, devotion and faith.

Meditation on the long form of *Gāyatrī Mantra*

Oṁ bhūr	1st *chakra* (*mūladhāra*)
Oṁ bhuvaḥ	2nd *chakra* (*svādhiṣṭhāna*)
Oṁ svaḥ	3rd *chakra* (*maṇipūra*)
Oṁ māhā	4th *chakra* (*anāhata*)
Oṁ janaḥ	5th *chakra* (*viśuddha*)
Oṁ tapaḥ	6th *chakra* (*ājñā*)
Oṁ satyam	7th *chakra* (*sahasrāra*)

Oṁ tat savitur vareṇyaṁ
bhargo devasya dhīmahi
dhiyo yo naḥ pracodayāt
I invoke the Earth Plane, the Astral Plane, The Celestial Plane, the Plane of Spiritual Balance, the Plane of Human Spiritual Knowledge, The Plane of Spiritual Austerities, the Plane of Ultimate Truth.
We meditate upon the splendour of the Divinity, the Spiritual Effulgence of That Adorable Supreme Divine Reality, the Source of the Physical, the Astral and the Heavenly Spheres of Existence. May That Supreme Divine Being enlighten our intellect so that we may realise the Supreme Truth.

Sit facing east or north in a comfortable and relaxed meditation posture, with the head, neck and spine aligned. Close your eyes and bring your focused attention to the midpoint between the eyebrows at the Spiritual Eye, on the Light of Truth.

Chant the *Gāyatrī Mantra* clearly and rhythmically without strain.

In this longer form of the *Gāyatrī Mantra* you can also concentrate on the *chakra* that correlates with each *mantra*. For example, chant *Oṁ bhūr* while concentrating on the first *chakra* (*mūladhāra*), and so on.

MANTRAS THAT AFFIRM THE TRUE IDENTITY OF WHO YOU ARE

You need to constantly remind yourself of your true identity and remain aware of your true nature, of the inner blissful Self, that is always pure Consciousness, eternal and infinite, unaffected by the phenomena of nature (*prakṛiti*). Remind yourself daily that you, the Self within (the pure principle of awareness in you), are distinct from the instruments that express your individuality – body, mind and intellect – and that you are and always will be a witness of their functions. Without the constant repetition of the knowledge of your true Self, you cannot be free from ignorance and doubt.

Sachara chara para purna
Shivoham, Shivoham
Nityananda svarūpa
Shivoham, Shivoham
Anandoham, Anandoham, Anandoham, Anandoham
I am that (Pure Consciousness) which prevails everywhere and is complete in itself.
I am Śiva (Pure Consciousness), I am Śiva
My essential nature is eternal Bliss
I am Śiva, I am Śiva (pure Consciousness)
I am Joy itself, I am Bliss, I am Bliss, I am Bliss.

'The Absolute Reality (*Brāhman*) is Consciousness and Bliss and that is our true nature.'

Brihadaranyaka Upaniṣad 3.9.28

ATMA SHATKAM (THE SONG OF THE SELF)

The following six Sanskrit verses of *Atma Shatkam* (also called *Nirvana Shatkam*) with English translation were spoken by the great Adi (first) Shankaracharya (eighth century CE) when he was only eight years old. As he wandered along a path in the Himalayas in search of his Guru, he met a sage who asked him the question, 'Who are you?' He answered with the six verses of the *Atma Shatkam*. The sage happened to be Swāmi Govindpada Acarya, the Guru he was searching for.

Every day it is important and essential to withdraw your sense of identification from the body, mind and intellect, and affirm your true nature. If you chant these verses and reflect or contemplate on their meaning daily, they will help you to reassert and affirm your true essential nature, dispelling the old habit of wrong identification with the mind-body-ego complex, and false separation. After chanting these verses slowly in a meditative mood a number of times, sit with your body and mind in the stillness of meditation, and with attentive awareness abide in the true blissful nature of your Self, the ever-present Reality, the ever-present awareness of 'I'.

manobuddyahamkāra chittāni nāhaṁ
na cha śotrajivhe na cha ghrāṇanetre
na cha vioma bhūmir na tejo na vāyuḥ
cidānandarupaḥ sivo'ham, sivo'ham
I am neither the mind, intellect, ego nor memory,
neither the ears nor the tongue nor the senses of smell and sight, neither ether, air, fire, water or earth.
I am the joy of pure consciousness and bliss. I am Śiva, I am Śiva ('the Pure One'; 'Auspicious One'; the transcendental Self).

na ca pranasajño na vai pamcavāyuḥ
na vā saptadhātur na vā paṃcakośaḥ
na vākpānipadam na copasthapāyu
cidānandarupaḥ śivo'ham, śivo'ham
Neither am I the energy (*prāṇa*), nor the five types of airs in the body (*prāṇa vāyus*), nor the seven material essences of the body (*Rasa*, *Rakta*, *Mamsa*, *Medas*, *Asthi*, *Majja* and *Shukra*), nor the five sheaths (*pañca-kośa*). Neither am I the five instruments of action (elimination, procreation, motion, grasping, or speaking).
I am the joy of pure consciousness and bliss. I am Śiva, I am Śiva.

na me dveśarāgau na me lobhamohau
mado naiva me naiva mātsaryabhāvah
na dharmo na cartho na kāmo na mokṣaḥ
cidānandarupaḥ śivo'ham, śivo'ham
I have no hatred or dislike, nor greed, nor delusion; I have no pride, envy, or jealousy. I do not need the four necessities of life: *dharma* (duty), *artha* (wealth), *kama* (desires), liberation (*mokṣa*). I am the joy of pure consciousness and bliss. I am Śiva, I am Śiva.

na puṇyaṃ na pāpaṃ na saukhyaṃ na dukhyaṃ
na mantro na tīrtham na vedā na yajña
ahaṃ bhojanaṃ naiva bhojyaṃ na bhoktā
cidānandarupaḥ śivo'ham, śivo'ham
I have neither virtue nor vice, neither pleasure nor sorrow, nor happiness or sorrow, I have no need for any *mantra*, sacred places nor scriptures (*Vedās*). Nor do I perform any rituals or sacrifice (*yajña*). I am neither the food nor the eater nor the act of eating (no distinction between the knower, knowing, and known). I am the joy of pure consciousness and bliss. I am Śiva, I am Śiva.

na me mṛtyuśaṃkā na me jātibhedaḥ
pitā naiva me naiva mātā na janmaḥ
na bandhur na mitraṃ gurunaiva śiṣyaḥ
cidānandarupaḥ śivo'ham, śivo'ham
I have no fear of death because I have no death, nor senility or old age. I have no father, mother or birth. I am not the relative, nor the friend, nor the guru or disciple. I am the joy of pure consciousness and bliss. I am Śiva, I am Śiva.

ahaṃ nirvikalpo nirākāra rūpo
vibhutvāca sarvatra sarveṃdriyāṇaṃ
na cāsangata naiva muktir na meyaḥ
cidānandarupaḥ śivo'ham, śivo'ham
I am all-pervading and exist everywhere. I am without any form. I am beyond all senses. I am free from everything and I have no desire for or attachment to anything, not to this world nor for liberation (*mukti*). I am the joy of pure consciousness and bliss. I am Śiva, I am Śiva.

Part 6

Rāja Yoga

6.1

THE ROYAL PATH

In the period of the late Sanskrit texts – *Upaniṣads*, *Yogatattva*, *Dhyānabindu*, *Nādabindu* and some other texts composed after the fifth century BCE – there was a tendency to consider that spiritual liberation could not be attained only by means of gaining intuitive knowledge, but it had to be experienced as a result of following a certain Yoga technique. The *Śvetāśvatara Upaniṣad* was composed around the fifth century BCE (the middle period of the *Upaniṣads*), and stresses that the absolute unity of the Self (*ātman*) or *puruṣa* is the ultimate consciousness. The pure spirit (*ātman*) is identical to the transcendental reality known as *Brāhman*. In the *Śvetāśvatara Upaniṣad* (2:8–15) this text had already described some instructions for holding the body steady, breath control for controlling the vital forces in the body, and concentration to achieve subtler states of the mind in order to perceive *Brāhman*. The *Śvetāśvatara Upaniṣad*'s systematic presentation of Yoga was still in a rudimentary stage of development at this time, and it took about another six or seven hundred years before there was a change.

Around the second or third century CE, a sage by the name of Patañjali brought together all the threads of these previous teachings of the *Upaniṣads*, and compiled and formulated them into a new *Yoga darśana*, and used them as a tool for achieving the goal of the *Sāṃkhya* metaphysics, the liberation of *puruṣa* from the bondage of *prakṛiti*. This new *Yoga darśana* of Patañjali was titled *Yoga Sūtras* (Yoga aphorisms), a spiritual and masterly exposition of *Aṣṭāṅga Yoga* (the Eight Limbs of Yoga). This system of classical Yoga from Patañjali's *Yoga Sūtras* became paired with *Sāṃkhya* philosophy, and was recognised as one of the six orthodox systems of Hindu philosophy (*Ṣad Darśanas*; *darśana* is from *dṛiś* – 'to see'; spiritual vision).

Patañjali's Yoga is *Rāja Yoga* (Royal Yoga), which encompasses the teachings of all the main Yoga paths: *Laya*, *Kuṇḍalinī*, *Kriyā*, *Mantra*, *Jñanā*, *Bhakti* and *Karma*.

Rāja Yoga is a practical, systematic and scientific discipline that leads one to realisation of Ultimate Reality. The vision of God, the cognition of the Ultimate Reality, union with the Absolute, is the ultimate aspiration and aim of Yoga. If this aspiration is inwardly absent, the practice of Yoga becomes a mere mockery and a waste.

Rāja Yoga takes into consideration every aspect of life, in a gradual process of unfoldment. It shows how to overcome the imperfections of the lower nature and how to gain complete mastery over the mind and senses, so that one can regain true awareness and realise once again his or her everlasting oneness with the Divine.

Unlike religion, which relies on unquestionable faith and teaches its followers what to do, *Rāja Yoga* guides us to discriminate wisely and teaches us how to *be*. *Rāja Yoga* is not merely a practice, or set of practices, but the science of Life and

Reality, and is scientifically designed to restore an individual to his or her Divine Heritage.

Meditation (*dhyāna*) is the pinnacle of *Rāja Yoga* and the consummation of spiritual endeavour. It is through direct and practical experience of deep inner meditation that the aspirant can verify his or her true innermost nature as being divine, perfect and infinite. Through false identification with the body, mind, senses and the transient worldly forms, we have forgotten our true identity, which has limited us. It is this false identification which is the source of all our problems, suffering and unhappiness.

To break this bondage to our self-created illusions and identification with the false ego, Patañjali enlightens us on how to break the bondage in his *Yoga Sūtras*:

> *'Yogaś citta-vṛtti-nirodhaḥ.'*
> 'Yoga results from neutralising the vortices of feeling.'
>
> *Yoga Sūtras 1:2*

This is the basic definition of Yoga. The word *nirodhaḥ* can not adequately be translated. It does not really mean control or restraint, not in the sense of suppression or repression, yet it may include all these and more. *Nirodhaḥ* is a certain inner control, like the control over a motor car. Many of those practising Yoga, especially Yoga meditation, have a funny idea that Yoga means stopping thinking, making the mind totally blank and empty. Try it – it is impossible. Then how do I know what control means? In the case of a motor car, it implies knowing at what speed to go, where, when and how to apply the brakes, the clutch, etc. All this together constitutes control. It involves a deep understanding of what is involved. It does not mean making the mind blank. *Nirodhaḥ* is the kind of untranslatable word that you can paraphrase, comment on, or try to substitute a number of other words for, but if you have not experienced it, you cannot *know* what it is.

In the same *sūtra*, two more words were introduced – *citta* and *vṛtti*. These two words are explained here.

Just as light is reflected off a mirror back to its source, the soul-consciousness is reflected off the intellect or intuitive intelligence (*buddhi*) back to the soul (*puruṣa*). The intellect, the discriminating faculty (*buddhi*), which is centred in the frontal brain at the midpoint between the eyebrows, that is the liaison between *puruṣa* as pure awareness and the objects of the senses, functions like a mirror where sensations are reflected, so that the soul becomes conscious of its reflection in the intuitive intelligence. Images of the sense objects are received through the physical senses and are sorted by the recording mind (*manas*), the seat of thinking, which is the organising aspect of *citta* (feeling), which is centred in the heart. Due to the states of feeling in response to these images of objects presented to the intellect by the mind and senses, the reflection presented back to the soul becomes distorted and obscured by vortices of energy known as *vṛttis* (alternating vortices or eddies of thought impressions, desires, emotions, likes and dislikes that revolve around the ego). It is like looking into a mirror that is warped and covered in dust – you only see a distorted and clouded reflection of yourself. It is this mirror-distorted reflection that we may mistakenly think to be oneself. Similarly, the soul mis-identifies itself through the changing states of mind, the *vṛttis*.

Patañjali states, 'Yoga results from neutralising the waves of feeling.' Through Yoga meditation the mind is neutralised of the distorted reflection of the Spirit, leaving a clear reflection of the soul (*puruṣa*). Meditation stills the waves of feeling so that the Supreme Consciousness reflection as the blissful soul is clearly mirrored within.

Next, Patañjali states, 'Then (when the waves of thought and feeling are neutralised) the seer abides in its own true nature, the Self.' When the outward manifestations of consciousness, or vortices of feeling (*vṛttis*) are neutralised and made to be still, then Self-realisation occurs.

> *'Tadā draṣṭuḥ svarūpe vasthānam.'*
> 'Then the seer abides in its own true nature, the Self.'
>
> *Yoga Sūtras 1:3*

Yoga results from neutralising the vortices of feeling. Then when the vortices of feeling become still, the seer, or the perceiver (the subject, the conscious being) abides in its own true nature (the Self). Or in other words: the Self abides or dwells in the Self, the highest state of pure consciousness, *asamprājñāta samādhi* – 'superconsciousness beyond knowledge'. That is the highest state. Patañjali does not say that in this state one knows God, but only that the conscious being, the Self, exists in its own true nature. When this happens the mind turns inward and the *vṛttis* – the fluctuations and modifications of the mind which include thoughts, feelings and emotions – are reversed back and absorbed into the *citta*, the field of consciousness. The *citta* includes *manas* (recording mind that receives impressions through the senses), *buddhi* (intellect, the discriminating principle), *ahaṁkāra* (ego, the experiencer) and the storehouse of latent impressions (*samskāras*).

When there is a cessation of all *vṛttis* in the *citta*, the field of consciousness, what is left are only the *samskāras* (impressions) which remain as a residue of *asamprājñāta samādhi*.

The nature of the soul is pure consciousness. It has always abided in its own true nature, just as the nature of the sun is to shine – even when it is obscured by clouds it will always shine.

Patañjali then tells us that, at other times, when the seer is not established in its true nature, it becomes identified with the changing states of the mind.

> *'Vṛtti-sārūpyam itaratra.'*
> 'At other times the indwelling Self is identified with the changing states (modifications) of the mind.'
>
> *Yoga Sūtras 1:4*

When through the veiling power of *avidyā* (ignorance), the Self loses awareness and memory of its own true nature, it becomes identified and absorbed in the fluctuating thoughts and feelings of the mind. This creates the appearance as if the *buddhi* (intellect) and soul (*puruṣa*) are one; as if they appear to have only one perception. This misidentification creates the illusion that 'I am thinking and feeling', and creates in the *citta* and *buddhi* the feeling of a separate existence, an individual personalty that is separate from everyone, and from everything. Even though this illusion takes place, the soul (*puruṣa*), which is pure consciousness, and is beyond space, time and causality, remains unaffected and unchanged.

When the reflection of the Self in *buddhi* (intellect) is mixed together with the reflection of an object in the *buddhi*, it creates *vṛttis*, the vortices of feeling, and in turn these *vṛttis* create *samskāras* (latent impressions) which become stored in the *citta*, in the subconscious mind, where they lie latent, like seeds buried in the earth lying dormant until activated by favourable conditions.

The aim of Yoga is union of the individual self (*ātman*) with supreme Self (*paramātma*). To attain the aim of Yoga nothing is required externally; ultimate Reality and Truth is forever here and now. It is not found outside, for what we are seeking is within us.

The process of Yoga is to remove the obstructions in the mind or field of consciousness that veil us from realising our own true nature (Self-realisation). *Rāja Yoga*, the royal spiritual path to Self-realisation, leads one to the direct experience and awareness of one's true inner Self, and of the Self's eternal oneness with the Absolute, God.

The obstacle to realising our essential nature – the eternal, unmanifest and pure conscious Self – is the *vṛtti*, the thinking, feeling principle in the mind, which blocks the ever-present, ever-conscious, eternal reality.

6.2

INTRODUCTION TO AṢṬĀṄGA YOGA (THE EIGHT LIMBS OF YOGA)

Yoga unites the individual soul or Self to the supreme Reality, God, by means of the Eight Limbs of *Yoga*, which will be systematically explained. *Aṣṭāṅga* means 'eight limbs' (*aṣṭā* means 'eight'; *aṅga* means 'limb'). It is not unusual for Yoga teachers to use another terminology – the eight steps. When you look upon these as the eight steps it can give rise to a slight misunderstanding which is later condensed into a doctrine. When you climb a flight of steps you climb them one by one, so the Yoga teacher assumes that here in *Aṣṭāṅga Yoga* are also eight steps, that you must step up one by one.

However, if you look at this method as composed of eight limbs you see that one limb alone is incomplete, insufficient, inadequate, imperfect; and eight imperfections put together cannot lead to perfection. A human person is not an assembly of eight limbs – it's a person, the total being. Approached from that angle it suggests that on the very first day you are exposed to Yoga, or you practise anything concerning Yoga, you ensure that these eight limbs are all intact together. This is the essential difference between the two approaches. One teacher says that there are eight steps and unless you are fully established on the first two steps you are going to break your neck; and the other teacher says that unless you get together all the eight limbs at the same time, whatever you do is going to be imperfect. Yoga is integration and wholeness; only the eight limbs practised together constitute Yoga.

The eight limbs of Yoga that prepare us for the inward journey from the gross state of consciousness to the subtle, higher state, for realising our true nature, the Self, are as follows:

1. ***yama*** – self-restraints – social discipline
2. ***niyamā*** – fixed observances – individual discipline
3. ***āsana*** – posture
4. ***prāṇāyama*** – regulation of the vital-force (*prāṇa*) through the breath
5. ***pratyāhāra*** – withdrawing the mind from the senses
6. ***dhāraṇā*** – concentration
7. ***dhyāna*** – meditation
8. ***samādhi*** – absorption, superconsciousness.

In this complete system of Yoga, the eight limbs are the means to the final goal. The eight limbs are interdependent; they prepare different aspects of the mind and body for meditation and support the attainment of the superconscious or absorptive state of *samādhi*. The first five limbs – *yama*, *niyama*, *āsana*, *prāṇāyama* and *pratyāhāra* – are called external limbs (*bāhiraṅga*) and form the foundation for spiritual practice (*sādhana*), as the path of *Haṭha Yoga*.

The last three limbs – *dhāraṇā*, *dhyāna*, *samādhi* – are termed internal limbs (*antaraṅga*) that relate only to the activities of the mind. Together they are the path of *Rāja Yoga*.

When *dhāraṇā*, *dhyāna* and *samādhi* are performed together on the same object, it is termed *saṃyama*. This is a specific type of concentration in which *dhāraṇā*, *dhyāna* and *samādhi* alternate in rapid succession, resulting in giving profound knowledge of the object, and wisdom (*prājñā*).

In the *Haṭha Yoga Pradīpikā* (mid-fourteenth century) and the *Gheraṇḍa Saṃhitā* (late seventeenth century), two instruction manuals on Yoga, it is stated at the beginning of the first chapter of both books that the science of *Haṭha Yoga* leads to the superior science of *Rāja Yoga*.

Haṭha Yoga is only a means to the higher *Rāja Yoga*; they are both necessary and they support and complement each other. *Haṭha Yoga* is training the body with physical disciplines; this is the first step to training the mind or *Rāja Yoga*, that deals with the mind, consciousness and meditation.

Haṭha Yoga, when practised correctly, gives complete control over the physical body and the mind so that the yogi, staying in good health, will not be troubled when practising *Rāja Yoga* – meditation, leading to superconsciousness (*samādhi*), and beyond to final liberation (*kaivalya*).

These eight limbs of Yoga will be discussed in more detail in the following chapters.

In his *Yoga Sūtras* (2:28), Patañjali tells us that, by the consistent and sustained Yoga practice (*yogāṅganuṣṭhānād*) of these eight limbs, the impurities of the mind which are obstacles to Yoga – the five afflictions or *kleśas*: ignorance (*avidyā*), ego (*asmitā*), attachment (*rāga*), aversion (*dveṣa*) and clinging to life (*abhiniveśa*) – are removed, allowing the light and clarity inherent in *sattva buddhi* (pure state of mind) to manifest. This culminates in discriminative discernment (*viveka*).

The root cause and support of the *kleśas* is ignorance. It is like the bad root of a tooth causing pain to a person; until the root is removed, the person continues to suffer pain. Similarly, until ignorance is dispelled or removed, the five afflictions or *kleśas* continue to cause suffering. These *kleśas,* or psychological limitations, are the sources of psychological distress and self-ignorance. Yoga enables us to come to grips with ourselves, to see ourselves as we are in truth (not as we imagine ourselves to be) and by doing so remove the fundamental cause of psychological distress.

6.3

THE YAMAS AND NIYAMAS

The *yamas* (moral and ethical restraints) and *niyamas* (observances – personal and mental disciplines) are the foundation of spiritual life; without them, the other practices of *Yoga* and meditation have no power to take the aspirant to the ascent of spiritual realisation and illumination. These vows or commitments are universal. They have to be adhered to at all times, in all places, and under all circumstances. Then alone can one's impure conduct, habits and instincts, which contradict human nature and which have been established over years, generations and lifetimes, be overcome. In the absence of these vows of *yama* and *niyama* we become more and more enslaved to fulfilling our senses and fall into delusion, forgetting our divine nature.

Those who think Yoga is only for the purpose of performing Yoga postures, and that the aim of Yoga is to develop a beautiful, healthy, flexible and strong body, have only a partial view of what Yoga is. They are building their house on unstable foundations. We can build a sturdy house with bricks and mortar, but if it is not first standing firmly on strong and stable foundations, the house will collapse. For example, if a house is built on soft sand or soft mud the house will sink and collapse. Similarly, if our lives are not based on ethical principles and morality – non-harming, truthfulness, the wise use of one's energy (including sexual energy), non-stealing, and non-acquisitiveness – psychologically we become unbalanced and unsteady. We become ungrounded in our relationship with the environment, people and objects of the world we live in. The aim of practising true Yoga is: *yogaś citta-vṛtti-nirodhaḥ.* Yoga is the cessation of the fluctuating waves of thought and feeling (*vṛttis*) – the likes and dislikes that continually disturb the mind – obstructing you from realising your own true blissful nature (the Self). Yoga is also union of the individual self (*jīvātma*) with the supreme Self (*Paramātma*).

Yama and *niyama* are divided into ten principles or ten mental attitudes. They are universal human practices, and are the foundation of all true religions and spirituality.

The essential purpose of the *yamas* and *niyamas* is to promote moral and ethical principles in the individual and to limit the selfish expression of the ego. They are an integral part of Yoga practice and we cannot advance spiritually without practising them. The *yamas* and *niyamas* play an important part in purifying and preparing the mind for Yoga meditation.

The *yamas* and *niyamas* are not merely ethics and morality, but scientific requirements and logical stages, which are unavoidable in one's life. They are the means for self-adjustment with the state of affairs in which we are placed at the present moment. There is nothing unimportant, and nothing that can be neglected in this world; everything is of great value in some way. While living in the world we are all obliged to maintain a relationship with the environment, people and objects whether it be perceptual or conceptual. Our attitude to the people around us is the principal subject of the *yamas*. If we are to live a harmonious, peaceful, balanced and integrated life, we must first cultivate right attitudes towards others and towards oneself. The *yamas* apply both to the way we act in external relationships, and to our internal states of mind and body.

THE RELATIONSHIP BETWEEN *YAMA* AND *NIYAMA*

Yama and *niyama* have an intimate relationship – *niyama* safeguards *yama*. For instance, if one has contentment (the *niyama*: *santoṣa*) one will not steal (the *yama*: *asteya*), tell a lie (the *yama*: *satya* – 'truth') or harm others (*ahiṃsā* – 'non-violence'). Another example is if one has internal purity (the *niyama*: *śaucha*), one can achieve chastity, or conserve energy.

6.3.1 THE FIVE *YAMAS* (RESTRAINTS)

Ahiṃsā – non-harming, non-violence

Satya – truthfulness

Asteya – non-covetousness

Brāhmacarya – conservation of one's vital energy

Aparigrahā – non-possessive, non-attachment.

The word *yama* means 'restraint' – restraint with regard to one's behaviour, self-restraint. *Yama* basically means 'to refrain' from actions, words and thoughts which cause distress and harm to others. In Yoga these restraints must be self-chosen and self-imposed. The aspirant following the path of Yoga must be prepared to alter his or her way of life and to give some time each day to Yoga practice. It is important to begin with being aware of one's own behaviour, particularly from a moral and ethical point of view; therefore, discrimination is necessary.

Yama is also the name of the King of Death. In this context, *yama* means there must be a dying to ignorance, which is the source of egoism, attachment, hatred, greed and desire.

Patañjali tells us in his *Yoga Sūtras* (2:31) that the five *yamas* (*ahiṃsā*, *satya*, *asteya*, *brāhmacarya*, *aparigrahā*) are universal in their application, and that they are supreme, because they describe the absolute values of life. Because the *yamas* are absolute values, they do not require any modification – they apply to everybody in any and every country, at any and every time. Once we are able to see the interrelatedness of life, where every expression is interrelated to every other as part of the wholeness of life, then we will accept the *yamas* as absolute truths. We will incorporate them naturally into our lives without any struggle or effort of will.

The *yamas* are not commandments or rules that are determined by an Almighty God, who punishes us if we break the rules. No, the *yamas* or self-restraints are simply commitments that remind us to bring awareness to our actions of body, speech and mind. We need to remember that everything we think, say or do has an effect on those around us. Our reactions to things are our relationships, and our reactions evoke return reactions from people in a corresponding manner. The *yamas* are here for us to restrain harmful urges and impulses, and unwholesome thoughts.

Yoga is a gradual development of personality towards self-integration, which is achieved by the adjustment and adaption of oneself with the environment in which one lives. The *yamas* are very important because they limit the ego in its selfish attitude to life. The *yamas* (five restraints) regulate one's attitudes in relation with other beings. It is important for an aspirant on the spiritual Yoga path to make a conscientious effort to regulate one's habits and have control over one's behaviour by following the *yamas* and *niyamas*. The *yamas* purify and steady the mind, and should be practised in thought, word and deed at all times, under all circumstances, wherever you are. If the moral nature of the aspirant following the path of Yoga does not cooperate with his or her efforts, there cannot be progress in Yoga. This is because morality is an insignia of one's essential nature. If we remain contrary to what we are seeking, there will be no achievement. To be moral is to establish harmony between our own nature and the nature of that highest Truth which we seek in life.

AHIṂSĀ (NON-VIOLENCE, NON-HARMING)

Ahiṃsā is the root of the restraints (*yama*) and observances (*niyama*). The *yama* and *niyama* are for strengthening this root.

Ahiṃsā literally means 'non-violence' or 'non-harming'. But this word *ahiṃsā* also has a deeper philosophical meaning. When someone commits an act of violence by hurting another, it is not committed impersonally. Hurting or harming another is the outcome of a personal attitude of the mind. The intention behind the performance of an action is the deciding factor in concluding a judgement whether a particular action violates *ahiṃsā* or not. When a person commits an action, what is his or her intention? That must be noted. For instance, what is the difference between a surgeon who performs an operation with a sharp knife or scapel, and an assassin who stabs someone with a sharp knife? The difference is only in the intention, and not in the outward act. The outward acts are the same – they both cut a body with a knife – but their intention, motive and purpose is different. The surgeon compassionately uses his knife to save a life, and the assassin uses his knife to violently harm or kill, to end a life. So, the term *ahiṃsā*, from the point of view of Yoga, has to be considered in the larger context of relationship of things, and not merely in a social, political, or even a personal sense.

Unless a person has an intention or desire to harm, injure, hurt or exploit another person, he or she will not try to exploit, or commit a harmful act to anybody. Exploitation itself is an injury, and perhaps it is the the major injury that we inflict on others. The desire to use someone, at the cost of that person, for one's own advantage and selfish desire, is the root of the further manifestation of it in the form of violence, either psychologically, verbally or physically. *Ahiṃsā* is not merely a spiritual practice (*sādhana*), but a commitment which you must take and adhere to, making yourself an embodiment of universal love, kindness, compassion and forgiveness, radiating joy and peace to all.

There are two other *yamas* that also relate to exploitation – *asteya* (non-stealing), and *aparigrahā* (non-greed, non-possessiveness, non-hoarding). A thief is one who has the intention of using somebody for their own selfish purpose at the cost to the other person being exploited. Just the intention in the mind makes exploitation a theft. The desire to possess more than what a person actually requires is both theft (related to *asteya*) and possessiveness (related to *aparigrahā*). From this you can see how the *yamas* are interrelated.

Violence in speech or actions first begins in the mind. When the mind moves, the *prāṇa* also moves. When the *prāṇa* moves, the energy also moves – one follows the other. A thought arises of dislike towards someone, stirring up feelings of anger and hostility. If it is not controlled then the feeling of anger intensifies and manifests as hatred, and takes action in an attack of violence towards the other. This may create a negative consequence of revenge from the other person, stirring feelings of resentment and the thoughts of retaliating with an equal attack of violence – a vicious circle of fear, resentment, hatred and violence is created. In some cases anger can be justified; for example, a mother may shout at her child and even slap his bottom to make him aware of the danger of playing with matches or fire. The mother is not doing it with hatred, but out of love and compassion to protect her child. But hatred cannot be justified, it is always destructive. We need to be able to recognise and ensure that our initial negative thoughts and emotional responses do not translate into destructive verbal and physical action. We need to divert the mind from the source of irritation and defuse the negative emotional reaction before it explodes into anger.

The goal of Yoga is to realise that all life is One. If we are to truly live in that realisation, we must affirm that Oneness and unity by being kind, compassionate and respectful to all living beings in thought, word and actions. We must refrain from causing or wishing harm, distress or pain to any living being, including ourselves and the environment. It would also be equally wrong to approve of another person's harmful actions. Violence is destructive at all levels. We must not only refrain from violence against living beings, but against all forms – there can be violence in slamming a door closed in anger, or in picking a rare wild flower, or in polluting the environment. These expressions of violence are basically on the gross level, caused by ego, desire and attachment, but the mind also needs to be watched for the more subtle expressions of violence or harming that arises in one's own thoughts, feelings and emotions.

> 'You are all gods, if you only knew it. Behind the wave of your consciousness is the sea of God's presence. You must look within.'
>
> *Yogananda 2010, p.129*

Those who become established in *ahiṃsā* achieve equanimity, inner peace, and inner and outer happiness. With perfection of *ahiṃsā* one realises the unity and oneness of all life and attains universal love, peace and harmony.

SATYA (TRUTHFULNESS)

Satya, 'Truthfulness', the second of the five *yamas*, is very simple and easy to understand, because untruth is nothing but exploitation. God is truth; anything that contradicts truth contradicts God and denies God.

To exaggerate, pretend, distort, or lie to others, or to manipulate people for our own selfish concerns, is against our essential nature. Our essential nature is truth, and living in truthfulness means to be anchored in the awareness of God. Honesty with oneself is the first step to self-improvement. Without integrity in a relationship with others there can be no trust, and without trust no credibility or mutual respect. Dishonesty is due to selfishness and the fear of loss of reputation, to which one loses claim by being a hypocrite.

How can you ever achieve any success in self-realisation or self-knowledge by sending out false messages about yourself? If you tell lies, you construct a personality which consists of nothing but lies, and you deceive yourself. You can never know what truth is if you are immersed in lying or untruth.

To be truthful is not to be tactless. Thoughtfulness is essential to the usefulness of truth in relationship to others.

If you live in truth you will have peace of mind, free from fear, anxiety and worry. When you are true to yourself and to others in thought, word and actions, people will respect you from all walks of life. Those that live in truth have the power of the universe behind their thoughts and intentions. It is said that if a person makes truth the main focus of their life, every word that they speak will come true, because such a person is incapable of untruth.

The practice of truthfulness means being truthful under all circumstances, even if it is inconvenient. For example, there are some people returning from holidays abroad that avoid paying tax duty on expensive goods that they have brought back. They lie to the customs officers and walk through the green light that says 'nothing to declare'. Others tell lies and act dishonestly when they have to fill in their yearly tax returns. Trying to reveal something partially and keeping something back is also a kind of dishonesty. Thinking something inside while appearing to be something else outside is also a contradiction of truth. But on occasion that can also be an act of kindness and compassion. In order to uphold *ahiṃsā*, temporarily you may have to slightly deviate from truthfulness. For example, you see a beggar on the street who has a disfigured face due to a fire accident. Perhaps you feel revolted inside, but for fear that you might hurt this person's feelings if you turn away in disgust, you put on a calm appearance, smile from your heart and kindly give him a small monetary offering to help him. In this way you avoid hurting his feelings by not outwardly showing your revulsion. It is not wholly an expression of truth, but it becomes justifiable, because you have managed to uphold the higher *dharma* of compassion, of *ahiṃsā*.

Truth that harms is considered equal to untruth. We have to see the consequence of our conduct and behaviour before we can decide whether it is virtuous or not. When truthfulness endangers the lives of innocent people, should we be truthful? There is a story in the Hindu epic scripture, the *Mahābhārata* that covers this point.

THE STORY OF KAUSHIKA

Kaushika lived in a hut in the forest. He was an ascetic, who practised intense spiritual austerities. Kaushika had taken the vow of truthfulness and was true to his vow of truth.

One day he saw some frightened people running quickly towards him. As they reached him, he saw the terrified expressions on their faces. 'What is wrong?' he asked.

'We're being chased by robbers who want to kill us. Please, please let us hide here!' They then quickly hid themselves in the dense forest close to Kaushika's hut.

Soon afterwards, the robbers arrived, and seeing the ascetic, they immediately went up to him and asked if he had seen a group of people passing his way. Now, because Kaushika was avowed to truthfulness, he could not lie, so he said, 'Yes, I've seen them,' and pointed in the direction of the forest. 'They are hiding there.'

The robbers searched the forest, and found the terrified and innocent people, and killed all of them.

In this story from the *Mahābhārata*, it is said that Kaushika eventually died, and was sent to hell for causing the death of innocent people by his truthfulness. If he had told the robbers that he had not seen the people that the robbers were chasing, he would have told a lie, but that untruth would have saved his own life and also the lives of those innocent people.

Now, the moral of this story is that, under the circumstances, it would have been better for Kaushika to have lied to protect and save those innocent people, because in this case lying is as good as speaking the truth. By understanding the deeper meaning of righteousness, one will not see any unrighteousness in one who tells a lie in order to save innocent lives.

There were similar scenarios that happened during the Second World War when the Nazis were persecuting the Jews. There were many incidents that happened in concentration camps and ghettos, where innocent Jews were betrayed by their fellow inmates or informers, sending the innocent to the gas chambers. Perhaps some of the innocent Jews could have been saved if their inmates had lied to protect them.

In such extreme cases there is no harm in lying: telling a lie is as spiritually beneficial as speaking the truth, and being truthful is as spiritually harmful as telling an untruth. From the point of view of the *yamas*, it should be understood that unless the situation is extreme we must never lie. The general rule is that if telling the truth causes harm or injury to another's life or feelings, it is to be regarded as untruth, even though it looks like truth in its outer form. Our actions and thoughts should have a relevance to the ultimate goal of life. Only then do they become truths. There should be a harmony between the means and the end.

It is important to discern if our words and actions will result in harm or harmony. Before telling the truth or telling a lie we should examine our thoughts in case they cause harm to another. We should determine if the desire to act is motivated by an interest in the welfare and benefit of others or by a selfish need to protect oneself, or to punish another person.

Yoga morality is deeper than social morality or even religious morality. Our nature has to be in conformity with the form of Truth. As Truth is universal, any conduct which is not in harmony with the universal cannot ultimately be moral, at least in the sense that Yoga requires it. We have to become honest before Truth, and not merely in the eyes of our friends. It is this openness before the Absolute that is the meaning behind the *yamas* (moral restraints), as a course of self-discipline which is not imposed upon us, but as what one imposes upon oneself for attaining that moral nature consistent with the demands of Truth. When one knows the Self, he or she is no longer bound in delusion and ignorance, and so such a person no longer has any need of rules of behaviour, because he or she transcends all moral imperatives and acts spontaneously from the awareness that everything is his or her own Self. Love, compassion and truth is his or her nature.

ASTEYA (NON-STEALING)

Asteya is non-stealing or non-appropriation of what does not lawfully belong to oneself. These definitions have a negative connotation, but we need to read between the lines and see the positive attitude hidden behind them. Not everybody is a burglar or a thief in the sense of breaking into someone's house or going into a shop to steal a camera, but inwardly one can be a thief, in a different sense altogether. A thief can be someone who has the intention of using somebody for their own selfish purpose at the cost of the other person. Even if one entertains the intention in the mind, it is a theft.

If a person possesses more than what he or she is expected to possess, under the circumstances in which he or she is placed, that also becomes theft. To be earning undeclared income or receiving unemployment benefit that is given by government when you have no intention of working is also theft. Accepting a bribe is theft. On a more subtle level we can steal people's time, affections, attentions, ideas and thoughts, to win or gain attention and fame for ourselves.

Stealing out of necessity cannot be justified because it means violating another's right to keep what he or she has earned or inherited. *Asteya* means not depriving others of what belongs to them. In the case of someone who is homeless and steals a loaf of bread because they are hungry and have no money, the individual should be accountable for the crime first of all, while society should take necessary measures to treat the cause.

Stealing also breaks the *yama* principles of truthfulness (*satya*) by lying and dishonesty to conceal the theft; non-violence (*ahiṃsā*) because stealing disturbs the mind of the victim of the theft; and non-attachment (*aparigrahā*) by stealing with greed. Hoarding too much of anything is also stealing.

The main reasons for stealing are insecurity, selfishness, greed, poverty consciousness (the feeling that 'I am poor'), out of desperation ('I *must* have that'), and envy.

Greed and desire are the source of stealing. Desire keeps one continually looking to the future for one's fulfilment, instead of realising that perfection is attainable in the present, here and now. The mind is constantly turning outward, because it believes fulfilment lies in the external world. To try to gain satisfaction by fulfilling the endless desires that arise in the mind is an utterly futile endeavour; it will only cause unhappiness and sorrow. Desire arises from the ego, from the thought of 'I', 'I want', 'I need', 'I must have'. Examine your desires and you will find that what you are really wanting or seeking is eternal happiness and joy, eternal peace and eternal love. To experience this we must look within; it cannot be found outside of our Self. Jesus the Christ says: 'The Kingdom of God is within you' (Luke 17:2). The Kingdom of God is not a place that you can enter, it is your real essential nature; it is the Self. There is no one outside the Self – where is the other to find it? When you come to know your Self, which is identical to the absolute Reality, to God, then your true essential nature will be known. To know the Self one has to be still. The constant production of thoughts, feelings and images produced by the mind have to become neutralised, so that the mind becomes still. By meditation, focusing within on your Source, your essential Self, you will eventually become aware of yourself as pure Being, Existence, Consciousness and Bliss.

Once you attain love, joy and peace from within, it will also come to you from without. 'Seek ye first the Kingdom of God and all these things will be added unto you' (Luke 12:31).

It is through forgetfulness of our true identity and separation from God, the ultimate Truth, that we feel lost and experience unhappiness. The Spirit of God dwells within us, but until we have a conscious awareness of God's presence within, it cannot bear fruit in our experience.

BRĀHMACARYA (NON-SENSUALITY)

Brāhmacarya is the sum and substance of Yoga. The Sanskrit word *Brāhman* is the name given to the Ultimate Reality, the all-permeating Supreme Intelligence. *Carya* is derived from the root *car*, meaning 'to walk, to move, to live'. *Carya* means 'the way of living'.

Brāhmacarya means 'living with the inner consciousness flowing constantly towards Truth, the Absolute (*Brāhman*)'. *Brāhmacarya* is living in the awareness of the Absolute, God.

The word *brāhmacarya* has been misunderstood and mistranslated by many students, teachers, and even surprisingly by some *swāmis*. They generally understand *brāhmacarya* to mean celibacy. But celibacy is very restricted; it is an incorrect interpretation. Celibacy means abstinence from sex, sexual relations and sensual desires, and is generally thought to be practised by monks, priests and nuns. However, the word *brāhmacarya* is not limited to celibacy, though that maybe regarded as one definition of it. Morality is not a rigid formula of mathematics. No standard of it can be laid down for all times, and for all situations. Yoga considers *brāhmacarya* from all points of view, and not merely in its sociological and religious implication. Yoga morality calls for *brāhmacarya* of the purest type, which has a deeper significance. It requires a purification of all the senses, and what *brāhmacarya* really refers to is wise use of one's energy, especially with regard to the sexual impulse, because sexual excess leads to the dissipation of vital energy that is needed to attain higher states of consciousness.

Brāhmacarya means to conserve vital energy or force for the purpose of meditation. It is conserving one's power for a higher purpose – Self and God-realisation. All practices that successfully conserve and convert the sex energy into a higher form and utilise it for a higher spiritual purpose are included in the broad meaning of the term *brāhmacarya*. Therefore, *brāhmacarya* is not only a single act of restraint; it is a whole way of life, that involves moderation in all your activities and a wise restraint of all your senses.

To be *brāhmacarya* one does not have to be an unmarried celibate. There is no need to become self-righteous by judging others on this point. One can be in *brāhmacarya* in married life or a sexual relationship while following the path of Yoga. This is perfectly normal and part of a healthy balanced life. Of course, if the sex impulse becomes insatiable, compulsive, obsessive, addictive, perverted or abnormal, and we become attached to that desire, then it is not using the senses moderately and wisely. Over-indulgence in any of the senses depletes vital energy that could be used for attaining deeper states of consciousness. There must be a balance between the extremes of over-indulgence and repression.

Repression and suppression of sensual and sexual impulses can cause more harm because it leads to frustration and abnormal states of mind and behaviour. Therefore, *brāhmacarya* involves moderation in all your activities and wise restraint of your senses. When sex energy is wisely conserved and preserved, it gradually becomes transformed into a rarefied and subtler energy available for higher intellectual pursuits and meditation.

For one who has truly transcended sensual cravings for the aim of Self-realisation, sex is not an obstacle. Those who realise the greatness of a higher spiritual goal, and understand the necessity of the important *sādhana* (spiritual practice) of self-control in order to attain that goal, do it willingly and voluntarily. There is no question of suppression or repression forced upon you by circumstances beyond your control, by social environment, by religion, by an organisation, or through taboo.

Brāhmacarya in married life

If *brāhmacarya* only meant celibacy then married people who wanted to have children would not be able to practise Yoga. *Brāhmacarya* has a wider meaning than the restraint of the sex impulse, otherwise there could not have been householder saints and yogis with children. One such yogi was Lahiri Mahasaya (1828–1895), guru of Swāmi Sri Yukteswar (Paramhansa Yogananda's guru), who was initiated into the ancient technique of *Kriyā Yoga* by the immortal yogi-master Mahavatar Babaji in the foothills of the Himalayas in 1861. Lahiri Mahasaya was a householder yogi; he and his wife had five children born to them some years after Lahiri was initiated by Babaji.

It is interesting to note that during ancient times many saints were householders. They would bring up families while continuing their practice of Yoga and leading a spiritual life. To them, there was no conflict between sex and God. It was only later that asceticism and celibacy entered into the Indian religious tradition.

In most religious traditions sexuality is regarded as an obstacle to spiritual life; this has become ingrained in the human consciousness, causing feelings of guilt, shame and having sinned. Such wrong notions about the sex energy are all the result of a failure to understand the sublimity of this force.

Sex energy

Sex in itself is neither pure nor impure, it only becomes impure if it is used without discrimination, understanding, respect, care, love and responsibility. There is nothing to be ashamed of or to feel guilty about – we were all born from sex. Consciousness does not take birth without sex. God created sex for the purpose of procreation and creativity, not merely for sense-gratification and selfish pleasure.

The energy within you is a part of the Cosmic Energy, the great infinite Cosmic Force or *Mahā Śakti* that enlivens and sustains this universe. It is a manifestation and a dynamic expression of *Brāhman* (God). Cosmic Energy individualised in the human being is manifested in many aspects. A very important aspect in the physical biological aspect is sex energy. Sex energy is part of the one indivisible Cosmic Power present in every human individual. In its gross biological aspect, it is called sex energy; and in its subtle aspect, it is the energy of discrimination, that gives the power of the intellect to analyse and enquire. In a more subtle aspect it is the power of the *kuṇḍalinī*. In its supreme aspect, it is *ātma śakti*, because *Brāhman* (The Absolute, Infinite Consciousness,) and *śakti* are the static and dynamic aspects of one and the same principle. Therefore, the sex energy is nothing but the presence of the Divine Mother in all human beings. The sex energy is divine; it is a sacred process for cooperation with *Brāhma*, the Creator. It is the function of reproduction which is present in all nature and all life. Its supreme function is to keep the universal process going, for without this subtle power of duplication or reproduction, all species will become extinct.

Importance of the vital essence

A tree draws its essence from the earth, which is then circulated through the tree to its twigs, branches, leaves, flowers and fruits. The colour and vital life in the leaves, flowers and fruits is due to its essence (*rasa*). Similarly, semen (*vīrya* – 'potency'; *śukra* – 'seed'), that is manufactured out of the blood by the cells of the testes in the male, gives colour, lustre and vitality to the human body. The two male testes located in the scrotal bag are called secretory glands. And just as bees collect honey drop by drop in the honeycomb, so also the cells of the testes collect the semen drop by drop from the blood. The vital fluid is then carried by spermatic cords (*śukra-vahasrotases*) to the urethra. If the mind and body become sexually excited and a sexual act is performed, this vital fluid or semen which contains sperm is ejaculated by the ejaculatory ducts into the urethra, where it is mixed with the prostatic juice, and then suddenly ejected in orgasm out of the body.

Semen secretion starts during adolescence at about 14 to 16 years of age, depending on maturity. In *Āyurveda*, sex is contraindicated in children below the age of 16 years and above 70 years, because it has a depleting effect on the *ojas* and the body tissues. In males before attainment of age 21, and females before age 18, *ojas* is vitally needed to support and nurture the body system while it is still growing and developing. That is why traditionally in India celibacy is practised up to these ages. During old age (*vata* period starts at 70 years of age) catabolism is pronounced and one should abstain from sex to conserve one's own energy, and preserve the body tissues.

Semen (*vīrya* or *śukra*) nourishes the physical body, heart and intellect. The Yoga tradition states that to produce one drop of semen it takes 60 drops of blood, and to make one drop of blood it takes 60 morsels of food. According to *Āyurveda*, the secret of health lies in the preservation of this vital force contained in *śukra*. One who wastes this energy cannot have physical, mental, moral and spiritual development. The science of Yoga also teaches similar principles to *Āyurveda* in conserving vital energy for higher spiritual development. The yogis discovered that whenever the seminal secretion was conserved and reabsorbed into the body system, it went to the enrichment of the blood and strengthening of the brain, giving bodily, mental and spiritual vigour. Both the mind and the nerves are invigorated, and all the bodily systems renovated. Just as oil flows up a wick and burns steadily with a glowing light, so also does *śukra* or semen flow up by the scientific practice of Yoga and is converted into *tejas* or *ojas*, and is stored in the brain as *ojas shakti*. The brain cells are nourished, and the *ojas shakti* or spiritual energy is used for the higher practices of meditation. When this happens the yogi shines with Brahmic aura or lustre in his or her face. The very advanced yogis who practise *brāhmacarya* are able to get control over the astral nature of semen (*vīrya* or *śukra*) and prevent the formation of the actual semen fluid of the body. The science of Yoga informs us that semen exists in a subtle state throughout the body. It is withdrawn and turned into its gross form in the sexual organs under the influence of the sexual will and sexual excitement. But a very advanced yogi who has transcended sensuality and sexuality does not merely prevent the emission of gross semen already formed but actually prevents its formation as gross seed. In such a yogi, the semen dries up and the seminal energy ascends to the higher brain centres. He or she becomes established in both physical and mental *brāhmacarya*.

Āyurveda, 'The Science of Life' that dates back to about 5000 years, teaches us that this reproductive fluid, semen (*śukra*) is the most precious and potent substance in the human body. In *Āyurveda* it is one of the *Sapta Dhātus* (seven basic tissues). The Sanskrit word *dhātu* literally means 'to support' or 'to nourish'. These seven bodily tissues are composed of all five elements (*bhutas*), but only one or two elements predominate in each tissue. *Dhātus* promote the growth of the body and provide structure and nourishment to it. *Dhātus* are actually the material results of the functions of the three humors or *doṣas* (*vata*, *pitta*, *kapha*), the vital forces that influence all of the body's functions, which includes biological processes and mental functions.

Ojas

The generative counterpart of semen (*śukra*), sperm, is an ovum (*bījarakta*) in females and is termed variously as *puṣpa*, *phala* or *bījarakta*. The Sanskrit word *puṣpa* means 'flower', *phala* means 'fruit' and *bīja* means 'seed'. All these terms indicate that it is this generative cell which takes part in conjugation with sperm and formation of a fertilised ovum.

Though the sperm and ovum contain all the five basic elements, sperm (*śukra*) is cold and contains predominantly water element (*ap*), whereas an ovum (*bījarakta*) contains predominantly energy element.

The female gonads, the ovaries (*antahphala*), the corresponding part of the testes in the male, produce, develop and mature the precious, vital force like semen. This is the ovum. The ovum and the hormones secreted by the ovaries are essential for the maximum physical and mental wellbeing of a woman. Although the woman does not actually lose this precious vital force out of her body, as the man loses his semen when he ejaculates, it does leave the ovaries and is taken up in the process of conception to form the embryo. Child-bearing is a strain and drain on a woman's strength. Repeated depletion of this vital force and the strain of childbirth, and the intense sensuous excitement of the act, can shatter the nervous system and drain both the mental power and the body of energy. For these reasons women should also preserve this precious vital force.

The essence of semen is *ojas*, which vitalises the whole body. *Ojas* is a very fine and subtle material in the body; it is the purest form of all the tissues. It is the subtle essence of all *kapha* or water in the body, particularly the essence of the reproductive fluid. *Ojas* gives vitality, energy, lustre, strength and immunity to the whole body. Excessive sexual indulgence with great loss of the reproductive fluid and *ojas* takes its toll on the physical body. Losing its vitality, the body's immunity becomes imbalanced and more prone to loss of strength and disease. The digestive fire (*agni*) becomes weakened due to diminished *ojas*. With weakened *agni*, digestion becomes less effective, leaving the undigested and partially digested materials that *Āyurveda* terms *ama* (accumulated impurities and toxins). Creativity and joy are dampened, and the mind becomes weak and restless. Wandering aimlessly, the mind is unable to concentrate properly. For an aspirant practising Yoga and meditation, this is a great obstacle. A mind filled with desires and sexual fantasies is unable to meditate. Therefore, moderation and restrained sexual activity is recommended for physical and mental health.

According to Yoga and *Āyurveda*, a person with abundant *ojas* is vital and vibrant, with a strong, firm and flexible body; the skin is smooth and clear with radiance or lustrous glow; the eyes are bright and sparkling. He or she has a sharp and clear mind, increased memory, spiritual power, intelligence, health, vital energy, love, and joy that radiates outward with an inner glow. *Ojas* is responsible for psychological stability and provides resistance, protection and strength to endure emotional conflicts.

The life-sustaining essence *ojas* can be decreased not only through sexual excess but also, according to *Āyurveda*, through anything that aggravates or increases *vata dosha*, such as irregular schedule and *vata*-increasing foods. Over-consumption of too many spices and bitter herbs, and eating food tasting of only one flavour, can also reduce *ojas*. As also can excessive exercise, fasting too long or too often (causing dryness, wasting and emaciation of the body), anxiety, anger, worry, grief, sorrow, depression, stress, excessive discharge (of semen, blood, mucus), time factors (old age), illness, injuries to the body, alcohol, smoking and stimulant drugs.

For regulating and redirecting sexual energy

For those who are practising Yoga and meditation who would like to regulate their sexual activity, it is advised to become vegetarian (red meat stimulates the sexual appetite), and abstain from garlic, onions, hot spices and alcohol, as all of these stimulate the sexual appetite.

The energy of the sex impulse can be regulated by channelling it into physical exercise, sports, nature hikes, and into creative outlets such as art, playing a musical instrument, craft-making and writing. This creative energy of the sex impulse can also consciously be withdrawn from the lower *chakras* and redirected to the higher centres in the brain in meditation, using the power of concentration, breath and *mantra*.

A meditation for redirecting sexual energy for males and females

Sit in any comfortable meditation pose, with the head, neck and spine aligned. Close the eyes and relax the whole body. Keep the body still and bring your attention and awareness to the area in your body where the sexual organs are located. Now begin to inhale slowly and deeply in *ujjayi* breath (breathing with a slight contraction of the glottis in the throat to produce a soft hissing sound), feeling a cool sensation with a suction effect of drawing the current of life energy upward in the spine. Imagine that the breath starts from the sexual organs, and redirect it inward towards the spine, and then upward through the spine to the midpoint between the eyebrows, at the Spiritual Eye, the seat of spiritual consciousness. Then holding the breath in, concentrate at the Spiritual Eye and mentally chant *Oṁ* three times, feeling that you are transmuting the energy as you do so. Then exhale and relax, and feel that you are transmuting the sexual energy into *ojas* and spiritual energy – giving vitality, energy, lustre, strength and immunity to your whole body.

Repeat this method of meditation six to 12 times until you feel inwardly calm. Then remain in the state of the present-moment stillness and deep inner calmness. Dissolve all sense of individuality and separateness… Expand your consciousness into the Infinite and feel that Oneness with all that is God… Mentally affirm that the infinite presence of the Divine is ever within you: '*I am resting in the calm stillness of eternal peace and eternal love that is God. I am free, I am free, I am free.*'

Restoring vitality after sexual intercourse

Āyurveda recommends that the best time for engaging in sexual intercourse is during the two hours between 10 pm and midnight. It is advised not to perform sex at dawn, midday, dusk or midnight, because at these times *vata* and *pitta* are increased, and one cannot take adequate rest after sexual intercourse.

To help restore vitality that may be depleted after engaging in sexual intercourse, *Āyurveda* recommends the following drink recipe. Mix into a mug of warm milk a spoonful of ghee (clarified butter), a few ground almonds or cashews, a teaspoon of raw sugar, and a teaspoon of the deeply nourishing herbs Ashwagandha (*Withania somnifera*) and Shatavari (*Asparagus racemosa*), Āyurvedic herbs in powder form. Shatavari is particularly good for women.

APARIGRAHĀ (NON-POSSESSIVENESS; NON-COVETOUSNESS)

The Sanskrit word *apara* means 'of another' and *agraha* 'to grasp or crave'. *Pari* means 'things'. *Aparigrahā* means 'without craving for what belongs to another'. It can also mean 'not hoarding or accumulating'. *Aparigrahā* also has another meaning: living a life of simplicity, not being unnecessarily extravagant and luxurious, because the more you live an extravagant and luxurious life the more things you will want. Your desires to possess become endless, bringing enmity and jealousy, leading to inner restlessness, frustration, disappointment, and loss of contentment and peace of mind.

The difference between non-covetousness and non-greed is that non-covetousness means not to desire what is not rightfully one's own, whereas non-greed means not to be attached even to what already is one's own. In fact, non-greed is more appropriate in connection with *aparigrahā* than *asteya* (non-stealing).

Possessiveness has exclusiveness, there is an attachment to it – an ego-sense of 'I'-attachment ('It's mine, I own it, it belongs to me'). Possessions themselves are not the problem, it is our attitude towards them that creates problems. It is not that we have to deny ourselves of all material possessions, obviously while we are living in the world we need food, clothes, a house to live in and provisions for our health. These are accepted essentials that we have to acquire in order to live. The problem of possessiveness arises only when we become attached to our possessions or when we desire and crave more. If we become attached, addicted or dependent on our possessions, we bring suffering and pain to ourselves. There is a difference between acquisition for utility according to one's needs, and acquisition for possessiveness – to use with attachment or exclusiveness.

As well as material objects and other people, possessiveness also applies to what the ego identifies with – our own body, thoughts, feelings and emotions. We can become grasping and possessive with fame, power and knowledge. Possessiveness can also motivate us to keep something that is no longer useful to us, or prevent someone else from having it.

If we go to the root of 'grasping' and possessiveness we can understand that from attachment arises fear, and the root cause of fear is *avidyā* (ignorance). Fear is the key word here. We are afraid of not having something when we need it. Fear of not having enough to live on. Fear of losing our health and our wealth. Fear of not being loved, fear of being alone. And ultimately we fear death; we cling to life and all its entrapments. We are afraid of the unknown. We fear because we have forgotten our true essential nature, the eternal inner Self, which is *Sat-chit-ānanda* (Ever-Existing, Ever-Conscious, Ever-New Bliss), and so in our ignorance and through mis-identification we look outside ourselves for the support we crave, and become disconnected or separated from our true Divine Source within.

6.3.2 THE FIVE *NIYAMAS* (OBSERVANCES)

Practising the *yamas* alone is not enough. They are necessary and indispensable to stop you going in a downward direction into delusion and impurity, but at the same time, you must also make an effort to progress in a positive upward direction towards spirituality and divinity. Therefore, the great yogic sage, Patañjali, formulated the five *niyamas* or obligatory observances.

The yogic discipline of practising the *yamas* and *niyamas* is the foundation of spiritual life. They help to purify the mind and develop one-pointed concentration. The *niyamas* are the personal observances. They are similar to the *yamas* as far as their importance is concerned, but there is a difference in that the *niyamas* have a greater connection with the individual personally than the *yamas*, which have a particular reference to one's attitude towards, or relationship with the society outside.

There are five principles of *niyama*:

Śauca – purity, cleanliness

Santoṣa – contentment

Tapas – austerity

Svādhāya – study leading to the knowledge of the Self

Īśvara praṇidhāna – devotion to the Supreme Lord.

ŚAUCA (PURITY, CLEANLINESS)

Any entanglement of consciousness in things or circumstances which have no constructive relationship with the goal of Yoga are to be regarded as an impurity. This is the essential meaning behind the term *śauca*. Purity means both inner and outer cleanliness of the body and the mind. *Niyama* is purity of conduct, internally and externally. It is not only the physical body that has to be kept pure, but also the *prāṇas*, the mind, the senses and the intellect, all have to be kept pure. Purity implies freedom of oneself from everything which cannot be set in harmony with the aim of Yoga. This also implies non-contact with those objects which communicate impurity or exert an unhealthy influence. Association with undesirable company should also be avoided.

Purity means being pure in body, mind and speech. For most people, physical purity is comparatively easy to maintain. Purity of speech is difficult, but more difficult than these is maintaining mental purity. In human society, even those who have high social status, and keep themselves and their house physically clean, can still behave badly and have impure thoughts. One can cause harm to another person by a wrong attitude of speech, and even a jealous glance. Again, we can see how *ahiṃsā* (non-harming) is connected with *śauca*. *Ahiṃsā* is the supreme virtue, and all the other principles of *yama* and *niyama* come under *ahiṃsā*.

The inner light of the soul within you is the same light in all people, but it appears to shine more brightly in some people than others. If you have two oil-burning lamps that give the same amount of light, but the glass window of one lamp is covered with dust and soot, then the other lamp will shine more brightly. It is not a matter of more light, but of cleaning or clearing away the impurities that are blocking the light. To allow the soul's light within us to shine freely and brightly we need to cleanse our physical body both internally and externally; purify our mind and emotions, and keep the environment in which we live clean and orderly.

In the Bible – the Gospel according to Matthew – Jesus says: 'Blessed are the pure in heart, for they shall see God' (Matthew 5:8).

Pure heart is actually the pure mind. Physical eyes are not necessary to see God, for even a blind person can perceive and experience God with the inner eye of the pure mind.

Internal purity is more important than external purity, because when the mind is pure and one-pointed, one is able to see clearly and purely. Without cleanliness and purity (*śauca*), *brāhmacarya* cannot be attained. *Brāhmacarya* and *śauca* work together.

According to Patañjali (*Yoga Sūtras* 2:40), physical cleanliness helps one to reduce lustfulness, and this is the primary reason why physical cleanliness has to be observed. The yogi reflects on the nature of the physical body, and sees that no matter how many times it is washed and cleaned, it becomes dirty again. Every day one has to clean the body of waste products: body odours, sweat, mucous, phlegm, bile, dead skin cells, urine, faeces, blood or menses (in females), and other bodily secretions. The yogi having observed the impure nature and impermanence of the body gradually develops a dispassion for the body as a source of pleasure. This leads to an awareness of the unclean state of other people's bodies, and a distaste develops to engage in intimate sensual or sexual contact with the bodies of others. However, this dispassion for the physical body does not make one become apathetic, unfriendly, unloving or unaffectionate towards others. The yogi rises above physical sensuality and lustfulness, but keeps the body clean and healthy, so that it may be a fit vehicle of enlightenment. The yogi sees his or her body as a temple of God.

> 'The food that we eat is transformed in three different ways: the gross part of it becomes waste matter, the middle part is transformed into flesh, and the subtlest part goes to form the mind.'
>
> *Chandogya Upaniṣad 6.5.1*

Cleanliness and purity also applies to the food you eat. For a yogi, purity means eating food that is *sattvic* in nature. Because the food we eat affects both the body and the mind, it must be pure, fresh and wholesome and vegetarian. The food should not be stale and rotten, nor must it be extremely spicy.

> 'The foods that promote longevity, vitality, strength, health, happiness and a good appetite, which are filled with flavour and nourishing, substantial and agreeable, are liked by the *sāttvika* person.
>
> The foods that are very bitter, sour, very saline, excessively hot, pungent, dry and burning are liked by the *rājasika* person. Such foods are unhealthy and disease producing.
>
> Those foods which are stale and tasteless, putrid, foul-smelling, impure, and the leftovers of others, are the foods liked by the *tāmasika* person.'
>
> *Bhāgavad Gītā 17, 8–10 (Author's translation)*

The food you consume, the people you associate with, the environment that you live in, the thoughts that you harbour, and the things that you read all need to be considered if you are to live, behave and move in purity.

When the body is clean, and the mind purified of all worldliness, the mind becomes *sattvic* and one attains cheerfulness (*saumanasya*). From this arises one-pointedness (*ekāgra*) – the mind is able to concentrate on one object during meditation. This, in turn, leads to control of the senses, subjugating both *rajas* (activity, passion) and *tamas* (inertia). Then with the mind established in purity (*sattva*) and all mental content stilled, one is fit to perceive the Self (*ātman*), which is pure, undifferentiated consciousness.

SANTOṢA (CONTENTMENT)

The Sanskrit word *santoṣa* has its root in the word *tush* meaning 'to be pleased'. *Santoṣa* is a psychological discipline and also a metaphysical discipline. It not only helps to liberate you from your present condition of false personality and sense cravings, but also helps you to become more established in your permanent and divine state of *puruṣa*, the blissful Self.

> 'As a result of contentment one experiences supreme happiness.'
>
> *Yoga Sūtras 2:42*

True contentment is attained only when the mind has been freed from the qualities of *tamas guṇa* and *rajas guṇa*. There is a predominance of *rajas guṇa* (quality of activity and passion) in the mind that keeps it constantly occupied with thoughts of external things, people, and objects outside of our own self. The desire and endless wanting to obtain them generates excitement, anticipation and intense longing in us. And our ego says, 'I will be happy when I get what I want.' For example, when a person falls deeply in love, he or she finds that just the mere presence of the other individual is joyfully intoxicating. Just to look at the other individual is a mesmerising experience. For a while this makes one feel happy and content, but after one gets to know the other individual intimately, it seems impossible to sustain that same level of joyful intoxication. One may still find the other individual attractive, and feel tremendous affection for them, but that special something, that magic, is gone. One has invested all their happiness in the other, but what one is left with is discontentment.

To the ego and the personality, happiness is equated with the excitement of wanting to possess and acquire something or someone for oneself. When we possess a desired object, we experience pleasure, and there is a form of happiness in that pleasure. But even when the object of desire has been obtained, the enjoyment of the object, and the happiness attained from it, is short-lived. We quickly become discontented and new desires arise in the mind for something else. *Rajasic* and *tamasic* desires are always projected into the future, and so happiness and contentment cannot be present here and now. When the mind is free of desires, it is true contentment, which brings inner and outer happiness.

If we consider the truth of our own personal experience we recognise that our moments of greatest joy, happiness and contentment were actually those moments when we desired nothing and wanted nothing, absolutely nothing at all, from anyone or anything. In that moment of not wanting or desiring, we were perfectly content, happy, and at peace within.

In contentment there is no competition and no comparativeness. *Santoṣa* is a sense of contentment that arises when you do not compare yourself with others, or compare your acquisitions with what others have.

Contentment is a state of happiness and equanimity, accepting things as they are and being satisfied with what one has. To be content is also to have a true understanding and knowledge of one's own powers and limitations. Being content is accepting every moment as it is, without thinking that it should or could be different. In the contented state one affirms:

> 'My happiness is complete by itself. I am sufficient as I am. My happiness is not dependent on the senses and their gratification. I am not the sense, nor the body, nor the mind, I am *Sat-chit-ānanda*, the ever-conscious and eternal blissful Self.'

When your consciousness is established in its own pure natural and spiritual state, you know yourself as you truly are, and do not feel yourself to be something you think yourself to be.

Contentment is not a passive acceptance of one's physical and psychological circumstances and unnecessary sufferings and pain, or resignation to life. It does not mean that we should not make future plans, but rather that plans grow from our present reality, living in the present moment, rather than from dreaming and longing.

Live with awareness in the present moment; have no desire to know the nature of the next moment. Wishful thinking and anticipation often lead to disappointment, causing anxiety and tension, which drain one's energy.

When we are content, we are happy. Happiness is a state of mind which is independent of circumstances, and does not depend upon any external conditions at all. Our happiness should not be conditioned by what we have or do not have. Happiness and unhappiness are states of mind. The mind that is constantly changing and not content cannot be satisfied or fulfilled permanently with anything. If a person is not content, their mind will restlessly wander, and they will find it impossible to concentrate and meditate.

> *'Yogas citta-vṛtti-nirodhaḥ.'*
> 'Yoga (union) is neutralising the vortices of feeling.'
>
> *Yoga Sūtras 1:2*

When all conflict and confusion in the mind is resolved, the vortices (*vṛttis*) subside and become calm. The mind becomes still, and from this stillness of thoughts and feelings arises contentment, which brings a continuous flow of happiness and inner peace. The light of the soul, the Divine Self, reveals itself without any distortions when the vortices (*vṛttis*) of feeling formed by countless desires and attachments subside.

Contentment (*santoṣa*) is closely related to equanimity (*samata*), which means being equal-minded, calmness of mind, freedom from attachment and aversion.

In the *Bhāgavad Gītā* there are references to both contentment and equanimity. Krishna says:

'That person of action is free from karma who accepts with contentment whatever comes to them, who is free from jealousy, and has transcended all dualities of life, and who is balanced in success and failure.'

Bhāgavad Gītā 4:22 (Author's translation)

'Those whose minds are established in equanimity (equal-mindedness) are free from the relativities of existence (birth and death, pleasure and pain), even in this world. They are flawless like the Supreme Reality. With even mind they are already situated in pure consciousness...

Being fixed in deep inner communion with the Supreme Truth, with unwavering discrimination and free from delusion, they are neither falsely elated by pleasant experiences or depressed by painful ones.'

Bhāgavad Gītā 5:19–20 (Author's translation)

TAPAS (AUSTERITY)

The Sanskrit word *tapas* is derived from the root *tap* 'to heat' or 'to burn'. *Tapas* literally means 'that which generates heat'. When there is heat, there is also energy. *Tapas* is energy that is concentrated or focused with conscious willpower on a specific point, so that it releases power and sets it in motion. The practice of *tapas* through self-disciplined training of the body, mind and senses enables one to strengthen a firm resolve to overcome the egoistic nature of the mind, and direct the power of the mind for higher spiritual aims and purposes. This is likened to concentrating the sun's rays through a magnifying glass over a piece of paper. The heat is concentrated and intensified into a single fine beam of light, which produces a powerful energy of heat to burn the paper.

The practice of *tapas* enables one to strengthen a firm resolve and develop a strong willpower to overcome the egoistic nature of the mind. *Tapas* helps one to control and direct the power of the mind and body for higher spiritual aims and purposes.

A person who has *tapas* is full of spiritual fervour. The heat of strength, or power, or energy is generated and increased in one's system by the restraint of the senses and the mind. There is a burning zeal for Self and God-realisation. Essentially, *tapas* is restraint of the senses and the mind. *Tapas* or austerity is the practical application of the *yamas* and *niyamas* through such acts as simple living, that is, free from sensual indulgence, maintaining an occasional fast, maintaining a vow of silence, practising *prāṇāyama*, practising deep meditation, chanting the names of God, subjecting the body to occasional strain and hardship for spiritual reasons, and so on. A person who practises *tapas* has greater strength and willpower than one who does not practise it. One who performs *tapas* has a glow in his or her face, a lustre in their eyes, an aura around their personality, a strength in their speech, and a capacity in their body on account of the austerity that he or she performs. Every word that he or she speaks will have tremendous force and will carry conviction. *Tapas* is austerity of the whole personality – body, speech, senses and the mind.

Three types of austerity

The *Bhāgavad Gītā* (17:14–16) classifies three types of austerity which are *sattvic* in nature:

> **Austerity of the body.** Worship of God; adoration for holy people, gurus (spiritual teachers) and the wise; maintaining physical purity; straightforward behaviour; sexual restraint; harmlessness (refraining from committing violence) – these are considered the austerities of the body. Physical austerity also contributes to developing mental strength and willpower.
>
> **Austerity of speech.** Speaking words that are truthful, inoffensive, pleasant and beneficial, as well as the repetition of *japa* and recitation of the sacred texts: these are considered the austerities of speech.
>
> **Austerity of the mind.** Calmness, Even-mindedness, cheerfulness, gentleness, silence, and self-restraint. Purity of heart, and meditative communion with the inner Self: these are considered the austerities of the mind.

Tapas or austerity in Yoga is not mortification or self-torture, as implied in extreme acts of asceticism, such as lying on a bed of nails, flagellation of the body, walking on hot coals, or standing on one leg for years (the leg becomes shrivelled and useless for lack of use). In the *Bhāgavad Gītā*, Krishna clearly states that austerity which is performed with deluded understanding and torture to the mind, senses and body, or undergoing penances with the aim of causing injury to another, is declared to be *tamasic* (ignorance; darkness). In fact, it is the subtle force of their attachment to sense pleasure that moves them to such severity!

> 'Those ostentatious austerities which are practised with the object of gaining respect, honour and admiration are said to be rajasic (in the mode of passion), unstable and transitory.
>
> Austerities which are practised foolishly, with self-torture, or for injuring others, are said to be *tamasic* (in the mode of ignorance).'
>
> *Bhāgavad Gītā 17:18–19 (Author's translation)*

It is important to understand that *tapas* is not an end in itself. *Tapas* should be practised with intelligence and discrimination. To torture the body and mind, and make the senses dull and unresponsive, is not the purpose. *Tapas* practised in the true spirit of Yoga is not penance (an act performed through feelings of regret that one has committed a sin). To flagellate one's own body or lie on a bed of nails is not part of the yogic attitude towards life; this is denying life in a negative way. The ascetic pursues pain to avoid pleasure and the worldly person seeks pleasure to avoid pain. In both, pain is inseparable from pleasure.When we pursue pleasure or pain, we deny ourselves freedom, peace and joy in life. We have to find a balance between indulgence and abstinence.

> 'Those who eat too much or eat too little, who sleep too much or too little do not find success in Yoga… Those that are regulated and balanced in eating, sleeping, work and recreation find an end to sorrow through Yoga.'
>
> *Bhāgavad Gītā 6:16–17 (Author's translation)*

Through Yoga disciplines we can train our bodies and senses to be useful instruments of selfless service to others. In this way our minds become purified and we can make a positive contribution to life.

When we have control over the mind and its modifications, and the senses are naturally and spontaneously regulated, the body and mind become clear channels for the soul within to express itself naturally and clearly. The object then of *tapas* is to train the body, mind and senses to become steady and balanced so that they work naturally, spontaneously and selflessly for the soul to express itself purely.

SVĀDHYĀYA (SELF-STUDY)

> 'By self-study one is united with that loved aspect of divinity.'
>
> *Yoga Sūtras 2:44*

Sva as a prefix means 'oneself', 'one's own'; *dhyāya* means 'to study'. *Svādhyāya* means 'self-study'.

Svādhyāya (self-study) in combination with *tapas* (austerity) and *Īśvara praṇidhāna* (devotion to the Supreme Lord) work together as tools for weakening the five afflictions (*kleśas*): ignorance; egoism; attraction; repulsion; and clinging to life, or fear of death.

Svādhyāya is study that leads to the true nature of one's own Self, connected with the goal of life – Self- and God-realisation. Self-study is not an intellectual process, but simply a perceptive awareness of the movements of the mind, which arise through our distraction from moment to moment. When we recognise our distraction or lack of awareness we can discover our true identity, and reality as it is.

Patañjali also says:

> 'Austerity, self-study, and devotion to God is *Kriyā Yoga*.'
>
> *Yoga Sūtras 2:1*

Svādhyāya can also mean the study of sacred or scriptural texts and the silent or mental recitation of *mantras* to oneself. The mental recitation of *mantras* in this way is called *japa*. By repeating the *mantra*, inevitably your consciousness takes on a certain subtle form. Both the study of scriptural texts and *mantra japa* are to be practised in a meditative and concentrated state of absorbed awareness. If they are practised mechanically and without an understanding, then they have a negative value.

Such sacred texts as the *Bhāgavad Gītā*, Patañjali's *Yoga Sūtras* and *The Gospels of the New Testament* can be recited every day, with concentration and contemplation on their meaning, and absorbing one's mind in them. We can also be inspired by reading the writings of the great saints such as St Francis of Assisi, and by reading works written by sages, yogis and spiritual Masters, such as *Autobiography of a Yogi* by Paramhansa Yogananda (1946). We can study their inspired expositions and ourselves be spiritually inspired by them. This helps us by awakening the spirit of enquiry within us, and by directing our thoughts and energy in the right direction, preventing us from reading false lessons from our life's experiences.

The basis for self-study is concentrated within all the *yamas* and *niyamas*. These confront our involvement with all of life around us and then slowly centre in a study of our inner self. When one has become established in the first three *niyamas* – *śauca* (purity), *santoṣa* (contentment) and *tapas* (austerity) – then one is ready for self-study, self-introspection or self-awareness. In self-study one learns not by gaining intellectual or material knowledge but by self-inquiry (*ātma-vichāra*), a method of reflection and discrimination for investigating the nature of the Self. It is observing with awareness our own thoughts, feelings, behaviour, desires, motives and attitudes, so that we can see the delusions, false attachments and ignorance that prevent us from realising our true inner Self.

The practice of *svādhyāya* helps to reduce the obstacles of desire, selfishness and attachment that keep us bound in ignorance and delusion. *Svādhyāya* encourages spiritual awakening in us, so that we can realise our divine nature and the reality of God.

At the deepest level of our inner being we are pure consciousness, made in the image and likeness of God. If we do not know this, it is because of self-forgetfulness and ignorance due to identification with the mind and the objects of the senses. All our problems in life ultimately stem from our separation from the source of our divinity, which is the Ultimate Reality, God.

Most people live primarily for themselves and their families; their vision seldom reaches higher than that. Society (politicians, teachers, parents, the advertising media) teaches and conditions us to look outside of ourselves for happiness and fulfilment. But the great spiritual Masters tell us differently. Jesus said: 'The Kingdom of God is within you' (Luke 17:21). He also stated: 'But seek ye first the Kingdom of God, and His righteousness; and all these things shall be added unto you' (Matthew 6:33). And in the *Bhāgavad Gītā* (9:22) Krishna reflects a similar message: 'To those who meditate on Me as their very own, ever united to Me by incessant devotion, I provide their deficiencies and make permanent their gain.'

The Kingdom of God, which is Infinite Intelligence, wisdom, love, joy and inner peace, is within each one of us. These qualities are within us because they are in God, and we are made in His image. Each one of us is an expression of God-consciousness, using God-faculties and expressing God-qualities. Until we awaken to this fact of life, and experience the presence of God within, knowing that we have free will to choose and can direct our mind, control our emotions, senses and body, we will continue to remain unaware in a conditioned state of sleep. In this state of somnolence or ignorance, the Spirit of God dwelling within us cannot express itself in all its light and glory; the soul's potential is in effect thwarted. In this conditional state of ignorance we are delayed in attaining our perfect and complete experience of superconscious union with God.

The practice of svādhyāya

When you awaken to your true nature within, your innermost consciousness or Self, you will grow into the light, which will remove all darkness and unknowing from your mind and consciousness. With soul-awareness you will be able to control your own destiny, living a life guided by the divine Spirit within, governed by truth.

The Absolute Reality, God, cannot be completely understood or realised through the intellectual process. Understanding refers to *indirect* knowledge, whereas Self-realisation refers to *direct* knowledge. Self-study must begin with awareness and an understanding of the mind's movements, the study of the nature of thought and the thinking process. What is thought? How does it arise? What are its functions and limitations? Self-study is simply a perceptive awareness of the movements of the mind. When we recognise our distraction or lack of awareness we can discover our true identity and reality as it is. All that is needed is attention to what is happening in us and around us in each moment. Whatever we are doing, whether we are breathing, meditating, working, studying, cleaning the dishes or eating a meal, if we do it with attentive awareness, each moment will be a freeing experience in which we will see and understand something new.

Life requires of us to be constantly in clear awareness, with a quiet mind which is full of energy, love and compassion – a mind which is free from past conditioning, reactive behaviour patterns, subconscious motivations, habitual ego-centred behaviour, sense-urges, negative emotions and negative attitudes. In the quiet, aware and alert mind there is true freedom from tension, conflict and sorrow. There is a direct perception of life without distortion.

Without attentive awareness and alertness, our consciousness becomes clouded, we become sleepy and our senses lose their sensitivity and become dull. When our attention and sensitivity are sharpened and heightened with awareness, our perception becomes clear. In this state of observation we are able to perceive and recognise those limiting conditions within our minds that prevent us from fulfilling our true potential and destiny in life. With inner awareness we can understand why the mind is distracted and inattentive. In unbroken, clear awareness we can decondition and dehypnotise the mind of its subconscious motivations, ignorance, addictions and bad habits.

Self-awareness begins with you here and now in this present moment, in every moment of your life. When you live every moment in that awareness, you will experience the Eternal as a living reality.

The average person only uses a tiny fraction of awareness in his or her everyday living. We go from one day to the next throughout life in a state of distraction, unawareness and restlessness. Half-heartedly we go through all the activities of the day in a somnolent state of unawareness, and the beauty of life escapes us. In this conditioned state of mind we are mostly attentive to our subconscious motives, and therefore our perception is distorted. We are not even aware or mindful when eating our meals, cleaning our teeth, or listening attentively when someone is talking to us. Perhaps you go to the bathroom or kitchen and leave it untidy or dirty, burn the toast, leave water running from the tap, or forget to switch the light or heater off before you go out of the house. They may be small activities in your life, but the way to Self-realisation requires sensitivity, awareness, care and attention to all that we do in thought, word and action, no matter how small it may seem. We need to live each moment of life completely, carefully observing all the details with constant awareness and attention. It is only when we perceive clearly and live truly in accord with life's processes that the Divine Reality is glorified through us.

It does not matter how long you have been sitting in the dark; when light is brought in, the darkness disappears. It is our responsibility to awake in the light, to consciously realise our true nature and reality as the Self. With knowledge, understanding and mastery of our mind, body and senses, we can direct our lives intelligently, expressing ourselves in a balanced and fulfilling way on all levels of our being.

Removing the ignorance that obscures the Self

Self-knowledge or Self-awareness is not a goal to seek. The Self is knowledge. Self-awareness cannot be divided from awareness, which is the Self.

Self-knowledge is the awareness of the immortal reality within us, which sets us free from the bondage of ignorance, the cause of all our sorrows. This knowledge and awareness, which is the Self, is ever present here and now. It has never ceased to be, and so is not a goal that we have to go in search of.

There is no mystery to it. All we need to do is remove the obstacles, dispelling the ignorance that obscures the Self as knowledge. The sun is always shining, but when it is obscured by dark clouds we do not see it. When the clouds disperse then the sun becomes visible and the light shines.

Patañjali instructs us how to remove ignorance effectively:

> 'The practice of uninterrupted awareness and discriminative discernment between what is real and what is unreal, removes ignorance.'
>
> *Yoga Sūtras 2:26*

The intelligent practice of the first seven of the eight limbs of Yoga with uninterrupted awareness gives us the basic methods in removing ignorance (*avidyā*). When ignorance is removed, *puruṣa* (Self, soul) is established in its own true nature.

If we are to remain in the light of Self-knowledge, then we need to be vigilant, constantly awake, alert and aware in every moment. This is no part-time exercise; the practice of Yoga, once taken up, involves your entire life. This total approach to life reveals your sincerity and commitment to awakening in absolute Awareness, pure Consciousness. If we are unmotivated, uncommitted and are practising only half-heartedly, we cannot expect complete success and Self-realisation in this life. We must sincerely want to awaken from our ignorance, and become actively involved in our own spiritual unfoldment.

The nine obstacles that distract the mind

The practice of Yoga is basically the removal of obstacles and obstructions from the mind and body, so that the inner light and joy of the Self that is within us (but is not shining because of obstructions, ignorance and forgetfulness) can shine in perfect Self-awareness.

In his *Yoga Sūtras* (1:30), Patañjali lists nine main obstacles or impediments (*antarāyāḥ* – from *aya* 'move'; *antara* 'make a gap' in one's practice) that distract the mind (*citta*), and obstruct progress.

While these distractions (*vikṣepas*) remain in the mind, one cannot enter one-pointed concentration (*ekāgratā*).

These nine obstacles are:

1. Disease
2. Dullness
3. Doubt
4. Carelessness
5. Laziness (physical and mental)
6. Attachment to sense-pleasures
7. False perception
8. Instability
9. Non-attainment of a yogic state/lack of perseverance.

Disease (*vyādhi*)

'A healthy body is the guest chamber of the soul; a sick one is its prison.'

Francis Bacon, Augmentis Scientarum: Valetudo

Disease means loss of ease, balance and harmony; it means there is tension within. If the body and mind are in balance, disease will not occur. Our spiritual progress can be restricted by a dis-eased mind and body. For example, if you are ill, and your body is in pain and feeling weak, and lacking in energy, it is very difficult to sit calmly in meditation. Your mind is distracted by the physical pain and discomfort, and you are unable to concentrate or become focused clearly in meditation.

Āyurveda (Science of Life), the sister science to Yoga, tells us that health and disease are relative to the normal and abnormal states of the three *doṣas* – *vata* (air), *pitta* (fire) and *kapha* (water). These three body constitution qualities that move throughout the entire body, influencing all of the body's functions – biological and psychological – can produce either health or disease, depending on whether they are in balance or aggravated and imbalanced (*vikriti*).

Āyurveda gives this definition of health:

'One whose *doṣas*, *agni* and functions of *dhātu* and *malas* are in a state of equilibrium, and who has a cheerful mind, intellect and sense-organs is termed as *svastha* (healthy).'

Suṣruta Samhita, Sūtrasthana 15:41

Doṣas

The three principal forces – *vata*, *pitta* and *kapha* – governing the biological processes in the body in the normal state of equilibrium constitute health, and are referred to as *dhātus*, 'supports'. When the *dhātus* are in disequilibrium the three are referred to as *doṣas* ('faults'; from *duṣ* 'to spoil', 'to impair').

Dhātus (the seven basic body tissues)

Dhātu means 'to give support'. The *dhātus* are the seven basic tissues of the body: plasma (*rasa*); red blood cells (*rakta*); muscle (*mamsa*); fat (*meda*); bone (*asthi*); bone marrow and nervous tissue (*majja*); and reproductive tissue (*śukra*). A person's immunity is based on the strength of his or her *ojas* – a very refined and subtle material that nourishes the whole body. It is derived from *śukra* (reproductive tissue) after having gone through a sequential forming of the seven tissues or *dhātus*. *Ojas* is the end product. It promotes immunity, mental and physical health, and vitality. As the seat of *śukra* is throughout the body, this *ojas* is also produced in every part of the body, but only collects in the heart (*hridaya*). If *ojas* becomes weak or reduced, vitality is lowered, which in turn can cause disease. This is why it is important to follow a balanced lifestyle according to your body type. According to *Āyurveda*, the three pillars of life and good health are: proper nutrition; adequate rest; and conservation of sexual energy through moderation.

Agni (digestive fire)

From a health point of view, *agni* (digestive fire) is also important. According to *Āyurveda*, most diseases stem from an unhealthy digestive system. When the digestive fire (*agni*) is weakened, digestion becomes less effective, leaving undigested and partially digested food materials, referred to in *Āyurveda* as *āma* (accumulated toxins or impurities that clog the body systems). This results from an unhealthy diet and lifestyle, poor digestion and elimination, and a high intake of toxins into the body.

Nirāma (without *āma*) is the state of normal health, indicated by such signs as proper appetite and elimination.

Malas

The *malas* are the waste products of the body's elimination system: sweat, urine and faeces. These waste products are transported and eliminated through tubular canals of circulation called *srotas* (from the Sanskrit root *sru* 'to flow'). The *srotas* also aid in the production and transport of nutrients both to and between the cells, *dhatus*, and the organs of the body. In Āyurvedic terms, the *srotas* or channels for sweat, urine and faeces are:

svedavaha srotas – sweat

mutravaha srotas – urine

purishavaha srotas – faeces.

For optimal health these *srotas* need to be flowing naturally and normally. Abnormal working of the *srotas* can take the form of excessive flow, deficient flow, obstructed flow, diverted flow, and abnormal direction of flow.

Prerequisites of natural immunity to disease and wellbeing

- Live in harmony with natural laws.

- Maintain a clean, healthy bloodstream. This comes from pure nutrition, pure water, pure air, good digestion and efficient elimination.
- Practise both Yoga and *Āyurveda*. These two ancient sciences from India complement each other. *Āyurveda* (the Science of Life and longevity – the study and practice of preserving and restoring health and preventing disease) provides a system of health incorporating the factors of lifestyle, diet, seasonal regimen, cleanliness, physical purification, herbal treatments, massage, and cultivation of knowledge and attitudes that sustain wellbeing.

  Āyurveda's aim is also in attaining the four *puruṣārthas* or principles of life: *dharma* (righteousness), *artha* (prosperity), *kāma* (enjoyment), and *mokṣa* (liberation).

  Health and wellbeing are important in Yoga, but spiritual liberation is its aim. The primary subject of Yoga is consciousness and the uniting of the individual self (*puruṣa*; *ātman*) with the universal Self (*Brāhman*).
- Take regular daily exercise (aerobic and Yoga postures). Exercise strengthens, stretches, gives stamina and energy, and tones the internal body organs and systems.
- Breathe properly, and learn the Yoga techniques of *prāṇāyama*.
- Take sufficient rest, sleep and relaxation.
- Meditate regularly every day.
- Maintain a positive attitude and enthusiasm for life. Have a cheerful outlook on life in all circumstances.

Do the best you can in any circumstance and leave the rest to God.

Dullness (*styāna*)

Dullness is a quality *of tamas guṇa* (inertia), and relates to the mind. Through lack of interest and energy the mind is disinclined to make an effort; it becomes mentally lazy or languid. The mind also becomes restless and loses its focus. It becomes distracted, and this restless wandering and distraction becomes an obstacle to concentration and meditation. When the mind is restless and distracted it is called *vikṣepa*. There are two main causes for *vikṣepa*: lack of purpose and the mind being turned outwards and distracted.

To overcome this obstacle:

- Establish your priorities.
- Give conscious attention to important matters such as meditation.
- Determine your current life priority and direction, then live with intention.
- Identify those habits that are preventing you from giving attention to important priorities, purpose and direction in life.
- Be more purposeful, willing and enthusiastic. Develop an interest in all that you do.

- Be disciplined with interest and enthusiasm in your daily routines and spiritual practices. Develop a keen interest in pursuits that will help you attain self-mastery.
- Develop the power of concentration and clear thinking. A person with a distracted, restless mind cannot achieve anything. Tremendous power flows into us when we concentrate and are one-pointed.
- Do not put off what you can do now. If you procrastinate you will never achieve your aims in life. Change your mental attitude and become motivated and willing to make the effort now. Never accept failure – if you do so, you will become a failure and deny the power of God within you. Be determined and resolve never to cease trying to do your best. If you are making a continuous effort now, you cannot fail.
- Make good use of your time, for every moment is precious. Do not waste your time and restrict your spiritual unfoldment by being idle. Remember, life is very short, there is no time to lose in awakening to God-consciousness. Be clearly aware of your true purpose for being here and make the most of every available opportunity.
- Practise introspection. Keep a mental diary of what you are doing and thinking throughout the day. Constructively analyse your bad habits and find the cause. Why is it that you are lazy or are procrastinating? How did you acquire the negative traits? Be discriminating and recognise your weaknesses, then remove them from your consciousness. Resolve to make a positive change in your life and affirm aloud with firm conviction:

  > 'Today I make a firm commitment to move willingly in a purposeful direction to fulfil my spiritual aim in life. I make wise use of my time, energy, and talents. I am positive! I am energetic! I am enthusiastic!
  >
  > I consciously and attentively practise necessary disciplines in my daily routine to attain self-mastery and realise my unity with the Supreme Realty, God.'

- Create more energy. Paramhansa Yogananda said: 'Willpower directs energy, and energy in turn acts upon matter. The stronger the will, the greater the force of energy.' Energy is an important key to spiritual life. All matter, including human beings, is in reality energy. This energy is infinite, it has no limitation and we can tap into it and draw from this universal supply as much as we want to.

Yogananda also said: 'Joy and energy go hand in hand.' If you have high energy you cannot be sad, and if you are joyful, you have energy. Look at those people who are depressed. Everyone who is depressed has low energy, and one of the most difficult things psychologists have to do with people who are depressed is to get them to do something about it. There is no energy flowing in a depressed person, but people who are joyful are full of energy and vitality.

Unwillingness, boredom, moodiness, and fear of failure are all mental energy blocks that we should work to overcome.

When we bring our will in attunement with God's Will we become unlimited; in this way willpower makes us divine. The greatest use for willpower is to use it to meditate, to discover the Divine Heritage within you.

Doubt (*samśaya*)

Doubts are our worst enemy. When the mind is in doubt it wavers and becomes undecided, uncertain, and even disbelieving. The mind becomes torn between different possibilities, jumping restlessly from one to the other, and becomes more and more confused.

If you have doubts about the existence of God, the scriptural sacred texts, the tradition of your guru and his teachings, or your own inner reality and your purpose in life, then clear your confusion and resolve your doubts by developing the opposite of doubt, which is faith (*śraddhā*). Faith brings clarity and calmness to the mind. It is developed by interest and attraction towards knowledge of the true reality. Knowledge removes doubt.

Depending on one's attitude, doubt can be positive and expand our awareness, or negative and destructive, resulting in a depressive mood. When you are in doubt, ask yourself, 'Am I in doubt so that I will not have to act, enabling me to escape from responsibility and commitment; or am I in doubt because I intuitively feel that something is not quite right?' Positive doubt that stimulates genuine inquiry can expand our awareness. Negative doubt created through restlessness and impatience arising from the ego decreases our awareness.

Meditate deeply, so that you develop your power of intuition. After meditation remain calmly seated with your concentrated gaze at the Spiritual Eye, at the midpoint between the eyebrows, and in the silence pray to God for faith, strength and inner guidance to overcome your doubts. When your emotions are settled and your mind is free from restlessness and confusion, then you will be able to clear your doubts.

Carelessness (*pramāda*)

Carelessness or negligence is lacking in careful attention to both those things that are important in life and those which are considered unimportant. In Yoga and meditation, if there is a lack of conviction, attention, concentration, enthusiasm and persistence in your practice, the mind weakens and becomes careless preventing progress and success on the spiritual path.

Negligence is failing to be consciously attentive, and being uninterested in your spiritual practices and disciplines. To overcome *pramāda*, cultivate a sincere interest in your spiritual unfoldment. To create a firm foundation for spiritual growth, be intentional in your spiritual practices and disciplines. Resolve now to be committed to living perfectly with clear understanding and resolve to express Divine will.

If you are aware of higher realities but are still continuing to act from conditioned and habitual ways, your spiritual growth will be restricted and limited.

Laziness (*alasya*)

Laziness is failure to progress spiritually due to lack of perseverance, willingness and enthusiasm, with an extreme lack of energy or vitality (or in the state of *tamas*).

There is a mammal called a sloth, which is of a sluggish, slow-moving nature, that inhabits tropical parts of Central and South America. There are also human beings who are sluggish, physically and mentally. Disinclined to exertion, they move slowly and pass their time in idleness. This is the *tamasic* state that Krishna mentions in the *Bhāgavad Gītā*, chapter 17.

Paramhansa Yogananda once said: 'I can forgive the physically lazy person, but not the mentally lazy person.' What he meant by this was that sometimes the physically lazy person can be excused if the laziness is due to ill health, but mental laziness is inexcusable for those who choose to be unwilling, unmotivated, with no self-effort.

To overcome inertia and laziness one needs to purify and energise the physical body and mind to rise to the *sattvic* state. The mind and body are inseparable – if the body is not nourished with a healthy balanced vegetarian diet, the mind is affected. A diet of heavy food, meat, alcohol, drugs and cigarette smoking causes inertia, heaviness and dullness in the body and mind. Overeating, sleeping for longer than necessary, and lack of exercise also cause lethargy. In this state of *tamas*, one is unwilling to meditate.

Attachment to sense-pleasures (*avirati*)

Our desire or need for someone or something apart from God creates a sense of separation from our true Source of joy and happiness. It makes us believe that we could be satisfied without the power and presence of the Supreme Self. The more we desire, the more we become attached. Attachment deepens our desires. Attachment to sense-pleasures prevents us from concentrating on our spiritual reality. When our mind is distracted by strong ego-desires and needs, and outer sources of sense stimulation, we lose our self-awareness, and become mentally restless, confused and emotionally unsettled. The happiness and joy that follows from the satisfaction of a desire is not the result of the return of consciousness to itself, under certain circumstances which prevail on the fulfilment of a desire. The mind is under an illusion when it imagines that it is necessary to move towards an object for gaining some kind of satisfaction or fulfilment. Satisfaction does not come from this contact.

Think of this gross example: if your skin is itching, to relieve the irritation of the itching sensation you would normally scratch the skin. The relief that you feel by scratching the itching skin is not the result of merely scratching, though it may appear that scratching gives some relief and happiness. The relief comes due to the movement of the blood to that part of the skin, which for some reason was previously deprived of that blood supply because of the ailment of the skin. The activity of scratching is not the cause of the satisfaction; the movement of blood is the cause. Similarly, something like this happens in the mind itching for enjoyment from the objects of the senses. The satisfaction that one gets by means of contact with a sense object is something like the satisfaction that one gets by scratching the itch. The scratching does not bring relief. Likewise, the contact of the mind with the object does not bring satisfaction and happiness. The joy or happiness that we experience is due to a resting of consciousness in itself, due to the Self (*ātman*, *puruṣa*) resting in itself, as a consequence of the cessation of this activity of coming in contact with the external object.

The strong attraction of the senses for worldly objects and pleasures prevents us from one-pointed concentration and meditation, therefore we need to regulate our sense-pleasures and bring them into balance. This requires careful discrimination and complete, clear understanding of our emotions, so that we can withdraw energy from them and neutralise them.

False perception (*bhrānti-darśana*)

Due to false perception, ignorance, ego-sense, and lack of understanding we may totally reject philosophical truths that great saints, sages and sacred texts like the *Bhāgavad Gītā* and the *Yoga Sūtras* have taught us.

If we are mentally confused and have misconceptions about the spiritual path of Yoga, or misunderstand the nature of the inner Self, the Absolute or Ultimate Reality, we can improve our understanding by developing devotion and faith (*śraddha*) in God and the great Self-realised Masters. We can develop an understanding of Truth through learning. Study the teachings of the great respected Spiritual Masters: Jesus Christ, Krishna, Adi Shankara, Patañjali and Paramhansa Yogananda, to name a few. Read and study the great classic scriptures: *The Gospels of the New Testament*, *Bhāgavad Gītā*, *Yoga Sūtras* and the *Upaniṣads*. Read also Paramhansa Yogananda's *Autobiography of a Yogi* (original 1946 edition). This classic Yoga book has inspired thousands of Truth-seekers.

Instability (*anavasthitatvā*)

The obstacle here is that one may gain a higher stage of Yoga, but fall from it, or be unable to maintain oneself there due to the unsteadiness and inattention of the mind. It is only when the state of *samādhi* is attained that the mind attains stability (*sthiti*).

To overcome this inability to maintain a certain level of concentration, and a stable state in meditation, one needs to persevere with enthusiastic effort and further intensify one's practice of meditation. Then when the *tamasic* and *rajasic vṛttis* (vortices of feeling) are neutralised, the *sattvic vṛtti* flows uninterruptedly to the object of concentration.

Non-attainment of a yogic state (*alabdha-bhūmikatva*)

We may fail to make progress to the higher stages of Yoga, even though we have been practising the proper practices. This failure to make progress to the next stage can cause distraction to the aspirant, disturbing the equanimity of the mind. To overcome this obstacle one needs inexhaustible patience, and the willingness to achieve success in Yoga by persistent effort of the will, with respect and devotion. This persistent practice (*abhyāsa*) – the effort required to become firmly grounded in one-pointed concentration – is needed to overcome the strong pull of the *saṃskāras* (latent impressions) on the mind that distract us from the meditative state.

Patañjali says:

> 'That practice becomes firm in ground only when spontaneous awareness continues with consistent efforts without interruption for a long time.'
>
> *Yoga Sūtras 1:14*

To become firmly grounded in our practice of Yoga, there are three things we need to do:

- Practise for a long time.
- Practise without interruption.
- Practise with respect, faith and devotion.

Four secondary obstacles as symptoms of a distracted mind

Patañjali identifies four secondary obstacles as symptoms of a distracted mind:

> 'Suffering; despair; trembling or restlessness; irregular inhalation and exhalation.'
>
> *Yoga Sūtras 1:31*

These four conditions or symptoms of a distracted mind represent the four stages which follow one another when the mind is in *vikṣepa* (distraction), and interfere with the practice of concentration and meditation.

Duḥkha (pain, suffering and sorrow)

This is the first symptom of a distracted mind. When you experience pain, unhappiness or sorrow, the mind is attracted to it. The mind is distracted from that which is beyond pain – the inner Self. One is unable to meditate when the mind is distracted by painful memories, emotional hurts, and painful unfulfilled desires.

There are three kinds of pain:

- *adhyatmika* – within oneself (physical, mental and emotional)
- *adhbhautika* – caused by other beings (including wild animals and insects)
- *adhidaivika* – caused by natural forces (sound, air, fire, water, earth, heat, cold and planetary forces).

Daurmanasya (despair, frustration)

This is the disturbance of the mind that arises when one's desires are obstructed. When pain is combined with the frustration of not being able to remove it quickly and effectively it leads to despair and restlessness (*vikṣhipta*).

Meditation is disturbed by the mind being distracted by negative moods, frustration, negative thoughts, anxiety and disturbed emotions. Moods are the result of low energy. Change the energy level and its direction, and you will develop a positive state of mind.

Paramhansa Yogananda once told one of his disciples, who was inclined to be moody: 'If you want to be unhappy, no one in the world can make you happy. But if you make up your mind now to be happy, no one and nothing on earth can take that happiness from you.'

Aṅgam-ejayatva (unsteadiness of limbs)

Despair then leads to nervous agitation, which is an outer physical symptom of despair. The restless mind causes nervous agitation in the body. The body twitches, shakes, and makes unnecessary movements, causing it to become unsteady.

Śvāsa-praśvāsa (disturbed inhalation or exhalation)

Nervous agitation then affects the breathing, creating irregularities in the flow of *prāṇic* currents in the body. Uneven inhalation and exhalation is caused by fluctuations of the mind and emotional instability. If you are attentive to your breathing, you will be aware of the degree of distractedness of the mind. The less distracted it is, the calmer the breathing is; the more distracted, the more restless and irregular the breathing is.

If you want to know what total absorption of the mind is, exhale and suspend your breathing. It is the breath (or the movement of the *prāṇa*) that enables your mind to think. If you suspend the breath, or slow the breathing to a minimum, the mind loses its fuel and becomes quiet and still. This is what happens in deep meditation, where there is total absorption of the mind.

How to remove these disturbances and accompanying symptoms

In the next *Yoga Sūtra*, Patañjali tells us how to remove these disturbances and their accompanying symptoms that distract the mind:

> 'To eliminate those (disturbances and their accompaniments) practise one principle (of one-pointed concentration).'
>
> *Yoga Sūtras 1:32*

The average person lacks not only concentration of purpose but also the capacity to focus the concentration of the mind within. Those who are following the spiritual path of Yoga have to not only pursue a spiritual objective with energy, willingness, and perseverance, but also the objective must be *within*.

When concentration of purpose has been developed sufficiently, then the elimination of the obstacles that distract the mind follows naturally.

The stability of the *ekāgra* state, or one-pointed concentration of mind, is required for attaining the higher levels of *samādhi* (absorption). To achieve this, the mind needs to be steadily focused and concentrated on one truth or principle (*eka tattva*), in other words the object of meditation, such as the Supreme Self or God. The most effective way to practise one-pointed concentration is to bring your attentive awareness to the midpoint between the eyebrows at the fifth *chakra*, which Paramhansa Yogananda referred to as the Spiritual Eye, the seat of spiritual consciousness. Yogananda said that the physical body has two eyes, but the astral body has only one eye, like a *flame of fire*. It is the one astral flame of fire which pours into the two eyes, giving them power and manifesting them as two. For this reason, when the two eye currents are concentrated and reflected back in the medulla oblongata by focusing the eyes on the midpoint between the eyebrows, they are perceived as one single Spiritual Eye of light. And this is what was meant when Jesus said: 'If therefore thine eye be single, thy whole body shall be full of light' (Matthew 6:22). When the two physical eyes manifest as the single Spiritual Eye, then one can perceive, by continuous spiritual development, the physical body as filled with the super-lights of the astral body. The light of the Spiritual Eye observed in deep meditation is seen as a circle of golden light representing the astral universe. Within this circle of golden light is dark blue light representing the causal universe, and within the dark blue light at its centre is a radiant silver-white, five-pointed star, which represents the Supreme Spirit beyond Creation.

With the inner gaze calmly focused at the Spiritual Eye, begin to watch the natural breath flowing in and out at the midpoint between the eyebrows. First inhale deeply, then slowly exhale. Then as the breath naturally flows in of its own accord, mentally follow it with the seed-syllable *mantra Hong*. As the breath naturally flows out, mentally follow it with the *mantra Sau*. Remember, this is not a breathing exercise, you are only witnessing the natural breath flow in and flow out. When your attentive awareness focuses naturally on the flow of breath in the nostrils, concentrate on the breath while simultaneously gazing into the Spiritual Eye, and identify the breath with the *mantra Hong Sau*. This seed-syllable *mantra Hong Sau* means 'I am He', the inner Self, Pure Consciousness.

Practising the *mantra Hong Sau* while looking into the Spiritual Eye will deepen your concentration, making it one-pointed. It will bring deep inner calmness, and therefore, eliminate the distractions and accompanying symptoms of the mind.

Purifying the mind

The mind is impure when it is tainted by the six impurities (*kāluṣhya*):

1. *Rāga* (attraction or attachment)
2. *Īrśhya* (jealousy)
3. *Parāpakāra chikīrśhya* (malevolence)
4. *Asūya* (anger)
5. *Dveṣa* (aversion or hate)
6. *Amarśha* (vengeance).

In his *Yoga Sūtras* 1:33–34, Patañjali instructs us in two methods of how to purify the mind from the *rajasic* and *tamasic* tendencies. The two methods are prerequisites for attaining steadiness, calmness and one-pointedness (*ekāgratā*) of the mind, preparing it for meditation.

> 'The mind becomes calm and serene by cultivating the attitude of friendship towards those who are happy, compassion towards those who are suffering, delight towards those who are virtuous by nature, and equanimity towards those who are non-virtuous.'
>
> *Yoga Sūtras 1:33*

Cultivating the inner attitude of friendliness (*maitrī*) means friendliness towards those who are our equals. This feeling of equality is a spontaneous expression of the inner attitude of equanimity in which the yogi is established. Friendliness is the opposite of animosity and such negative emotions as jealousy and envy are removed from the mind when we are established in friendliness.

Compassion (*karuṇā*) is an attitude of sympathy, empathy and warmheartedness towards those who are sorrowful, or who are suffering in any way. Compassion is not just sharing the experience (empathy) with others, but genuinely wishing to see them relieved of their suffering. We have only to understand that we would expect the same for ourselves if we were suffering or in distress. By compassion towards those who are suffering, the impurity of the desire to cause harm to others is removed from the mind.

By cultivating cheerfulness, joy and delight (*muditā*) towards those who are successful and spiritually advanced, the yogi does not suffer the discontent aroused by another's possessions, success, spiritual elevation or happiness, for in the attitude of equanimity and a balanced mind he or she is happy in the happiness of others.

At other times, certain circumstances arise in which we are placed in a situation or presence of a non-virtuous (*apuṇya*) or impious person, whose consciousness and energy is spiritually lower than ours. This lower consciousness can have a negative effect on your consciousness, disturbing your inner calmness. If you cannot practise friendliness, compassion and cheerfulness towards others who engage in actions that you do not approve of, then, do not ignore them or be judgemental, but remain impartial and even-minded, neither accepting nor condemning their attitude. By equanimity towards the non-virtuous, the impurity of intolerance is removed from the mind.

Try to keep in the company of, and associate with, those persons who uplift your consciousness in positive and spiritual ways, rather than those who think negatively and who are loud, aggressive and restless.

> 'Or by exhaling and retaining the breath (the mind becomes calm and steady).'
>
> *Yoga Sūtras 1:34*

The word 'or' (*vā*) at the beginning of this *sūtra* is actually in relation to the following *sūtras* 1:35–1:39, not to the previous *sūtra* 1:33.

The breath and the mind are intimately connected. When the breath becomes calm, the mind also becomes calm and steady. Irregular breathing indicates a disturbance in the mind or the heart, affecting our emotional state.

> 'Just as a bird tied by a string, after flying in various directions without finding a resting place elsewhere settles down at the place where it is bound, so also the mind, after flying in various directions without finding a resting place elsewhere settles down in breath, for the mind is bound to breath.'
>
> *Chandogya Upaniṣad 6:8.2*

To understand the connection between the stilling of the mind and the breath, you can practise an experiment now. Inhale deeply, then exhale deeply and without strain hold the breath out for 15 seconds.

In those 15 seconds both the mind and the breath were in a suspended state. The thoughts, and the vortices of feeling (*vṛttis*), had become still. During those 15 seconds your mind became one-pointed, fixed on the breath alone.

There were no thoughts! What made you take your next breath is *prāṇa* (life energy). It is the movement of *prāṇa* that enables your mind to think and your lungs to breathe. But if you suspend the breath even for a few seconds, the mind becomes still. If the breath is subdued, so is the mind, because they are closely connected.

In deep meditation the pauses between each breath become longer, resulting in the 'breathless state', This happens naturally and spontaneously when the mind is absolutely calm, the *vṛttis* stilled, and the concentration is one-pointed (*ekāgratā*). Paramhansa Yogananda's *Hong Sau* Technique is good for deepening the concentration to enter the 'breathless state'.

Developing stability of mind

Patañjali, in his *Yoga Sūtras* 1:35–39, gives several methods of bringing steadiness and stability to the mind by using different objects of meditation.

> 'Or concentration on the subtle sense perceptions also firmly establishes the steadiness of the mind.'
>
> *Yoga Sūtras 1:35*

This *sūtra* is referring to the spontaneous manifestation of subtle sense perception. It is in the subtle realm of the senses (*tanmātra*) in the astral body that the mind is captivated, destroying doubt, and making the mind become one-pointed. In meditation we can concentrate on the higher subtle sense of listening to the inner sounds of the *chakras* and to *Aum*. In deep meditation with the eyes closed, concentrating at the midpoint between the eyebrows (Spiritual Eye), we can see the inner light. Other subtle manifestations can be experienced by concentration on the subtle sense perceptions such as fragrance, taste and touch, leading to the subtle nature of the object. Through the direct experience of deep concentration, inner knowledge and dispassion for the lower stages of concentration is attained.

> 'Or (the mind becomes calm and steady) by concentrating on the supreme, ever-blissful light within, that is beyond sorrow.'
>
> *Yoga Sūtras 1:36*

This *sūtra* is a continuation of the preceding *sūtra*, in the sense that it causes steadiness and calmness of the mind. The previous *sūtra* relates to concentration on the subtle senses and subtle elements (*tanmātra*). This *sūtra* (1:36) is referring to the internal objects as the manifestation of the light of *sattva*. Only the awareness of 'I am' is experienced (*asmitā mātra jyotishmatī*).

This subject-focused meditation is different from the concentration on the subtle sense perceptions, which have an external object such as fragrance or taste, since the object is the *puruṣa* (Self, soul) itself. Sorrow (*viśokā*) is an indicator of distracted attention; when our calm attention is one-pointed concentration on the inner light (the luminous Self within), which is free from *rajas* and *tamas*, steadiness and calmness of mind is attained. We become freed from all mental distractions, and sorrow.

> 'Or (the mind becomes calm and steady) by attunement with the consciousness of an enlightened being who has transcended desire and attachment to sense-objects.'
>
> *Yoga Sūtras 1:37*

To gain inner stability of the mind you can also meditate on an enlightened being who is perfectly established in the principle of non-attachment (*vairāgya*). Such a pure enlightened being or true guru, beyond ego-consciousness, is free from conditioning, desires, attachments, likes and dislikes. By attuning your will to the guru's will you can be guided by his or her wisdom to find perfect freedom in God. The guru and his teachings are a channel for the Divine Will, or Supreme Being, to reach the Truth-seeking soul. When you are in attunement with the guru, you connect your life with Supreme Consciousness. The guru will guide you and help you to remain steadfast in the spiritual principles that you need to succeed on the spiritual path.

By remaining loyal and attuned to the wise, enlightened guru your mind will develop dispassion for the objects of the senses. The mind will become steady, and when you meditate you will be able to enter deep within the calmness of your true inner Self.

Attune yourself to the enlightened guru by keeping him ever in your heart. Be one with him in principle. Visualise your guru or take a picture of him, and sitting still with no other thoughts, concentrate on his eyes or his Spiritual Eye. Meditate on his omnipresence, the spiritual consciousness beyond his physical form. Feel that you are seated in his divine presence, that he is meditating with you. Pray to him: 'Divine Master, bless me, guide me, and protect me, show me the true path to Self-realisation.' Become absorbed in that one prayerful thought then, in the silence and inner communion, wait for an answer by listening and feeling his presence in your own heart. You will be guided by soul-intuition from within and pointed in the right direction.

My guru, Paramhansa Yogananda, said that without a guru it is very difficult to find God. It requires 25 per cent of devoted practice of meditation, 25 per cent blessings of the guru, and 50 per cent grace of God. But if you remain steady in your efforts to the end, God will appear before you.

> 'Or (the mind becomes calm and steady) by concentration on the insightful wisdom (*prajña*) gained in dream or deep sleep states.'
>
> *Yoga Sūtras 1:38*

In sleep you forget the world; even the 'I-am-the-body' awareness does not exist. The 'I' experience does not exist in sleep. When you are asleep, you are not consciously aware that you are sleeping; you do not say 'I sleep'.

During the dream state (*svapna*) the experiencer of the dream is only conscious of internal objects. The senses are quiet and absorbed in the mind. The consciousness of the individual is withdrawn from the physical senses and becomes identified with the subtle body, the waking state temporarily disappears and the consciousness enters the dream state. In this dream state, the individual consciousness is restricted to the *antaḥkaraṇa*, the fourfold inner instrument, consisting of the *manas* (deliberation), *buddhi* (determination), *ahaṁkāra* (egoism or 'I-ness') and *citta* (recollection).

The dream state and images are projected inwardly upon the mental screen from impressions seen during the waking state. When these impressions and the external objects are modified and left in the mind the individual experiences dreams.

In the dreamless deep sleep state (*suṣhupti*) there is an absence of mental activity; there is no thinking, feeling or sensory perception. The individual is not conscious or aware of anything. But this is not negative, or a state of non-existence, for on waking we are happy and conscious of having slept a sound and restful sleep. We feel we existed even during sleep. In comparison to the waking and dreaming states of mental activity, whose characteristic is the presence of a knower and a known, or a thinker and a thought, in dreamless sleep the principle of consciousness remains and exists without its seeming to assume the duality of a conscious subject and object. Consciousness is continuous.

In deep dreamless sleep (*nidra*; *suṣhupti*), the mental functions cease altogether – there is no thinker to think thoughts, there is no awareness of thoughts or 'I', there is no ego and no world. The Self recedes even from the mind. Both the five organs of perception, and the mind, remain hidden and latent, suspended in a state of ignorance (*ajñāna*), within the the blissful sheath of the causal body.

During dreamless sleep the soul is united with consciousness, the nature of absolute bliss. But this is not the transcendental state or the fourth, known as *turīya*, in which the consciousness merges into the *ātman* (Self). This union is only apparent, it is only a reflection; it is not the true union or superconsciousness that follows the knowledge and realisation of the Self. The sleeping individual returns to the consciousness of the waking state and returns to his conditioned personality, with the same habits, desires and attachments. The individual self remembers that it had a happy and sound sleep. This recollection results from experience, therefore there must be experience in the deep dreamless sleep (*nidra*; *suṣhupti*).

The recollection of the pleasant and joyful feeling from deep dreamless sleep brings an experience of inner calmness and peace, which can be used as an object of meditation in the wakeful state (*jāgrat*).

In the dream state (*svapna*) one can have a spiritual dream or a superconscious dream in which a revered guru, saint or deity appears. Awakening from such a spiritual dream brings peace and joy to the mind and heart. By recollecting and remembering the spiritual dream one can become absorbed in that vision; then the mind becomes calm and steady in meditation. Insights gained in the *svapna* and *nidra* states can calm and steady the mind.

In 1982 when I first met Swāmi Kriyananda (a direct disciple of Paramhansa Yogananda) in London, I had a superconscious dream in which Paramhansa Yogananda appeared personally to me. The purpose of him appearing in the spiritual dream to me was to remove any doubt that he was my guru. Yogananda stood before me and in his calm but authoritative voice said: 'Fear not, for I am Paramhansa Yogananda, your true guru. This is your spiritual path, come follow me!'

In the morning when I awoke from the dream, I felt a great sense of joy and happiness and peace within. The memory of my dream was vivid and clear in my mind; it felt very real and meaningful. I was so inspired that Yogananda had appeared to me that my mind remained in a joyful, calm and steady state throughout the whole day. Now whenever I remember that dream experience, my mind turns inward and becomes stabilised in the *sattvic* state of calmness, peace, joy and devotion.

> 'Or by meditating on any chosen object that is spiritually elevating, one attains steadiness of mind.'
>
> *Yoga Sūtras 1:39*

In this *sūtra*, Patañjali concludes this subject of the six methods for stilling the mind by saying that we may choose any object of meditation according to our preference. In other words, any method or object that is agreeable to the mind, that brings steadiness and calmness and one-pointedness to the mind, can be used for meditation.

According to our temperaments, and the particular spiritual tradition that we follow, we may have different inclinations towards a particular object or method of meditation. For example, one who has an emotional temperament may find a natural preference for the method given in *sūtra* 1:37. This may be the image of Krishna or Jesus Christ, or a revered guru such as Paramhansa Yogananda.

ĪŚVARA PRAṆIDHĀNA (ATTUNEMENT TO THE PRESENCE OF THE SUPREME CONSCIOUSNESS)

Īśvara praṇidhāna is the last of the five *niyamas* (observances or personal practices) given by Patañjali in *sūtra* 1:23.

> 'Or (*samādhi* can be attained) by a self-offering in attunement to God.'
>
> *Yoga Sūtras 1:23*

The word *Īśvara* is derived from the Sanskrit root *īsa*. *Īśate rajate iti Īśvarah*. *Īśate* means 'to permeate'. *Īśvara* is that which permeates everything. *Īśvara* is the eternal all-permeating Supreme Consciousness that is omnipresent, omnipotent and omniscient. In the concept of Yoga the Supreme Consciousness or God is known both as pervading all that exists and as residing within us. Attunement to the presence of the Supreme Consciousness means to inwardly attune yourself to the all-permeating presence of God.

In meditation we can attune our consciousness in an attitude of devotion towards the Supreme Consciousness by becoming absorbed in God through His manifestations or qualities of Light, Sound, Power, Wisdom, Calmness, Peace, Love and Joy. By practising the inner presence of God the sense of 'I', the ego, is removed and faith (*śraddhā*) is developed.

The word *praṇidhāna* is usually translated as 'surrender' in other commentaries on the *Yoga Sūtras*, but the word 'surrender' does not convey the real sense of the meaning. It makes God look like a policeman or an armed soldier, and makes us look as though we have to passively give in to Him. Surrender means to give in to an opponent, to give up, or to hand over – but what will you surrender? What will you hand over or give to God? The only thing that needs to be given up is ignorance (*avidyā*) the false identification of the *puruṣa* (the Self) with *buddhi* (intellect, the discriminating aspect of the mind). Self-ignorance is the root cause of our suffering – it keeps us in delusion, and egoism (*asmitā*) the sense of 'I, me, mine', is what sustains it. The ego-sense of individuality creates a sense of separation.

So if it is surrender, it is self-surrender, transcending *avidyā* and ego. It is not passive but a constant and dynamic self-offering and attunement to the omnipresent Consciousness, the Supreme Self within.

The ego is a strong opponent – it is the one thing we must *not* give in to. In this life your ego has been constructed and conditioned by your thinking, ideas, education, family, friends, culture, tradition, and even religion. It requires great faith and dedication to renounce and transcend the ego, and that is why it is important to have a strong and steady foundation on the path of Yoga by applying sincerely the *yamas* and *niyamas* to daily life. The *yamas* and *niyamas* prepare the mind for the next stage of the Eight Limbs of Yoga: *āsana* (posture).

6.4

ĀSANA (POSTURE)

Āsana is the third limb of Yoga. Patañjali deals with the subject of *āsana* (posture) in only three *sūtras* (2:46–48), and here he is really referring only to the meditative *āsanas* such as *Sukhāsana* (Easy pose), *Siddhāsana* (Adept pose) and *Pādmāsana* (Lotus pose).

> *'Sthira-sukham āsanam.'*
>
> *sthira* – steady, stable; *sukham* – comfortable, easy, pleasant; *āsanam* – posture
>
> 'The posture should be steady and comfortable.'
>
> *Yoga Sūtras 2:46*

> *'Prayatna-śaithilyānanta-samāpattibhyām.'*
>
> *prayatna* – (through) effort; *śaithilya* – relaxation; *ānanta* – the Infinite; *samāpattibhyām* – absorption of the mind
>
> '(Posture becomes firm and steady) by the relaxation of effort and by absorption in the Infinite.'
>
> *Yoga Sūtras 2:47*

> *'Tato dvandvānabhighātaḥ.'*
>
> *tataḥ* – consequently; *dvandva* – by the dualities; *anabhighātaḥ* – undisturbed
>
> 'Consequently, (the mind is) undisturbed by the dualities.'
>
> *Yoga Sūtras 2:48*

Aṣṭāṅga Yoga (Eight Limbs of Yoga) is comprised of three groups of spiritual methods that are a gradual succession of refinements towards inner stillness.

The first group are the *yamas* and *niyamas*, which cultivate the aspirant in ethical behaviour essential to the pursuit of the spiritual goal of Yoga.

The second group consists of the external practices (*bahiranga*) that focus primarily on physical disciplines that strengthen the physical body, increase and expand *prāṇic* life-force, and calm the mind:

> *Āsana* (posture), *prāṇāyama* (regulation and expansion of the life-force) and *pratyāhāra* (withdrawing the mind from the senses).

The third group is known as *Rāja Yoga*, which includes the internal practices (*antaranga*), which prepare the aspirant for the final higher stages of Self- and God-realisation: *dhāraṇā* (concentration), *dhyāna* (meditation), and *samādhi* (superconscious absorption).

ĀSANA IN *HAṬHA YOGA*

In the two ancient principal treatises on *Haṭha Yoga* – the *Haṭha Yoga Pradīpikā* (a mid-fourteenth century treatise by Svatmarama Yogendra), and the *Gheraṇḍa Saṃhitā* (late seventeenth century) – it is said that Lord Śiva (the Lord of the Yogis and founder of *Haṭha Yoga*) taught all the 84,000 *āsanas* to his consort Parvati. Throughout the centuries this great science has been passed down in disciple succession. Lord Śiva initiated Matsyendranath, who in turn taught his disciple Gorakshanath, and so on. The *Haṭha Yoga Pradīpikā* lists 35 great *Haṭha Yoga siddhas* or masters. As time went by the many thousands of *āsanas* were greatly reduced and modified, until there were no more than a few hundred, of which only 84 are generally known and are of importance. Out of these, only 32 are thought to be commonly useful today in giving achievement, accomplishment and perfection (*siddhi*). These 32 suitable and useful *āsanas* are named in the *Gheraṇḍa Saṃhitā* as:

> *Siddha, Pādma, Bhadra, Mukta, Vajra, Svastika, Siṃha, Gomukha, Vīra, Dhanur, Mṛta, Gupta, Matsya, Matsyendra, Gorakṣa, Paścimottāna, Utkaṭa, Saṅkaṭa, Mayūra, Kukkuṭa, Kūrma, Uttānakūrmaka, Uttānamaṇḍūka, Vṛkṣa, Maṇḍūka, Garuḍa, Vṛṣa, Śalabha, Makara, Uṣṭra, Bhujaṅga* and *Yogāsana.*

It is interesting to note that half of these *āsanas* are named after living creatures of nature, such as animals, fish and birds, and the other half are sitting postures. The early yogis and sages took their inspiration from the natural world. For example *Vṛkṣa* means tree; *Matsya* means fish; *Maṇḍūka* means frog; and *Garuḍa* means eagle.

The oldest known evidence of *Haṭha Yoga* being practised dates back to about 2500 BCE. In archaeological excavations at Mohenjo-Daro, a north Indian civilisation, a fired clay seal belonging to the ancient Indus Valley civilisation (Chalcolithic Age) was found, which is often pointed to as an indication of how old the science of *Haṭha Yoga* really is. It portrays a three-faced human figure sitting in the meditative posture *bhādrāsana* (gracious pose) – the ankles are placed under the buttocks on either side of the perineum and the soles of the feet are pressed together. This posture is also known as *Gorakṣāsana*.

THE PURPOSE AND AIM OF *ĀSANA* (POSTURE)

In the *Haṭha Yoga Pradīpikā* it states:

> '*Āsana* is the first stage of *Haṭha Yoga* and should be practised first. It gives steadiness, health and lightness of the body.'
>
> *Haṭha Yoga Pradīpikā 1:17*

This is the purpose of *āsana* (posture) in *Haṭha Yoga*: to give steadiness, health, firmness, flexibility and lightness to the body. The body needs to be a fit vehicle for the higher stages of *Rāja Yoga*. *Haṭha Yoga* is a process through which purification and control of the body is foremost. The *prāṇic* energy channels (*nāḍīs*) are cleared of blockages and purified of toxins by *Haṭha Yoga* practices, enabling the *prāṇā* to flow freely throughout the body. The *chakras* are opened and balanced, and the energy in the spine is awakened for the purpose of raising it to the higher centres in the brain.

The Yoga aspirant becomes fit for the higher meditational practice of *Rāja Yoga* only after the successful completion of *Haṭha Yoga*. The *Haṭha Yoga Pradīpikā* states:

> 'All the techniques of *Haṭha Yoga* are used to attain success in *Rāja Yoga*.'
>
> *Haṭha Yoga Pradīpikā 4:103*

> 'In the course of *Haṭha Yoga*, various *āsanas*, *prāṇāyama*, *mudras* and *pratyāhāra* should be practised until success in *Rāja Yoga* is attained.'
>
> *Haṭha Yoga Pradīpikā 1:67*

Although *āsanas*, or postures, are not the goal of Yoga, they are tremendously useful for the Yoga aspirant in the effort to overcome the distractions and weaknesses of the physical body: disease, pain, stiffness in the muscles, joints and spine, lack of energy, inertia and restlessness. Yoga *āsanas* are beneficial for the flexibility of the spine and joints, and toning and firming the muscles. All the body systems are benefited: cardiovascular, lymphatic, nervous, respiratory, glandular and digestive. The practice of *āsanas* assists in the elimination of toxins from the body, the internal organs are massaged, and circulation and glandular function are improved. The entire nervous system is brought into balance, bringing harmony stability, and clarity to the practitioner's mind.

Through regular and consistent practice, the beneficial effects of practising *Haṭha Yoga* begin to appear: radiant health, greater energy and vitality, a feeling of wellbeing, the disappearance of minor ailments and irritations, improved digestion and elimination, deep restful sleep, deeper relaxation, improved breathing (slower and deeper), increased awareness, focused attention and concentration, a sense of contentment, clarity of mind, and a feeling of inner freedom, harmony and peace.

The breath and awareness both play an important role in the practice of Yoga. When the breath is coordinated with movement of the body, the Yoga practice becomes harmonious, the breath deepens and the circulation and metabolism are stimulated. Yoga postures should always be practised with awareness and coordinated with the breath. The breath can be used to enhance muscle relaxation by concentrating on tense areas of the body and with awareness consciously relaxing those parts with each exhalation.

Stress and anxiety cause rapid and shallow breathing, and poor posture with the spine bent also causes shallow breathing. Poor posture and bad habits in the way we stand, move, sit and sleep place undue pressure on the spine, resulting in muscular tension, causing neck, shoulder and back pain. Strong and flexible muscles form an important protection for the spine and joints. The practice of Yoga postures with awareness can be a very beneficial discipline in removing these problems to strengthen the body, and to make it healthy, toned and supple. In the science of Yoga the body is seen as the vehicle of the soul, or Self, and with this in view it must be kept in perfect condition so that the mind may not become restless and distracted. There needs to be a balanced integration between a healthy body and a calm, clear mind to be able to meditate deeply and go into stillness.

Over the years of practising Yoga and meditation I have seen many meditators who are uninterested in the *Haṭha Yoga* practices of *āsana*, *prāṇāyama*, *mudrā* and *bandhā*. For whatever reason they dismiss *Haṭha Yoga* and Yoga postures, thinking them to be unnecessary if one is following the path of meditation. This is a mistake, because *Haṭha Yoga* is a great and beneficial aid towards making the body calm and steady and fit for the practice of meditation. It is a necessary preparation for the higher practices of meditation in which the mind, emotions, and the subtle energy currents of the body are brought under complete control.

The full training of *Haṭha Yoga* is best taken up during one's youth. After the age of about 40, it can become more difficult to practise. If one takes the practice up early and is consistent and regular in the practices of *āsana*, *prāṇāyama*, *mūdra*, and *bandhā* over many years, the benefits are tremendous. To truly understand this it has to be experienced; it is of no avail to intellectualise and argue about it.

Haṭha Yoga gives power and energy to *Rāja Yoga*. It aids in helping one to attain inner stillness more rapidly. In the beginning, physical discipline and bodily health through the practice of *Haṭha Yoga* assume greater importance, but in the higher stages of Yoga more emphasis is given to mental discipline and meditation.

MEDITATION *ĀSANAS* (POSTURES)

In the *Tejobindu Upaniṣad* it states: 'When *āsana* (posture) remains steady for three hours, it is adequate for the practice of Yoga.'

The aim of perfecting or mastering *āsana* is the attainment of an uninterrupted state of bodily equilibrium without pain or discomfort. A state in which one goes beyond body-consciousness, beyond the dualities of opposites such as the sensations of hot and cold.

Āsana-jay (mastery of *āsana*) is achieved when the Yoga aspirant is able to sit effortlessly, maintaining undisturbed stability in a meditation posture for three hours without experiencing any pain or discomfort.

For most of us this may seem impossible to attain. Even after sitting in a posture for 30 minutes one can experience restlessness as well as aches and pains in the lower back, knees, neck and shoulders. Just as the mind is distracted and unable to concentrate on any particular thing for a protracted period of time, so the body too has difficulty sitting in one particular posture.

Concentration implies bringing all your energy to focus on a certain point; but the mind wanders away with extraneous thoughts and so you have a perpetual conflict between the desire to concentrate, to give all your energy in trying to meditate, and the mind which is wandering, which you try to control. The body, mind and *prāṇa* are all related – if anything happens to one of them, then the others are also affected. Whatever *āsana* we choose for the purpose of Yoga, it has to bear a relationship to the mind's purpose, which is meditation. The intention is concentration of the mind, therefore, any seated posture which will help in the concentration of the mind should be regarded as that which is steady, pleasant and comfortable.

The degree of difficulty in assuming a Yoga *āsana* will depend on the nature of the posture itself. The most advanced and difficult meditation pose is *Pādmāsana* (Lotus pose). The most comfortable and the most excellent of the seated meditation postures is *Siddhāsana* (Perfect pose). The *Haṭha Yoga Pradīpikā* highly praises and recommends this posture:

'Of the eighty-four postures, one should always practise *Siddhāsana*. It purifies the 72,000 *nāḍīs* (subtle prāṇic channels). The yogi who meditates on the Self, follows a moderate diet, and practises *Siddhāsana* for twelve years, attains perfection (*siddhi*). When Siddhāsana is mastered, and the flow of *prāṇa* is stabilised, there is spontaneous 'breathlessness' or spontaneous breath retention (*Kevala kumbhaka*), of what use are the various other *āsanas*?'

Haṭha Yoga Pradīpikā 1:39–41

'When *Siddhāsana* is mastered, the three *bandhas* naturally occur without any effort. There is no *āsana* like *Siddhāsana*, no *khumbhaka* like *Kevala*, no *mūdra* like *Khechari*, and no *laya* (absorption of the mind) like *Nāda* (subtle inner sound).'

Haṭha Yoga Pradīpikā 1:42–43

The three *bandhas* (meaning 'lock', 'bind' or 'tie') are: *Uḍḍīyāna* (abdominal retraction lock), *Jālandhara* (throat lock) and *Mūlabandha* (root lock). These physical exercises 'bind' the *prāṇic* life-energy in certain vital areas of the body, and they form a very important aspect of Yoga practice. The yogi uses the *bandhas* to control the *prāṇic* life-force in the body (see section 6.5.1).

Khecharī is a *mūdra* ('a seal', 'sealing', 'closing'). The highest stages of Yoga are attained through the subtle process underlying this practice of *Khecharī mūdra*, which is accomplished when the yogi reverses the tongue and effortlessly inserts it into an opening located above the nasopharynx in the skull, causing complete absorption of the mind.

SITTING POSTURES FOR *PRĀṆĀYAMA* AND MEDITATION

Sitting for meditation or for *prāṇāyama* requires a stable posture that is relaxed and comfortable; a posture in which you can maintain the natural curves of the spine, and can remain seated in for a significant amount of time without any movement. When the body posture is held without effort, the breath is steady, quiet and subtle, the mind is perfectly calm, then you will be able to enter a deep state of stillness.

When sitting for meditation or for practising *prāṇāyama*, it is necessary and important to sit with the upper body straight. To sit steadily and comfortably for any length of time the head, neck, spine and pelvis must be in alignment directly over the base of the spine. The neck, shoulders, back muscles, hips, knees and legs need to be relaxed. To maintain the natural curve of the lumbar spine, you need to sit up on the front of your sitting bones, not slumping back or arching forward. To sit in a cross-legged posture on a cushion or folded blankets, you need to sit high enough so that your knees are lower than your hips. This creates space in the front of the groin, making it easier for the pelvis to tilt into proper alignment.

A balanced spine supports the relaxation of the whole nervous system. If there are any imbalances and misalignments of these body structures, they will create discomfort, tension and pain. These imbalances can also impede or block the natural flow of *prāṇic* energy in the *suṣumnā nāḍī.*

Regular practice of Yoga postures will help enormously to improve alignment and comfort in the sitting poses by developing flexibility in the legs, hips, knees and spine. The Yoga postures will also help in strengthening the lower back and opening the chest, developing and maximising your breathing.

Apart from *Virāsana* and *Vajrāsana*, all the other sitting poses listed below are cross-legged poses. These have the advantage of drawing the energy inwards towards the body and directing it upwards in the spine. It is also easier to apply *bandhas* (locks) in the cross-legged poses.

There are seven classical Yoga sitting postures for meditation:

1. ***Sukhāsana*** – Comfortable or easy pose (cross-legged)
2. ***Virāsana*** **–** Hero pose
3. ***Vajrāsana*** – Diamond pose or Thunderbolt pose
4. ***Siddhāsana*** – Adept pose
5. ***Svastikāsana*** – Auspicious pose
6. ***Ardha Padmāsana*** – Half-lotus pose
7. ***Padmāsana*** – Lotus pose.

1. Sukhāsana (Easy pose)

For those who have difficulty in sitting for long periods in *Siddhāsana*, *Vajrāsana*, *Ardha Pādmāsana* or *Pādmāsana*, you can sit in *Sukhāsana* (Easy pose). This is simply sitting cross-legged.

Sit on a firm cushion at an appropriate height for you to make the posture comfortable. Sitting on a firm cushion helps in stimulating and directing subtle energies. To avoid straining the back muscles try to keep the knees lower than the level of the hips, or at least at the same level. This allows your thighs to relax downward, reducing tension in the hips, and frees the spine to lengthen upwards. If you have a knee injury then support both knees with firm cushions, bolsters or rolled blankets under them.

Cross both legs and place the right foot under the left thigh and the left foot under, or in front of, the right calf on the floor. If it is more comfortable, cross the legs in the opposite way. Sit upright with the weight of your body towards the forward edges of your sitting bones. Align the upper body and shoulders directly over the base of the spine. Lengthen the spine and open the chest, and draw your shoulders back. Place your hands relaxed on your knees or thighs.

Sitting on a chair

If you are unable to sit comfortably and painlessly in *Sukhāsana* (Easy pose) then sit on an upright chair that has no arm-rests. (If your feet do not touch the floor, then support them with folded blankets.) The most important points are that the body is straight and in alignment, with the natural curves of the spine supporting the actions of the body; that the body is comfortable and relaxed; and that the body can remain still throughout the duration of the meditation or *prāṇāyama* practice.

When sitting on a chair for meditation, sit with your back away from the back of the chair. Sit on the forward edge of the chair, with the soles of your feet flat on the ground and your spine upright. Gently round and arch the lower back a few times, tilting the pelvis forward and back, until you have centred your spine and sitting bones. When you feel that your head, neck, spine and pelvis are aligned, then slightly lower your chin and lift the back of the skull to create space at the base of the occiput, where the head meets the neck.

For your comfort, make sure the chair is padded, or place a small cushion or folded blanket on it. Place the feet hip-width apart on the floor, with the lower legs perpendicular to the floor. You may find it useful to have your hips slightly higher than the knees, so that the thighs slope slightly downward to minimise strain in the legs. A cushion can be used to raise the height of the seat if necessary. If you wish, you may place a woollen or silk cloth over your chair and extend it on to the floor, for your feet to rest on. According to the yogis, wool and silk insulate against the subtle magnetic currents in the earth, which tend to pull the energy down.

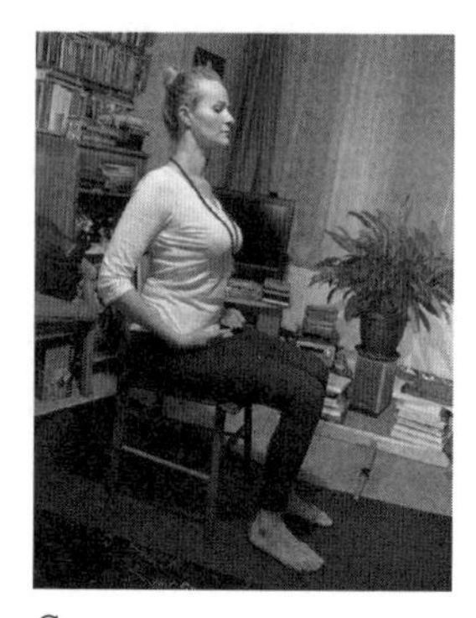

Sitting for meditation on a chair

Place the hands relaxed, palm upwards, at the junction of the thighs and abdomen (palms turned down you feel more grounded; palms turned up you feel more energised). Lift your shoulders, roll them up and back, and then drop and relax them. Keep the chest up. Lift up through your spine to the top of the head, so that your head, neck and spine are aligned, so that there is no impediment to the flow of subtle energy ascending in the spine to the higher brain centres.

Sitting on a meditation bench

Another useful prop for sitting is to use a wooden meditation bench with a slanting seat that allows the pelvis to tilt forward and provides support and lift to the spinal column. The meditation bench stands approximately eight inches high from the floor, and is padded for comfort, or a small cushion is placed on it.

To sit on the meditation bench you need to go into a kneeling position with the buttocks sitting on the bench and your legs folded underneath with your shins resting on the floor. Keep the thighs parallel and straight out from the hips. Place the hands relaxed on the upper thighs, and keep the head, neck and spine aligned.

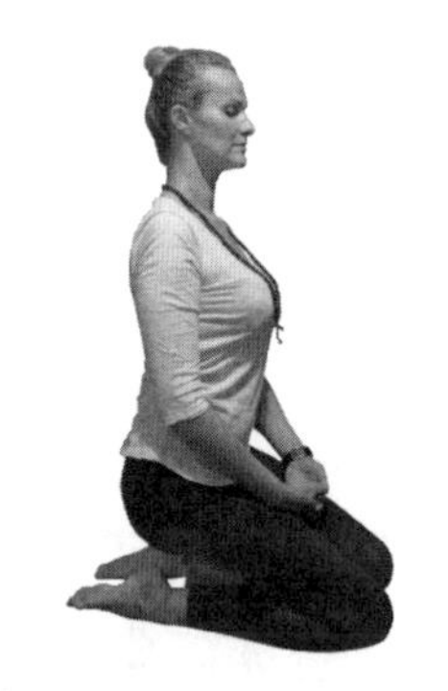

Sitting for meditation on a meditation bench

The sitting postures for the adept

For those of you who have more flexibility and suppleness in your body, and are are not suffering from knee injuries, sit in any of the following postures: *Siddhāsana*, *Vajrāsana*, *Virāsana*, *Ardha Pādmāsana* or *Pādmāsana*. These postures present a greater challenge to your hips, knees and ankles.

2. *Virāsana (Hero pose)*

For this sitting pose you will need one or two brick-shaped rubber blocks or folded blankets for a sitting support. Kneel on the floor with your knees about 4 inches (10 cm) apart with your feet separated slightly wider than your hips. The tops of the feet rest on the floor pointing straight back. Position the support block(s) between your feet with the long side of the block placed horizontally between your ankles. Make sure that both of your sitting bones are balanced evenly on the block and comfortably supported.

If you are comfortable sitting on your heels without the block, then lift up enough to allow you to use your hands to pull your outer calf muscles away from the thighs, before you sit down between your heels.

Place the hands palms down on your thighs close to the abdomen. To come out of the pose, lean forward onto your hands and slowly straighten the knees, walk back and stand up.

Caution: *Virāsana* puts a slight twist in the knees, so if you have a knee injury be careful, and practise with awareness only under the competent guidance of an experienced teacher.

3. *Vajrāsana (Diamond or Thunderbolt pose)*

This pose is also used by Muslims and Zen Buddhists as a position for prayer and meditation.

Come up on to the knees (knee stand). Place the legs together, tilt the upper body forward and sit back by lowering the buttocks onto the inside surface of the feet with the heels touching the sides of the hips. Cross the right big toe over the left, or alternatively have the big toes touching each other.

Keep the trunk upright and place the hands palms down, relaxed, on the thighs. The head, neck and back should be kept straight and relaxed.

4. *Siddhāsana (Adept pose; Perfect pose)*

Siddhā means 'perfected', 'accomplished'. A *siddhā* yogi is one who is perfected or accomplished in Yoga, or adept (skilful) in Yoga. *Siddhāsana* is considered as the foremost meditation posture and a favourite of adept yogis.

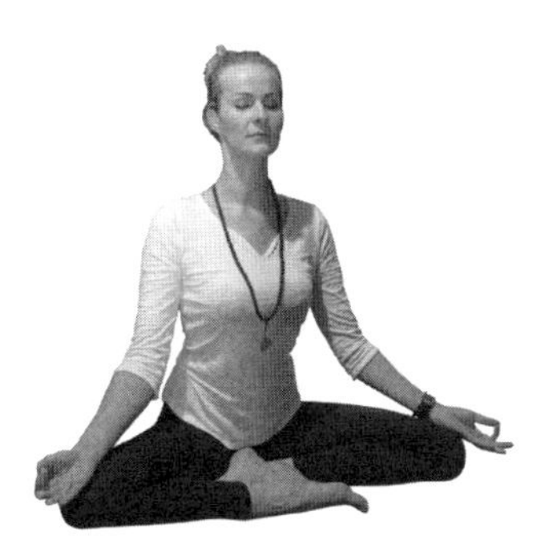

SITTING IN SIDDHĀSANA (ADEPT POSE; PERFECT POSE)

Sit on the edge of a firm cushion or a folded blanket. Bend your right leg and place the sole of the foot flat against the inner left thigh with your heel pressing against the perineum (the area midway between the genitals and the anus), sitting on top of the right heel. Then bend your left leg and place the left ankle directly over the right ankle so that the ankle bones are touching and the heels are positioned one above the other. Press the pubis with your left heel directly above the genitals. Push the outer edge of the left foot and the toes between the right calf and thigh muscles. Grasp the right toes and pull them up in between the left calf and thigh.

Note: In men the base of the penis rests against the bottom heel. Lift the penis, scrotum and testes up and out of the way, and then place the left heel close to the pubic bone.

Sit with the head, neck and spine in alignment, and with the knees touching the floor. Close the eyes, and place your hands on your knees or thighs with the palms either downward in *jñanā mudrā* (gesture of intuitive knowledge) or palms upward in *chin mudrā* (gesture of consciousness). In both *mudrās* the tip of the index finger and thumb touch. The other three fingers are extended and relaxed.

Chin mudrā represents the union of the cosmic with the individual consciousness. The index finger represents individual consciousness and the thumb, cosmic consciousness, The three remaining fingers symbolise the three *guṇas* (*sattva*, *rajas* and *tamas*), the three fundamental qualities of Material Nature (*prakṛiti*). The goal of the yogi is to transcend the three *guṇas* and to unite with the Cosmic Self.

Both *mudrās* help to activate the lower lungs and encourage diaphragmatic breathing, and stimulate the grounding effects of *apāṇa vāyu* (functions in the region of the navel to the feet). *Chin mudrā* also stimulates *prāṇā vāyu*.

In this pose, the pressure of the heel against the perineum stimulates *mūlabandha*, and the pressure against the pubic bone stimulates the *svādhiṣṭhāna*, directing the *prāṇic* flow of energy from the lower *chakras* upward through the spine, stimulating the brain and calming the entire nervous system.

Note: Women, like men, should position the heel against the inner surface of the inferior pubic rami. But this means that the heel will have to be placed directly against the soft tissues of the genitals, well in front of the fourchette (the fold of skin which forms the union of the lower ends of the labia minora). The heel will be more intrusive in the female because the upside-down V formed by the pubic rami is shallower than in the male. If women sit directly on the floor without a cushion, the back of the lower heel will be in the exact place where both the urogenital and pelvic diaphragms are interrupted by the vaginal introitus.

The posture used by women is called *Siddha Yoni āsana*. Sit with the legs straight in front. Bend your right leg and place the sole of the foot flat against the inner left thigh. Place the heel of the right foot firmly against or inside the labia majora of the vagina. Bend the left leg and position the left heel directly on top of the right heel so it presses the clitoris, and tuck the left toes down between the calf and thigh. Hold the toes of the right foot and pull them up between the left calf and thigh. The knees should be firmly on the floor, and the head, neck and spine aligned. The hands are placed on the knees in either *jñanā mudrā* or *chin mudrā*.

Benefits: Channels and directs the *prāṇic* life-energy to the *ājñā chakra*. Controls the nervous and *prāṇic* energy from *mūladhāra* and *svādhiṣṭhāna chakras*. Prevents blood pressure from falling too low during meditation, and helps to maintain the inner body temperature. It also stabilises the cardiac function. The two lower *chakras*, *mūladhāra* and *svādhiṣṭhāna*, are stabilised and the *prāṇa* is redirected upward towards the higher *chakras*.

5. Svastikāsana (Auspicious pose)

The symbol of the *Svastika* represents the different corners of the earth and universe, the spokes, and their meeting point and centre of consciousness. *Svastikāsana* is the third most important classical meditation posture, after *Siddhāsana* and *Pādmāsana*. The Auspicious pose (*Svastikāsana*) does not involve as much strain on the leg joints, so it can be managed for a long period of sitting.

Sit on a the edge of a firm cushion or two folded blankets with the legs stretched forward. Bend the left leg and place the sole of your left foot against the right inner thigh. Take your right foot by the ankle and place it on top of your left calf and position the outer edge of the foot and the toes in between the thigh and calf muscles. Place your hands relaxed on the knees with the thumb and index fingers touching, positioned in either *jñanā mudrā* or *chin mudrā*. Keep the head, neck and spine in alignment.

The difference between this pose and *Siddhāsana* is that in *Svastikāsana* the heels are not in line with each other. This makes it slightly easier as it requires less hip flexibility than *Siddhāsana*. In *Siddhāsana* and *Svastikāsana*, both knees come close to the floor. This supports the lower back by creating a natural inward tilt to the sacrum, giving a slight arch to the lower back.

Svastikāsana activates and rejuvenates the entire nervous system.

6. Ardha Pādmāsana (Half-lotus pose)

This posture is recommended for those unable to sit comfortably in the Full Lotus pose (*Pādmāsana*).

Sit on a the edge of a firm cushion or two folded blankets with the legs stretched forward. Bend the right leg and place the foot very close to the body on the floor. Then bend the left leg and bring the foot very close to the body on top of the right thigh. Keep the head, neck and spine in alignment, and both knees resting on the floor.

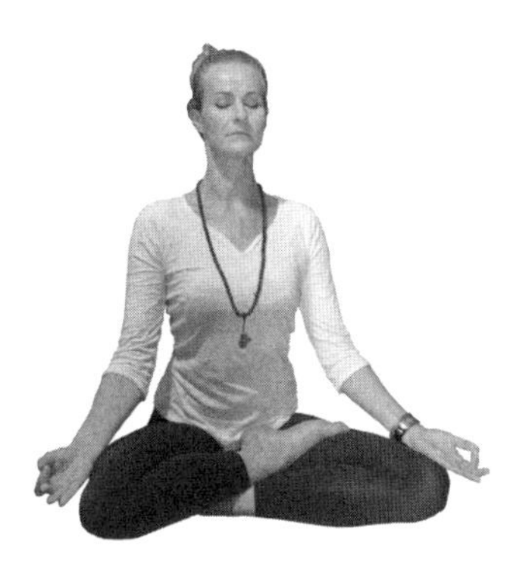

SITTING IN ARDHA PĀDMĀSANA (HALF-LOTUS POSE)

Ardha Pādmāsana can also be practised by bending the left leg first and bringing the right foot on top of the left thigh. To prevent imbalances in the hips and pelvis it is good to regularly change the crossing of the legs, so that both hips remain equally open. This principle also applies to the other crossed-legged postures.

7. Pādmāsana (Full Lotus pose)

Pādmāsana is the classic Yoga sitting pose for meditation that has a balancing influence on all the *chakras*. In pictures we see the great yogi masters such as Mahavatar Babaji, Lahiri Mahasaya, Swāmi Sri Yukteswar and Paramhansa Yogananda sitting in the superconsciousness state of *samādhi*, while sitting in the Full Lotus pose.

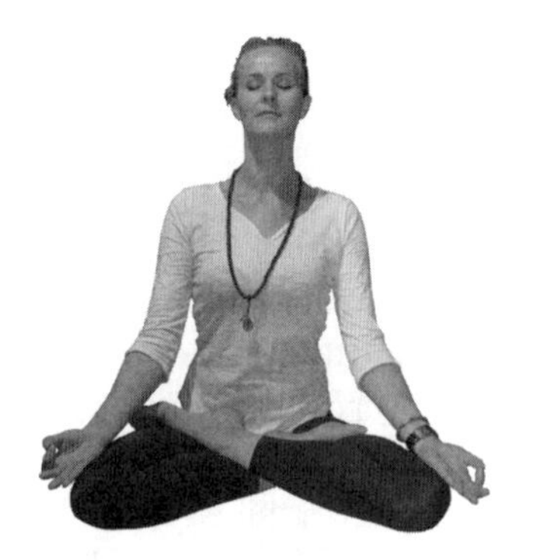

Sitting in Pādmāsana (Full Lotus pose)

But for most Westerners it is one of the most challenging poses to perform and so it is not practical as a meditation pose. It places stress on the knees and hip joints; it demands a very strong external rotation of the thigh bones in the hip sockets; and if the hip joints are tight, this pose can place enormous stress on the knees. The knee is a hinge joint with a limited capacity to rotate, and it is usually the intra-articular structures of the knee such as the cruciate ligaments and menisci ligaments (which act as pads for the knee joint) that get torn in an injury.

It is essential first to be able to perform a full range of motion of the ball and socket hip joint to protect the hinged knee joint. So, unless you have practised it in your childhood and youth, it is not likely to work satisfactorily. But for those adepts who have mastered this beautiful looking pose, it is said to bring an incomparable feeling of repose and calmness to the mind.

If you are going to practise *Pādmāsana,* do not force yourself into it, but carefully learn progressively with appropriate warm-up stretches and modifications under the guidance of an experienced teacher who is able to practise it competently and safely. Avoid this pose if you have knee problems or varicose veins.

If *Pādmāsana* or the Full Lotus pose can be practised properly and correctly, and one is able to sit in it comfortably, it gives great stability and strength to the lower back while locking the legs securely in place. It is difficult to fall over even if you were to fall asleep; this is why it is the chosen pose by yogis for going into the superconsciousness state of *samādhi.*

Benefits: *Pādmāsana* purifies all the systems of the body, and brings calmness and joy to the yogi. It increases *sattva guṇa* (purity).

Warm-up for Lotus pose

It is good practice before any exercise where the knees are to be rotated into advanced sitting poses, such as *Pādmāsana*, to take time to warm and relax them by rubbing the sides of both knees with the palms of your hands. Rub vigorously using a rotating motion. This allows the bursae located around the joint (which function to cushion the knee) to lubricate, protecting the knees from sudden forcible flexion. The aim of Lotus warm-ups is to increase movement in the hip and knee joints, and stretch the thigh muscles. Therefore, exercises where you work both inward and outward rotation are helpful in augmenting the multidirectional range of motion in the hips.

When you come out of *Pādmāsana*, straighten the leg, raise the kneecap, and pull the toes towards the body, so as to elongate the hamstring and relieve any cramps in the muscles.

First warm-up: Half Butterfly pose

Sit with your back and legs straight. Breathing normally, place the right foot with the sole of the foot facing upward, on top of the left thigh as close to the hip as possible. (If this leg position is difficult, then place the foot on the floor alongside the inside of the thigh close to the body.)

Hold the toes of the right foot with the left hand, and with slight pressure move your knee up and down ten times with the right hand.

Return to the starting position and perform the exercise with the left leg.

Benefits: Stretches the muscles of the inner hip and thighs and encourages blood circulation into the hips.

Second warm-up: Full Butterfly pose

Resting firmly on your sitting bones, sit on a cushion on the floor. Bring the soles of the feet together and draw the heels close into the groin. Clasp the feet with interlocked fingers and pull against the feet for leverage. Open the knees and press them towards the floor.

Inhale, lift the lower back and, extending the sternum, elongate the spine to the crown of the head. Exhale, creating a shoulder-blade squeeze, and slightly arch the lower spine, and work to lower the thighs towards the floor.

Third warm-up: Cradle pose

From the same sitting position as before, outstretch your right leg. Take hold of the left leg, and keeping the left foot up high, place it into the crook of the right arm at the elbow. Bring the left arm around and interlock the hands, creating your cradle (like holding a baby). Inhale, elongating and straightening the spine by extending the sternum upward. Exhale as you rock the cradled leg from right to left.

Inhale, elongating the spine again. Exhale, this time hugging the leg closer to your chest. Hold the position and feel the stretch in the thigh. Repeat the process with the other leg.

Full Lotus pose (Pādmāsana)

Sit with the legs extended straight in front of you. Then, slowly and carefully bend your left leg, holding the left foot with your hands. Turn the foot around so that the sole is facing you. Place the instep up high on the thigh as you lower the knee to the floor. The heel should be close to the pubic bone.

Bend the right leg. Holding the right foot with your hands, place the instep up high on the left thigh.

In the final position, both knees should ideally touch the floor. The head, neck and spine must be aligned with the shoulders relaxed, and the hands relaxed on the knees in either *jñanā mudrā* or *chin mudrā*. Close the eyes and relax the whole body.

A comfortable alternative to the Lotus pose

Pādmāsana is an excellent posture for stability – it locks the pelvis into a perfect vertical position, keeping the spine upright and aligned. The pelvis is moved into the vertical position by the pulling of the gluteus medius muscles. The sitting bones are positioned correctly and the knees are rooted firmly to the floor.

For many Yoga practitioners the Lotus pose is extremely difficult to accomplish, because in order for the feet to rest high on the thighs without injuring the knees, the thighs have to rotate outward about 116 degrees in the hip sockets, and the knees have to move closer together. There is a considerable amount of strain on the knee joints; forcing oneself into this pose can easily injure a knee by tearing the meniscus ligament. But there is an alternative substitute – a comfortable, steady, supported version that combines the balance between the stability of *Pādmāsana* (Lotus pose) and the ease and comfort of *Sukhāsana* (Easy pose) to create stability, comfort, and ease.

Preparation

To begin your practice you will need to sit against a wall on a carpeted floor to cushion your ankles (or you can fold a Yoga mat). You will also need three or four folded blankets to sit on and another blanket rolled into a long roll to place over your feet. Place the three or four folded blankets parallel against the wall.

Method

1. Sit on the folded blankets with your back upright against the support of the wall. Then cross your legs and bring the right leg in so that your shins contact each other, and each foot rests on the floor under the opposite thigh.
2. Adjust the height of the knees until they are parallel to the floor.
3. Place the long rolled blanket over the tops of both feet and adjust it to support the legs.
4. Tilt your pelvis forward by leaning your upper body forward, then sit upright with your back against the wall. Rest the backs of your hands on your thighs, so that the hands are relaxed.
5. Roll the tops of your shoulders back and lean your head gently against the wall.
6. With the head, neck and spine in alignment keep the chest lifted and relax your abdomen and diaphragm muscle as you breathe slowly and rhythmically.

ĀSANA FOR RELAXING THE BODY FOR MEDITATION

To practise meditation the body needs to be free of tension. It needs to be able to relax the tensions that build up in the muscles of the neck, shoulders, back, and the joints of the body. These tensions create agitation, restlessness and disturbance in the nervous system, the mind and the breath, which is a distraction to meditation. The body, mind and breath are closely connected. For the body to relax, the mind has to relax and become calm, and the breath has to become slow, steady and even. When all three – body, mind and breath – are in harmony and attuned with each other, then the inner environment for meditation is ready. Yoga *āsanas,* when practised with the breath, awareness and concentration, relax the body of all tensions.

Relaxation and awareness are the first preparations towards meditation and the state of inner calmness and stillness. A Yoga pose that is calm and relaxed helps in inducing a calm state of mind. Forward bending *āsanas* such as the seated forward bend *paścimottānāsana* (posterior stretch) have a great soothing effect on the brain. Inverted postures also have a calming and relaxing effect, such as *sarvāṅgāsana* (shoulder stand) which soothes and nourishes the whole body. *Viparīta Karaṇī mudrā* (Reverse Action pose) is another inverted posture which soothes and relaxes the mind and body. The ultimate posture for relaxation is *Śavāsana* (Corpse pose), which is done in the lying down position.

ĀSANA FOR AWAKENING ENERGY IN THE SPINE FOR MEDITATION

It is important to relax the mind and body to enter into a calm state of meditative stillness, but one also needs energy to meditate. The spine needs to be awakened. Energy needs to be flowing upward in the spine towards the brain and the higher centres or *chakras*. The connection between the mind and body is the *prāṇic* flow of energy, which flows through a network of subtle channels called *nāḍīs*. This energy transmits signal impulses from the senses to the brain, and from the brain to the body. If the flow of energy becomes obstructed or imbalanced, then both the mind and body go out of harmony. This can cause a stagnation of energy, resulting in tiredness, fatigue, lethargy and dullness in both the body and the mind, making them unfit for meditation.

Changing the inner level of one's energy can create a very positive effect on the quality of one's consciousness and mental awareness. Paramhansa Yogananda said: 'The greater the will, the greater the flow of energy!' When we think positively the energy flows upward, and when we think negatively there is a corresponding downward flow of energy. By conscious, positive willing you can draw *prāṇic* life-energy into the brain, the spine, and the body through the medulla oblongata (located at the top of the brain stem at the back of the brain). It is the strength of our willpower and concentration that is able to consciously draw life-energy directly from the Cosmic Energy into the body.

In practising Yoga *āsanas* to awaken energy in the spine, one can switch on willpower and concentrate on sending energy upward through the spine. The standing Yoga *āsanas*, forward and backward bending *āsanas*, and twisting *āsanas* are all good for energising the spine. The *Sūrya Namaskāra* (Sun Salutation) sequence, and the *Aṣṭāṅga Yoga Vinyāsa* Primary Series sequence are both excellent for awakening energy in the spine. These sequences, particularly *Aṣṭāṅga Yoga Vinyāsa*, strengthen and purify, rejuvenate and balance all the systems of the body.

Practise the *āsanas* with awareness, remain calmly centred and balanced within the spine, and as you concentrate, connect and synchronise your breathing with the movement of the *āsana*. Think of your *āsana* practice as movement in meditation.

6.5

PRĀṆĀYAMA

Prāṇāyāma is the fourth limb of *Aṣṭāṅga Yoga* (Eight Limbs of Yoga). The Sanskrit word *prāṇāyāma* is formed by two words: *prāṇa* means energy or subtle life force; *ayāma* has two meanings – to regulate, and to extend, lengthen or expand. *Prāṇāyāma* means regulating and harmonising the energy or subtle life force within the body. *Prāṇa* is not merely the breath, and *prāṇāyāma* is not just regulating or controlling the breath, but direct perception of the life principle.

By the process of *prāṇāyāma*, individual energy and consciousness are expanded into universal energy and consciousness.

RĀJA YOGA DEFINITION OF *PRĀṆĀYĀMA*

The perfect state of *prāṇāyāma*, in which one identifies one's inner Self with the Supreme Consciousness, is attained in the state of concentration in which the movement of the heart for inhalation and exhalation is suspended.

Advanced *prāṇāyāma*, in which the meditator identifies oneself with Supreme Consciousness, is the state of concentration in which the movement of the chest for inhalation and exhalation is forgotten and unknown to the meditator.

HAṬHA YOGA DEFINITION OF *PRĀṆĀYĀMA*

That state which leads one to the above-mentioned states is when the respiratory system is trained by regulating the inhalation and exhalation; it is called the breathing practices of *prāṇāyāma*.

> 'On that (*āsana*) being accomplished, *prāṇāyāma* follows: regulation of the life-force through stilling the breath.'
>
> *Yoga Sūtras 2:49*

Patañjali says we should have a steady posture (*āsana*) before attempting *prāṇāyāma*, because when you practise, the *prāṇa* vibrates more powerfully. The posture has to be steady and comfortable, and the mind concentrated on the Infinite. When this is accomplished, the body and mind become stable. Then the breath can be easily suspended for extended periods of time.

> 'The variations in prāṇāyama are external, internal or suspended. The interval is regulated by space, time and number, and becomes progressively prolonged and subtle.'
>
> *Yoga Sūtras 2:50*

In this *sūtra* Patañjali describes three types of *prāṇāyama* on the basis of the nature of the interval that causes a temporary suspension of the breath:

External breath retention (*bāhya kumbhaka*) – a pause after a very slow and prolonged exhalation.

Internal breath retention (*ābhyantara kumbhaka*) – a pause after a deep, prolonged inhalation.

Suspension of breath (*stambha vṛtti*) – natural and spontaneous suspension of both the external and internal breath. The chest remains standing still like a straight pillar, or a motionless jar full of water. Therefore it is called *stambha vṛitti prāṇāyama* (*stambha* – 'pillar'; *vṛitti* – 'similar'). This can take place any time when the breath becomes very subtle and the mind is totally one-pointed in concentration on the infinite.

In this method of *prāṇāyama*, Patañjali says the interval is regulated by space (*deśha*), time (*kāla*), and number (*saṁkhya*). Space (*deśha*) refers to where the breath is held (external, internal or suspended).

The importance of *prāṇic* energy is also given in the ancient scripture *Bhāgavad Gītā*:

'One practice of Yoga offers the incoming breath (*prāṇa*) into the outgoing breath (*apāṇa*), and the *apāṇa* into the *prāṇa*, thereby, through *prāṇāyāma* (control of the energy), rendering the breath unnecessary.'

Bhāgavad Gītā 4:29

'The muni (one for whom liberation is the sole purpose of life) controls his senses, mind, and intellect, removing himself from contact with them by neutralising the currents of prāṇa and apāṇa in the spine, which manifests (outwardly) as inhalation and exhalation in the nostrils. He fixes his gaze in the forehead, at the point midway between the two eyebrows (thereby converting the dual current of physical vision into the single, omniscient Spiritual Eye). Such a one attains complete emancipation.'

Bhāgavad Gītā 5:27–28

WHAT IS *PRĀṆA*?

Prāṇa is not breath in its gross form. The air that we breathe through the nostrils cannot be identified with what is called *prāṇa*. Although the air that we inhale and exhale is inseparably connected with what we regard as *prāṇa*, the two are not identical with each other. Similarly, an effect (such as turning on a light switch) produced by electricity cannot be regarded as electricity itself, though one cannot be separated from the other.

The breathing process – the breath that we can feel in the form of air moving in and out through the nostrils and lungs is an outward indication of the internal movement of the forces of vital energy or life force called *prāṇa*. This vital energy or *prāṇa* is superior to air or oxygen which activates the lungs. Respiration is an outward effect of an internal activity of *prāṇa*, it is not the activity of *prāṇa* itself. *Prāṇa* is subtle, it is situated in the subtle body, which is also known as the the astral body (*sūkṣhma sarira*). The *prāṇās*, the senses, the mind and the intellect are all in the subtle body.

The manifested universe is composed of *prāṇa* (energy). *Prāṇa* is the universal force of nature and the energy that pervades the entire physical system that acts as a medium between the body and the mind. *Prāṇa* is more subtle than the physical body but grosser than the mind. *Prāṇa* acts but does not think; the mind is more subtle. Although we can not see *prāṇa*, its existence can be inferred by the process of our breathing, for air is drawn in and out of the lungs by the action of *prāṇa*. In reality, this vital energy we call *prāṇā* is one energy, but appears to be more than one when viewed from the standpoint of its different functions.

THE VITAL AIRS: LIFE FORCES OF THE BODY

Prāṇa is the cause of movement in the body; without *prāṇa* the physical body would become inert. In the *Kaushitakibrahmanopaniṣad* it is stated:

> '*Prāṇa* is the span of life and the span of life is synonymous with *prāṇa*. *Prāṇa* is immortality; only so long as there is *prāṇa* in the body is there life.'

Prāṇa is known as *vayu*, or 'vital air', when it operates within the human body systems. In both the subtle and gross bodies, *prāṇa* has been differentiated into five major and five minor *prāṇas*, the only difference being that of subtle and gross according to the bodies. When the subtle body permeates the gross body, the subtle *prāṇas,* like the gross ones, are also present in the subtle body. After the death of the physical body, it is this *prāṇa* that sustains and takes the subtle body to the astral plane.

Without *prāṇa*, no activity can take place in the subtle body, nor any support of life. Subtle *prāṇa* performs all actions in every part of the body. It is *prāṇa* that is responsible for respiration, digestion, activity, movement of energy in the body, and the acquisition of the five *tanmātras* – *shabda* (sound), *sparsha* (touch), *rupa* (colour/form), *rasa* (taste) and *gandha* (smell), the subtle components of the ultra-atomic particles that form the nuclei of the physical world.

From these five subtle *tanmātras* evolve the generic gross elements, the five *mahābhūtas* – *ākāśha* (ether), *vayu* (air), *tejas* or *agni* (fire), *apas* (water) and *pṛithvī* (earth). The *mahābhūtas* are the essential 'states' of matter; they are not visible, and so they should not be confused with the periodic chemical elements known to modern science.

Prāṇa is differentiated into five major vital airs (*prāṇa vayus*) and five minor *vayus*, which should not be identified with the air that we breathe. The *prāṇa vayus* are the intelligent life forces which are manifested in the astral body. These subtle powers that sustain the systems of the subtle body of the human organism derive their power direct from the source of life-energy that manifests in the body by virtue of the presence of the *puruṣa*, Self. According to the ancient philosophical system of *Sāṃkhya*, these vital airs (*prāṇa vayus*) are the products of *rājasic ahaṇkāra* (active ego) that evolves out of *prakṛiti* (nature). All creations and all life processes are dependent on the hierarchical evolution of the 23 metaphysical and physical categories (*tattvas*) of *prakṛiti* as according to the *Sāṃkhya* system of philosophy.

Both the philosophical system of Yoga and the *Vedānta* system are in agreement with *Sāṃkhya* philosophy, and accept the reality of *prāṇa*.

The five major *prāṇa vayus* that function in designated areas of the body are: *prāṇa*, *apāṇa*, *samāna*, *udāṇa* and *vyāna*.

The five minor *prāṇa vayus* are: *nāga*, *kūrma*, *kṛkala*, *devadatta* and *dhanañjaya*.

It must be noted again that the vital airs (*prāṇa vayus*) are not synonymous with the air, oxygen and other gases that we breathe. The *prāṇa vayus* work on the subtle plane in the astral body, not the physical. They can only be understood through the yogic practice of *prāṇāyāma*. To be able to control the body and mind one needs to learn to master and guide the activities of the subtle *prāṇa vayus*.

These *prāṇic* currents flow through subtle channels known as *nāḍīs*. The Yoga practice of *prāṇāyāma* – regulating the *prāṇic* flow of energy – helps to remove impurities from the three planes of existence: physical, astral and causal bodies, and also from the five sheaths (*koshas*) that contain and envelop the soul within the body. These five sheaths that represent different levels of consciousness are: *annamaya kosha* (physical sheath); *prāṇāyāma kosha* (vital force sheath), that connects the physical body to the astral body; *manomaya kosha* (mind sheath); *vijnanmaya kosha* (intellect sheath), that connects the astral body to the causal body; and *anandamaya kosha* (bliss sheath), that is identified with the spiritual consciousness of the causal body.

THE FIVE MAJOR VITAL AIRS

Prāṇa vayu

Prāṇa vayu ('ascending vital air') derives its name from the generic *prāṇa*. It functions in the chest region, and is seated in the heart. It uses the autonomic nervous system controlling speech, the respiratory muscles, blood circulation, and body temperature. *Prāṇa* is the colour of a red diamond, or a rose pink like that of a coral.

In the respiration, the exhalation is the activity of *prāṇa vayu*, and the inhalation is the activity of *apāṇa vayu*.

Samāna vayu

Samāna vayu ('equalising vital air') functions in the region between the heart and the navel. It controls the all the metabolic activity involved in digestion through the sympathetic part of the autonomic nervous system. *Samāna* is the colour somewhere between that of milk and crystal, which shines.

Apāṇa vayu

Apāṇa vayu ('descending vital air') functions in the region from the lower abdomen to the soles of the feet. The seat of *apāṇa* is in the anal region. *Apāṇa* has a downward movement normally, but carries the *kuṇḍalinī shakti* upwards in the *suṣumnā* (the central subtle channel in the astral spine) to unite with *prāṇa*. *Apāṇa* controls the function of the kidneys, excretory system and reproductive system through the autonomic nervous system. *Apāṇa* is a dark red colour.

Udāṇa vayu

Udāṇa vayu ('elevating vital air') functions in the body from the throat to the top of the head. It controls the automatic function of the cephalic divisions of the autonomic nervous system. It controls speech, swallowing, the sense of balance, memory and the intellect. It also encourages growth, lightness and agility of the body, and is responsible for taking us to sleep when we are tired or exhausted. *Udāṇa* has an upward movement – it carries *kuṇḍalinī* to the *sahasrāra chakra*, and separates the astral body from the physical body at the time of death. *Udāṇa* is a pale white colour.

Vyāna vayu

Vyāna vayu ('pervading vital air') is the force that pervades the entire body, and so does not have a specific seat in the body. *Vyāna* is the aura around the body. It is responsible for the movement of the blood circulation and the movement of oxygen that we take in through the capillaries of the lungs. *Vyāna* helps all the other *vayus* to harmoniously function properly. It controls both the voluntary and the involuntary movements of the muscles and the joints, and keeps the whole body upright by generating unconscious reflexes along the spine. In addition to this, it controls the physical nerves and the subtle astral channels (*nāḍīs*). *Vyāna* is the colour of a ray of light.

THE FIVE MINOR VITAL AIRS

The five major functions (*samanyakaran vrutti*) of *prāṇa* that 'balance the activity within' is its principal form. It has also five minor vital airs (*upaprāṇas*) that function in secondary importance with such activities as opening and closing of the eyelids, yawning and causing hunger.

Naga vayu – Controls the functions of belching and hiccoughing. It also gives rise to consciousness.

Kurma vayu – Controls the function of opening and closing the eyelids and causes vision.

Karikara vayu – Controls sneezing and induces hunger and thirst.

Devadatha vayu – Controls yawning.

Dhananjaya vayu – Causes the decomposition of the body after death. At the time of death all of the *prāṇic vayus* depart from the body except the *dhananjaya vayu*.

Yogendra Svatmarama states:

> 'When there is *prāṇa* in the body, it is called life; when it leaves the body, it results in the death. So one should practise *prāṇāyāma*.'
>
> *Haṭha Yoga Pradīpikā 2:3*

PRĀṆA AND THE *CHAKRAS* AND *NĀḌĪS*

Within the subtle body there are seven main energy centres known as *chakras*, through which the *prāṇic* energy is distributed throughout the body via a network of subtle channels (*nāḍīs*). *Prāṇa*, the all-permeating force which vibrates though all life, is the link between the gross and the subtle world. If there is an imbalance of *prāṇic* energy in any of the *chakras*, a corresponding imbalance will occur in the physical body. Disturbance of the *prāṇa* in the body is the primary cause of many mental and physical diseases. *Prāṇāyāma* is important for maintaining this balance. Each of the *chakras* is a centre for *prāṇa*, but the main dynamo where *prāṇa* is generated is in the navel centre (*maṇipūra chakra*), and for the purpose of distribution, *prāṇa* is stored in the *ājñā chakra* (the centre that is at the midpoint between the eyebrows).

Just as there is a vast network of veins, arteries and capillaries that transport blood throughout the physical body, so there is also a vast network of subtle channels (*nāḍīs*) in our astral bodies that carry *prāṇic* energy in the form of currents of bright light. There are 12 major *nāḍīs* that branch off into 72,000 mid-sized subtle channels. From these, a vast number of finer channels branch off, bringing the total to 350,000 *nāḍīs*.

In the astral body of the pelvic region, between the anus and the root of the genitals, just above the *mūladhāra chakra*, is an egg-shaped structure that is about three inches (7.6 cm) wide and seven inches (17.8 cm) long. It is known as the *kand chakra*, and from it originates nine major *nāḍīs* that distribute *prāṇic* energy to certain areas of the body. In the *BrihadĀranyaka Upaniṣad*, the oldest of the *Upaniṣad* texts (800 BCE), it states that the *nāḍīs* are as fine as a hair split into 1,000.

Of the 12 main *nāḍīs*, the three that are most important to the yogi are the *iḍā*, the *piṅgala* and the *suṣumnā*.

The Sanskrit word *Haṭha* (as in *Haṭha Yoga*) refers to the movement of energy in the two subtle energy channels:

> *Ha* is the upward movement of energy on the left side of the spine called *piṅgala* (positive pole; solar energy).
>
> *Tha* is the downward movement of energy on the right side of the spine called *iḍā* (negative pole; lunar energy).

The main central subtle channel (*suṣumnā*) originates near the root of the spine, passes through the *kand chakra*, and then continues upwards in the spinal column (*merudanda*) to a cavity in the brain (*Brāhmarandhra* – 'Gateway to Supreme Consciousness').

The *iḍā nāḍī* emerges from the left side of the *suṣumnā* and spirals upward around the *suṣumnā* to the left nostril, and branches out to the *ājñā chakra* (positive pole: Spiritual Eye; negative pole: medulla oblongata).

The *piṅgala nāḍī* starts from the *kand chakra* on the right side of the *suṣumnā* and spirals upward in a reverse pattern to the right nostril, and also branches out to the *ājñā chakra*.

The balance between these two currents of energy strongly influences our inner and outer experiences through the mind and senses. The upward flow of energy in the left subtle channel (*iḍā nāḍī*) corresponds with the inhalation of the breath, and the mind is drawn outward to the objects of the senses. The downward flow of energy in the right subtle channel (*piṅgala nāḍī*) corresponds with the exhalation. If there is a strong downward movement of energy in the spine, the exhalation will also become stronger. Notice how we sigh with a deep exhalation when we feel depressed or 'down'. Whereas when we are feeling positively joyful, we inhale with a surge of upward energy and vitality.

The yogi learns to consciously bring these two currents of energy (positive and negative poles) back into balance – in which both flow equally in the *suṣumnā*.

PRĀṆA AND THE MIND

Both *prāṇa* and the mind are interdependent; they influence each other. When the flow of *prāṇa* in the *chakras* and the body is disturbed, the mind is also disturbed; and when the mind is disturbed, the *prāṇa* is disturbed. In *Rāja Yoga*, calming the mind is of primary importance, especially in its feeling and emotional aspect. This is more important than merely holding the breath to calm the mind, because the mind is the internal mechanism behind the movement of the breath. So it is necessary to be more aware of the mental processes than their outward expression in the form of the movement of *prāṇa*.

When the mind becomes calm and steady, the *Prāṇa* becomes settled of its own accord. Paramhansa Yogananda taught a wonderful *Kriyā Yoga* technique for calming and concentrating the mind. It is called the *Hong Sau* (pronounced 'hong saw'), which is a *mantra* meaning 'I am He', or 'I am the Self'. This seed-syllable *mantra* is the inner sound of the inhaling and exhaling breath. It corresponds to the *prāṇic* currents in the spine, in the *iḍā* (upward flow) and the *piṅgala* (downward flow) *nāḍīs*.

Hong Sau is practised by sitting in a meditation posture, with the eyes closed and the inward gaze looking into the Spiritual Eye (at the midpoint between the eyebrows). Then as the breath naturally flows in, one mentally pronounces the *mantra Hong*. As the breath naturally flows out, one mentally pronounces the *mantra Sau*.

Hong Sau is not a breathing technique but the *awareness* of watching the breath. The concentration is on the breath while keeping the focused attention at the midpoint between the eyebrows.

Prāṇa is intimately related to the mind and mental processes; one cannot move without the other also moving. When there is turbulence in the mind, the breath becomes restless and vice versa.

We need only become aware of emotions such as anger, fear, hatred and jealousy to feel what effect it has on our breathing. When we become angry or emotionally upset, our breathing is markedly changed in its rate and depth. For example, when we become angry, we breathe faster and lose control over the breath and mind. Such negative emotions as anger agitates and shatter the whole nervous system, and can lead to hatred, which is even worse; for when the heart is attuned to hate it is impossible to feel attunement with God, who is love.

The emotions and the mental processes are related to the nervous system and through it they change our breathing. That is why it is important to develop and affirm attitudes and positive thoughts, and to change or overcome unwanted negative or destructive tendencies and behaviours. How? By developing the virtues we associate with divine qualities: love, inner joy, compassion, selflessness, kindness, generosity, loyalty, gentleness, forgiveness, peacefulness, calmness and inner contentment. When these virtues are naturally and spontaneously expressed, then the energy naturally and continuously flows in abundance. The *prāṇa* in an upward flow permeates the entire body, elevating the consciousness. Conversely, if we become negative in our thoughts, attitudes and behaviour, or suppress our natural feelings, the *prāṇic* flow of energy sinks downward and becomes concentrated in the lower part of the body and the lower three *chakras*. The body and mind become depressed and the breath unstable.

> 'By the proper and careful practice of *prāṇāyāma* one can attain health, a calm, steady mind, and a firm and lustrous body free from disease.'
>
> *Haṭha Yoga Pradīpikā 2:16–18*

The practice of *prāṇāyāma* helps in transforming the total personality by clearing mental obstructions; purifying the subtle channels (*nāḍīs*) through which the currents of *prāṇa* flow; awakening dormant forces in the body; focusing the attention; developing concentration; and improving overall health and vitality.

PRĀṆA AND THE SENSES

> 'The senses are said to be superior to the body; but greater than the senses is the mind. Superior to the mind is the discriminating intellect; and the inner Self (the innermost principle of the intelligence of all beings) is superior to the discriminating intellect.'
>
> *Bhāgavad Gītā 3:42 (Author's translation)*

The intention behind the practice of *prāṇāyāma* is the restraint of the senses. The 11 senses (*indriyas*) are: *manas* (the thinking or recording mind), the five *jñānendriyas* (organs of perception: the ears, eyes, skin, tongue and nose), and the five *karmendriyas* (organs of action: the vocal cords, hands, legs, reproductive organs and anus). The *prāṇa* operates through the instruments of the senses in any direction of any particular object or goal in one's outward life, which is a means of satisfaction to the mind. The mind is the dynamo generating the energy passing through the *prāṇā*, which flows through the instrument of the senses to particular objects of sense.

The senses are restrained by regulating the *prāṇā*, which is greatly achieved by subduing the mind in deep meditation.

PRĀṆĀYAMA PRACTICE

Before beginning *prāṇāyama* one should strengthen and purify the body and the subtle *prāṇic* channels (*nāḍīs*) by practising the following five purifications. This will also make your *prāṇāyama* practice more effective and lay the foundation for awakening energy in the spine. In addition to the four classical purifications you can also practise *jala neti,* which cleanses the nasal passages, the pharynx and the sinus cavities.

THE FIVE PURIFICATIONS

In addition to the classical *Haṭha Yoga shatkriyas* (six methods of purification) there are four purification techniques based on these which were devised by yogis to simplify and make safer the methods of purification. These five techniques can be practised instead of the classical Yoga *shatkriyas* for purifying the *nāḍīs* (subtle *prāṇic* channels), and for awakening the *chakras* and the life energy in the body.

The five purifications are practised in the following order:

1. *Jala neti*
2. *Nāḍī śodhana*
3. *Kapālabhāti*
4. *Agnisāra kriyā*
5. *Aśvinī mudrā*

Practice time: To prepare the body and purify the *nāḍīs* for the practice of *prāṇāyama*, the five purifications are practised over a period of two to three months. This is important for those who are beginners, who have had no previous experience of practising *prāṇāyama*.

1. Jala neti (water nasal cleansing)

Jala neti can be practised daily, but once a week should be enough. It should be practised particularly when the nasal passages are congested.

The practice of *jala neti* promotes a balance between the left and right nostrils, balancing the right and left hemispheres of the brain and the entire central nervous system. It gives mental clarity and helps in creating a balanced flow of *prāṇa* in the three *nāḍīs*: *iḍā*, *piṅgala* and *suṣumnā*. It activates the *ājñā chakra* (Spiritual Eye).

On the physical level, *jala neti* helps in preventing and eliminating sinusitis and sinus headaches by promoting drainage of the sinuses, preventing stasis of mucus and keeping them clean and functional. It maintains healthy secretory and drainage mechanisms of the entire ear (including the eustachian tubes) in the nasopharynx, nose and throat area. This helps to ward off colds, coughs, catarrh, hay fever and tonsillitis.

Jala neti also strengthens the eyes, through stimulation of the blood vessels of the eyes and nose. It exerts a relaxing and irrigating effect upon the eyes by stimulating the tear ducts and glands.

On an emotional level, *jala neti* releases tensions and is beneficial in depression, anxiety and hysteria.

Preparation

To practise *jala neti* you will need a special pot for the purpose of pouring water into the nostrils, called *neti loṭā* or *neti* pot. In India it is made from copper, brass, steel or clay and looks like a small teapot. In Europe and the USA you can buy a modern version made of plastic. The spout is designed to fit the nostril. The water must feel comfortable when used. Mix one level teaspoon (5 ml) of salt into half a litre of lukewarm water until it dissolves.

Caution: Too little salt will cause an unpleasant sensation, while too much will cause a burning sensation in the mucus membranes.

Method 1

Check your nostrils to feel in which nostril the flow of air is more predominant. You will pour the water through the nostril that is breathing more freely.

Stand with your legs apart and lean forward over a bath or wash basin if you are inside a building. Outside, you can stand in the garden. Keep the whole body relaxed. Take the *neti* pot of lukewarm salt water, and hold the spout to one nostril while tilting the head slightly forward and to one side. Breathe through your mouth. Let the water run in one nostril and pass out through the other. If the head is tilted properly, the water will easily flow down and out of the lower nostril. Now with the head centred again, blow the nose to clear the nostril of water. Then repeat the process using the other nostril.

Method 2

After both nostrils are clear, raise your head and tilt it back. Pour water into the left nostril and allow the water to flow down into the oral cavity. Then lower your head and spit the water out through your mouth (do not swallow the water). Repeat the process using the right nostril.

Method 3

Fill your mouth with water and inhale deeply through both nostrils. Hold the breath in, bend forward slightly, lower your head and exhale deeply through both nostrils. As the air from the nostrils is expelled, the water held in your mouth will slowly come out through both nostrils.

After practising *jala neti* you may find that you still have some water left in your nasal passages, to drain it out, stand with your feet about hip-width apart and bend forward from the waist, so that your head is lower than your waist. Remain like this for one or two minutes to allow excess water to trickle down and drain out of the nostrils. Then closing one nostril with your thumb, blow the air out with the water in short, sharp bursts, while still keeping your head lower than your waist. Repeat the same process with the other nostril.

Afterwards, sit kneeling on your heels in *Vajrāsana* (Thunderbolt pose) and practise a few rounds of *bhastrikā* (bellows breath).

Jala neti can also be practised using oil or clarified butter (*ghee*). With a clean glass dropper a few drops of almond oil or clarified liquid *ghee* are poured into both nostrils and then are inhaled with force. These liquids help to remove problems related to the brain, hair and respiratory system.

Caution: Before practising *jala neti* consult the guidance of an expert or Āyurvedic physician.

2. Nāḍī śodhana (subtle channel purification)

The breath is a vehicle for deepening concentration and bringing the mind to a state of calm and inner stillness. Alternate Nostril Breathing (*nāḍī śodhana* or *anuloma viloma*) is an excellent primary revitalising Yoga breathing practice that relaxes the mind, deepens self-awareness in preparation for meditation, opens the flow of *prāṇic* energy in the *nāḍīs* (subtle energy channels) and purifies the *nāḍīs* of impurities, balances the left and right hemispheres of the brain, and equalises the flow of energy in the *iḍā* and *piṅgala nāḍīs* – the left lunar and right solar subtle energy channels located on either side of the central channel (*suṣumnā nāḍī*) that twines upward through the spine, intersecting at each *chakra*. *Iḍā* ends in the left nostril; *piṅgala* terminates in the right.

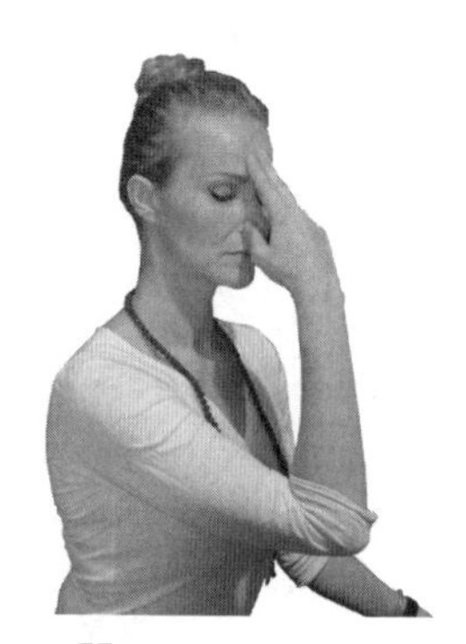

HAND POSITION FOR NĀḌĪ ŚODHANA (SUBTLE CHANNEL PURIFICATION)

Śodhana (pronounced 'shodana') in Sanskrit means 'to purify'. This is the alternate nostril breathing *prāṇāyama*, that maintains an equilibrium in the catabolic and anabolic processes in the body. It purifies the blood and the brain cells. It brings consistency and regularity to our patterns of breathing, and it has a calming effect on the nervous system.

A smooth and unobstructed flow of *prāṇa* is needed for concentration and meditation. For the yogi it is usual to make the breath flow equally in each nostril. When the flow of air is equal in each nostril, then the flows in the *iḍā* and *piṅgala nāḍīs* are also equalised – they become balanced. Under these balanced conditions, *prāṇā* begins to flow in the central main *suṣumnā nāḍī*, influencing all the *chakras*, and the mind becomes centred and still for the purpose of entering into meditation – calm awareness of the inner Self.

Method

Sit in any comfortable meditation pose, with the head, neck and spine aligned. Close the eyes and relax the whole body. Keep the body still and bring your attention and awareness to the midpoint between the eyebrows at the Spiritual Eye (*ājñā chakra*).

Place your left hand palm upwards relaxed on your left knee. Raise your right hand (in *Viṣṇu mūdra*, an energy seal that helps to contain *prāṇā* within the body) with the palm in front of your face, and fold down your middle and index fingers into the palm, keeping the thumb, ring and little fingers extended. Alternatively, you can place your hand in *nāsikāgra mudrā* (with the index and second finger positioned at the eyebrow centre, use the thumb to open and close the right nostril and the third finger to open and close the left nostril).

Exhale and close the right nostril with your thumb. Inhale slowly, smoothly and deeply through the left nostril. Pause. Close the left nostril with the ring finger and slowly exhale through the right nostril. Pause. Inhale through the right nostril. Pause. Close the right nostril with your thumb and exhale through the left nostril. This completes one round.

Begin with five to ten rounds and over a period of time gradually increase to 20 rounds. Practise twice daily – morning and evening, on an empty or light stomach. When doing a complete Yoga practice session, practice alternate nostril breathing just after *āsanas* and prior to meditation.

Breathing ratios for beginners

It is advised to start with a 1:2:2 breath ratio for a few months before taking up the advanced ratio 1:4:2. For beginners this means that the breath retention is twice that of the inhalation, and the duration of exhalation is the same as that of the retention. For advanced students it means that the breath retention is four times that of the inhalation, and the duration of exhalation is twice that of the inhalation.

The minimum starting proportion for a beginner is 4:8:8. After having practised this ratio for one month, then increase the ratio to 5:10:10. Then increase gradually until you reach 8:16:16. On no account should you increase this proportion until you are able to practise it with comfort and ease. You must never force, strain or interrupt the overall rhythm of your breathing practice – to do so could cause strain and injury to the physical body. If your next breath is gasping or hurried, then you have certainly held the breath for too long. Always seek advice from an experienced and qualified teacher who practises *prāṇāyama*.

Breathing ratios for advanced students

As you progress with these ratios, you will be able to change to the advanced ratio of 1:4:2, gradually increasing the ratio to 8:32:16. It could take up to two years of practice to reach this level.

Note

Note that when the breath retention (*kumbhaka*) is longer than ten seconds, then it is important to hold *jālandhara bandha* (chin lock, see page 295).

If you feel any discomfort while practising then reduce your breathing ratio – under no circumstances should you force the proportion of the breathing. It is a gradual practice, the breath should flow gently and naturally, there should be absolutely no strain or tension in breathing. If you have a medical condition such as high blood pressure then please consult your medical doctor or consultant before attempting to practise breathing ratios. Do not practise if you have a severe headache, a fever, a seizure disorder, are tired and unable to concentrate, or are very restless and agitated.

3. Kapālabhāti

In Sanskrit, *kapāla* means 'cranium' and *bhāti* means 'light', 'splendour' or 'to shine' ('cranium-shining' effect) by means of cleansing or purifying. *Kapālabhāti* is one of the six *Haṭha Yoga shatkriyas*; a powerful frontal brain cleansing, clearing and energising technique that invigorates the brain and its entire circulation, including the pineal and pituitary glands, awakening the dormant centres which are responsible for subtle perception. It is an excellent technique in preparation for meditation. The *ājñā* and *maṇipūra chakras* are particularly awakened with *prāṇic* energy by *kapālabhāti*.

Method

Sit in any comfortable meditation pose, with the head, neck and spine aligned. Close the eyes and relax the whole body. Keep the body still and bring your attention and awareness to the midpoint between the eyebrows at the Spiritual Eye.

Bring your awareness to your navel – the chest is not activated, only the abdominal muscles are activated in *kapālabhāti*. The strong contraction of the abdominal muscles causes the short, quick and rhythmic expulsions of breath. In *kapālabhāti* there is no resistance to breathing. Both the nostrils and the glottis are wide open. The muscles of the neck and the face are kept relaxed so that the air escapes smoothly.

Exhale fully, and then inhale deeply through the nose to fully expand your chest. Keep the chest expanded and passive throughout the active round of breathing. Also, keep your shoulders steady and passive, and your face, jaw and neck relaxed. As you exhale and inhale (about every one to two seconds or the speed of an eye-blink) rapidly and lightly with a series of short, light breaths through both nostrils, emphasise the exhalation with a short, forceful contraction of the abdominal muscles (moving the navel towards the spine). The abdomen contracts, and presses upwards against the diaphragm, pushing the breath out through the nose. The inhalation comes as a natural reflex, with the downward release of the diaphragm as the abdominal muscles relax after contracting to exhale.

Beginners' level of practice

Beginners can practise three to five rounds of ten *kapālabhāti* breaths. After each round, inhale and exhale deeply twice, using the complete yogic breath. Then, after completing three to five rounds, return to normal breathing and sit still for meditation. Maintain your awareness at the Spiritual Eye, at the midpoint between the eyebrows.

If this is your first time practising *kapālabhāti*, you may feel dizziness, caused by hyperventilation. If this happens then stop the practice and lie down on your back and relax. So you don't experience dizziness again, make sure that only your abdomen is moving when you practise *kapālabhāti*, not the chest. The abdomen should contract and move inward every time you exhale. Do not pump too fast, as this may also cause dizziness.

Intermediate level of practice

In the intermediate practice of *kapālabhāti*, practise ten breaths. On the tenth breath exhale slowly and fully, emptying the lungs of carbon dioxide. Then inhale and exhale with a full yogic breath, and return to normal breathing. Sit for meditation, maintaining your awareness at the Spiritual Eye, at the midpoint between the eyebrows.

Practice five rounds of ten *kapālabhāti* breaths. Over a period of time you can gradually increase the number of breaths and rounds.

Advanced level of practice

In the advanced practice, breath retention can be added. After completing your last round of *kapālabhāti* exhale fully, allow a natural pause to take place, then inhale with a full yogic breath (use *ujjayi* breath – slight contraction of the glottis in the throat). Lower your head and apply the chin lock (*jālandhara bandha*) with your chest and shoulders fully open. Without any unnecessary tightening in the throat, neck and shoulders, hold the breath (*kumbhaka*) in for as long as comfortable. Do not force or strain.

To exhale, first, release the *jālandhara bandha* by lowering the shoulders and raising the head, and slowly and smoothly exhale with *ujjayi* breath. Then inhale and exhale with a full yogic breath, and continue with the next round. You can gradually increase the speed and number of breaths up to a total of 120 exhalations per round.

After completing a number of rounds of *kapālabhāti*, sit still and calm in the inner silence of meditation. With your eyes closed, fix your whole attention with your relaxed inward gaze at the midpoint between the eyebrows, at the Spiritual Eye. Expand your consciousness into infinity and experience that ineffable peace that is God within you.

Benefits

Kapālabhāti stimulates the nerves, which in turn activate the *nāḍīs*, which activate the *prāṇās*. The *prāṇās* then gravitate towards the area where the action is taking place in the frontal lobes of the brain. This brings an awakening to the Spiritual Eye (*ājñā chakra*).

Kapālabhāti purifies the *iḍā* (upward current on left side of spine) and *piṅgala* (downward current on right side of spine) *nāḍīs* and stimulates every tissue in the body by eliminating large quantities of carbon dioxide, making the blood rich with oxygen. It helps in awakening the *kuṇḍalinī* power and induces alertness and inner awareness, preparing the mind for concentration and meditation. The fast abdominal breathing in *kapālabhāti* has a soothing and calming effect on the central nervous system (CNS) and the autonomic nervous system (ANS).

Kapālabhāti cleanses and drains the sinuses, and opens the lungs and its breathing passages. The overall breathing efficiency is increased by the strengthening and toning of the diaphragm. The heart is given a gentle massage.

Caution

There should be no undue strain on the breathing mechanism at any stage of the practice of *kapālabhāti*. In the beginning, practise carefully under the expert guidance of a qualified teacher. *Kapālabhāti* is best practised in the morning before meditation. Do not practise at night, since it activates the brain and nervous system and may prevent you from sleeping when you go to bed. Do not practise if you have high blood pressure, epilepsy, lung disease or heart disease. Do not retain the breath longer than is comfortable. If you feel dizzy or feel that you are going to faint, stop the practice and calmly return to normal breathing.

4. Agnisāra kriyā (fire purification)

In Sanskrit, *agni* means 'fire', the elemental quality for digestion, and transformation. *Sara* means 'essence'. *Kriyā* means 'action'. *Agnisāra kriyā* means 'cleansing with the essence of fire'. *Agni* (fire) is the presiding element of the *maṇipūra chakra* at the navel centre. The subdivisions of *prāṇā* function with the *maṇipūra chakra* to nourish and sustain the body.

Method

The best time to practise *agnisāra kriyā* is in the early morning after emptying the bowels. It is easier and safer to practise with an empty stomach, so you can practise before meals and during your *āsana* practice. Allow at least three hours after a meal before you practise *agnisāra kriyā*.

First stage: akunchana prasarana (stomach squeeze)

Stand comfortably with the feet slightly wider than hip-width apart. Bend your knees and rest your hands on the thighs. Lean forward slightly to bring the weight of the torso over the straight arms so you can relax the deep muscles of the abdomen which support the lumbar spine. Lengthen the spine and the back of your neck, tuck the chin in, and look down at your lower navel.

Inhale, then exhale deeply, emptying the lungs as much as possible. Hold the breath out and contract the lower abdomen back, forming a hollow. Tuck in the tail bone, and contract the sphincter muscles and the pelvic floor, drawing inwards and upwards. While contracting the lower abdomen and the pelvic floor, hold the breath out for as long as comfortable. Then inhale and reach the tailbone back, release the muscle contractions, and completely relax. Repeat the practice five to ten times.

Benefits: Massages the internal organs, improves digestion and elimination, increases and improves the circulation of the lymph and blood in the abdominal area, gently massages the heart and lungs, tones and improves the abdominal muscles.

Second stage: abdominal pumping

From the same standing position as before, inhale, then exhale deeply, emptying the lungs as much as possible. Hold the breath out and contract the pelvic floor and the lowest part of the abdomen just above the pubic bone. Then contract and pull the lower abdomen firmly inwards and upwards, draw the diaphragm up under the ribs. Immediately release the diaphragm, abdomen and pelvic floor and begin to inhale. In quick succession repeat this rapid in-and-out movement of the abdomen while the breath is held out without strain.

Begin with three to five repetitions and increase gradually to ten, beginning with 20 pulls and increasing to 60 in each breath. Practise daily.

Third stage: nauli (abdominal massage)

The Sanskrit word *nauli* comes from the root *nala* or *nali*, which means a 'tubular vessel' or 'pipe', referring to the pipelike appearance of the abdominal recti as they are contracted. *Nala* is the term for the *rectus abdominii* muscles. *Nauli* is also known in Sanskrit as *lauliki karma*. *Lauliki* comes from the Sanskrit root *lola*, which means 'rolling and agitation'. The *Haṭha Yoga* technique *nauli* rolls, rotates and agitates the whole abdomen with all its associated nerves and muscles. In this technique the abdominal muscles are isolated by contraction, and are rotated.

Before attempting *nauli* the practices of *agnisāra kriyā* and *uḍḍīyāna bandha* should be perfected. *Nauli* should be practised only when the stomach is completely empty. Allow at least five hours after meals. That is why the best time to practise *nauli* is in the morning after emptying the bowels and before breakfast.

Madhyama nauli (middle isolation)

Stand as you did in the previous two stages, with the feet slightly wider than hip-width apart. Bend the knees slightly, lean forward and place your hands on the thighs with the arms straight and the fingers pointing towards each other. Exhale fully and perform the two locks *uḍḍīyāna bandha* (abdominal lock) and *jālandhara bandha* (chin lock) while maintaining external breath retention (*bahir kumbhaka*).

Then contract the *rectus abdominii* muscles so that they form a vertical tubular shape along the centre of the abdomen. This is called *madhyama nauli* (the middle isolation). Hold the contraction with the breath held out for only as long as comfortable. Do not strain.

Release the contraction and *bandhas*, raise your head and return to the upright standing position. Inhale slowly and deeply, and relax the whole body. Allow the breath and the heartbeat to return to normal.

Start with five rounds of *madhyama nauli* and gradually work up to ten. When *madhyama nauli* has been mastered, then you can proceed to try practising *vama nauli*.

Vama nauli (left isolation)

Follow the same instructions as for *madhyama nauli*, to contract and isolate the *rectus abdominii* muscles so that they form a vertical tubular shape along the centre of the abdomen. Then isolate the *rectus abdominii* muscles to the left side by pushing down on the left thigh, so that they form a vertical tubular shape only on the left side of the abdomen. Hold for as long as comfortable without strain, and return to *madhyama nauli*. Release the abdominal contraction, raise your head and return to the upright position. Inhale slowly and deeply. Completely relax, allowing the breath and heartbeat to return to normal.

Dakshina nauli (right isolation)

Now repeat the practice in the same way, by isolating the *rectus abdominii* muscles on the right side of the abdomen.

Once you have mastered isolating the middle, left and right *rectus abdominii* muscles, then you can proceed to practise abdominal rotation.

Abdominal rotation or churning

Practise rotating the *rectus abdominii* muscles first to the left, then to the right, and back to the left in a continuous rolling or churning movement several times. To begin with, practise three continuous rotations. Release the abdominal contraction, raise your head and return to the upright position. Inhale slowly and deeply and relax, allowing the breath and heartbeat to return to normal.

Start with five to ten rotations, gradually increasing to 25 rotations over a period of months.

Benefits

Agnisāra kriyā is an invigorating practice that works on the deep muscles of the lower abdomen, and has a beneficial effect on all the physiological functions of the abdomen. It strengthens the muscles of the pelvic floor and abdominal wall. Internally, *agnisāra kriyā* tones, activates and cleanses the digestive and eliminative systems in the body.

According to the life science of *Āyurveda*, many diseases start from stagnation and toxins (*āma*) that build up in the digestive tract, so the practice of *agnisāra kriyā* can help to a great extent in keeping the digestive tract and the other organ systems in the body functioning healthily. Contractions of the lower abdominal muscles massage the bladder. The lymphatic vessels in the lower abdomen and pelvic area are massaged and flushed, stimulating healthy functioning of the immune system. *Agnisāra kriyā* improves the circulation to the reproductive organs in the pelvic area, and other organs in the abdomen.

On more subtle levels, *agnisāra kriyā* creates a strong upward movement of energy, increasing one's vitality. It strengthens *uḍḍīyāna bandha*, and creates heat at the navel centre (*maṇipūra chakra*), which purifies the *nāḍīs* and stimulates the digestive system. *Agnisāra kriyā* stimulates the five *prāṇās* (*prāṇā*, *apāṇa*, *samāna*, *udāṇa* and *vyāna*), especially *samāna prāṇā*, which connects two main *chakras* – *anāhata chakra* and *maṇipūra chakra*. *Samāna prāṇā* is strengthened through the practice of *agnisāra kriyā* and *nauli*. The most effective technique for awakening *samāna prāṇā* is *Kriyā Yoga*. The practice of *Kriyā Yoga* warms the entire body. This is due to the rising *of samāna prāṇā*.

Nauli stimulates and purifies the *maṇipūra chakra*, the storehouse of *prāṇā*.

Caution

Do not practise *agnisāra kriyā* if you have high blood pressure, cardiovascular disease, hiatal hernia, acute duodenal or peptic ulcers, kidney or gallstones, chronic diarrhoea, during menstruation (*agnisāra kriyā* stimulates an upward flow of *prāṇic* energy that is counter to the cleansing downward flow during menstruation) or pregnancy.

5. Aśvinī mudrā (horse gesture)

Aśvinī is the Sanskrit word for 'horse' and *mudrā* means 'seal' or 'lock'. *Mudrās* are practised to awaken and direct the flow of *kuṇḍalinī*, to induce stillness and strength, and to 'lock in' the benefits resulting from the other practices.

Aśvinī mudrā is so called because, after a horse has evacuated its faeces, it then dilates and contracts the anus several times. During defecation, peristaltic waves in the colon push faeces into the rectum, which triggers the defecation reflex. Contractions push the faeces along, and the anal sphincters relax to allow them out of the body through the anus.

The practice of *aśvinī mudrā* is a preparation for *mūlabandha*.

Note: *Mūlabandha* (root lock or perineum lock) differs from *aśvinī mudrā* (horse gesture) in that there is no alternate contraction and dilation of the anal sphincter. In *mūlabandha* the actual point of contraction is the centre point of the perineum, a diamond-shaped region of muscles between the anus and the genitals. *Mūlabandha* is a gentle contraction of the pelvic diaphragm and the muscles of the urogenital triangle. It does not counter intra-abdominal pressure so much as it seals urogenital energy within the body, controlling and restraining it during *prāṇāyama* and meditation. Whereas in *aśvinī mudrā* the pelvic diaphragm, the anus and the gluteals are strongly activated.

Aśvinī mudrā can be used as a preparatory practice for *mūlabandha*.

Stage 1

Sit in a comfortable meditative pose with the head, neck and spine aligned. Close the eyes and relax the whole body.

Become aware of your natural breath, then after a few minutes, breathing normally, focus your attention on the anus, and practise contracting the anal sphincter muscles, slowly and smoothly with maximum contraction for a few seconds. Then, without straining the muscles, totally relax them for a few seconds. Then repeat the whole process evenly and rhythmically a few more times, gradually increasing the speed at which you contract and relax the sphincter muscles.

Stage 2

Sit in a comfortable meditative pose with the head, neck and spine aligned. Close the eyes and relax the whole body.

Inhale deeply and hold the breath in. Contract and release the anal sphincter muscles rapidly and repeatedly for as many times as you can comfortably hold your breath. Then relax the contraction and exhale.

Start with three rounds of 30 contractions each, gradually increasing this number to ten rounds of 60 contractions each. End the practice by allowing the breath to return to normal. Sit calmly with the eyes closed in meditation.

Benefits

Aśvinī mudrā strengthens the anal muscles and pelvic floor, preventing prolapse of the rectum and uterus. It prevents constipation by stimulating intestinal peristalsis, and tones up the seminal glands and nerves in the pelvic area. It strengthens *mūlabandha* and redirects the *prāṇa* upwards.

Caution

Do not practise *aśvinī mudrā* if you suffer from high blood pressure, a heart condition or fistula.

THE YOGA WAY OF BREATHING

Yogis have stated that a person who breathes shallowly in short, sharp gasps is expected to reduce his or her lifespan, compared with a person who breathes slowly and deeply. So sure were they of this principle that they measured a person's lifespan not in years but by the number of breaths. They considered that each individual is allocated a certain number of breaths in their lifetime, with the number varying from person to person. Therefore if a person breathes slowly and deeply, they will not only gain more energy and vitality, but they also optimise their experience of life.

The ancient yogis who lived in the forests of India, or in secluded hill or mountain regions, had intimate contact with nature all around them. In this natural environment they were able to observe and study the wild animals in great detail. They discovered that animals with a slow breathing rate, such as snakes, crocodiles, elephants and tortoises, have a long lifespan. Conversely, they noticed that animals with a fast breathing rate, such as birds, cats, dogs and rabbits are short-lived. It was from this observation that they realised the importance of slow breathing.

It is also interesting to note that the respiration is directly related to the heart beat. Slow respiration occurs with a slow beating heart, which is conducive to a long lifespan. For example, a whale's heart beats about 16 times a minute, and an elephant's approximately 25. Both these mammals are renowned for their longevity. In comparison a mouse's heart beats approximately 1000 times a minute, making its lifespan very short.

For the human being it is important to understand that stress, anxiety, nervousness, tension, pain, and negative emotions such as anger and fear restrict our natural breathing, causing it to become irregular, rapid and shallow; we contract our consciousness. Whereas, when we breathe with a quiet, regular rhythm, breathing slowly and deeply with joy and positive feelings, it has a calming effect upon the body and mind; we expand our consciousness. The mind and the breath are deeply connected; whenever the mind changes, the breathing changes. One has only to be aware, and to observe the mind and the breath, to witness how they affect each other. If you change your breathing, you change your thinking.

Through learning and experiencing the yogic way of breathing we are made aware of our irregular breathing rhythms. By consciously being aware we can begin to change them, and return to the natural breath of breathing with awareness, and embracing life in the moment.

The practice of Yoga begins with the awareness of the breath and how to breathe properly. Then when the body, mind and breath are prepared, the practices of *prāṇāyāma* can begin.

Diaphragmatic (abdominal) breathing

Anatomy

The diaphragm, a large, strong muscular and fibrous elastic wall, simultaneously separates and connects the two principal cavities of the torso – the abdominal cavity and the thoracic cavity. The origin of the diaphragm is where it attaches along a rim that begins at the bottom of the sternum, and extends around the base of the ribcage to the front of the lower spine. The 'insertion' of the diaphragm is the top of the flattened 'dome' it forms.

The top of the diaphragmatic dome is situated at the level of the fourth and fifth ribs or slightly higher than the xiphoid process. At the back, the top is at the level of the seventh thoracic vertebra.

The base of the lungs, which are covered by pleural membranes, rest on the diaphragm. The heart, wrapped in a serous membrane (pericardium), rests on the central tendon of the diaphragm. Every time the diaphragm moves, it directly influences the internal organs – the kidneys, spleen, pancreas, abdominal aorta, and the flexures of the large intestine, lungs and heart.

Diaphragmatic breathing is the most important aspect of effective breathing and breath control, because it increases the suction pressure created in the thoracic cavity of the torso, and improves the venous return of blood, which reduces the load on the heart and enhances circulatory function.

In the diaphragm's piston-like action it coordinates with muscles below it. Tight or overstretched abdominal muscles, front and back, connected to the lumbar vertebrae, hamper the action of the diaphragm.

Diaphragmatic inhalation

During inhalation, the diaphragm and external intercostal muscles (muscles between the ribs) contract to expand the chest cavity, pulling the lungs downwards. This creates a lower air pressure within the lungs than outside the body, causing air to be drawn into the lungs.

Diaphragmatic exhalation

During exhalation, the diaphragm and external intercostal muscles relax, causing the chest cavity to decrease in size. The lungs rise towards the top of the thorax and tend to pull the diaphragm upwards.

Diaphragmatic breathing is the most efficient

Diaphragmatic breathing is not synonymous with abdominal breathing. The relaxed expansion and contraction of the chest is equally diaphragmatic. In the Full or Complete Yogic Breath, three parts of the torso are used – the abdomen, mid-chest and upper chest – in which the diaphragm moves. Of the three types of breathing, diaphragmatic breathing is physiologically the most efficient, particularly when one is in the upright position. Chest breathing requires more work to accomplish the same blood/gas mixing than does slow, deep, diaphragmatic breathing.

Technique one: Diaphragmatic breathing (lying down)

1. A simple way to learn diaphragmatic breathing is to lie down on your back in the Yoga relaxation pose (*shavāsana*), with the arms alongside the body, palms upward, and with the legs about hip-width apart. Completely relax the body.

2. Feel the movement of the breath by placing your right hand on your abdomen, just above the navel, and the left hand over the lower edge of the ribcage. Inhale, and visualise the diaphragm sheet of muscle flattening out and pushing down on the abdominal organs below it. Feel the lower edge of the ribcage expand, and the abdomen rise. As you breathe in this way, there should be hardly any movement in the chest.

3. Then, as you exhale, the diaphragm relaxes and arches upward into a dome-shaped position in the chest or thoracic cavity. Feel your abdomen, navel and ribs relax downward and inward.

Technique two: Diaphragmatic breathing (sitting), 1:1 ratio

1. Sit in a comfortable and relaxed position with the head, neck and spine held upright in alignment. For a few minutes relax the body by becoming aware of the natural breath, without trying to control it in any way.

2. Then begin diaphragmatic breathing by inhaling to a count of four and exhaling to a count of four. The breath should be relaxed, smooth, even, and regular. Practise for five minutes.

The Complete Yogic Breath

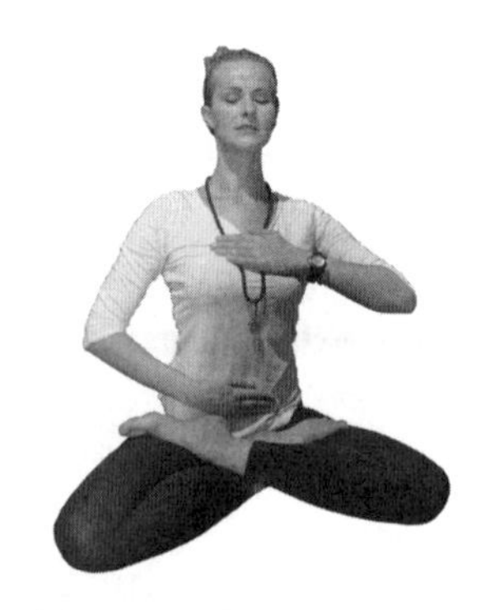

The CompleteYogic Breath is the foundation and the first main practice of *prāṇāyāma*. It is important and necessary to learn this technique properly before progressing on to other *prāṇāyāma* techniques.

The Complete Yogic Breath combines the three modes of breathing into one complete harmonious and continuous movement. In this form of respiration the entire respiratory system is brought into use: all the respiratory muscles including the internal and external intercostals and abdominal muscles; the ribcage; every part of the lungs and their air cells; and the diaphragm. It is this type of breathing that we are interested in developing, since only yogic breathing can give the maximum inhalation and exhalation of breath.

The Complete Yogic Breath can be classified into three parts:

1. Abdominal or diaphragmatic breathing (lower breathing)

2. Intercostal or mid-chest breathing (middle breathing)

3. Clavicular or upper chest breathing (upper breathing).

Mechanism of abdominal breathing

We have covered this above.

Mechanism of mid-chest breathing

In intercostal breathing the movement of the ribs is brought into play. During expansion of the ribcage outwards and upwards by muscular contraction, the lungs are allowed to expand. This results in air being drawn down into them from the front side and inhalation takes place. The intercostal muscles control the movement of the ribs – when they are relaxed, the ribs move downwards and inwards. This movement compresses the lungs and exhalation takes place.

Mechanism of upper chest breathing

In upper chest breathing, inhalation and deflation of the lungs is achieved by raising the upper ribs, shoulders, and collarbones (clavicles). This method requires maximum effort to obtain minimum benefit. Very little air is inhaled and exhaled, since this movement cannot change the volume of the chest cavity very much.

Upper breathing or chest breathing is common in Western society, owing to the modern lifestyles we have adopted, particularly in the cities and large towns where we are more susceptible to stressful conditions – pollution; noise; smoking; central heated and air-conditioned rooms and offices that contribute to unhealthy breathing; and chairs that are badly designed for the posture. We get into a state of anxiety or we immobilise our diaphragm in an attempt to contain our stress and fears of anger, aggression and other deep emotional feelings, causing us to breathe shallowly in the upper chest.

Technique one: Complete Yogic Breath (lying down)

1. Lie down on your back in *Shavāsana* (Corpse pose). Relax the feet outwards, hip-width apart. Position the arms slightly away from your sides with the palms turned upwards to encourage an opening to your shoulders and upper chest. Close your eyes and relax.
2. Place one hand on your abdomen and the other hand on your chest. As you inhale, first feel the abdomen rise, and then the chest.
3. As you exhale, feel the chest lower first and then the abdomen.
4. Now place your hands on the side of the ribs (fingers point towards the centre of the chest) and feel how far the ribs expand and contract beneath your hands as you inhale and exhale.
5. Next, place your hands just beneath the collarbones and feel the movement of the chest in this area as you inhale and exhale.
6. Practise breathing in this way, quietly and gently for a few minutes. With attentive awareness, observe how the movement of the breath gradually becomes slower and the exhalation becomes longer with the deepening relaxation.

7. Return your hands to relax palms upward by your sides. Relax in *Shavāsana* for one to two minutes observing the normal and natural flow of the breath.

Note: This technique can also be practised lying down with the legs bent with the soles of the feet on the floor.

Concentration: On the whole body and the breath.

Benefits: Deepens the breath and leads to physical and mental relaxation. Calms and revitalises the whole body.

Technique two: Complete Yogic Breath (sitting)

The Complete Yogic Breath consists of breathing continuously and progressively in a smooth and uninterrupted transition from the abdomen, to the mid-chest, and then to the upper chest.

Inhalation

1. Sit in a meditative posture with the head, neck and spine aligned. Close your eyes and relax the body.
2. **Abdomen:** Exhale deeply, contracting the abdomen to squeeze out all the air from the lungs.
3. Inhale slowly, keeping the lower part of the abdomen contracted while expanding the abdomen above the navel slightly.
4. **Mid-chest:** At the end of the upper abdomen expansion, start to expand your mid-chest with the action of the diaphragm.
5. **Upper chest:** Continue drawing the breath into the higher lobes of the lungs, so that it lifts and expands your upper chest, causing your collarbones and your shoulders to raise upwards. Your lungs should now be completely filled with air.

Breath retention

6. Hold the breath in for a few seconds, with the head forward in *jālandhara bandha* (throat or chin lock), This is practised by gently dropping the head forward so that the chin rests in the notch between the collarbones. Do not strain or force your neck into the position, but keep the neck and throat muscles soft and relaxed. Move your chest upwards to meet your chin as you bring it down, then you will not strain the neck or throat. Only hold *jālandhara bandha* for a few seconds or for as long as is comfortable while holding the breath.

Exhalation

7. Release *jālandhara bandha* by raising your head.

8. **Abdomen:** Begin your exhalation with the release of your diaphragm so that it presses in and upward. Your lower ribs begin to soften inward as your diaphragm moves upward.
9. **Mid-chest:** Continue exhaling by relaxing your mid-chest.
10. **Upper chest:** Now smoothly exhale from the upper chest, so that the collarbones and shoulders lower naturally back into their normal relaxed position.

Concentration: On the whole body and the breath.

Benefits: Increases lung capacity and oxygenation; deepens the breath and leads to physical and mental relaxation; calms and revitalises the whole body; promotes alertness and clarity of mind.

There should be one continuous, smooth movement of breathing in the Complete Yogic Breath. Each of the three phases of breathing merges harmoniously into the next, without there being any obvious transition point. There should be no strain or jerky movements with the body or the breath. The body should remain relaxed throughout the practice. With practice you will find that the whole process will occur naturally with no undue effort.

The reason for practising *jālandhara bandha* (chin lock) is to retain the pressure of the air within the lungs so as to reduce any pressure in the brain and regulate the flow of blood and *prāṇa* to the head, heart and thyroid glands in the throat.

This practice develops good healthy lung tissue which resists germs, making you much less susceptible to disease. The blood receives a good supply of oxygen and every organ in the body is nourished by it. Digestion and assimilation are improved, and bodily energy and vigour are increased. The nervous system and the brain benefit through the blood being properly oxygenated, making them more efficient instruments for generating, storing and transmitting nerve currents. Clarity of thought is improved.

To develop yogic breathing as an automatic and normal function of the body, develop the habit of consciously breathing with awareness. If you feel tired, depressed, angry or anxious, then become centred within yourself and sit down, or lie down, and practise yogic breathing. Breathe slowly and deeply with your concentration on the breath. Feel that you are inhaling not just air, but joy, peace, strength, courage, or whatever positive quality you want especially to affirm. As you exhale, breathe away any negative qualities that your mind may be holding on to. Then your mind will become calm and revitalised.

Bhastrikā prāṇāyāma (bellows breath)

The Sanskrit word *bhastrikā* means 'bellows'. Just as a blacksmith's bellows blow air vigorously and rapidly to fan the flames of the fire, so in this practice the practitioner inhales and exhales rapidly in a series of quick and successive forceful breaths, to stoke the *prāṇic* fire to purify the body of its impurities.

Bhastrikā prāṇāyāma is one of the most powerful breathing practices in Yoga. It helps in the activation of the *kuṇḍalinī* energy if the *nāḍīs* (subtle *prāṇic* channels) and nervous system are purified.

Within the *suṣumnā* (central subtle channel) in the subtle or astral spine are three *granthis* (subtle knots). These knots or energy blocks prevent the free-flowing movement of the *prāṇa* (energy) in the *suṣumnā*. The three *granthis* are:

Brāhma granthi located at the *anāhata chakra.*

Rudra granthi located at the *viśuddha chakra.*

Viṣṇu granthi located at the *ājñā chakra.*

To free the *prāṇic* current and break these subtle knots, one needs to perform *bhastrikā prāṇāyāma*. When they are broken, the *kuṇḍalinī* energy is free to rise gradually towards the *sahasrāra chakra* (crown centre), the subtle counterpoint of the brain.

The difference between *kapālabhāti* and *bhastrikā prāṇāyāma*

The difference between *kapālabhāti* (skull shining breath) and *bhastrikā prāṇāyāma* is that in *bhastrikā* the breath is retained at the end of each round with the three *bandhas* (locks) to unite the *prāṇa* and *apāṇa*. In *kapālabhāti* there is no breath retention.

Kapālabhāti also differs in that the inhalation is effortless and spontaneous, without the diaphragmatic muscle activity contracting, and the exhalation is forceful and rapid; whereas in *bhastrikā*, the pace is more vigorous. The inhalation is forceful, produced by an active contraction of the diaphragm, and is as rapid as the exhalation, with no pause before the inhalation.

Method

1. Sit in a comfortable meditation posture, with the head, neck and spine aligned. Beginners can sit in a simple crossed-legged pose or in the kneeling pose (*Vajrāsana*). More advanced students can sit in *Siddhāsana* (Adept pose) or *Swastikāsana* (Auspicious pose). Relax your chest and shoulders and close your eyes. Allow the movement of this *prāṇāyāma* to be only in the navel area.

2. Begin by taking a slow, deep inhalation through both nostrils, then with the lungs full, immediately inhale and exhale vigorously and rapidly, so that the expulsions of breath follow one another in rapid succession. This will bring into rapid action both the diaphragm and the entire respiratory apparatus. One rapid inhalation and exhalation completes one *bhastrikā* breath. For this bellows action of the breath to work properly one needs to coordinate the action of the diaphragm and abdominal muscles so that air moves rapidly in and out of the lungs like a bellows. As the abdominal muscles relax at the end of an exhalation, the diaphragm actively contracts to begin inhalation. As the diaphragm begins to release its contraction after the peak of inhalation, the abdominal muscles begin to contract.

3. Practise ten breaths, exhaling completely on the tenth expulsion. Then take a long, slow, deep inhalation through both nostrils.
4. Hold the breath in for as long as comfortable without strain, applying *jālandhara bandha* (chin lock) and *mūlabandha* (anal lock), with your awareness and concentration on the *kuṇḍalinī* in the *mūladhāra chakra* at the base of the spine. (See section 6.5.1 for detailed descriptions of the locking techniques.)
5. Slowly release the chin lock, then the anal lock, and exhale slowly and smoothly through both nostrils.

This completes one round of *bhastrikā prāṇāyāma*. Take a short rest between each round by taking a few deep diaphragmatic breaths, or do three complete yogic breaths, and then let your breathing gradually return to normal.

Bhastrikā variation

After practising one round of *bhastrikā prāṇāyāma*, close the left nostril and inhale deeply through the right nostril. Then hold the breath in and apply the *mūlabandha* (anal lock), and *jālandhara bandha* (chin lock). Hold the breath for as long as comfortable, then slowly release the chin lock, then the anal lock, and exhale slowly and smoothly through the left nostril. Repeat this cycle three times.

Levels of *bhastrikā* practice

Mild: Practise one or two rounds of *bhastrikā*. Begin with 10 breaths for each round, at the speed of one breath per second. As you progress, gradually increase to 25 breaths for each round.

Moderate: Practise two or three rounds of *bhastrikā*. Begin with 10–15 breaths. As you progress, gradually increase to 50 breaths for each round. You can also increase the speed of practice to two breaths per second.

Intermediate/advanced: Begin with 15–20 breaths per round, then increase by five breaths per week to a maximum of 120 breaths per round. You can also gradually increase the vigour and speed of the practice to two breaths per second. After each round exhale completely, then inhale fully and apply the *mūlabandha* (anal lock), and *jālandhara bandha* (chin lock). Hold the breath for as long as comfortable, then exhale slowly and smoothly.

Benefits

The practice of *bhastrikā* burns up the impurities that have settled at the entrance of the *suṣumnā nāḍī*, and activates the *kuṇḍalinī śakti* (serpent power energy) in the spine. One will benefit more from *bhastrikā* if the *nāḍīs* (subtle energy channels) are purified first by the practice of alternate nostril breathing (*nāḍī shuddhi*). After purification has taken place *bhastrikā* can break the three *granthis* (subtle knots) in the *chakras*. *Bhastrikā* uses both nostrils equally, so the energy is balanced on both sides of the *suṣumnā*.

Bhastrikā also activates the *ājñā chakra* and *sahasrāra chakra*, and induces tranquillity to the mind, preparing the mind for meditation.

This practice increases the supply of blood to the brain, tones the entire nervous system, increases the gastric fire and gives warmth to the body. It is good to practise during the winter months.

Bhastrikā clears the nasal passages, sinuses and lungs. It massages the abdominal organs, stimulating the liver, spleen and pancreas. It mildly stimulates the cardiovascular system.

Caution

Sometimes, for beginners new to this practice, *bhastrikā prāṇāyāma* causes them to hyperventilate. The carbon dioxide levels in the bloodstream drop more rapidly than their body can handle. The body responds by decreasing the blood supply to the brain, resulting in temporary dizziness and anxiousness, usually with accompanying tingling sensations in the lips and fingertips. If this happens then stop the practice and simply return to slow diaphragmatic breathing. Similarly, if you experience a 'stitch' in your side or a sharp pain under the ribs, like a cramping feeling that marathon runners sometimes get, then stop the practice and return to slow diaphragmatic breathing.

Persons with high blood pressure, heart ailments, hiatal hernia or vertigo should not practise *bhastrikā prāṇāyāma*. Because this *prāṇāyāma* increases abdominal pressure, it is also not recommended for women during menstruation or pregnancy, or for women using a contraceptive intra-uterine device (IUD).

Śitalī prāṇāyāma (cooling breath)

Śitalī (pronounced 'sheetali') is a cooling breath. It cools the body and induces relaxation by soothing the nervous system, giving tranquillity to the mind. *Śitalī* removes extra heat from the body, such as stress and low fever; reduces agitation, anger and anxiety; purifies the blood; improves digestion; and relieves thirst.

Method

1. Sit relaxed in a comfortable meditation posture with the head, neck and spine aligned. Rest your hands on the knees in either *jñanā mudrā* or *chin mudrā*, and close your eyes and relax the whole body. Focus your attention at the Spiritual Eye, at the midpoint between the eyebrows.
2. Extend your tongue so that it rests between your lips without protruding beyond them, and curl or roll it lengthways to form a tube shape. Inhaling, suck the air in through this channel slowly and deeply, with a hissing sound, feeling the breath cool the entire length of your tongue, until your lungs are filled completely. This will draw the air into your body producing a cooling sensation, and a cooling effect in the throat, oesophagus and stomach. Concentrate on the cooling sensation and feel that it is spreading throughout your brain, spine and nervous system.

3. Withdraw your tongue, close your mouth and retain the breath and perform *jālandhara bandha* (chin or throat lock) for as long as comfortable without any strain.
4. Release *jālandhara bandha* and exhale slowly through both nostrils and relax.

This technique can be practised daily in the morning, beginning with ten rounds and gradually increasing to 40 rounds. It is best practised after *āsanas* and *prāṇāyama* practice. Since it is a cooling breath, it should not be practised during the cold winter months, and especially not if the body is feeling cold.

Śitkārī prāṇāyāma (cooling-hissing breath)

Śitkārī (pronounced 'sheetkari') is also a cooling breath, and gives similar benefits to *śitalī*.

Method

1. Fold your tongue back so that the tip of the tongue touches the upper palate. Bring your teeth together, and with your jaw soft and relaxed, open your lips as much as is comfortable and inhale slowly and deeply with a hissing sound (sounds like 'shee') through your gently clenched teeth.
2. Then, close your mouth keeping your tongue touching the upper palate. Retain the breath while holding *jālandhara bandha* (chin lock) for a few seconds.
3. Release *jālandhara bandha* and raise your head and slowly exhale through your nostrils. Feel the cool sensation of breath spread throughout your brain, spine and nervous system.

Śitkārī can also be practised daily in the morning, beginning with ten rounds and gradually increasing to 40 rounds.

Differences between *śitalī* and *śitkārī prāṇāyāmas*

The positioning of the tongue is different in each of the *prāṇāyāmas*: in *śitalī* the tongue forms a tube, and the awareness is focused on the cooling sensation of the breath; in *śitkārī* the tongue is not curled and awareness is focused on the hissing sound through the teeth.

Bhrāmarī prāṇāyāma (humming bee breath)

> 'By this yogic practice of *Bhrāmarī*, yogis with their minds absorbed in bliss, feel an indescribable joy in their hearts.'
>
> *Haṭha Yoga Pradīpikā 2:68*

Bhrāmarī comes from the Sanskrit word *bhramara* meaning 'bumblebee'. This is because the humming breath sounds like the drone of a male bee. Through concentration on this sound the mind reaches a state of self-absorption.

The practice of *bhrāmarī prāṇāyāma* calms the nervous system and the mind, and has a direct effect on the *viśuddha chakra*. According to Tantric texts, there is a subtle centre called *talu chakra* which controls the pineal and pituitary glands. When the nerve endings in the upper part of the throat and the roof of the mouth are stimulated by *bhrāmarī*, the *talu chakra* is affected too. *Bhrāmarī* promotes concentration, and prepares you for meditation, bringing you into contact with your inner Self.

Practising *bhrāmarī* involves vibrating the vocal cords as in humming, but with the additional resonance in the nasal cavity. As the tongue is slightly pressed towards the roof of the mouth, the sound shifts from the throat to the nasal cavity. The sound is produced by air being expelled through the lungs, which passes through the voice box (larynx). The larynx supports the two fibrous bands known as the vocal cords. When the muscles attached to the vocal cords tighten as air passes by, they vibrate to create sound. If the tension of these muscles increases, the sound pitch rises.

Method

1. Sit relaxed in a comfortable meditation posture with the head, neck and spine aligned. Rest your hands on the knees in either *jñanā mudrā* or *chin mudrā*, close your eyes and relax the whole body.
2. Inhale deeply through the nose using *ujjayi* breath, creating a mild suction effect in the throat. Feel a cool sensation in the throat and relate the cool sensation to the spine as you draw the current of energy up from the base of the spine to the medulla at the top of the spine.
3. Hold the breath in and apply *mūlabandha* (anal lock) for five seconds. While holding the breath in, bring your focused attention and awareness to the midpoint between the eyebrows at the Spiritual Eye. Raise your hands to the level of your ears. Close off the ears with your thumbs by pressing the ear-flaps closed, and rest the fingers of each hand on your forehead.
4. Then, simultaneously release your hands and the anal lock, and slowly exhale with your mouth and lips closed, but with the teeth slightly separated. Make a long, deep, continuous, steady humming sound like that of a bee for the duration of your exhalation. Feel the humming bee sound vibrating throughout your brain.

Take one or two normal breaths in between each round. Practise five rounds increasing to 12 rounds as you progress with this practice.

Now the body is still and relaxed. The perception of God begins when the body and mind are still. Continue to sit in the stillness with your eyes closed and your inner gaze at the Spiritual Eye, at the midpoint between the eyebrows. Feel the resonance and vibration from the practice of *bhrāmarī* in your brain. Feel this vibration expanding to the crown of the head, then to about three inches above your head.

Meditate in the tranquil silence being aware of your Self as pure, existence-being. Remain in this still state of absorbed meditation for as long as it persists. Mentally affirm: '*The Spirit of God vibrates and resonates within me as pure joy.*'

Ujjayi prāṇāyāma (victorious breath)

The Sanskrit prefix *ud* means 'to rise upwards', and *jayi* means 'victory'. *Ujjayi prāṇāyāma* helps one to have victory or overcome derangement of the vital energy known as *udāṇa*, the upward flowing *prāṇa* (flows from the heart to the head and brain), and the accompanying physical and psychological disorders that occur when *udāṇa prāṇa* is out of balance.

Ujjayi breathing creates the expansion and upward movement of the *prāṇic* energy through the *suṣumnā nāḍī*, the central *prāṇic* energy channel. The two distinctive characteristics of *ujjayi* breathing are: an action in the throat that produces a soft snoring-like sound of 'haaa' in the vocal cords and epiglottis in the throat; and a smooth and even flow of the breath in both the inhalation and the exhalation. This is a very soothing and calming breath that keeps your awareness and attention on the breath. It promotes interiorisation of the senses (*pratyāhāra*), and develops awareness of the subtle body. To breathe in *ujjayi*, close your mouth and breathe in through the nose, so that your breath moves upwards along the back of your throat with the smooth, continuous and steady 'haaa' sound, and out through your nose with a continuous and steady, sibilant sound of 'saaa'. The purpose of the *ujjayi* sound is to attune your attentive awareness to each breath. *Ujjayi* breath warms and filters the air entering the nostrils, producing a calming and relaxing effect in the brain. The practice of *ujjayi* is especially recommended for persons who have insomnia, mental tension, anxiety, depression and hypertension. It helps in regulating the blood pressure, endocrine secretions and gastrointestinal activity, removes phlegm from the throat, and cools the head. On a subtle level it generates *prāṇic* energy within the body and induces meditation.

Ujjayi prāṇāyāma can be practised at any time and in all positions – Yoga postures, standing, lying down and walking – safely without breath retention. To balance the *prāṇa* and *apāṇa*, keep the length of the inhalation and the exhalation the same, and breath through both nostrils.

Method

1. Sit in a comfortable and stable meditation posture with the head, neck, and spine aligned. Relax the mind and body by taking a few deep breaths. Inhale deeply and tense the whole body, then exhale and let go of all tension from the body and completely relax. Place your hands palms down on the knees in *jñānā mudrā* (gesture of knowledge). Close your eyes and relax, with your awareness on the natural breath.
2. Now inhale slowly with a smooth, deep and continuous *ujjayi* breath (close the mouth and inhale through the nasal passages with the glottis partially closed; the glottis is the opening between the vocal cords, at the upper part of the windpipe). This causes the air to rush past the partly closed glottis,

producing a soft sound within the throat. The passage of the incoming air is felt on the roof of the palate and makes an 'aaah' sound or the aspirate sound of 'ha'. During the inhalation keep the abdominal muscles slightly contracted. Completely expand the lungs with air, by raising and expanding the ribs until the chest is expanded forward like a victorious warrior.

3. Now exhale slowly with a smooth, deep and continuous *ujjayi* breath through both nostrils. The outgoing breath makes a sibilant 'sa', 'so' or 'sau' sound. During exhalation the abdominal muscles will naturally be more contracted. The duration of the exhalation is always longer than the inhalation, usually in the proportionate ratio of 1:2. This means that if you inhale for five seconds, exhalation should be ten seconds.

Practise five to 20 rounds of *ujjayi prāṇāyāma*, starting with five and increasing by two rounds each week until you reach 20.

Advanced *ujjayi prāṇāyāma*

Advanced practitioners can apply *mūlabandha* (anal lock) and *jālandhara bandha* (chin lock) with breath retention (*kumbhaka*).

1. Sit in a comfortable and steady meditation posture with the head, neck and spine aligned. Relax the mind and body by taking a few deep breaths. After inhaling in *ujjayi*, feeling the breath in the throat, completely close the glottis and apply *mūlabandha* (anal lock) and *jālandhara bandha* (chin lock). Hold the breath for as long as is comfortable.
2. After comfortably holding your breath (*kumbhak*), first release *mūlabandha*, followed by *jālandhara bandha*.
3. Exhale through your left nostril, by closing the right one with your thumb. (This traditional way of exhalation through the left nostril requires less effort to breathe in the 1:2 ratio. This is because exhalation through one nostril will require double the time of inhalation through both nostrils, provided the force of breathing is constant.)

This completes one round. Repeat the practice a further 3–5 times.

Ujjayi prāṇāyāma variation using Hong Sau mantra in the spine

1. Sit in a comfortable and steady meditation posture with the head, neck and spine aligned. Relax the mind and body by taking a few deep breaths. Place your hands palms upward on the knees in *chin mudrā* (gesture of consciousness). Close your eyes and relax, with your awareness on the natural breath.
2. Now as you inhale, smoothly and continuously in *ujjayi* breath (close the mouth and inhale through the nasal passages with the glottis partially closed), mentally follow the breath with the *mantra* ***Hong*** (rhymes with 'song'). Feel

a cool current of *prāṇic* energy slowly rising up the spine from *mūladhāra*, the root *chakra* at the base of the spine, to the medulla oblongata at the base of the brain, and then through the brain to the midpoint between the eyebrows at the Spiritual Eye.

3. While gazing with your attentive awareness into the Spiritual Eye, mentally chant ***Aum*** three times, and then breathing smoothly and continuously in *ujjayi* breath, mentally repeating the *mantra* ***Sau*** (rhymes with 'saw'), slowly exhale and feel a warm current of *prāṇic* energy descending back down through the spine to *mūladhāra chakra*.
4. In this way, continue several times breathing up and down the spine with the *mantra Hong Sau* until you feel the warmth and sensation of a tingling current of energy in the spine. Then, on the next inhalation, draw the breath up the spine to the medulla, and then through the brain to the Spiritual Eye, at the midpoint between the eyebrows.
5. Now with the body and mind still, breathe normally. With closed eyes and without straining, gently lift your gaze upward to the midpoint between the eyebrows, and with steady concentration and calmness look into the Spiritual Eye. Feel the natural breath flow in and out of the nostrils. Feel the sensation of the breath, and try to feel where the flow of breath is strongest in the nostrils. Once you have found it, then concentrate on the breath there.
6. Then begin to feel the breath higher in the nostrils, up by the midpoint between the eyebrows, at the seat of concentration. Inhale deeply, then slowly exhale. As the next inhalation naturally arises and flows into the nostrils, feel the breath where it enters the nostrils, and mentally follow the breath with the *bīja* (seed-syllable) *mantra Hong*. Imagine that the breath itself is making this sound. And as the breath flows out naturally of its own accord, mentally pronounce the *mantra Sau*.
7. Make no attempt to control the breath, just allow its flow to be completely natural. The process of *Hong Sau* is not a breathing technique; it is simply being consciously aware with the concentration on the *Hong Sau mantra* as the breath flows. Feel that the breath itself is silently making the sounds of *Hong Sau*. Continue gazing into the Spiritual Eye, the seat of spiritual consciousness, and as the breath naturally flows in mentally pronounce the *mantra Hong*. As the breath flows out, mentally pronounce the *mantra Sau*. By concentrating on the breath, the breath gradually diminishes. This gradual refinement leads naturally to an interiorised meditative state.

Hong Sau means 'I am He', 'I, the manifested Self, am He, the Unmanifested Spirit (the Absolute).' By consciously repeating mentally the seed-syllable *mantra Hong Sau*, in conjunction with the concentration on the breath, we affirm that the ego-self is one with the Infinite Spirit. *Hong* as the inhaling breath represents the contraction of consciousness into finitude. *Sau* as the exhaling breath represents the expansion of consciousness and the reabsorption of differentiation into pure unity.

6.5.1 *BANDHAS* (LOCKS)

Bandha means 'lock', but can also refer to a posture in which certain parts of the body are controlled or contracted in some way. *Bandhas* are restrictive positions or muscle contractions that protect the body from injury by restraining the flow of energy. In the practice of a *bandha*, the energy flow to a particular area of the body is temporarily blocked with a 'lock'. When the *bandha* is released, the energy flows more strongly through the body with an increased pressure. *Bandhas* are the inner actions that direct the subtle power of the breath or *prāṇa*, and help in removing the obstruction in the *suṣumnā* (central subtle channel) to promote a free flow of *prāṇic* energy through it.

There are four types of *bandha*:

Jālandhara bandha – throat or chin lock

Uḍḍīyānabandha – abdominal lock

Mūlabandha – anal lock

Maha bandha – great lock (practice of all three bandhas together).

> 'These three *bandhas* are the best of all and have been practised by the masters. Of all the means of success in the *Haṭha Yoga*, they are known to the yogis as the main ones.'
>
> *Haṭha Yoga Pradīpikā 3:75*

It is very important to use *bandhas* in advanced *prāṇāyāma*, for without them you could injure the nervous system and possibly cause a *prāṇic* short-circuit in your body. To understand this, you need only a basic knowledge of an electrical circuit. Electricity is sent through a circuit, which can work well and cause no harm so long as it has transformers, fuses, conductors and switches. Without these, the electric current going through it could be lethal. The *bandhas* 'lock in' the *prāṇa* to prevent it being dissipated and direct the *prāṇic* energy or current to its destination, according to the concentration of the yogi. The *bandhas* also help to unite the upward and downward vital energy forces (*prāṇa* and *apāṇa*) and direct this powerful *prāṇic* current into the *suṣumnā nāḍī*, to awaken the *kuṇḍalinī śakti*. What actually happens is that the *prāṇa* is prevented from flowing upwards by the yogi applying the chin lock (*jālandhara bandha*); and the *apāṇa* is prevented from flowing downwards by the anal lock (*mūlabandha*). This causes the two vital energies *prāṇa* and *apāṇa* to unite and flow into the *suṣumnā* (central subtle channel) in the astral spine.

The *bandhas* also have a beneficial effect on the physical body by toning the internal organs, toning the central and sympathetic nervous systems, invigorating centres in the brain, and improving coordination between the voluntary and involuntary nervous systems. *Bandhas* also have a beneficial influence on the *nāḍīs* and *chakras*. The energy channels are purified, blockages released and the exchange of energy is greatly improved.

JĀLANDHARA BANDHA (THROAT OR CHIN LOCK)

> 'It tightens the *nāḍīs* and stops the nectar (from the Soma or Chandra in the brain) from flowing downward from the hole in the palate. It is therefore, called the *Jālandhara bandha* – the destroyer of a host of diseases of the throat.'
>
> *Haṭha Yoga Pradīpikā 3:70*

Jala means 'net', 'web' or 'network'. In the neck there is a network of nerves and arteries which go to the brain. *Dhara* means 'holding up' or 'supporting'. *Jālandhara bandha* (chin lock) supports the *uḍḍīyāna bandha* (abdominal lock) to effortlessly hold the lifted *nāḍīs*.

When *jālandhara bandha* is applied, the internal and external carotid arteries, which are situated on both sides of the neck and carry blood to the brain, are squeezed under pressure. *Jālandhara* also places pressure on the carotid sinus nerve. These pressures influence the blood pressure, slow down the heart rate, and slow down the nerve impulses to the brain. This brings calmness to the mind and *prāṇa*, and so prepares the mind for meditation.

Jālandhara bandha awakens the inner energy centres, especially the *vishuddhi chakra*. It improves the concentration and the ability to retain the breath for a long period of time. It tones the thyroid, parathyroid and thymus glands.

From an esoteric point of view there is a subtle nectar that flows from the *sahasrāra chakra* through the hole in the palate to the *maṇipūra chakra* and is consumed by the gastric fire (*agni*). *Jālandhara bandha* prevents this nectar from falling and so the elixir of life is stored and life itself is prolonged.

Method

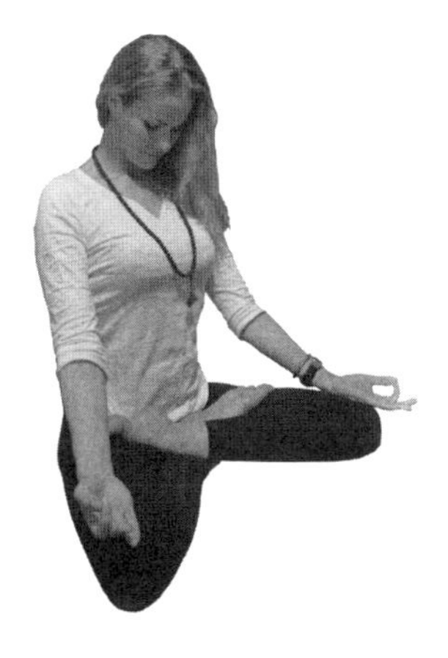

1. Sit in a comfortable and steady meditation posture, preferably *Siddhāsana* (Adept's pose), so that the knees are firmly on the floor. Place your hands palms down on your knees. Close your eyes and relax.
2. Inhale deeply and retain the breath. Lift your shoulders and stretch the spine, back and neck, and tilt your body forward slightly, keeping the back straight. Apply *jālandhara bandha* (throat or chin lock) by pressing your chin firmly into the hollow of your throat (jugular notch) between the collarbones so that the windpipe and oesophagus are firmly closed. This gives a good stretch to the cervical vertebrae, which stimulates the nervous centres, frees the cranial nerves and beneficially affects the thyroid gland.
3. Concentrate on the *vishuddhi chakra* and hold the breath for only as long as comfortable.

4. Release the chin lock by slowly raising your head, then exhale and return to the starting position.
5. In this position relax all efforts and breathe normally.

Practise up to ten rounds, gradually increasing to 20.

Note: *Jālandhara bandha* can also be practised from the standing position, with the feet positioned about hip-width apart, the trunk leaning forward with the palms just above the knees and the arms straight.

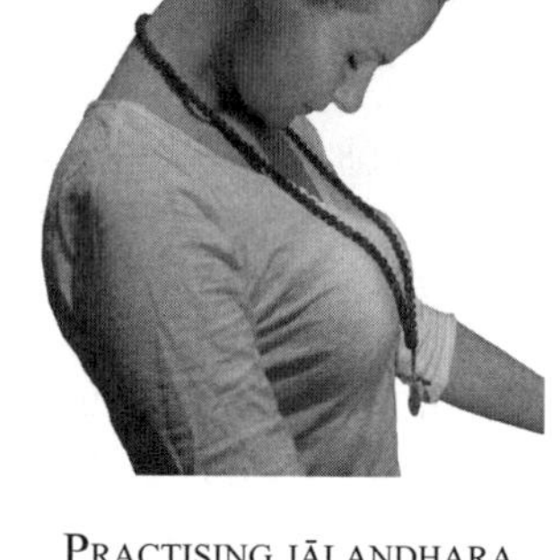

Practising Jālandhara bandha (throat or chin lock)

Caution

It is important not to inhale or exhale until the chin lock has been released and the head is upright.

Jālandhara bandha should not be practised by persons with high intra-cranial blood pressure or heart ailments without expert guidance.

UḌḌĪYĀNA BANDHA (ABDOMINAL LOCK)

Uḍḍīyāna comes from the Sanskrit root *ud* and *di*, which means 'flying up', 'upward lift'. The *prāṇic* energy flies up through the *suṣumnā nāḍī* from the *maṇipūra chakra* to the higher *chakras*. In the practice of the abdominal lock, the abdominal organs are simultaneously pulled in and lifted upwards.

Uḍḍīyāna can be practised sitting, lying down, standing, and in inverted postures. For beginners it is best to start practising from a standing position, because it is easier to accomplish in this position.

Uḍḍīyāna activates the *maṇipūra chakra* and solar plexus, and encourages the *prāṇic* energy to flow upwards through the *suṣumnā* subtle channel. It increases the gastric fire (*agni*); the abdominal organs and glands are invigorated and toned; it stimulates intestinal peristalsis and improves the function of the digestive and eliminative systems; it stimulates the liver, pancreas, kidneys and spleen; it balances the adrenal glands; it strengthens the immune system; and it tones the spinal nerves in the coccygeal and solar plexus regions. It balances the mind, and soothes irritability and anger.

Seated method

1. Sit in a comfortable and steady meditation pose in which the knees touch the floor (*Pādmāsana* or *Siddhāsana* are best), and place your palms on the knees.
2. Exhale completely and hold the breath out.

3. Contract the abdominal muscles, pulling strongly inward towards the spine and slightly upward, which causes the diaphragm to rise up into the thorax.
4. Hold the breath out while maintaining the contraction of the abdomen for as long as comfortable without strain. Concentrate on the *maṇipūra chakra.*
5. Then, relax the abdomen releasing the *uḍḍīyāna bandha*, and inhale.

Rest for a few moments breathing normally and then repeat the practice four more times.

Caution

Practise only on an empty stomach. Allow three to four hours after a meal before practising. The ideal time to practise is early morning after evacuating the bladder and the bowels. Women should not practise during pregnancy or menstruation. Those suffering from heart problems, high blood pressure and stomach ulcers should also not practise.

Standing method

1. Stand with your feet about two feet apart, and with your knees slightly bent, grip the middle of your thighs with your hands and lean your trunk forward from the waist.
2. Look forward as you inhale deeply, then exhale completely. Slowly lower your head forward and apply the chin lock (*jālandhara bandha*) by resting your chin in the hollow of your throat.
3. Contract and pull your lower abdominal muscles, then your upper abdominal muscles, back towards the spine, lifting the abdomen slightly upwards. Raise your lumbar and dorsal spine forward and upwards.
4. Hold the breath out while holding the *uḍḍīyāna bandha* for as long as comfortable. On no account strain or go beyond your endurance. Concentrate on the *maṇipūra chakra.*
5. To release *uḍḍīyāna bandha*, relax the abdominal muscles first. Then slowly raise your head and inhale slowly. Return to normal relaxed breathing for a few breaths, then repeat the whole process again.

In the beginning practise three to five abdominal lifts, gradually increasing to ten in each held breath.

MŪLABANDHA (ANAL LOCK)

The Sanskrit word *mūla* means 'root' and refers to the region between the anus and the genitals (the perineum). It is from this base root that the yogi creates an energetic lift that rises up through the spine and the subtle channel of the *suṣumnā nāḍī.*

Mūlabandha is practised in conjunction with *prāṇāyāma* and *mudrās*. In the practice of *mūlabandha*, the *apāṇa* (downward flowing energy) merges with the *prāṇa* (upward flowing energy), resulting in generation of a great amount of energy that helps in activating the serpent energy known as *kuṇḍalinī*.

On the physical level, this practice strengthens the reproductive glands; strengthens the muscles of the pelvic floor; stimulates the gastric fire (*agni*); relieves constipation and haemorrhoids and congestion in the pelvic area; and calms the autonomic nervous system and the mind.

Method

1. Sit in a comfortable and steady meditation posture, preferably *Siddhāsana* or *Siddhā yoni āsana* (for women), because these postures improve the effect of the *bandha* by the heel being pressed against the perineum. This stimulates an automatic contraction, creating an upward pressure in this region of the body. Place your hands on the knees.
2. Inhale slowly and deeply.
3. Apply *jālandhara bandha* (throat or chin lock) and retain the breath for as long as comfortable without strain.
4. Simultaneously contract the internal and external sphincter muscles. This may seem difficult initially, but if you first bring your awareness to the anus and contract it, then concentrate on a point just above the sphincter muscle (perineum) and contract it, you will find that it is not so difficult. At the same time, draw the *apāṇa* upward by contracting the abdominal muscles.
5. The breath is retained internally while holding both *mūlabandha* and *jālandhara bandha* in order to unite the *prāṇa* and *apāṇa*. Concentrate on the *mūladhāra chakra*.
6. Release the contraction of both the internal and external sphincter muscles. Then slowly release *jālandhara bandha*, by raising the head and exhale. Relax and breathe normally for some time.

Practise three to five rounds.

Mūlabandha can also be practised with external breath retention. The breath retention, internal or external, is held for as long as comfortable without strain.

Caution

Do not practise if you have high blood pressure or heart problems.

MAHĀBANDHA (GREAT LOCK)

Mahābandha is also called *tribandha* (triple lock) because it is the combination of all three locks – *jālandhara*, *uḍḍīyāna* and *mūlabandha*. These three locks are held simultaneously during the external retention of the breath in *prāṇāyāma*.

Mahābandha combines all the benefits of the three individual *bandhas*. The *prāṇic* energy flow is stimulated, vitalising the whole body with *prāṇa*.

Method

1. Sit in a comfortable and steady meditation posture, preferably *siddhāsana* or *siddhā yoni āsana* (for women), with your palms on your knees.
2. Inhale deeply and then exhale deeply through the mouth.
3. Perform *mūlabandha*, *uḍḍīyāna*, then *jālandhara,* in that order.
4. Hold your breath in external retention, holding the three *bandhas* for as long as comfortable without strain.
5. Release the *bandhas* in reverse order: *jālandhara*, *uḍḍīyāna*, then *mūlabandha.*
6. Inhale slowly, relax, and return to normal breathing.

6.6

PRATYĀHĀRA (WITHDRAWAL OF THE MIND FROM THE SENSES)

In the preceding chapters we have studied four of the eight limbs of Patañjali's Yoga. Let us briefly review them:

The practice of *yama* – five restraints – which have a particular reference to one's mental attitude and relationship towards other beings.

The practice of *niyama* – observances – individual discipline.

Yama and *niyama* help to remove restlessness, desires, delusions, wrong attitudes, unsettling emotions, and attachments from the mind. They are ideals towards which an aspirant following the spiritual path works with sincerity.

The practice of *āsana* (posture) trains us to make the body steady with ease and comfort, in order to ensure that the mind becomes still and quiet in preparation for meditation. *Haṭha Yoga*, which includes *āsana*, is also a necessary auxiliary and essential to *Rāja Yoga*. It ensures physical health, harmony, vitality, and energy – prerequisites for concentration and meditation.

The practice of *prāṇāyāma* purifies the subtle channels (*nāḍīs*), and purifies and removes distractions from the mind.

Each limb of Yoga forms a progression of bringing one into stillness. The *yamas* and *niyamas* help to bring stillness to the mind by removing mental and emotional disturbances; *āsana* is stillness of the body; *prāṇāyāma* is stillness of the breath; *pratyāhāra* is stillness of the senses; *dhāraṇā* (concentration), *dhyāna* (meditation) and *samādhi* (absorption) are stillness of the mind.

Now we come to the fifth limb of Yoga, called *pratyāhāra*. This is covered in only two *sūtras* by Patañjali:

> '*Pratyāhāra* is the interiorisation of the mind, by reversing the senses' outward attention from external objects to their source within (the divine Self).'
>
> *Yoga Sūtras 2:54*

> 'By conscious interiorisation of the mind, the senses function intelligently and in harmony without ego-mind interference. One attains complete mastery over all the senses.'
>
> *Yoga Sūtras 2:55*

The practices of *yama*, *niyāma*, *āsana*, *prāṇāyāma* and *pratyāhāra* are concerned with the body and brain. They constitute the outer phase of Yoga. The final three limbs – *dhāraṇā*, *dhyāna* and *samādhi* – constitute the inner phase of Yoga, and are concerned with the reconditioning of the mind.

The Sanskrit word *pratyāhāra* is a combination of two words: *prati* ('reverse', 'opposite direction'), and *ahar* ('removing', 'taking away', 'withdrawing'). *Pratyāhāra* means to withdraw in the reverse direction. It is withdrawal of the mind from the five senses and their respective objects in the world. As a result, the mind becomes interiorised. *Pratyāhāra* is an indispensable prerequisite to concentration, so inner Yoga is impossible without first becoming well established in *Pratyāhāra*. If the mind is not withdrawn from the senses and their objects and interiorised, it becomes externalised and scattered over many things, making concentration extremely difficult. The senses are turbulent, they are outward going, they draw the mind outwards, and through the mind the *puruṣa* becomes completely involved and identified in *prakṛiti*.

Pratyāhāra is a state in which the attention does not externalise itself. Usually as you look at something, listen to some sound, or smell or touch something, your attention is drawn out of yourself. In *pratyāhāra* the attention is directed inwards.

Through the practice of *āsana* and *prāṇāyāma* one turns the mind's attention within, being totally aware of where the impulse to breathe in and breathe out arises. Total attention and awareness of that is itself *pratyāhāra*, or drawing one's attention into and within oneself.

Pratyāhāra is an automatic process that occurs when the mind is interiorised and concentrated.

THE MIND AND THE SENSES

We are all seeking happiness and want freedom from sorrow and suffering. Most people generally seek it through external activities, in objects, people, or in anything that gives pleasure through sense enjoyment. The seeking is external; it is not ultimately fulfilling because the external objects of the senses have a changeable, temporary and transient nature. When we try to find happiness through our desires and the senses, the mind becomes restless, unsteady, discontented and unfulfilled. There may be some temporary satisfaction and happiness when the desired object, person or thing that we wanted is attained, but the mind does not remain happily content for long – happiness seems fleeting. All actions are motivated by desire and activated by *rajas guṇa* (activity, desire, passion). Without *rajas guṇa* or desire there is no movement of the senses; they remain still. When we control desire we restrain the senses.

Indulgence in the senses can only give us temporary gratification, it can never give us real happiness that is fulfilling and lasting. True happiness and freedom from sorrow and suffering is only possible when the desires and restlessness of the mind cease. All desires are our longing for the divine Self within, and until we look within we will never find real happiness, for the external world is not the source of our spiritual fulfilment. The infinite, all-pervading universal Self is the ultimate source of happiness, peace and joy.

An electricity power point can become weakened from loss of its voltage if there are too many electric connections that take it beyond its limit. Likewise, the mind can become weak by connecting itself too much to the objects of the senses. But when all the connections are cut off, the power point meter immediately shows a rise in voltage. Similarly, one can perceive a rise in the voltage of the strength in the mind, the moment the connections of the senses with their respective sense objects are cut off or disconnected. Patañjali says in his *Yoga Sūtras* (2:54) that *pratyāhāra* is that state where the senses separate from the mind and appear to be one with the mind. They are no longer outside the mind, but have assumed the form of the mind itself.

THE SENSES – A MEANS FOR GATHERING EXPERIENCE

The five components of creation – ether, air, fire, water and earth – have given us our five senses: hearing, feeling, sight, taste and smell, respectively.

The soul (the true Self) shines by its own light; it is the true source of intelligence which gives life to the body, mind and senses. Without the life force of the Self, the body, mind and senses cannot function at all.

Primarily (as young children prove) the senses are the first instruments to gather knowledge or perception from the external world. The reason I use the expression 'to gather' is because awareness of sense perceptions arises only if the information delivered by the senses reaches the mind. Without mind there is no recorded perception and so the senses become useless as instruments.

When the mind receives the collected information from the senses it examines, analyses and discriminates what it has received and acts upon it. But what makes the senses go out and gather information? It is curiosity. So curiosity has to exist in the mind to determine it to send the senses out to gather information to satisfy that curiosity. But the more you try to satisfy your mind's curiosity, the more curiosity is generated, because each piece of information triggers more questions.

The mind has this inborn curiosity because it is searching for meaning. It wants to enlarge the whole informational picture until it makes sense. So curiosity, or the desire to find out and know things, is a search for meaning.

So why does the attempt of the mind and senses to find meaning in life fail so often? The senses are the means for gathering experience. Experience may be divided into pleasant and unpleasant, like and dislike. Each sensory experience leaves an impression (*samskāra*) on the mind. For example, when you first perceive an apple and touch it, smell it and taste it, you have knowledge of an apple. An impression (*samskāra*) is immediately formed in the subconscious mind, and at any time this *samskāra* can generate a memory of the object – the apple and knowledge of the apple.

After accumulating a number of experiences that are alike, the mind forms an idea about them. So now the ego, the 'I-maker' which is born of ignorance (*avidyā*) intervenes, disregarding the truth or the reality that all these experiences come and go.

The ego says: 'That was beautiful, I want to keep it. That is ugly I want to avoid it.' But neither of these is possible. If the beautiful thing we saw is not present, the mind which registered the experience as memory goes on wanting it; and what is even more unfortunate, the mind also remembers an unpleasant experience and goes on fearing it. It is not there, but you know it might come again. It also might not return, but the mind retains the impression of that momentary experience of pleasure or of displeasure, and out of these are born desire, like and dislike. When the momentary experience of pleasure born of sense contact is allowed to leave an impression on the mind, the mind becomes coloured by it, so that afterwards wherever you look, that thing continues to rotate in the mind – 'I want that, I must have it,' or 'I want to have that, but I fear it may not happen.'

Gradually the obstinate efforts to repeat pleasurable experiences and avoid unpleasant ones leads to abandoning the initial search – the search for meaning. Instead, one becomes addicted to sense pleasure and comfort, not understanding that pleasure is not in the objects but in the condition of the mind, and that happiness is not in the objects but within one's inner Self. Our lives become ruled by desire and attachment, and the need to defend what we think belongs to us.

WHAT MAKES THE SENSES FUNCTION?

When you open your eyes, they see, and in that sight there is no love or hate. The sight also sees different colours. To some sights the eyes respond without blinking, and to some sights the eyes immediately want to close. These are natural, and the word 'natural' means that they are inherent in all living beings. If the senses are to function naturally, they must function as decided by life and intelligence.

Does this experience, this impulse for expression, arise in life and intelligence, or is there an ego interference in it? Put simply, did this impulse, or this action, or experience, arise from the intelligence or from the mind? The mind is the ego, the ego sense, and the ego is the mind. When the question arises, a sudden change takes place within you – that is called *pratyāhāra*. That is, you are looking at something and you say, 'Ah, that is beautiful, I love it,' and immediately the question arises, 'Is this from the mind or the intelligence?' When the question arises, the whole thing immediately turns back. Something that was externalising or flowing out immediately turns back. It is as simple as that.

Then that intelligence and that awareness itself is capable of ensuring that the experience or the expression is not ego-motivated. The ego need not make any effort to shut out all these, so it is not as though when I see a beautiful face: 'No, I don't want to see!' That being an activity of the ego is useless to Yoga. If it is ego-motivated rejection, it is still rejection, and if the ego finds it convenient, it will take it back some time later. It is the intelligence that raises this question 'Does it arise in the intelligence or is it ego-motivated?' and that can eliminate all ego-motivated expressions and experiences.

So the awareness is aware merely of the source of the action or the experience. This is *pratyāhāra* in a very different form of control. You will see change taking place in your behaviour and in your experience, but not because the ego decides that this is better than that, and not because the ego decides this is good and this is not good. A natural change takes place, and that change brings you into total alignment with the inner intelligence, and that is precisely how *pratyāhāra* is defined in the *Yoga Sūtras* (2:54): '*Citta svarūpānukāra*'.

That is, the senses function in total alignment with the inner intelligence, which means there is no mind or ego interference. When that happens, of course the ego reveals its nature. The awakened intelligence sees the countless ways in which the ego tries to step in and pollute actions and experiences.

DULLING OF THE SENSES

The other intervening phenomenon is a dulling of the senses due to over-indulgence and repetition. The drug addict starts with marijuana and goes on to take stronger and more dangerous drugs such as cocaine and heroin. The smoker smokes more cigarettes. The drinker drinks more, and ends up becoming an alcoholic. The relationship that becomes more and more sexual, based on physical self-gratification without love, soon becomes dull and repetitive, and so one or both partners continually look for more stimulating and exciting forms of sex with other partners, who become mere objects of stimulation.

Whether it is drugs, alcohol, sex, smoking, coffee or sugar, indulgence in any pleasure dulls the sensitivity of the senses and the nervous system. In the end it will either bore you or enslave you, and in that there is no freedom, beauty or joy. The initial stimulus is no longer strong enough to cause pleasure. The initial sharpness and awareness of the sense-experience wears off and the senses need a stronger one in order for the ego to have the kind of pleasure it expects.

THE EGO'S RELATION TO EXPERIENCE

The way the ego relates to experience is also wrong, in that it wants to possess the objects of attachment. The ego is frustrated by the fleetingness of pleasure and wants to externalise it through possession. In fact, possession is a delusion. We do not even own what we eat. We just recycle energies, and even that process is not a conscious one. Possessiveness 'freezes' the relationship with the object or person.

Instead of using our senses to discover the meaning at the interface of any process of relating, we want to 'have' this or that experience out of it. What gets lost again is the meaning, the teaching that we receive. We unwittingly refer to the ego rather than the real *Self*.

FALSE IDENTIFICATION WITH THE OBJECT OF THE SENSES

> 'Egoism (*asmitā* – I-am-ness, sense of individuality) is the false-identification of the Seer (*puruṣa*, Self) with the instrument of cognition (*buddhi*, intellect or mind).'
>
> *Yoga Sūtras 2:6*

The body, mind and senses are the non-Self (unconscious principle) that are evolutes of *prakṛiti* (material nature). The Self (*puruṣa*) is the eternal conscious principle.

Although the Self (*puruṣa* – the subjective power of consciousness) and the intellect-mind (*buddhi* – the instrument of cognition) are completely different, when the mind is covered by ignorance (*avidyā*) they appear as if they are the same. The reflection of the Self on the intellect-mind produces the separate ego sense of 'I'. Due to ignorance (*avidyā*) the intellect-mind acts as if it is the Self. This delusive affliction is known as *asmitā kleśa* (affliction of ego).

It is not the object that binds or enslaves you. It is the false identification of the thought with the object that causes desire, possessiveness, attachment and fear. It is the identification and labelling of things as 'desirable' and 'undesirable' by the ego that causes all the problems. The mind labels a sensation or experience desirable, which automatically makes its opposite or absence undesirable – pleasure creates pain. The sensation becomes a feeling at the point when thought arises to label the sensation. The labelling creates division between the thought and the experience. In pure experiencing there is no labelling. In the state of pure awareness, the mind is undivided and steady. If the mind seeks the experience of something other than the inner joy and inner peace of the Self, the awareness of its own nature is lost or hidden.

When the futility of desire and the pursuit of sensory objects is seen, the mind is left with the feeling that something is lacking or missing. It is forgetfulness of our true essential nature – the blissful Self within. That which is missing is the inner joy and inner peace of Self-fulfilment. We have lost the memory and awareness of our original blissful state. Through mis-identification with the ego-self we try to find happiness and fulfilment with the fleeting joys of sensory pleasures. The reason we search with continual determination for true happiness and joy is that we have the memory of our true nature. The individual soul is inwardly conscious of losing its blissful contact with the Supreme Consciousness, the source of all joy, peace and love, the one and only Reality of our being, and can never remain satisfied with the limited pleasures of the senses. Eventually, every soul must awaken to their true Divine nature and return to Oneness.

THE ART OF BEING DETACHED INWARDLY

Pratyāhāra is an art that needs to be practised all the time, because it is not only confined to just sitting in meditation but is also a process that needs to be constantly practised throughout your everyday activities. Your Yoga practice will never succeed if you only confine it to centring yourself in the inner Reality when you sit for meditation, while the rest of the time is spent in allowing your mind and senses to roam outwardly in the perception and enjoyment of the senses. Without constant awareness of your inner Reality or the Self, the mind and senses will move restlessly towards sense-objects and become absorbed and entangled in them to such an extent that you will lose awareness of your inner Self.

Most spiritual seekers who are practising Yoga are not living in an isolated Himalayan cave, but are living in villages, towns and cities. They have a social life, they work or study, and they may be married with children to care for. This is their *dharma* or duty to fulfil while living in the world. So, *pratyāhāra* is very important in its aspect as a continuing daily process throughout the waking hours. It is the art of being in the world and yet not being in it. This means living in the world but not being affected by it, not getting entangled in the world of objects and all its distractions. You need to be like the beautiful lotus flower that grows in the lake, rising above the mud and the water so as not to be affected or contaminated by it.

In this constant awareness while in the midst of life's activities you can be centred in your inner Self even while performing your duties. This process of *pratyāhāra*, of being inwardly aware, alert, and keeping your discrimination constantly active supports you in remembering your inner divine nature and your true aim or purpose in life. So that when you come into contact with sense objects, they will not disturb your mind. They will be unable to have an impact on your inner consciousness.

This *pratyāhāra* process of remaining alert, inwardly aware and discriminating wisely also has the positive effect of not creating new *saṁskāras* (imprint of past actions in the mind) and *vāsanās* (desires, latent impressions of past action). If you become so attracted to and absorbed and entangled in external activities and sense objects due to your desires, then every experience and sense contact that you engage in will create new *saṁskāras* and *vāsanās*, which will become submerged in your subconscious mind and cause distracting *vṛttis* (thought waves and feelings to revolve in the mind) to rise within your mind when you sit to meditate.

THE THREE SPIRITUAL COMPANIONS TO *PRATYĀHĀRA*

The three spiritual companions of *pratyāhāra* are:

Vichāra – reflection, enquiry

Viveka – discrimination

Vairāgya – dispassion.

Withdrawal and detachment in the midst of active involvement in the objective world is only possible if you are constantly aware of the illusory nature and the transient happiness of sense enjoyment. This requires both *vichāra* and *viveka* for *pratyāhāra* to be successful. When these two are brought into operation, the inner consciousness remains calmly centred within, even when you come into contact outwardly with sense objects. Your mind is undisturbed, and so you no longer create any new *saṁskāras* and *vāsanās*.

Also, to be successful and effective in *pratyāhāra* you need to develop dispassion (*vairāgya*), which is only possible when *vichāra* and *viveka* are sustained. To develop this further you can keep *vichāra* and *viveka* active and alive by supporting them with daily practice of *svādhyāya* (Self-study, study of the scriptures), *satsanga* (fellowship with those who embody spiritual values and truth), *brāhmacharya* (keeping the presence of God; control of vital energy), and *tapasya* (discipline, austerity). In this way, in this process of *pratyāhāra*, you will be able to progress and advance spiritually by keeping your mind always interiorised, not moving towards the senses but moving towards the calm presence of the blissful inner Self, so that your consciousness remains steadfast.

Pratyāhāra needs to be a continuous state of mind even in the midst of your daily activities. Your higher discrimination should always be active and your philosophical enquiry present. You need to raise your mind to a state of perpetual awareness of the presence of the Divine at all times, in all circumstances and surroundings, and amid all activities. Once the mind has become established in the supports of *pratyāhāra* – *vichāra*, *viveka* and *vairāgya* – the senses come under the influence of the mind and acquire a state of repose and become internalised in their respective centres. The senses no longer distract and agitate the mind. The Yoga practitioner then becomes ready and able to practise the process of concentration (*dhāraṇā*).

THE GOAL OF *PRATYĀHĀRA*

The ultimate goal of Yoga is complete control of the mind. It is to remove the impurities (*kleśas*) of the mind that are the root causes of bondage of the embodied soul (*puruṣa*). When the *kleśas* are removed, so are sorrow and suffering. The mind becomes purified from *rājas guṇa* (passion, desire, activity) and *tamas guṇa* (darkness, inertia) so that the *puruṣa* can be released from bondage. In that pure state of consciousness the mind becomes illuminated. The yogi realises that *puruṣa* (the Self) is his or her true essential nature, which is clearly perceptible from the body, mind and the senses.

An untrained mind that is extroverted and restless, and *puruṣa* is conditioned by the world, is unable to control the endless flow of desires and worldly phenomena bombarding the senses. Mental equilibrium becomes impossible for one whose ego-driven mind is constantly ruled by the senses and attached to its external objects. The mind's energy is dissipated, making it incapable of concentrating deeply for meditation.

The goal of *pratyāhāra* is to 'withdraw' the senses from their respective external objects and to interiorise the attention within. By withdrawing the senses we remove ourselves from attachment to the duality of pleasure and pain which causes us distress.

Unless the senses are withdrawn from their respective objects in the external world, the mind will not be still. To bring stillness and self-awareness to the mind, we need to reverse the outward flow of mental energy, so that all the senses focus their attention on the mind; they imitate it and become identified with the nature of it.

MASTERY OF THE SENSES

Krishna teaches us in in the *Bhāgavad Gītā* that if the senses are not controlled, the mind will be distracted and captivated by attachment to sensory experiences, leading to forgetfulness of one's true essential nature – the Self.

> 'Just as a tortoise draws in its limbs within its shell, the wise yogi, fixed in higher consciousness, disconnects the senses from their objects of perception at will, resulting in steadiness of mind.
>
> Those who deprive the senses from experiencing their objects experience that they still crave for them. These sense cravings only come to an end when one attains a higher knowledge and realises the Self.

Having brought the senses under control one should be joined in Yoga with the mind ever established in Me. The wisdom of one who has mastered the senses becomes steadfast and unwavering.

The senses become attached to an object when it is continually thought of. As a result of such involvement, the desire to enjoy the object arises. When such a desire is unfulfilled or obstructed, anger arises.

Anger clouds discrimination and one falls easily into illusion, losing the memory of one's own true Self. From loss of memory one loses the faculty of discrimination and eventually from the confusion of intelligence misses the goal of human life – Self-realisation.

However, those who can supervise the involvement between the senses and sense objects by exercising self-control, and who become free from craving and false repression attain inner calmness and peace.

In that inner calmness and inner joy comes the end of all sorrows. For the intelligence of the calm-minded soon becomes firmly established in the Self.

For one whose mind and senses are unsteady, there is no knowledge of the Self. When the mind is restless it cannot concentrate or meditate; it has no peace. Without inner peace, how can there be joy?

Just as a boat on the sea is carried away by the wind in a storm, so can a person's intelligence and understanding be carried away by the force of sense desire.

Therefore, one whose senses are completely mastered, becomes firmly established in wisdom of the Self.

Just as the vast ocean remains calm and unperturbed, even though many rivers flow into it from all sides, so a person should remain undivided by the continued arising of sense desires. One who is controlled by desire cannot attain true peace.

True inner peace arises when all sense desires are transcended and orientated to higher levels of consciousness; and when one acts free from identification with the false ego and the illusion of the sense of "I" and "mine".'

Bhāgavad Gītā 2:58–71 (Author's translation)

THE PRACTICE OF *PRATYĀHĀRA*

The difference between a Master of Yoga and an ordinary worldly person is that the yogi experiences true joy, inner peace and contentment by inwardly reversing the searchlight of perception from the senses to the divine source within, consciously at will. The worldly person, whose ego-mind identifies with and is attached to the senses, becomes disunited from the inner source of joy and peace – the Self. Instead, the worldly person suffers restlessly with anger, fear, and loss of inner peace and joy.

The worldly person can only disconnect the mind from the senses in the subconscious state of ordinary sleep; the life-force that connects the mind with the senses reverts back to the Self-conscious force of the soul. In this state of sleep there is no consciousness of 'I'. There is no desire to experience, there is no ego-sense. In sleep you are not aware that 'I am', otherwise you are awake! What remains is pure experiencing – there is no contact with the objects of the senses, and since there is no contact, the mind is not divided. That is why you do not experience pain or suffering at all during sleep.

In the dream state during sleep, the senses of perception are still and absorbed in the mind. It is only the mind that is actively operating during dreaming; it becomes both the subject and the object. During the wakeful state objects exist independently of the mind. Whether you are asleep or awake the objects are always there. However, in dreams the objects exist only as long as there is the mind to create them and for as long as the dream lasts. When you awake from your sleep all the dream objects disappear.

In sleep there is no time, no space, no objects other than you. You have gone to sleep, your mind and senses have withdrawn inward. The outer world of objects and people vanishes, but an inner world of images arises from within you. A world that seems real as a dream while you sleep, but unreal when you awake from that dream.

That same world that projects your dream experiences in sleep can become very active when you sit for meditation and try to concentrate your mind by disconnecting it from the outer world (*prakṛiti*) experience. The inner world or inner *prakṛiti* arises in the form of countless *saṁskāras*, *vāsanās* and memories that are submerged and latent in the *citta* (field of consciousness). Thoughts and feelings spontaneously arise in the mind and distract you as you try to concentrate. As a distracting thought arises, you become associated with that thought and the thought current begins to flow in numerous directions. And, losing your concentration and Self-awareness, you get swept away in that distracting thought current.

The reason why these distracting thoughts arise when you sit to concentrate for meditation is because when you are engaged in other daily activities and experiences on the outer plane, or engaged in some process that requires your attention, your mind is drawn outward and gets engaged in that process. So the inner process of *saṁskāras*, *vāsanās*, and memories taking the form of *vṛttis*, mental modifications, becomes restricted. Whereas when you are sitting for meditation with your mind and attention withdrawn from the outer world, a vacuum is created in the mind, which invites from deep within your subconscious the submerged and latent *saṁskāras*, *vāsanās*, memories and seeds of suppressed and unfulfilled desires, which are stimulated by *rāga-dveṣa* (attraction and aversion).

YOGA NIDRĀ: THE PSYCHIC SLEEP OF THE YOGIS

Yoga nidrā is one of the best techniques for developing awareness, purifying the mind, interiorising the mind (*pratyāhāra*), and bringing complete rest and relaxation to the body. It harmonises the various body systems and balances the body.

Nidrā means 'sleep', but not in the ordinary sense of the word as we know it. *Yoga nidrā* is conscious sleep or sleeping with awareness. Ordinary sleep is like being unconscious, there is no awareness. *Yoga nidrā* is more like meditation. It is practised lying down in the relaxation pose – *Śavāsana* (Corpse pose).

Yoga psychology realises that relaxation is a natural behaviour and can be relearned by those whose faulty living and thinking habits have caused unnatural, neurotic, over-reactive behaviour. Yoga techniques develop the faculty of concentration as well as bringing about relaxation. Concentration, the ability to focus the mind on one thought form, is a very effective way of removing the mind from worrying and anxiety-provoking thoughts. *Yoga nidrā* is therefore not only a powerful form of relaxation, but its repeated practice aids in the development of the mental faculties as well. Since relaxation is the first step in the development of meditation, *Yoga nidrā* is the ideal first practice of *pratyāhāra* for the student of Yoga.

In the *Yoga nidrā* state one is completely and totally relaxed on all levels – physical, mental and emotional. In this state the brainwave pattern changes and becomes slower than the usual busy, waking, beta level to the deeper, slower alpha level.

In *Yoga nidrā* one does not actually sleep in an unconscious way. The body, brain and nervous system are completely relaxed, while the consciousness remains totally alert, awake and aware. In this state of consciousness, which is on the borderline between sleep and wakefulness, there is contact with the subconscious and unconscious mind – the deeper layers of your personality. Through the practice of *Yoga nidrā* we are able to recognise, release and eliminate our suppressions, fears, phobias, neuroses and deep-rooted tensions – all things that condition our conscious thoughts and experiences in a negative way.

The main elements of *Yoga nidrā* are:

- **Body relaxation/awareness and rotation of consciousness:** The consciousness is rotated through the different parts of the body a number of times to reduce the mind's attention on external stimuli, thus interiorising the mind and relaxing the physical body.
- ***Pratyāhāra*:** The mind is very rebellious; it does the opposite of what you want it to do. So in *Yoga nidrā* we deliberately focus our attention on external things with complete awareness. In this way the mind loses interest in the external things and naturally withdraws and goes within.
- **Breath awareness:** With breath awareness, there is no attempt to force or change the breath. You just silently watch your natural breath flow in and flow out. This practice takes you into a deeper state of physical relaxation.
- **Awareness of feelings or emotions:** Through the practice of visualisation, using stories and images, we are able to awaken or recall, and voluntarily bring to the surface, suppressed and deep-rooted feelings and emotions from the subconscious and unconscious levels of our minds. When these deep-rooted fears and anxieties rise to the surface, we watch them with awareness, detachment and dispassion – we recognise them, then release them. This process can be useful to cleanse unwanted patterns from the mental field and emotional life.
- **Affirmation:** Having released the negative feelings and impressions from the subconscious it is important to implant a positive affirmation. During the deep relaxation of *Yoga nidrā*, the deeper layers of the subconscious are very impressionable to suggestions from the conscious will. Affirm with conviction, faith and deep concentration the statement of truth which you aspire to absorb into your life.

THE PRACTICE OF *YOGA NIDRĀ*

Practise *Yoga nidrā* in a quiet, clean, warm room. Wear loose, comfortable clothing. Lie down on your back on a Yoga mat with a blanket over it (or use a thick rug to lie down on). Keep the body warm by covering yourself with a blanket. In the classical Yoga relaxation pose (*Śavāsana*), position the feet about hip-width apart, and allow them to fall and relax to the sides. Move the arms slightly away from the sides of the body, and have the palms of the hands facing upward with the fingers relaxed (naturally curling in towards the palm). Keep the head, neck and spine in alignment.

Once the practice of *Yoga nidrā* has begun there must be no physical movement. One must remain completely aware and awake throughout the whole practice.

You can either be guided through the practice by an experienced Yoga teacher, who instructs clearly and slowly in a relaxed tone of voice, or you can be guided by listening to a *Yoga nidrā* cassette tape that has been recorded for this purpose.

OTHER *PRATYĀHĀRA* PRACTICES

Savitri prāṇāyāma (rhythmic breath)

Savitri prāṇāyāma is a rhythmic, harmonising breath, using a four-part breath ratio. The inhalation and exhalation are the same and the internal and external breath retentions are half that of the inhalation and exhalation.

The conventional ratio is 8:4:8:4. This is the best rhythm to strengthen and rejuvenate the body, and it promotes optimum health.

This rhythm is used as the basis of *pratyāhāra* (withdrawing the mind from the senses) and *dhāraṇā* (concentration). It brings calmness to the mind.

Method

1. Sit and relax in a meditative posture with your head, neck and spine aligned. Close your eyes.
2. Inhale slowly through both nostrils for a count of eight.
3. Retain the breath internally for a count of four.
4. Exhale slowly through both nostrils for a count of eight.
5. Retain the breath externally for a count of four.

This completes one round. Practise nine rounds, then gradually over time as you progress increase to 27 rounds. The duration of inhalation and exhalation can also be gradually increased over time, according to your strength and capacity, but do not force or strain the breath in any way.

6.7

DHĀRAṆĀ (CONCENTRATION)

Dhāraṇā (concentration) is the sixth limb of Patañjali's *Rāja Yoga*. The Sanskrit word *dhāraṇā* comes from the word *dhri*, 'to hold firm'.

When the senses have been mastered through *pratyāhāra*, they can be restored to serve the realisation of the Self, instead of being misguided in serving the ignorance of the ego. Then the mind is ready for the next stage – interiorisation of the mind. Calmly focusing the full attention of the mind and consciousness on one point to the exclusion of everything else – this is *dhāraṇā* (concentration).

The mind can be compared to a lake, and the thoughts that arise from the mind are compared to the waves of the lake. You can see your reflection clearly in the waters of the lake only when the waves on the surface of the water completely subside and become still. Similarly, you can realise the inner Self only when all the thought-waves and vortices of feeling (*vṛttis*) in the mind-lake are stilled. In *dhāraṇā* there is only one wave in the mind-lake. The mind assumes the form of only one object at a time – all other operations are suspended. When the *vṛttis* are controlled and reversed back and absorbed into the field of consciousness (*citta*), that is called Yoga. *Nirodhaḥ* (control, restraint, to stop) is the operative factor in causing the mind to leave its external activities and turn inward to become aware of its source.

In Patañjali's *Yoga Sūtras*, concentration (*dhāraṇā*) is simply described in only one *sūtra*:

> *'Deśa-bandhaś cittasya dhāraṇā.'*
> 'Concentration is the fixing (or binding) of the mind's attention (focused awareness) to one particular point (to the exclusion of everything else).'
>
> *Yoga Sūtras 3:1*

Patañjali is not referring to concentration on external stimuli, which stir up restless thoughts, desires, emotions, moods and attachment. He is not referring to concentration as generalised attention, where the mind is still engaged in thought-processes, but to the Yoga technique of 'one-pointed' (*ekāgrata*) concentration: a continuous flow of consciousness inwards, either on an internal object (*antara-visaya*), or an externalised object (*bahya-visaya*). The internal objects refer to points within the body – the navel, the heart, the midpoint between the eyebrows, particularly the higher *chakras*. The external object is an idea or image of an object that the mind's attention is calmly focused on from within.

Dhāraṇā is focusing the attention on a limited area. Even there you will begin to see the play of the ego. There is all this memory stored and the ego has a whole lot of hopes and fears, likes and dislikes; and even during the period when you are trying to focus your attention on something, all these come and try to distract your attention. This is likely to happen especially if the concentration itself is ego-motivated. That is also why Patañjali suggests that *prāṇāyāma* makes the mind qualified for concentration. In *prāṇāyāma* we already had a glimpse of something beyond the ego-self, and so when it comes to concentration there is virtually no effort, especially when it is done after practising *prāṇāyāma*.

The practice of concentration and *prāṇāyāma* are interdependent. If you practise *prāṇāyāma* you will also achieve concentration. *Prāṇāyāma* removes the veil of ignorance (*avidyā*) and inertia (*tamas*) that cover the pure state. It purifies the subtle channels (*nāḍīs*) and makes the mind steady, preparing it for concentration. One who can sit and hold a steady posture (*āsana*), and has purified his or her *nāḍīs* (subtle *prāṇic* channels) through the control of breath, will be able to concentrate easily.

For practising Yoga one must proceed on the spiritual path in gradual stages. First the spiritual foundations *yamas* and *niyamas* – right conduct and observances – along with steady posture (*āsana*), regulation of breath (*prāṇāyāma*), and withdrawing the mind from the senses (*pratyāhāra*) need to be regularly practised. Only then will the superstructure of concentration and meditation be successful.

INTEREST AND ATTENTION

There can be no concentration without *interest* and *attention*. Interest develops attention. We all know that it is difficult to focus the mind on an uninteresting object or an object in which we have no interest at all. Our minds have not been trained to endure prolonged attention. The mind becomes bored with monotony and wants to run towards a pleasing and interesting object. If you are sitting listening to a lecture by a professor on a subject that does not interest you, what do you do? You very quickly become bored and your attention fluctuates; you cannot pay attention to an uninteresting subject. But supposing that same professor was to give a lecture on your favourite subject – you would be able to listen with rapt attention. All the rays of your mind would be focused on listening with attention.

So, one has to be interested in the metaphysical subject of Yoga and meditation before one can be attentive to it. Interest and attention are interdependent.

Attention is of two kinds, voluntary and involuntary. When we direct our attention towards an object by determined effort of the will it is called voluntary attention. Involuntary attention is when there is no effort of the will. We see a beautiful sunset or a beautiful object and our attention is naturally and spontaneously drawn to it.

When you observe something you are attentive. Creative people such as artists and photographers can be more attentive because they are constantly observing with visual interest. This attention to visual observation makes one more aware and helps to sharpen the memory and perception. Through attention you can attain a profound knowledge of objects. When you listen or look, you receive fully because the attention is steady. When you perceive, there is steadiness, so you take in more things; when you listen, you are steady, so you take in more things.

What is attention? It is the focusing of consciousness. It is the focusing of awareness upon a single object or idea to the exclusion of all else. Simple attention to our lack of awareness is the awakening of awareness.

Our concentration can either be focused or diffused. If you focus the scattered rays of sunlight into a single beam through a magnifying glass, it can burn a piece of paper, whereas the diffused rays are too weak to burn the paper. Similarly, the mind's mental rays are usually dissipated on various objects and thoughts, but if they are collected and brought into sharp focus and clarity as a powerful single beam of concentration, it can burn away all the impurities (*samskāras*) of the mind.

Attention and concentration is necessary in all actions if we are to achieve anything successfully and safely. You can understand the importance of safety if you imagine what could happen if you were driving along a busy road with your attention scattered on other things, or if you imagine your dentist drilling your teeth with his head turned talking to his nurse!

Even in the simple actions of everyday living, our concentration and awareness is often lacking. Our attention is distracted and we forget that the bread is toasting under the grill and find it is on fire! We awake in the morning to find that we left the tap dripping all night or a light left on. The art of memory is attention. Those people who are inattentive usually have bad memories.

The difficulty in understanding the term 'concentration' in the yogic sense is that, commonly, concentration is associated with effort and tenseness. One concentrates in order to defend, possess or achieve something. In this sense, concentration is ego-motivated; it is an outward effort of the will, charged with the energy of the feelings, instead of a steady effortless flow of willpower. So in concentration the less effort the better!

ACHIEVING *DHĀRAṆĀ* (CONCENTRATION)

How do we have to change our approach to *dhāraṇā*?

- **Relax the mind and body.** The less tension there is in the mind and body, the easier it is for the mind to focus its attention. Relaxing the body in the correct posture is necessary for concentration because it allows the energies in the spine to flow upward to the higher brain centres without obstruction. Relaxation – the gate to openness and receptivity – helps to counteract the contractive force of the self limited ego-sense.

- **Steady the mind and body.** A steady pose gives concentration of mind. The practice of Yoga *āsanas* will enable you to regain steadiness of the body and mind, so that without distraction, the attention may be focused upon the object of concentration.

- **Calm the breathing.** If you pay attention to your breathing, you will come to know the degree of distractedness of the mind. The less distracted it is, the calmer the breath. The practice of *prāṇāyāma* brings calmness and equilibrium to the mind, enabling it to concentrate without distraction.

- **Cultivate willingness.** Remember that *dhāraṇā* has nothing to do with achieving a mundane goal, so there is no practical immediacy, there is no deadline, no effort. There is a willingness rather than an ego-motivated will that starts operating.

- **Cultivate interest and attention.** Concentration also requires interest and attention. We have to create interest to induce attention, because the mind finds it difficult to focus on an uninteresting object but easy to focus on an attractive one.
- **Focus on one idea alone.** Train your mind to concentrate on God or the blissful Self within through the daily practice of deep meditation. Then as the mind experiences immense joy from the practice of one-pointed concentration, it will not be distracted by external objects. The more your mind is fixed on God or the Self within, the more inner strength and energy you will acquire.
- **Discipline your mind with daily *sādhana* (spiritual practice).** Concentration increases by reducing your activities; watching the mind and through enquiry into the nature of the Self; observing silence for one or two hours daily; remaining in seclusion for one or two hours daily; practising *prāṇāyāma*; cultivating mental non-attachment; self-restraint; and increasing the time sitting in meditation.
- **How do we know when the mind is concentrated?** It happens when there is no sense of time. When we are deep in concentration, time passes by unnoticed. If we are reading a book and are interested in it, we give it all our attention, to the extent of not noticing the time at all, or even our surrounding environment. It is only when we stop reading and put the book down that we are surprised to find that a few hours have passed unnoticed. The mind is concentrated when one's interest and attention are sharply focused on a limited area (without the reference to thoughts) in the present moment – not the past or the future, but now.

It is stated in the yogic scripture *Kurma Purāna* that if the mind is continuously concentrated on one point for 12 seconds, it is *dhāraṇā* (concentration). Twelve *dhāraṇās* make a *dhyāna* (meditation), and 12 *dhyānas* will be a *samādhi* (absorption, superconsciousness).

THE STORY OF THE BOY WHO CONCENTRATED ON A BUFFALO

There is a story from India that is often told to Yoga students by *swāmis* to demonstrate the aim of concentration and meditation.

One day a boy was inspired by the peace radiating from a holy man and asked to learn meditation from him. The guru taught him to meditate on a deity, but after some time had passed, the guru noticed that his disciple was not making progress in his meditation, so he asked the boy what *interested* him most. The boy immediately told him that his buffalo was closest to his mind and heart. With this knowledge, the guru told the boy to go and sit in the meditation room and concentrate with his total attention on the buffalo.

The next day the guru knocked on the door of the meditation room and asked the boy to come out. For a few seconds there was no reply, only silence. After a short while the boy replied in a deep voice, 'I'm sorry master but I cannot leave the room, as the door is too narrow for my large horns to go through!'

The guru then realised that the boy had achieved such deep concentration and meditation that it had caused him to enter the superconscious state of *samādhi*, in which he had lost his individuality and had become one with the buffalo.

It is not a real loss of one's nature, but it is as if one's personality has been completely taken over by the object of meditation. For the time being the boy really thought that he was the buffalo he had concentrated on. Therefore it is suggested that one concentrates and meditates upon something that inspires and elevates the consciousness, so as to grow into the likeness of the image. The moral of this story is that deep concentration on something that interests us and that we love unites us with it.

FIXING YOUR MIND ON THE DIVINE SELF

When all your mental energies are centred and concentrated on one single thought or idea, the senses become still, and the mind becomes calm and steady. The dissipated rays of the mind are collected and focused only on that one thought or idea. This is one-pointedness (*ekāgratā*) of mind. When the mind is confined and fixed steadily on a certain idea or object for a prolonged period that state is called *dhāraṇā* (concentration). As this state deepens, the practitioner gradually loses awareness of his or her surroundings. As the concentration is continued it leads to the state of meditation, in which the meditator forgets even his physical form. Concentration is the master key that opens the door to meditation, and ultimately to the superconscious state in which the meditator experiences divine bliss.

We all have the ability to concentrate on something that interests us, whether it is a painting, a photograph, reading a book, watching a film or driving a car. But there are few people who can concentrate or fix their interest and attention on God or the inner Self. During the 24 hours of the day the rays of the mind are mostly scattered in every direction except our own natural blissful state within – the Self. This blissful state or inner joy is our true nature, it is our true heritage. The Sanskrit word for bliss or joy is *ānanda*, which is another name for the Self, for God – the one and only Reality of our being. The more we concentrate on our inner Self the more we are connected with *ānanda*, our own natural joyful state of being. Those who experience in deep meditation their identity with God or Self know the fullness of that joy.

If you kept a journal of how much time your attention was given to God, you may be surprised that out of 24 hours, it could be less than five minutes! Are we really that busy that we cannot think of God? What stops us from giving more attention to the Divine? Is it lack of faith or interest? Throughout the day the mind cannot see anything beyond self-interest (ego-sense); its identification and attention is mostly with the sense of ego ('I am this body-mind-personality'). The mind concentrates on acquiring wealth, fame, power and indulging in worldly pleasures to the exclusion of the most important aim in life, Self-realisation, to realise the true source of life – the Ultimate Reality, God. This Supreme Reality who is the Eternal Truth is Ever-Existing, Ever-Conscious, Ever-New Bliss (*Sat-chit-ānanda*). It is without cause and is the cause of all causes. It is the Source of each one of us. To live without the conscious awareness and presence of God is to live a limited life in which the mind seeks for worldly pleasure, but finds pain, suffering and sorrow.

If our consciousness is not attuned to the presence of God within us, if we are not centred in the conscious awareness of God, but are identified with the mind, which is limited to time, space and causation, then we do not experience that true lasting inner peace, harmony, divine love and inner joy or bliss that we are all seeking.

The individual soul-consciousness that we are, contains all the qualities of the Divine – love, peace, joy, light, wisdom – and we have only to become aware, awake, to know and realise it. Our true purpose in life is to take up the one idea of awakening to our divine nature within and remaining in that conscious awareness and presence of the reality of God, and until we do then we will never feel inner contentment, true fulfilment and completeness in ourselves. Paramhansa Yogananda said, 'True happiness is lasting happiness because it is spiritual in nature, whereas the "happiness" based on sense pleasure soon turns to sorrow.'

> 'One-pointedness reveals the Self as being Infinite and blissful… The only thing that matters is that you see the Self. This can be done wherever you remain. The Self must be sought within. The search must be steadfast.'
>
> *Maharshi 2014, pp.24–37*

> 'Most people live almost mechanically, unconscious of any ideal or plan of life, and without any apparent knowledge of spiritual truth. You must never forget that an important part of your equipment is your purpose in life. The whole world stands aside for the person who knows where he is going and is determined to get there. When you have resolved definitely upon a purpose in life, you must make everything serve that purpose.'
>
> *Yogananda 2008b, p.74*

THE STORY OF AN ARCHERY CONTEST

There is a story in the great Hindu epic the *Mahābhārata,* of which the *Bhāgavad Gītā* is a small part, that gives the idea of what *dhāraṇā* is. King Pandu had five sons – Yudhisthira, Bhima, Arjuna, Nakula and Sahadeva. Their teacher was Dronacharya, who was the greatest archery teacher of that time.

One day when Arjuna (who excelled in archery) was with Ashwathama, Yudhistira and other some students, Dronacharya was criticised for favouritism towards Arjuna. They complained that they were not less skilful in archery than Arjuna.

To settle this dispute, Dronacharya decided to test their skill in an archery contest. So the next day, he hung a carved wooden bird with a painted eye on a high branch on a distant tree. Then he asked his students to take their bows and arrows and prepare to aim at the eye of the wooden bird.

The first student he called to aim and shoot at the bird was Yudhisthira. Drona asked him, 'What do you see?'

As Yudhisthira stretched his bow-string he replied, 'I see the sun, the clouds and the trees.' He released the arrow, which whizzed through the air and landed some metres from the tree.

The next student, Ashwathama, then took his position and withdrew an arrow from his quiver and placed it in his bow. 'What do you see?' asked Drona.

'I see the bird, its legs, the twigs on the branch on which the bird sits, the small mango behind the bird, and the leaves surrounding the bird,' replied Ashwathama.

Everyone in the crowd that was watching was amazed at how much detail he could see from such a distance. Ashwathama shot his arrow through the air, but it missed the bird and landed close to the roots of the tree.

The other students tried, but all failed to hit the mark. Finally, it was Arjuna's turn. He took up his bow and arrow and with focused attention and concentration carefully aimed at his target.

'What do you see. Arjuna?' asked Drona.

'I can see the eye of the bird.'

'Do you see the tree?' asked Drona.

'No.'

'Do you see the branch?' asked Drona.

'No.'

'Do you see the bird?' asked Drona.

'No.'

'Then what do you see, Arjuna?'

'I see only the round black eye of the bird.'

Dronacharya was very pleased with Arjuna's deep focused attention and concentration. Satisfied with Arjuna's reply, he said, 'Now, shoot at the eye of the bird!'

With one-pointed concentration aimed on the eye, Arjuna released his arrow, which shot forward at great speed and pierced the centre of the eye of the wooden bird.

Arjuna's concentration was one-pointed. His total attention was focused only on the target – the eye of the wooden bird. His attention was so great that there was only one object in his mind – the eye of the wooden bird. He was able to fix his mind on that one object to the exclusion of everything else around him. He could not even describe the bird, for what he saw was just the eye as a single limited point on which his attention was totally focused. Arjuna was successful in his goal to hit the target because he was not distracted by anything; his mind did not wander from the target.

Likewise, if we are to be successful, both in everyday living and in a spiritual goal, we need to focus all our attention and concentrate on the goal. Paramhansa Yogananda said that most people are suffocated by distractions and are unable to find the pearls of success, and that mental efficiency depends upon the art of concentration.

Usually, in our everyday living, our attention rapidly turns from one thing to another. The mind is never focused and still. It receives a stream of thoughts, feelings and images that are constantly changing, rather like the moving pictures on a video screen.

In the course of experience, the objects continuously appear and disappear, but every one of the objects is illuminated by consciousness. So, consciousness (the common principle that underlies all states of knowing) is always present. The light of consciousness underlies the changing states that appear and disappear. Consciousness remains always ever-present.

THE PRACTICE OF CONCENTRATION

Saṁyama (holding together, integration)

Āsana, yama, niyama, prāṇāyama and *pratyāhāra* constitute the external (*bahiranga*) Yoga. *Dhāraṇā*, *dhyāna* and *samādhi* are considered as the internal (*antaranga*) and true Yoga – everything else is an external accessory to it.

When *dhāraṇā*, *dhyāna* and *samādhi*, the different stages of the same mental process, are practised together on an object, the act of concentration is called *saṁyama* ('the inner discipline of holding together'). Each succeeding stage differs in the degree and depth of concentration which has been attained, and more complete isolation of the object of meditation from distraction. It is not such a simple matter for one to go straight into *samādhi*. The mind has to make a gradual progression from external awareness through focused attention, deep concentration, and deep inner stillness through the preceding stages of *dhāraṇā* and *dhyāna* before attaining *samādhi*. Each of the stages has to be mastered before moving on to the next stage – *dhāraṇā* progresses into *dhyāna*, and *dhyāna* into *samādhi*. When the mind is fixed on its object of concentration for 12 seconds, that equals one measure of *dhāraṇā*. Twelve measures of *dhāraṇā* equal one measure of *dhyāna*. If we look at it mathematically, we can see that when the mind is focused in concentration for 144 seconds (2 minutes and 24 seconds), it is called *dhyāna* (meditation). Twelve measures of *dhyāna* (uninterrupted concentration in meditation), for 28 minutes and 48 seconds, is *samādhi* (total absorption).

Dhāraṇā, *dhyāna* and *samādhi* integrate to become *saṁyama*. The analogy of a diamond shows the relationship between *dhāraṇā*, *dhyāna* and *samādhi*. If we choose a diamond as our object of concentration, what we see first is the clarity of the multi-faceted gem itself. At this stage, we are developing our ability to focus, and our attention on the object is drifting away and wandering. As the attention becomes more focused we become aware of the light glowing from the centre of the diamond. As our awareness of the light continues to grow, awareness of the diamond as an object diminishes, until there is only light, without object or source. When our concentration is continuous without any interruption, then *dhyāna* is occurring. When there is no perception of difference between ourselves and the diamond (object), the light expands everywhere, that is *samādhi*.

To enter deep concentration

1. Relax your body and maintain a comfortable, firm, and steady *āsana* (posture).
2. Relax your mind, calm and steady your breath. Regulate your *prāṇic* life force with *prāṇāyāma*.
3. With detached awareness (*vairāgya*), still your senses by reverting them back inwardly to their source through *pratyāhāra* (withdrawal of the mind from the senses). With your thoughts diminished, collect the rays of your mind and calmly focus them with interest and attention on one point of concentration. This is *dhāraṇā*.

Meditation (*dhyāna*) begins only when all the mental energies of the mind are focused continuously on one idea alone. It is when the mind is concentrated inwardly on the supreme Self within.

In deep one-pointed concentration there is no consciousness of the body, surroundings or time. There is an increase of energy which magnetises the spine and progressively rises to the higher *chakras*, taking one into an expansive state of consciousness, in which one can realise the omnipresence of the Ultimate Reality.

INTERIORISING AND CONCENTRATING THE MIND

Awareness of the breath

To overcome mental restlessness, sit in a comfortable meditative posture and concentrate with focused attention inwardly on your natural breath. Make no attempts to control your breath in any way; simply observe its natural inward and outward flow, as if you were watching the tide flow in and out on a beach. Do not allow your mind to wander; if it does, then gently bring it back to the awareness of watching your breath.

Concentration on the Spiritual Eye

Continue to observe the natural flow of your breath attentively. When it is calm, focus your concentration on the midpoint between the eyebrows (Spiritual Eye). Concentration on this point acts like a magnet, drawing the *prāṇic* energy flow upwards, interiorising the energy in the higher brain centres.

Concentration on a mantra

Sound vibration is the most powerful force in changing the mind; it is very easy for the mind to concentrate on. When the mind is totally absorbed in the transcendental sound of a *mantra*, it rises into a blissful state of superconsciousness. *Mantra* means 'that which protects or liberates the mind'. *Mantra* protects and liberates the mind from restless thoughts and negativity; it transforms the energy of the mind and elevates it to a higher level of consciousness. Each syllable of a *mantra* is empowered with divine spiritual power. When the *mantra* is repeated with concentration and meaning, it vibrates in the mind to produce harmony and balance. It also activates the *chakras*.

Of all *mantras*, *Aum* (*Oṁ*) is the nearest symbol of God for helping the concentration of the mind. Patañjali tells us in his *Yoga Sūtras* that the *mantra Oṁ* is a direct expression of *Īśvara* (Supreme Consciousness). He says that *Īśvara* is a special *puruṣa* that is untouched by sorrow, actions, their results, and desires. By repeating and listening to the eternal divine sound vibration of *Oṁ*, we can more easily connect our consciousness to *Īśvara* or Supreme Consciousness.

Hong Sau technique of concentration

An excellent technique for deepening the concentration, and calming the mind in preparation for deep meditation, is a technique in which you focus on the inhalation and exhalation with the two seed-syllable (*bīja*) *mantra*, ***Hong Sau*** (pronounced 'hong-saw'). This *mantra* works on a pure vibrational level by stilling the mental energy in the form of restless thoughts and purifying the ego. *Hong Sau* is the inner sound of the inhaling and exhaling breath. It also calms and interiorises the *prāṇa* in the body. (For the *Hong Sau* technique see section 7.6.1.)

Trāṭak (steady gazing)

Trāṭak means 'to gaze steadily with concentration at a fixed point without blinking'. *Trāṭak* is a process of concentrating the mind and curbing its restless tendencies. It is the final stage of *pratyāhāra* (withdrawal of the mind from the senses) and the first stage of *dhāraṇā* (concentration), and is said to be a link between the two.

Trāṭak is one of the practices of the *ṣaṭkarma* (the six purification processes) of *Haṭha Yoga*. For the mind to be purified, the thoughts and the senses have to be directed inwards. *Trāṭak* helps to purify the mind by focusing the attention and concentration from the outer world to the inner world; from the gross to the subtle.

There are two types of *trāṭak* – internal and external. In external *trāṭak*, the eyes remain open and they do not blink. In internal *trāṭak,* the eyes are closed and the eyeballs are kept still.

Benefits

The practice of *trāṭak* increases the supply of blood to the eyes, stimulates the nerve centres, and strengthens and cleanses the eyes, improving vision. *Trāṭak* steadies the wandering mind; it improves mental concentration, willpower and internal subtle energy. It is therapeutic in depression, insomnia, anxiety, poor concentration, and in encouraging strong, positive willpower and one-pointedness. It corrects minor eye ailments such as eyestrain, myopia and astigmatism.

Caution

This practice is not suitable for persons with psychic problems. Those who have a tendency towards schizophrenia or hallucinations should not practise *trāṭak*. Be careful not to strain or tense the eye muscles. If the eyes become tired and start watering, stop the practice, close the eyes and sit still to rest them for five minutes. You can also wash the eyes by splashing them gently with cold water. In the beginning one should only practise this exercise for one minute. Then gradually over a period of time of regular practice one can increase the duration every week, until you are practising for up to ten minutes.

Practice time

Trāṭak can be practised at any time on a daily basis. Practise on an empty stomach. The most auspicious time is between 4 am and 6 am after *āsana* and *prāṇāyāma* practice. Or it can be practised late at night before meditation and retiring to bed. The benefits of *trāṭak* result only after persistent, steady practice on a regular basis for a long period of time.

Method

Practise in a darkened room. Sit in a comfortable meditation posture, with your head, neck and spine aligned upright, but relaxed. Sit three feet away or an arm's length from a lighted candle in front of you, with the flame at the same height as your chest. If the candle is placed too high, it can create tension at the eyebrow centre, or produce a burning sensation in the eyes. The flame should be still, so make sure the flame is not flickering from a draught.

Throughout the practice, keep your body still and your mind calm and quiet. Fix both your gaze and mental focus at the midpoint of the flame, where it is brighter, for as long as possible without blinking and without strain until your eyes begin to water or become tired. In the beginning, practise for about one minute and gradually increase to a few minutes over a period of time. Then close your eyes and visualise the flame internally at the midpoint between the eyebrows for one minute. If the after-image of the flame moves, gently bring it back to the centre and continue gazing until the image disappears. Repeat the practice three times.

As you concentrate on the candle flame, do not allow your mind to wander. Observe your thoughts and feelings as they arise in your mind but do not become involved with them, just remain a silent witness to them.

When you have finished your practice, rub the palms of your hands together until they feel warm. Place the warm palms over your eyes to relax and soothe them.

Trāṭak: steady concentration on a picture of your guru

To practise *trāṭak* (steady gazing) on a spiritual picture or image of your guru, a saint, Jesus Christ, Krishna, Rama or Śiva, sit in a comfortable and relaxed meditation posture, and place the picture of your choice in front of you at eye level at a distance of one arm's length. With your eyes open, gaze steadily at the image (particularly the eyes and the eyebrow centre – the Spiritual Eye) with your total attention and interest. Then close your eyes after a minute or two and visualise the face and eyes of the Master, guru or saint you have been gazing at. Attune yourself to the consciousness of the Master, guru or saint by visualising them at the midpoint between your eyebrows at the Spiritual Eye. Attune yourself, not to the form or personality, but to the consciousness behind the form in the picture. Feel their spiritual presence, and the expansion of love, joy, light and energy within the lotus of your heart. As you commune deeply, magnetically draw towards you the guru's consciousness, and feel that you are becoming one with that consciousness. Feel that the presence of the guru or saint is guiding your thoughts and spiritually inspiring you.

Remember that no matter how much love you direct towards the personalised image (saint, guru, deity, etc.), the object of devotional concentration should always be regarded as just one expression of God, otherwise we cease to feel the unity behind the multiplicity of manifestations – the unmanifested godhead, that which is not limited to time or space or causation, that which is omnipresent, omnipotent and omniscient. We need to go beyond personality worship, whether it be a guru or a saint, or worship of any form, and attune ourself to the Divine Consciousness that gives and expresses the eternal qualities of love, peace, calmness, light, joy and wisdom through the form of personality. Through attunement to these divine qualities we can expand our consciousness.

6.8

DHYĀNA (MEDITATION)

6.8.1 THE NATURE OF THE MIND AND ITS FUNCTIONS

Before we study *dhyāna* (meditation), the seventh limb of Patañjali's Eight Limbs of Yoga, let us look at the mind from the psychology and science of Yoga.

SĀṂKHYA PHILOSOPHY AND THE ORIGIN OF THE MIND

The underlying dualistic philosophy of *Sāṃkhya* ('enumeration') by the great sage Kapila is the key to understanding the Yoga concept of mind. *Sāṃkhya* is one of the most prominent and oldest of the six Indian philosophies. The *Sāṃkhya* philosophy proposes that *prakṛiti* (nature; matter) is the material cause and the primordial substance behind the world. It is the first and ultimate cause of all gross and subtle objects including the mind.

Both *Sāṃkhya* and Yoga deal with the hierarchy of the basic *tattva* categories of Reality. The *Sāṃkhya* philosophy represents the theory, and Yoga represents the application or the practical aspects. *Sāṃkhya*, which means 'enumeration' or 'number', specifies the number and nature of the ultimate constituents of the universe, imparting knowledge of Reality.

Sāṃkhya is dualistic realism because it advocates two ultimate, eternal principles that cause creation. The two primordial principles are: *puruṣa* (consciousness, Self, Spirit), which is eternal, unmanifest and conscious; and *prakṛiti* (matter), which is eternal, manifest and unconscious. These principles cannot be known directly but their existence is inferred because everything that exists has these qualities.

Sāṃkhya deals primarily with the involuntary process which binds the individual soul into matter. Yoga philosophy deals with the evolutionary or reverse process by which a soul can attain release and liberation from the bondage of matter.

In *Sāṃkhya* philosophy the universe does not come into existence through divine volition, because pure classical *Sāṃkhya* is non-theistic and sees no need for a creator. In contrast to this, Patañjali in his *Yoga Sūtras* introduces the concept of *Īśvara* (Divine Being, ruler of creation, who is eternal, unborn, undying and unbound), a special kind of soul which is indicated by the sacred syllable *Oṁ*. The *Vedānta* philosophy presents a non-dualistic approach in which the two primordial principles *puruṣa* and *prakṛiti* are integrated into a higher conception of one ultimate reality known as *Brāhman*, which is identical to *ātman* (individual soul or self). Also, according to *Vedānta*, *prakṛiti* is unreal and non-existent. But *Sāṃkhya*, Yoga and *Vedānta* are in agreement that *puruṣa* or *ātman* becomes embodied in the subtle and gross elements of *prakṛiti* due to *avidyā* (ignorance), and is subject to *samsāra* (cycles of birth and death).

The universe evolves when *puruṣa* (the conscious Spirit principle) interacts with *prakṛiti* (nature), and through the activation of *prakṛiti*'s inherent three *guṇas* (energetic qualities of matter): *sattva*, *rajas* and *tamas*. It evolves into 23 additional categories of mind and matter (*tattvas*). The cause changes into the effect, which already exists in potentiality. This process of creation is essentially the movement from the absolute oneness of consciousness to the differentiation and diversity of all things mental and material, from the subtle to the gross.

The 23 *tattva* categories that enumerate and evolve from *prakṛiti* (nature; primordial principle of matter) are: *mahāt* (Cosmic Mind) or *buddhi* (intellect), *ahaṁkāra* (ego), *manas* (mind), five *jñānendriyas* (cognitive faculties), five *karmendriyas* (action faculties), five *tanmātras* (subtle elements), and five *mahābhūtas* (gross elements: earth, water, fire, air, ether) from which the gross elements arise that form the universe.

Buddhi (intellect) is the first manifestation of *prakṛiti*. It is an evolute of matter, and so it is unable to function by itself. It is aware only through *puruṣa*, from which it reflects consciousness.

Prakṛiti is dynamic in nature, which is attributed to its constituent *guṇas*: *sattva* (purity), *rajas* (activity) and *tamas* (inertia). The *guṇas* are the very essence of *prakṛiti*. The *guṇa* constituents are not only of *prakṛiti*, but are also intrinsic to all material objects, as they are produced by *prakṛiti*.

The evolutionary process is initiated by the activity of *rajas guṇa*, which activates *sattva guṇa*, and then these two *guṇas* overpower the inertia of the *tamas guṇa*. The universe remains in a potential state within *prakṛiti* for as long as the three *guṇas* remain motionless and undisturbed. In the unmanifested state of *prakṛiti*, the *guṇas* remain in perfect equilibrium (*saṁyavastha*). As soon as they are disturbed and set into motion, *prakṛiti* begins to unfold into the 23 *tattva* evolutes, resulting in the creation of the phenomenal universe.

Puruṣa (the conscious Spirit principle) is also known as *ātman* or *jīvātman* (individual soul or self). *Puruṣa* is the conscious principle within every living being. The philosophy of *Sāṃkhya* is not only dualistic but also pluralistic, for although it defines *puruṣa* as the true Self, it maintains that there are as many *puruṣas* as there are individual beings, that remain ever separate and distinct from one another.

WHAT IS THE MIND?

Electricity is generated from a great power point that flows into innumerable light bulbs to illuminate them. Similarly, *mahāt* or the Cosmic Mind is the source of consciousness and illumination that flows into all individual minds. The individual mind is a form of the Cosmic Mind or Universal Consciousness, that is an aspect of the Self. The mind is the subtle form of the body, and the body is a projection of the mind. When the mind turns outwards it takes on the form of the objects of the world, but when it turns within, it becomes pure Consciousness.

The word 'mind' is a general term in Western psychology, but in the psychology of Yoga, a more detailed analysis has been made. Usually, the Sanskrit word *manas* is translated as 'mind', but the meaning of these two words are not the same. In Yoga psychology *manas* is understood to be material and objective. *Manas* is made of subtle matter, and so at the time of death, it also departs from the body.

When we use the word 'mind', we need to be clear about what we mean, because there are two ways of using this word. Mind can either mean *citta*, that conscious awareness which is the background of knowledge; or it can mean *manas*, the activity of thought and images (projections of consciousness) that takes place against the background consciousness (rather than an actual entity that exists in and of itself).

In Western psychology the mind is either identified with the subject, or is associated with the physical body. It is used to signify a general operation of the psyche inside, including understanding willing and feeling. In Western psychology, the mind is often confused with the real Self, but in Yoga psychology, the mind is not the subject. The real Self, the Knower, is distinct from the mind, body and senses. The mind is not the Knower, but an object of knowledge. This can be proved by observing your own mind. You, the knowing Self, are distinct from all the organs of perception, and you, the Self, are also distinct from the mind, because you can observe your own mind directly through introspection. So the mind is an object of knowledge. You, the inner Self, are a principle that transcends all that is objective to you. So you cannot be the thinker, for the thinker is the object of consciousness and not the Self, otherwise you could not remember having thought. Whenever the principle of consciousness becomes identified with the body, the false notion of you being the thinker arises.

In Yoga psychology there is a metaphysical factor that Western psychologists do not know, something that is very subtle about the mind. The mind is present only when thought is present. When thought activity is not present, there is no mind, for thought activity is itself the mind. Your thought process and your mind are identical and inseparable; they coexist with each other. In Yoga terms your mind is a mass of *vṛttis* and *vāsanās*.

THREE TENDENCIES OF THE MIND

1. **Externalisation.** The mind's natural tendency is outgoing. In *pratyāhāra* (withdrawal of the senses from their respective objects), the yogi tries to control and overcome the outgoing nature of the mind by withdrawing or disconnecting it from the senses and interiorising it.

2. **Objectification.** The mind has an innate objectifying tendency. The mind has to be either active or asleep, therefore to overcome the mind's tendency to objectify you need to give your mind an internal object to focus upon. A focal point that you can keep your mind completely steady and concentrated on, to the exclusion of all other thoughts.

3. **Diversification.** The mind has the nature of always moving and being agitated and restless. The mind is not content to focus on any single point, or repose in the one – it is always scattered in the many. The mind is always continuously changing; it is restless and scattered.

   To overcome this, allow your mind to change, let it move, but discipline your mind by confining its restless wandering to one object and its related associations, so that your thoughts are only connected and related to one central object of concentration. For example, if I think of my guru, Paramhansa Yogananda, I can concentrate on his eyes and his face, and knowing the various stories of his life from his *Autobiography of a Yogi*, I can keep him in my consciousness by bringing to mind episodes of his life. For instance, I may bring to mind the image of Yogananda when he first met his guru, Swāmi Sri Yukteswar, or other meetings he had with great yogis and saints. In this way my mind is allowed to move among the many, but simultaneously it is spiritually focused on the one.

Then you may gradually focus your concentration to such an extent that you are only meditating on your guru's name, inwardly chanting it as a *mantra*, such as *Jai Guru* or *Oṁ Guru* repeatedly until your mind becomes unified with that one subject.

Or perhaps you may want to concentrate on God in Its formless aspect by meditating on the qualities and attributes of Divine Consciousness: love, wisdom, peace, calmness, divine power, infinity, eternity, limitlessness and omnipresence.

MEDITATION IS NOT MAKING THE MIND BLANK

Meditation is not making the mind blank or empty. How can we know this to be true? Because it is only through the thought process that we recognise the existence of the mind. If there is no thought process we would not even know that there is a mind. The mind cannot exist without thought, and thought cannot exist without the mind.

But the Yoga meditator must be careful not to have the misconception that concentration or meditation is trying to make the mind blank and empty. Passive, inattentive sitting is not meditation. On the contrary, Yoga states that making the mind blank or empty is an undesirable state, because if you try to do that you will become drowsy, you will lose your concentration and fall asleep. Your mind must either think or sleep. Meditation is alert, focused concentration on one's chosen object or ideal. Therefore to avoid drowsiness and sleep, which are *tamasic* states, you need to hold your mind on a focal point and keep it there continuously. For example, keeping your attention on the midpoint between your eyebrows while concentrating on the *mantra Hong* as your breath naturally flows in and *Sau* as your breath naturally flows out. This is *dhāraṇā* (concentration).

THE SEAT OF THE MIND

The mind is the seat of internal perception, that has many different functions. The principal functions are cognition, volition and emotion. The understanding, mind and intellect are all in the subtle body; they operate through corresponding centres in the physical brain. But the brain is not the mind, it is like a screen on which consciousness is reflected. The outer mind has its seat in the brain, through which it gains its experiences through the senses.

The inner subtle mind pervades throughout the body, but it has three main places in which it resides during the states of waking, deep sleep and dream. In the waking state the mind resides at the eyebrow centre in the *ājñā chakra*. During deep sleep the mind resides in a subtle state in the heart, *anāhata chakra*. In dream it resides in the throat, *viśuddha chakra*. In dreamless sleep there are no thoughts; the distracting world of duality temporarily disappears. As soon as you awake from deep and dreamless sleep, you, the real Self, continue to exist. You feel you existed even during deep sleep, because consciousness is continuous.

It is in the dreamless sleep state that we get a taste of the nature of absolute bliss. It is only the mind that creates differences, sorrow, duality and separateness. The inner mind or feeling nature is located in the heart.

THE FOUR FACULTIES OF THE MIND

It is impossible for us to be aware of something outside, unless there is an isolated thinking or individualising principle. In *Vedānta* psychology this principle is known as the *antaḥkaraṇa* (*antah* means 'internal'; *karana* means 'instrument'). *Antaḥkaraṇa* is the inner instrument or internal organ of perception, because it is through this instrument that you sense, perceive and reason. In Yoga psychology it is called *citta*. The interaction of *citta* with *manas*, *buddhi* and *ahaṁkāra* collectively form the *antaḥkaraṇa*.

This individualising principle is necessary in order to relate to the world or to anything that is outside.

Antaḥkaraṇa has four aspects to it:

Manas: that part of the mind that receives impressions through the senses from the external world; deliberation. *Manas* is centred in the head.

Buddhi: discriminating faculty; determination; contains intuitive wisdom. *Buddhi* is centred in the frontal brain between the eyebrows.

Ahaṁkāra: ego, the sense of 'I'. *Ahaṁkāra* is centred in the medulla oblongata of the lower brain.

Citta: subconscious mind; recollection; includes *manas*, *buddhi* and *ahaṁkāra*. *Citta* is centred in the heart.

All these four faculties of the *antaḥkaraṇa* are made from subtle unconscious matter. By themselves they are all devoid of consciousness; they are insentient. It is the reflected light of the Self (Pure Consciousness) on the mind and senses that enlivens them to function. It is like the light of the Sun which reveals itself to us directly and also reveals any object that its rays of light fall on. The mind receives the light of consciousness, and because of that appears to have the power of feeling. But it is not the mind that feels, it is the Self feeling through the mind. It is the light of consciousness that enables the mind to feel. Without cognition, or consciousness, there cannot be any feeling or willing. Both feeling and willing presuppose consciousness.

The sense organs cannot perceive their respective objects unless the mind is joined with them. Again, it is the Self that is permeated with the light of consciousness that perceives the object through the mind and the sense organs. It is because of this borrowed light of consciousness that the mind proves to be the main instrument of cognition.

A way of understanding the *antaḥkaraṇa*'s functions is to imagine an object at some distance under a large tree. You are unable to see the object clearly because it is in the dark shade of the tree. Your *antaḥkaraṇa* cognises the object but is unable to determine what the object really is. 'What is that? Is it a person sitting under the tree, a bear, or a rock?' When the *antaḥkaraṇa* has this vacillating cognition or function of deliberation it is referred to as *manas* (the thinking mind). Then you search within and recall some past impression that is related or similar to it. With this recollection you cognise the object as a bear. This faculty of reasoning (determinative faculty) to determine the true object is *buddhi*, which is usually inadequately translated as 'intellect'. The function of recollection and memory is *citta*. This leads to the cognition of the object, and you determine 'that is a bear (sitting under the tree)'. With the ascertainment 'that is a bear' arises the knowledge 'I know the bear'. When there is a factor of separation, for example when you are aware of being an individual different from everyone and everything else, that is called *ahaṁkāra* or ego.

In order to know something new you have to relate it to something already known. These four functions *manas, buddhi, citta* and *ahaṁkāra* represent four different states of mind (*antaḥkaraṇa*).

Manas

Manas is the thinking mind – it has thought, will and doubt. It is that part of the mind that receives impressions through the senses from the external world. The mind has only information and imagination about anything; it deals in mental activities – opinions, presumptions and conclusions – that misidentify as reality. It cannot actually know, because to know is to *be* that which is known. For example, to know about Yoga doesn't make one a yogi, or to know about India does not make one an Indian.

The mind is the 'I' of the self, which perpetuates the illusion of a separate personal identity.

Buddhi

Buddhi is the highest aspect of the *antaḥkaraṇa*. It is the discriminating factor that makes right determination or decision without doubt, and so represents complete knowledge or understanding. *Buddhi* discriminates between right and wrong, the real and the unreal, the eternal and the non-eternal, and between the Self and the non-self. *Buddhi* serves as the most effective instrument in raising one's consciousness. The light of the Self reflects in *buddhi*, transmitting the power to cognise objects and experience sensations.

Ahaṁkāra

Ahaṁkāra is egoism, the 'I'-sense, whose nature is to self-assert – 'I am the form' and 'I am the doer'. *Aham* literally means 'I', as undivided Consciousness, and *akara* means a shape or form. In this sense, *ahaṁkāra* means the formless unlimited Consciousness that appears as a form with limitations.

It is difficult for us to give up this sense of 'I' because the mind is dependent, it always attaches itself to something objective. For example, the moment we have the sense of 'I' we also have the sense of I am this, I am that, I am the other thing. I cannot think of myself as the pure 'I' in this present state. The mind reflects on some condition and it says 'I am happy' or 'I am sad'. The ego continually moves between identification with the body ('I am a man' or 'I am a woman') and identification with thoughts ('I am beautiful', 'I am intelligent').

The 'I' identifies itself with the function either of *manas* or *buddhi*; it does not seem to have any function of its own.

The ego self causes the real Self to appear as identical with the mind, body and senses. The personal pronoun 'I' always denotes the true Self, in which the totality of objective experience seems to occur. 'I think' really means '*I am conscious of* thoughts'; and 'I am happy' means '*I am conscious of a feeling of* happiness'.

The ego structure is dualistic; it divides the unity of Reality into opposites and contrasting pairs. *Ahaṁkāra* as the body-mind structure is the limitation that creates the illusion of a separate consciousness. It is our mistaken personal identification to the body, thoughts and feelings that keep us in ignorance of our real nature. The body, thoughts and feelings that produce a feeling of a personal self are continually changing, but we who claim them as our own are changeless. This ignorance causes us to personify the ego as our real Self. The ego sees and believes itself to be a personal, separate entity and the inferred source of its own existence. The ego fears dissolution and therefore resists giving up the illusion of a separate existence. When ego (*ahaṁkāra*) dissolves, both oneself and the world are experienced as appearing in the One Consciousness.

Citta

Citta is a comprehensive term, and like the word *manas* it may represent the whole of the mind. In *Rāja Yoga, citta* is usually termed 'mind field' or 'field of consciousness'. It is within this field of consciousness that all present actions, past memories and future visions take place. In *Vedānta* philosophy the subconscious mind is termed as *citta*.

The functions of *citta* are memory, attention, concentration and enquiry. Sensations from the sense organs communicate themselves first to that part of the mind called *citta*. So the first effort of the mind begins with the idea of gaining happiness and fulfilment outwardly through the senses. Part of its function is the search for happiness and fulfilment.

Citta is the conscious awareness with which we identify our being; it is the mind of the soul. *Citta* dwells in the spiritual heart, which is located on the right side of the physical heart. It is in this spiritual heart that deep feeling and knowing are working. The nature of *citta* is the capacity to feel; feeling through thought, emotion and sensation.

A thought is converted into a feeling because of some 'interference' somewhere. 'I like him', 'I don't like him', 'she looks beautiful', 'she looks ugly'. This judgement comes after thought formation. But where does all this take place? The material of which the sensations in their essential nature are made is *citta*. What is being said here is nothing but a string of words and more words. Yet *citta* still remains *citta*, and it will not be grasped by your mind, however intelligent you may be, until this thing that we call *citta* jumps in front of you and says 'I am *citta*.' The *citta* must be as true, as real to you, as your own body or as the chair you sit on, which you can see and touch. It must be as real as an ant crawling on your leg, felt externally, or the headache or anger experienced internally. Seeing the chair is a perception of a material object. Being aware of a crawling ant on your leg is a sensation, and the feeling of anger is an emotion. In one or all of these contexts the *citta* must become visible to you. You must experience it. It must be an existential, immediate reality for you. Not, 'I think once I experienced the self, or had direct vision of the *citta*.' If you had a headache six years ago, you cannot reproduce that same feeling now. No mother can relive the labour pains she had at the time of childbirth.

All the things we call meditation, *citta*, *vṛtti*, control, and so on, are irrelevant now, in terms of the *now*. These things do not mean anything to you here and now unless they actually exist in you at present. Just as you cannot experience a headache that is not actually there in you, you cannot meditate unless there *is* meditation, you cannot know what *citta* is unless *citta* reveals itself to you. You can do nothing about it. Until it happens, until life becomes intolerable to you, until all your desires, all your cravings begin to hurt you and the mind naturally turns upon itself, the understanding will not be there.

One cannot be false unto oneself. Only when it hurts will the mind detach from the cravings, the lust, the greed and the hatred. You do not have to detach from them at all. When you have developed sensitivity within yourself, then without any outside persuasion, the mind is ready to let them drop. Then the *citta* is seen, is experienced.

Meditation is coming face to face with *citta*, in that state of Yoga in which there is an inner understanding of the *vṛttis* and the *citta*. When this meditation, Yoga, takes place, then the *citta* has turned upon itself. The *citta* has become itself, and it remains in its own purity without any distortion whatsoever.

VṚITTIS

The nature of *vṛtti* is movement; thoughts and feelings are in constant motion, they are transitory and also ephemeral, and as a result of this they cause disturbance to the mind. The activity of mind or *manas* is like the ripples or waves on the surface of the lake of consciousness. Just as waves and bubbles arise on the surface of the lake, so also *vṛttis* arise on the surface of the mind-lake. In Sanskrit these ripples or waves are called *vṛtti*, from the verb root *vṛt* which means 'vortice; whirlpool, to revolve, movement'. Like waves ruffling the calm surface of a lake, the waves of feeling and thoughts disturb the calmness and peace of the mind or field of consciousness (*citta*). Just as the movement of wind creates waves on the surface of a lake, similarly objects (*pratyaya*) create *vṛttis* in the mind. When the wind becomes calm, the waves merge back into the water. Similarly, when the objects are removed from the mind, the waves of feeling and thoughts merge back into the *citta* (mind-field of consciousness).

We can also use the analogy of a clear, still lake into which a stone has been thrown, causing ripples to disturb the calm surface. The stone represents *avidyā* (ignorance). The clear, still lake is the consciousness of *citta*. The ripples created by the stone are the *vṛttis*: the vortices of feelings and thoughts that oscillate in the consciousness of *citta*.

Patañjali calls this state '*citta-vṛtti nirodhaḥ*', a state in which there is no movement in Consciousness. Consciousness becomes still and crystal clear, and in that state, the Seer (*draṣṭṛi*) becomes aware of Itself. The Seer or the Self becomes established in its own true nature.

> *'Yogas citta-vṛtti nirodhah.'*
> 'Yoga (the realisation of the Self) is the neutralisation of the vortices of feeling.'
>
> *Yoga Sūtras 1:2*

The meaning of Patañjali's teaching here is that to realise the universal Self or pure Consciousness, one must first calm the vortices of feeling that create the restless waves on the surface of the mind. Then one comes to the realisation that one's own mind is the universal Mind, and that one's self is the universal Self.

The five akliṣhṭa vṛttis

According to Patañjali's *Yoga Sūtras* (1:5) there are five categories of *vṛttis* or mental functions within us. Some cause pain (*kliṣhṭa*), and some do not cause pain (*akliṣhṭa*).

Pramāṇa, *viparyaya*, *vikalpa*, *nidrā* and *smṛiti* are the invisible causative factors behind our difficulties in life and are referred to as *akliṣhṭa vṛttis* or the non-pain-causing functions of the mind. They are non-painful because we do not feel the pain that they cause.

1. **Right knowledge; valid proof (*pramāṇa*).** This is accurate perception that has been verified by direct sense evidence, accurate inference, or by reliable testimony.
2. **Wrong understanding; mistaken conception (*viparyaya*).** *Viparayaya* is a false perception of any object, for example a mirage of water seen in a desert, or a rope mistaken as being a snake.

   Viparayaya includes all thoughts that are based on the sense of having a separate existence; the root cause being ignorance (*avidyā*).
3. **Imagination (*vikalpa*).** In imagination there is no direct cognition of an object. *Vikalpa* is fantasy or hallucination that is unrelated to any proven or assumed theories. There is no reality behind imagination.
4. **Sleep (*nidrā*).** In sleep the mind is not completely absent. If sleep were completely devoid of experience, one could not have recollection of it. The subject-object relationship remains during dream sleep. It is only in dreamless sleep that there is a state of non-duality, which is characterised by the absence of objective experience and the continued presence of the real Self (the principle of consciousness; self-existent Reality; the experiencer of the the three states of consciousness: waking, sleeping and dreaming). Sleep is a *vṛtti*, an obstacle to *samādhi*, therefore in order to attain superconsciousness (*samādhi*) this *vṛtti* needs to be controlled.

5. **Memory (*smṛiti*).** This is recollection of a past experience that forms an image. All memories are recollections of latent impressions (*saṁskāras*) caused by the five *vṛttis*. There are two kinds of *smṛiti*: memory of unreal objects and occurrences experienced in the dream state; and recollection of real objects and occurrences in the awake state.

These five *vṛttis* are universal, and they cover our entire life. All *vṛttis,* whether they are painful (*klishṭa*) or non-painful (*aklishṭa*), are the product of these five main *vṛttis*, which can be either positive or negative, and lead to either bondage or liberation – wherever there is ocean there are waves, wherever there is *citta* there is *vṛtti*. It seems to be clear, but when you view the ocean as one indivisible entity, there are no waves apart from it. The whole thing, with all the waves, *is* the ocean.

Air moves only in relation to something else, to something static. It is only when I do not move that I am aware of the movement of an object. There is no motion independent of another object or entity. Fire does not know heat. Fire does not burn itself. We talk of fire burning, but it is really we who burn when we go near the flames. Water does not wet itself. It is I and my dry clothes that get wet if I fall into the water. Wetting only occurs in relation to something not wet, and change, motion, ocean waves, ripples, currents are noted only in relation to it. Only when I am standing aside, apart from that motion and looking at it, am I aware of the motion, change or colossal goings on.

To the ocean itself there is no motion, no change, no waves, ripples or currents. Similarly, in the physical body there are millions of cells sparking off, all sorts of rivers flowing from the heart to the various parts of the body and back again, there is tremendous activity, yet because the organism *is* the activity, and there is no division, it is unaware of it. The wave is not different from the ocean. The ocean is the entire volume of water, including what we call the current, the wave, the *vṛtti*. The diversity arises because you and I have created it. There is nothing called the Pacific Ocean as distinct from the Atlantic Ocean. It is one indivisible mass of water. To the ocean it is all ocean – it does not know anything about individual waves, ripples, currents or parts. But somehow on account of that mysterious power called *Mayā* (Illusion), *avidyā* (ignorance), the ocean limits itself, and that self-limited ocean is referred to as 'wave'.

Without *vṛttis* the mind would have no existence. The function of a *vṛtti* in the mind is to cause the removal of ignorance (*avidyā*), which covers all objects. When this veil of ignorance is removed, then perception of objects becomes possible. So *vṛttis* are not necessarily bad – they can help us in our individual evolution until we attain spiritual perfection.

The five kleśas – the sources of afflictions that cause suffering

Kleśa, from the Sanskrit root *kliś*, means 'to torment', 'afflict', 'cause suffering'. *Kleśas* are also obstacles because they obstruct the mind from realising the nature of the true indwelling Self. *Kleśa* is also a synonym for *duḥka* (pain).

The modifications of consciousness, termed as *citta-vṛttis*, are innumerable and are of infinite variety. The sage Patañjali in his *Yoga Sūtras* classifies all *vṛttis* into two standards. According to one, the *vṛttis* or movements of the mind are divided into five categories; according to the other, they are classified into two groups: *klişhṭa vṛttis* (that which gives suffering) and *aklişhṭa vṛttis* (that which does not give suffering). *Klişhṭa* means 'detrimental', and is from the same Sanskrit root as *kleśa*. *Klişhṭa* is suffering, sorrow, or pain. *Klişhṭa vṛttis* are the root cause of all suffering, and are obstacles to the attainment of Yoga.

The experiences that lead us into bondage are the *klişhṭa* or painful *vṛttis*; the experiences that lead us into higher spiritual states, that free us from the limitations of the body, mind and senses, are the *aklişhṭa* or pleasurable *vṛttis*. But we have to be careful – even if a *vṛtti* is pleasurable at first but afterwards causes pain, then both the pleasurable and the painful *vṛtti* should be classified as *klişhṭa* (painful). On the other hand, if the *vṛttis* of the mind create pleasure immediately and also afterwards, or if they create pain in the beginning and lasting happiness afterwards, then both *vṛttis* of the mind are classified as *aklişhṭa*.

In the *Bhāgavad Gītā* it is said:

> 'That happiness whose cultivation leads to the end of all suffering, which in the beginning is like poison but in the end is like nectar, is said to be *sattvic* (pure).'
>
> *Bhāgavad Gītā 18:37–38 (Author's translation)*

This *sattvic* happiness results from spiritual practice, which in the beginning may seem painful, but afterwards one is full of joy!

> 'That happiness which at first through contact between the senses and their objects is like nectar but in the end is like poison is said to be *rajasic*.'
>
> *Bhāgavad Gītā 18:37–38 (Author's translation)*

And here the immediate pleasure or happiness one experiences through the senses is in the beginning pleasurable but very soon becomes painful, bringing unhappiness.

Vṛttis or movements of the mind are caused by the five *kleśas* (afflictions; impediments). These are the obstacles that stop us from realising our true nature.

> 'There are five kinds of *vṛttis*; some are painful and some are not painful.'
>
> *Yoga Sūtras 1:5*

> 'Ignorance, egoism, attachment, aversion, and clinging to life are the five obstacles.'
>
> *Yoga Sūtras 2:3*

The five afflictions or obstacles are:

1. ***Avidyā*** (ignorance)
2. ***Asmitā*** ('I-sense')
3. ***Rāga*** (attachment)
4. ***Dveṣa*** (aversion)
5. ***Abhiniveśha*** (clinging to life; fear of death).

Avidyā

> 'Ignorance is regarding permanence in the impermanent, purity in the impure, pleasure in suffering, and the Self in the non-self.'
>
> *Yoga Sūtras 2:5*

Vidyā in Sanskrit means Self-knowledge, or *adhyātma*, realising and knowing your true nature. *Avidyā* means ignorance, but not in the ordinary sense of the word of lacking general knowledge of the world. Rather, *avidyā* means ignorance about one's own true nature. Ignorance here refers to wrong identification with one's body, mind and senses. It is the identification with the sensation of the ego-self, of the 'Me' – 'I am the body', 'I am American', 'I am Catholic', 'I am a *swāmi*', 'I am hurt', 'This is mine!'

From a lack of understanding of the true nature of things – the nature of Reality – ignorance (*avidyā*) arises first. *Avidyā* is the root cause of the other four *kleśas* (afflictions; roots of sorrow and suffering). Suffering is inflicted by thought, which gives it continuity. When we say, 'I was insulted, my feelings were hurt', then there is suffering. It is the identification with it that gives the continuity. True understanding liberates; ignorance causes bondage.

Asmitā

> 'Egoism is identifying the power of the Seer (*puruṣa*) with the instrument of seeing (*buddhi*).'
>
> *Yoga Sūtras 2:6*

Asmi means 'I am'. *Asmitā* is the sense of individuality, the principle of egoism, 'I-sense', 'I-am-ness'. *Asmitā*, the effect of *buddhi*, evolves out of ignorance (*avidyā* – the root cause of all other *kleśas*).

Buddhi, the intelligence-awareness aspect of *citta,* is the primary instrument of *puruṣa* (the Self). Without *buddhi*, *puruṣa* would have no awareness of the *prakṛiti* (matter; nature) mind and body. *Asmitā* or the ego falsely identifies *buddhi*, the instrumental power of sight, with the *puruṣa*, the divine inner Self. In other words the ego mis-identifies the changing non-self with the changeless and eternal true Self (*puruṣa*) as a result of illusion.

When the 'I-sense' becomes falsely identified as having a separate existence and self-importance, it is known as the ego (*ahaṁkāra*). Due to ignorance (*avidyā*) and our conditioned consciousness we think of ourselves as 'having' a soul, whereas in fact we are the divine Self expressing through a body-mind. The *citta-vṛtti* that we perceive is the activity of your divine inner Self.

Egoism causes false identification with our body, mind, energy and senses, which are all subject to change and are non-eternal. This false identification causes us to say: 'I am happy', 'I am sad', 'I am angry'. This is mis-identification. We are falsely identifying with our mental states, not the true Self. It is only the mind that is happy, sad or angry. The indwelling Divine Self is beyond the emotional sates of duality, it is changeless and eternal. Its nature is joy or bliss.

Rāga-dveṣa

> '(Due to the identification with pleasurable experiences) attachment (*rāga*) arises with pleasure.'
>
> *Yoga Sūtras 2:7*

> '(Due to the identification with painful experiences) aversion (*dveṣa*) arises with suffering.'
>
> *Yoga Sūtras 2:8*

In its separation the ego experiences 'likes' and 'dislikes' – objects or persons appear either as attractive (*rāga*) or repulsive (*dveṣa*) to the ego-self. There is approval and disapproval. *Rāga*, which also means attachment, arises every time the mind recollects any type of pleasure or happiness connected with an object or person. Memory precedes attachment. It is the past impressions called *samskāras* that remain latent in the mind, causing it and the senses to be subconsciously pulled towards objects and persons that have given pleasurable experiences in the past. In the *Bhāgavad Gītā* it is said:

> 'When one contemplates the sense objects, attachment develops for them. From attachment arises desire, and from unfulfilled (frustrated) desire arises anger. Anger produces delusion. Delusion causes forgetfulness (of one's true nature – the Self). Confusion of memory causes loss of discrimination. From loss of discrimination, one's own self is lost. However, those who can supervise the involvement between senses and sense objects exercising discriminating self-control, and are free from desire, attachment and aversion, attain tranquillity of mind.'
>
> *Bhāgavad Gītā 2:62–64 (Author's translation)*

Dveṣa, or aversion and dislike felt for an object or person, arises from the memory of pain or unhappiness connected with an object or person. Attachment and aversion keep us continually bound to the limited level of mundane consciousness. They strengthen the ego, creating an unending flow of desires and habits that condition our behaviour, which in turn conceals the bliss of our true nature.

Everybody has a sense of individuality, which is daily affirmed, strengthened and protected, causing it to be more separated from its true divine nature within. The individual self (*jīvātma*) is always seeking pleasure, avoiding pain and sorrow, and clings to life, avoiding death. We do not have to give up or deny experiences, for they are opportunities for self-discovery. The senses were given to us for that purpose. Experience the sensation with awareness in the moment but never become attached, because attachment is the beginning of the cycle of sorrow and suffering. Similarly, aversion will also cause suffering. Attachment and aversion are opposites in the world of duality; they are constantly changing, there is no permanence.

Abhiniveśha

> 'The fear of separation by death from the body is inherent in both the ignorant and the wise.'
>
> *Yoga Sūtras 2:9*

The fifth *kleśa*, clinging to life and fear of death (*abhiniveśha*), is the tenacious clinging to life, not wanting to let go of the ego, that is resistant to change. Clinging to life is the habit of dependence on objective sources of enjoyment and happiness, and fear of losing them. This clinging to life is inherent in us all, including the wise, not only the ignorant, because latent within us are the stronger *saṁskāra* seed-impressions of death. It can only be completely eradicated by transcending the identification with being an individual.

The greatest fear is death, fearing that we will cease to exist and lose our identity. Due to ignorance (*avidyā*) the ego-self, the 'I', identifies with the mind-body and believes that the 'I' dies when the body dies. But the 'I', the true Divine Self which is of the nature of spirit, is eternal, it cannot die. Anything that is not self-luminous, nor self-aware, and does not have consciousness as its very essence, is non-eternal. Both the mind and the body are of a material nature that is subject to change, and therefore cannot be eternal. Though the mind is of a material nature, it is very subtle and can reflect the consciousness of the Self or Spirit. Consciousness is not inherent in the mind so it borrows the light of consciousness from the Self.

How to overcome the five afflictions (kleśas)

> 'These subtle afflictions are eliminated by resolving them back into their original cause.'
>
> *Yoga Sūtras 2:10*

The afflictions have their roots in ignorance (*avidyā*), which is their primal cause, and are not easily eliminated or destroyed. Even though the afflictions can be resolved back into their primal cause, if ignorance remains in any form, there is still the potential for the afflictions to return to their fully active states. It is only when one attains the perfection of *asamprājñāta samādhi* in *nirvikalpa-samādhi*, the final liberation (*kaivalya*), that there is complete freedom from the afflictions (*kleśas*).

If we use the analogy of a tree, our desires are like the leaves, twigs and branches. The branches are the strong central desires that branch out into less strong or weaker desires (desires that are known) in the twigs and leaves. The afflictions – ignorance, egoism, attraction, repulsion and clinging to life – are the roots of the tree and trunk of the tree. It is not enough only to remove the numerous leaves, to reduce desires the branches need cutting. Final liberation (*kaivalya* – absolute freedom) is attained when the roots of the tree are cut with discriminative wisdom and supreme dispassion. Then the mind (*citta*) and the afflictions (*kleśas*) are resolved back into their primal origin of *prakṛiti* (the matter principle) and no longer exist as being separate. The mind and afflictions completely dissolve and the mind ceases to function as a mind.

'These *vṛtti* states of mind produced by the afflictions are eliminated by meditation.'

Yoga Sūtras 2:11

In this *sūtra* Patañjali tells us that it is the *kleśas* (afflictions) that produce the *vṛttis* or vortices of feeling, and that meditation (*dhyāna*) eliminates the more subtle *vṛttis* or the seeds of these afflictions.

By themselves the *kleśas* cannot be weakened or eliminated without the methods of *Kriyā Yoga*. So, Patañjali has given us three Yoga actions or methods that weaken the cycle of desires and attachments, habits and selfishness of the ego, and prepare the mind for *samādhi*. The purpose of practising these three methods is to purify the mind by reducing gross manifestations of the *kleśas* (afflictions) with the aim of attaining *samādhi* (superconsciousness; absorption). If we do not remove these *kleśas* of the mind it will not be possible to attain *samādhi*.

These three practices of *Kriyā Yoga* are particularly suited to those who are already established in spiritual disciplines and practices, but who have not completely mastered the practice of concentration.

'Tapaḥ svādhyāya Īśvara-praṇidhānāni kriyāyogaḥ.'
'Disciplining and purifying the senses, Self-study, and feeling the presence of God constitute the practice of Yoga.'

Yoga Sūtras 2:1

The Sanskrit word *tapaḥ* or *tapas* in this *sūtra* literally means 'to heat up' or 'to burn'. *Tapas* is purifying, it burns the impurities and desires in the mind.

Tapas does not mean mortification, suppression, nor repression. *Tapas* is an austerity in the sense of a discipline, and willingly accepting discomforts that limit the sense of ego. It is training the mind, body and senses to live the truth of who you are in reality. It is having control over your mind, body, senses and *prāṇa* (life-force).

Svādhyāya (Self-study) can be interpreted in two ways. One way is to study the sacred scriptures. The other way is introspection, observing your own mind to understand who you really are in essence. It is investigating the nature of the Self through inquiry to discover its origin, the source of consciousness. Study and observation purifies the intellect of ignorance, imbalances and impurities.

Īśvara-praṇidhāna is constantly keeping the Divine Presence in the heart. It is an attitude of devotion, feeling the omnipresence of the Supreme Being. Through this practice one acquires steadiness of mind (*samāhita citta*) and ultimately the state of superconsciousness (*samādhi*).

Thus, the grosser aspects of the *kleśas* are eliminated by the three methods of *Kriyā Yoga*. The subtle aspects are eliminated by meditation (*dhyāna*), but the residual impressions of the *saṁskāras* are not completely extinguished until the mind and all its *saṁskāras* resolve back to their source, in the attainment of the final absorption in the Self (*puruṣa*), in *nirvikalpa samādhi*, which is synonymous with *asamprājñāta samādhi* – superconsciousness beyond all knowledge. The attainment of *asamprājñāta samādhi* burns the *kleśas* seeds so that they can never become active again. Thus, the primary affliction of ignorance (*avidyā*), from which the other afflictions originate, is eliminated.

ABHYĀSA AND *VAIRĀGYA*

> 'The stilling of the *vṛtti* states of mind is achieved by practice and dispassion.'
>
> *Yoga Sūtras 1:12*

The practice of *Kriyā Yoga* weakens the restlessness of the mind with all its desires and attachments, and prepares the mind for *abhyāsa* (regular practice of one-pointed meditation) and *vairāgya* (dispassion).

In the *Bhāgavad Gītā*, Krishna also teaches us how a restless and unsteady mind can be controlled:

> 'Without doubt, the mind is unsteady, and difficult to control. However, it can be controlled by practice and dispassion.'
>
> *Bhāgavad Gītā 6:35 (Author's translation)*

It teaches us that the restless and turbulent mind can be controlled by continuous practice (*abhyāsa*) and that the natural flow of the mind towards outer objects of sense-pleasure can be removed by dispassion (*vairāgya*).

When the mind becomes free from distractions caused by sense objects and is grounded in one-pointed concentration, then it is able to flow inward and become stable through the regular practice of meditation.

Abhyāsa means 'practice', and it also means 'repetition' – repeated or regular practice which does not become repetitive and dull. So *abhyāsa* can either lead to more vigilance and alertness, or less vigilance and more dullness and sleep. If the mind is dull, there is no zeal in it. Such a mind should never have taken up Yoga.

Vairāgya means 'dispassion'. It is the opposite of *rāga*. *Rāga* means inordinate affection, infatuation. *Rāga* is also a melody – it entertains you, pleases you. Anything that promotes your pleasure instinct is *rāga*. You see how one thing leads to the other. *Rāga* also means 'colouring' – colours are pleasing to the eye. What music is to the ear, colour is to the eye. Anything that pleases the senses is *rāga*, and its result is also *rāga*. When there is infatuation, or inordinate, irrational affection, that is also *rāga*. *Rāga* means all these and a lot more. Its opposite is *vairāgya*.

Vairāgya is to see where there is this inner conditioning that attracts. The mind is attracted by pleasure and by what it has already decided to consider as pleasure. So we must go right back to the source to see where the decision has been made that this is called pleasure. Unless it is dealt with there, the *vairāgya* is not going to happen. Merely meddling with it superficially will not do. We may find substitutes; for example, if I have been a heavy smoker and I want to give it up, I start chewing gum – the mouth has to be doing something. But until I go right back to the source of this surge of energy which sets this craving, the real thing is not had. The traditional teaching is to examine yourself, your life and your mind, see what you crave for and deliberately avoid it.

Abhyāsa and vairāgya – two sides of the same coin

There are times when the Yoga student seems to be leading a double life. There is some high degree of intelligence at one stage and then there is something else. Life has not been totally and completely integrated. There are moments of awakening, moments of dullness; moments of wakefulness, moments of sleep; moments of alertness, moments of non-vigilance. By persistent practice, *abhyāsa*, these moments of intelligence stretch further and further, and as this happens *vairāgya* is eliminated.

Abhyāsa and *vairāgya* are two sides of the same coin. The two are one. Neither *abhāsya* nor *vairāgya* can be practised independently. When Self-knowledge becomes well-grounded, ignorance is eliminated. When light spreads in the morning, darkness seems to recede. The two are one. It is not as though light penetrates darkness – it cannot. When the light comes, darkness seems to go away. But darkness does not go away – light spreads over the entire surface of the earth. When that happens, the darkness which was not there is seen to be not there. Light falls on an object, it is seen. Immediately light falls on this thing called darkness, it goes – which means it was never there.

Since we have accepted darkness as a reality, the doubt arises again and again. Therefore this practice of Self-knowledge, God-consciousness, or inner Light, or whatever you want to call it, is also made necessary again and again and again. You think you have seen it – but then doubt arises. When this happens you need to come back to both *abhyāsa* and *vairāgya*, for neither of them can be practised independently.

In India, years ago, a holy man who was a *swāmi* gave a beautiful meaning of the essence of *abhyāsa* and *vairāgya*. He said:

> '*Abhyāsa* (repeated practice) is to know that all is One, that God is omnipresent, and to be constantly conscious that God is omnipresent. *Vairāgya* is never to allow the idea of the world to arise in your mind.'

Unless one has the strength of this *vairāgya*, *abhyāsa* or practice of Yoga is not possible. One cannot attach oneself to the Absolute unless one practises dispassion, detachment to the false values of life. *Vairāgya*, or detachment from the false values, does not mean a physical closure of one's eyes to the existence of things. This has been very clearly indicated in such sacred texts as the *Bhāgavad Gītā*. Our problem is not the existence of things, but the nature of our our notion about the existence of things. Unless our current wrong notion about the existence of the things of the world, or the world as a whole, is transformed, a physical disassociation from objects may not help us much.

Patañjali defines *vairāgya* in a psychological manner. *Vairāgya* has nothing to do with the outward renunciation of a monk, and nothing to do with entering into a monastery. No outward exhibition in conduct is indicated in *vairāgya*. It just simply means an absence of desires. *Rāga* is desire or attachment, and *vairāgya* is the opposite – dispassion, detachment. It is not indifference or repulsion. *Vairāgya* is sometimes called detachment, but there is a difficulty here. Detachment implies that there was attachment. Like divorce – I got into a mess, I married, got attached, can I completely detach myself now? There is the lovely cliché, 'Forgive and forget.' Can I forget? When someone has abused me, quarrelled with me, and broken my arm, can I really forget this? I may claim that I am a spiritual person, that I forgive and forget, but next time that person is before me, I will remember, 'He broke my arm.'

The only way is not to register the insult, or the hurt, in the first place. Once I feel offended, I cannot forget it. Once I have become attached to you, I cannot forget and detach. I must not get attached to start with. If I am not attached at all, do not hate at all, do not register offence or other feelings, then there is no real detachment. That is Yoga.

What is called *vairāgya* is extremely difficult to define, because all definitions presuppose the opposite. Detachment implies having been attached. 'I love someone and when I discovered her to be unworthy of my love, I pulled myself away, and now I hate her.' *Vairāgya* is not that. It is not dislike, nor indifference. It is not aversion, not the verbal opposite of infatuation, love. It is totally opposite, the absence of it. In the *Bhāgavad Gītā*, Krishna gives us some clues to the development of *vairāgya*. He tells us to look within and note where approval arises within us, where this *rāga*, this attraction and affection, arises. When you put a hand on a burning stove, it will immediately withdraw because the nerve endings in the finger tips do not 'like' the heat. In a similar way, if during Yoga practice there is a soft towel under you, the back of the neck 'likes' it. If there is a rough Yoga mat, the neck does not 'like' it. We are discussing whether I like it or I do not like it. The back of the neck 'approves' of a soft material and 'disapproves' of anything rough.

This approval or disapproval belongs not to me, but to my sensations, to my senses, my body. The skin responds positively to a pleasant sea breeze and negatively to ice-cold wind or desert heat. That is understandable, natural. But when you say 'I love him', or 'I hate him', that is not natural. It does not exist in nature (what is natural is permanent) but is a perversion of nature. When you begin to see this, then your heart, mind or consciousness does not register the causative factors of *rāga-dveṣa* (attachment-aversion), whatever caused the attraction or aversion. That state in which your consciousness does not register these causes at all is *vairāgya*. There is no more registration of experiences. Let life flow on. The sensations, the body, the life-force, approve of certain things and disapprove of others. Let your consciousness not be tainted by this. Just as I lift my hand and the finger may intentionally or unintentionally poke my eye – it happens. Let it happen! There is no accusation, because the finger and the eye belong to the same organism. There is no aversion, no hatred against the finger. The inner consciousness is not modified at all by these experiences. There is no judging, no condemnation, and therefore no need to forgive and forget.

OUR PROBLEMS ARE OUR DESIRES

The desire for things or objects is to be offered up in a higher perception. Our problems are our desires, not the existence of objects. Our desires arise on account of wrong knowledge of things. We lack right understanding, and due to not seeing things as they are, we have developed wrong attitudes towards them. We either cling to them, become attached, or we have an aversion to them. In reality, there is no necessity to become attached nor to have an aversion towards them. Both these are unwarranted attitudes in the context to objects, things or persons, as they really are. Everything is as we ourselves are. There is a supreme subjectivity present in all things.

If we are more dispassionate in our analysis we will realise that it is not the persons or things outside that cause the problems we experience, but rather our own relationship with those persons and things or objects which constitute our problems. Our experiences, whether pleasurable or painful, are brought about by relationships among people and things. If there were no relationship between the subject and the object, there would be no experience of the object. So, the experience of pleasure or pain, the feeling of problems, is due to a particular type of relationship between oneself and others.

The relationship and attitude to things is our mental activity – the *vṛttis* of the mind are the problem behind all the difficulties. Until the operations of the mind are restrained and directed in the right channel, the problems will continue. So, *vairāgya* has to be achieved by stages of self-reflection and self-analysis. *Vairāgya* is a gradual process of attainment, it has to be practised continuously every day.

This persistent effort in the direction of the detachment of oneself from the false values of life is the essence of spiritual practice or *abhyāsa*. *Abhyāsa* and *vairāgya* is a twofold process – a concentration of our attention, our consciousness, on the nature of Reality, and detachment from the false perceptions and values of life.

Abhyāsa means 'to be established there'. All effort directed towards remaining established there, in Truth, is *abhyāsa*.

Vairāgya was described by that holy man I mentioned earlier, as dispassion in the sense of, 'Never let the thought of the universe as a material reality arise in you.' Therefore *vairāgya* and *abhyāsa* are but two sides of the same coin, as was said earlier. The beauty of this Yoga philosophy is that it does not restrict you to a set of practices, to the adoption of a particular technique or method, saying that this alone is the way to truth and everything else is useless nonsense. Whatever enables you to be established in this cosmic consciousness is *abhyāsa*, be it chanting a *mantra*, or meditating, providing you persist in the practice for a considerable length of time. This does not mean merely meditating for half an hour in the morning, while thinking, 'All is God', and immediately afterwards getting angry when you find someone looking at you in a way that you resent. If all is God, why should God not look at me like that? This is not *abhyāsa*. *Abhyāsa* requires integration of one's entire life. This is similar to the Hassidic teaching in that one's whole life is offered to God, given a God-ward direction. If that is not there, then there is no *abhyāsa*, no practice. One is merely taking one step forward and two steps back, with not even the suggestion of progress implied in taking two steps forward and one step back. You can keep walking for ever, as when you try to run up a sand dune. After several hours you are still at the bottom, even though you thought you were making some progress.

TRUE DISPASSION

When it comes to this mad clinging to life, to the desire to live, to enjoy, to have what we call pleasurable experiences, how does one overcome this? In the *Bhāgavad Gītā*, Krishna expands this idea. The first need is to perceive immediately that all life is tainted by old age, disease and death. This does not mean that one should not eat, nor marry, and stop doing this or that. But when this immediate, direct perception is there constantly, then one's consciousness will not be influenced by these experiences called pleasure and pain. It will no longer run after pleasure because it knows that it is temporary, not real. Neither will it masochistically look for pain. Pain is inherent in life – there is no need to search for some more. When all desires re-enter oneself, return to the source, there is true *vairāgya*, true dispassion – the total opposite of passion and craving.

DESIRES – WHY THE MIND IS RESTLESS

Restlessness of the mind comes because of desires. The eyes looked at the object or person – naturally it was beautiful – but the mind came in, registered it and took a mental picture. And now the mind is coloured by that picture, and that keeps recurring and creating a desire, a craving. The craving arises even when the object or person is not present. So is it possible for me to realise at that point, 'It is not here, what are you craving for?'

When you sit down for meditation and the same object of pleasure comes in front of your mind, tell the mind, 'This is not the time, that object is not here, I will see when it comes.' Then this tyranny of memory is gone. The colouring is still there but it does not bother you at odd hours.

The nature of the mind is unsteady and is ever looking outwards. Anything we do in our life, particularly when it takes the the form of desire, a wanting, a craving, leaves a deep and active impression on the mind. And this happens whether the desire has been satisfied or not. This is likened to seeds that fall into the ground. They appear to be passive or dormant but are actually active in a latent form. When the conditions and time are right the seeds will germinate and sprout into a plant. Similarly, these seed-like impressions lie latent in the mind until the right time comes for them to sprout into desires. These desires make the mind very restless, causing us to try to satisfy and fulfil them, but even when we satisfy a desire it is usually short-lived.

The life cycle of a desire

If the desire is not fulfilled, we become frustrated. This causes us to become angry, jealous, envious, resentful and hateful. A vicious cycle is created which starts from contemplating the objects of the senses – ego-centred thoughts flow towards an object or person → attachment → desire → anticipation → unfulfilled desire → frustration → anger → delusion → loss of memory → loss of discrimination → suffering.

The cycle begins with a stream of ego-centred thoughts flowing continuously towards an object or person that the mind was dwelling on. This creates an attachment to the object or person. As the attachment increases in its forceful flow, it creates desire (*kāma*) to possess the object or person. If the desire is not satisfied or fulfilled then it turns into frustration, and then anger, which clouds one's reason, resulting in confusion of the mind and delusion (*moha*). One's perception becomes false, and judgements wrong; one is unable to rationalise or to think clearly. From this delusion one loses the memories which comprise knowledge. Once the memory is lost, then one's power of discrimination (*buddhi*) is also lost, resulting in a total lack of self-control and loss of peace of mind. The seeds of desire that became impressed on the mind as a result of the mind's restlessness and dissatisfaction produced an extremely bad harvest of frustration and anger.

How desires and attitudes arise in the mind

All the desires, emotions and feelings that arise within us trace back to either the affirmation or the denial of our own true essential nature, which is *Sat-chit-ānanda* (Ever-Existing, Ever-Conscious, Ever-New Bliss). Due to forgetfulness of our true spiritual nature, we have identified ourselves with the mind and the body. God, or our own Self, is infinite being, but if anything in our experience seems to deduct from the infinity of our being, we tend to resist it, hate it, or fear it. Through conditioned habit we are so identified with the mind and body that we seek happiness and fulfilment erroneously in the temporary things and objects of the world. We think that by getting married, having children, gaining lots of friends, attaining university degrees, and gaining fame and success materially, then we will gain a great expansion of being and happiness. But this is not reality because it is all in terms of identification of one's mind and body with things that are temporary. Anything that is material or comes from matter is subject to change. It is impermanent, and so therefore can never give us true and lasting fulfilment, happiness and joy.

The origin of our desires arises from our search for that truth, that ever-lasting eternal joy or bliss, that is our own true essential nature – the indwelling divine Self. We continually repeat the same mistake of searching for that truth and eternal joy, and freedom from suffering, by seeking it in the material things of the world. But the things of the world that have never been dependable, or that cannot be possessed, have never given us complete and lasting fulfilment, and that is why the mind is discontent and restless.

This external search for the truth of who we are and the joy that we seek is like being kept in a dark room for ages. We have forgotten how to turn on the inner light. Conscious remembrance of our God Self can remove this condition in a single moment. Turn on your inner light and darkness will disappear. You do not have to tell the darkness to leave; you just bring in the light as the conscious thought and awareness of God into the mind, then the darkness or ignorance regarding truth will disappear. Meditation and practising the presence of God will keep you in the Light.

Patañjali tells us:

> 'Ignorance (*avidyā*) is mistaking the impermanent as being permanent, the impure as pure, the painful as pleasurable, and the non-Self as the Self.'
>
> *Yoga Sūtras 2:5*

> 'The cause of that unavoidable suffering is the misidentification of the Seer with the seen.'
>
> *Yoga Sūtras 2:17*

Methods to weaken desires and restlessness of the mind

1. **Meditation and practising the presence of God.**
2. **Repeated practice (*Abhyāsa*).**
3. **Dispassion (*Vairāgya*).**
4. **Concentration** – giving your full undivided attention to whatever you do. This will gradually quieten the mind. Concentration means not allowing the mind to become scattered in all directions but holding it to one point.
5. ***Japa*** – chanting the repetition of a *mantra* or the holy name of God. *Japa* enables one to gain control over the mind, purify it, and master concentration. For best results *japa* has to be steadfast in practising regularly and intensely for several years. Spiritual progress takes place steadily but imperceptibly.

SAṀSKĀRAS

The Sanskrit word *saṁskāra* comes from *saṁ* ('complete' or 'joined together') and *kāra* ('action', 'cause' or 'doing'). The Sanskrit word *vāsanā* also refers to past impressions or actions. *Vāsanā* is a behavioural tendency or karmic imprint which influences the present behaviour of a person. *Vāsanā* is a synonym for *saṁskāra*.

Saṁskāras are latent impressions, and inherent tendencies, that cause us to think and act in a certain way. Our past thoughts – positive or negative – remain stored in the subconscious mind and construct our personality and make up our conditioning. Repeating *saṁskāras* reinforces them, creating a groove that is difficult to resist.

Imagine a solid jelly (the sweet fruit jelly that you have as a dessert) sitting on a plate. If very hot water is trickled on the top the jelly, it will run off onto the plate, leaving behind a faint groove where the hot water melted the jelly. If more hot water is poured on the jelly, the water will flow into the same grooves as before. This is because these grooves offer the least resistance. If you keep pouring hot water over the jelly, these grooves will become deeper and deeper, making it impossible to get the water to run anywhere else but in the deep grooves. Our habits are formed in the same way. Our thoughts and desires leave deep imprints or seed-impressions in the mind, and they germinate, creating an impulse within ourselves to repeat the same experience of which they were the impressions. For example, every time we become irritated, angry, obstinate, express resentment or become inhibited, we are responding to our *saṁskāras*, which derive from decisions made in response to earlier incidents or episodes in our life.

These *saṁskāras* keep us locked into conditioned patterns of behaviour by influencing the way we perceive our experience in daily life. The *saṁskāras* or seed-impressions that are embedded in our subconscious mind are formed the moment the mind is experiencing something. This is an experience that one has in the sense-plane. It then sinks down into the subconscious mind and forms an impression. The experience leaves a *saṁskāra*, and the memory of a specific experience rises from the particular *saṁskāra* which was formed from that particular experience.

For example, when you perceive a strawberry and taste it for the first time, your senses give you the knowledge of a strawberry – its shape, size, colour, smell and taste. Immediately, an impression (*saṁskāra*) is formed in the subconscious mind. This *saṁskāra* can generate a memory of pleasure and knowledge of a strawberry at any given moment in time.

The memory of the pleasure can also create an attachment to the object of pleasure. The mind then plans and schemes and makes a great effort in possessing that object in order to enjoy it.

These *saṁskāras* in the mind can germinate in the mind through a thought. When you think of a strawberry, which you have seen and experienced before, you mentally repeat the word 'strawberry'. A mental image of the strawberry appears in your mind and a thought is formed, such as 'I love strawberries', or 'I want a strawberry'.

Just as a seed is the cause of a tree and the tree is the cause of a seed, similarly, impressions cause thoughts and thoughts cause impressions. From birth our mind is a storehouse of impressions or *saṁskāras* that lie dormant in the subconscious mind as latent tendencies. They are created not only in this life but come also from previous lives. Though the physical body dies, the thoughts, desires and *saṁskāras* of our thinking and actions continue to live on in the same mind, that our soul carries into the next life. They are only completely destroyed when one finally attains liberation in *asamprajnāta samādhi*.

How to eliminate saṁskāras

To eliminate *saṁskāras* the mind has to be one-pointed in concentration. Like a laser beam, a concentrated mind can penetrate the depths of the subconscious and dislodge the deep-seeded impressions or *saṁskāras*, through deep *Kriyā* meditation and/or through chanting the holy name of God or a *mantra* (*japa*). These spiritual practices help to draw up the accumulated subconscious seed thoughts to the conscious level of the mind, where the meditator can disinterestedly watch them, without any involvement with them. In this way most of the thoughts can be eliminated; the mind can be purified of its *saṁskāras*. Then, it is only the very subtle *saṁskāras* that need to be destroyed in *asamprajnāta samādhi*.

6.8.2 *KARMA* AND *SAṀSĀRA*

Indian philosophy teaches us that human existence is linked by the transmigrations of the soul from one life to the next. The Sanskrit term for this cycle of births and deaths is *saṁsāra* (not to be confused with *saṁskāra*, which is a seed-impression) which literally means 'becoming' or 'conditioned existence'. *Saṁsāra* is the wheel of ceaseless becoming, an endless cycle of impermanent and transient existences – birth, death and rebirth.

The embodied individual soul (*jīvātma*) retains the residual memories of its *karmas* (past actions), in the form of *saṁskāras* (subconscious impressions) that become embedded in the subconscious mind, waiting for the right conditions and time to sprout. These impressions form the tendencies that will subconsciously form the course of the next life.

Ignorance (*avidyā*) gives rise to the mind, and desires creating the motivation for their fulfilment perpetuate the mind's conditioned existence in *saṁsāra* by binding it with *karma*.

The mind's attachment to the pleasures of the senses, derived from the fulfilment of desires, creates new desires, enmeshing the soul in the web of *karma* and *saṁsāra*. Thus every individual is constantly accumulating within their subconscious mind the subtle impressions of the diverse *karma* they perform. An individual's character and outer condition are determined mainly by the subtle impressions of his or her thoughts, words and deeds, acquired by their own *karma*.

This *saṁsāra* cycle that rotates continuously from birth to birth can only be broken when the mind reaches a point of unfulfilment and dissatisfaction in either the present life or a future lifetime; when it finally awakens from the delusion of trying to find happiness and joy in the pleasure of the senses and worldly goals. Paramhansa Yogananda said, 'To get off the wheel (of *saṁsāra*), you have to desire freedom very intensely. Then only will God release you. Your longing has to be fervent. If it is, and if you are determined no more to want to play, the Lord has to release you.'

Due to ignorance (*avidyā*) we have forgotten our true essential nature – the boundless, eternal divine Self. Our existence has become conditioned by our desires and *karmas*, causing us sorrow and suffering. To break this chain of karmic bondage and transcend our conditioned existence we need to make a strong, persistent effort in our practice of Yoga and meditation. The mind, body and senses need to be disciplined; the life-energy (*prāṇa*) of the mind and body to be controlled. There needs to be purification and mastery of the mind. To master the mind you need to understand it.

The Sanskrit word *karma* means any action, either physical, verbal or mental, as well as its consequences and its accumulative effect. The word *karma* is often used as a synonym for work, but not in the same sense as the English word. The two terms cannot be used interchangeably. *Karma* is distinguished from work by the example of a person lying in bed pretending to be ill in order to avoid work – obviously he does not do any work, but he does *karma*. He may avoid having to work, but he cannot avoid *karma* and its effects or consequences. There is no effect without a cause. As is the cause, so is the effect. Our thoughts, words and actions condition and shape our lives.

The law of *karma* is the natural law of causation, that evolves towards balance as a whole. Any thought or deed causes an effect and can be called *karma*. For example, a seed is a cause for the tree which is the effect. The tree produces seeds and becomes the cause of the seeds.

Karma does not have the negative connotation of God's judgement, punishment, pain or penalty. The doctrine of predestination is a dogmatic version of fatalism. According to this all that happens to us is predetermined by God; some of us are fore-ordained to everlasting happiness and some to everlasting suffering. It makes God responsible for our vices and sufferings. But how can God be conceived as all-just and all-merciful in such a case?

God does not interfere with our individual freedom, and our freedom does not counter God's existence as the Supreme ruler that maintains order and harmony throughout the universe and makes the operation of laws possible. This can be explained by giving the example of the growth of vegetation. The sun encourages and helps the growth of vegetation. Without the sun nothing can grow, yet each plant grows according to its type and potency under the sun. Whatever potency or power we have is derived from that Ultimate Source, God. In God's natural law everything functions in its own way. All things and beings are held in their respective positions.

Karma is not about sin and being punished. *Karma* is a natural law, not a moral law. The Greek word translated as 'sin' actually means 'miss the mark' – an archer's term for not hitting the target. For those of us who are consciously seeking Truth, the Ultimate Reality, God, the target is Self- and God-realisation. Are you hitting the target? Or sinning by 'missing the mark'?

Paramhansa Yogananda said, 'Never call yourself a sinner, to do so is itself the worst sin.' The delusions, habits and desires that chain you in bondage to *saṁsāra* are not you. Never negatively affirm their reality. You are pure, eternal, boundless and divine. Always affirm your true essential nature as the pure, infinite and divine Self.

Karma is also not fate or destiny; nothing is preordained in a fatalistic sense. No supernatural power determines the events of our lives, and there is no scope for chance in human existence. *Karma* is ever associated with self-determination. No volitional action is possible without self-awareness. *Karma* means that you are responsible, you determine your circumstances. You are the architect of your present situation, past and future. To accept responsibility for your life gives you the power to move, change and grow. You are not a victim of circumstances. The circumstances of life are created by us to provide the opportunity to grow towards realisation of our true divine nature.

The key to growth lies in those situations and relationships that give us the most discomfort. These situations and relationships repeat themselves, not out of 'bad luck' or 'bad *karma*', but because uncomfortable situations and relationships represent the barriers to our freedom. Freedom comes when we overcome these self-created barriers.

Take the analogy of a flower that grows from a bulb. For the flower to bloom into its full colourful splendour and beauty, it requires certain conditions – soil, moisture and certain temperatures that need to be maintained for a period of time.

The flower bulb is simply what it is, and certain conditions are required for it to bloom into full expression of its splendid and perfect nature. Similarly, a human being is simply on a natural course towards expression of the perfect Self. Each of us is in just the right conditions for our growth towards perfection to occur. *Karma* is a way to express these conditions. We have free will to choose in which direction our lives will go. We create our lives, which are shaped from our individual deeds and fitted to our individual needs.

THE SOUL IS SUBJECT TO THREE MAIN MODES OF *KARMA*

The three main modes of *karma* operate under the following four classifications:

1. ***Sañcita karma*** ('stored up') – the accumulated *karma*, the stored-up latent impressions (*saṁskāras*) of the past created either in the previous or present life, that will fructify in a future life or lives. *Sañcita karma* remains in a dormant seed state and has not yet started to mature.
2. ***Prārabdha karma*** ('commenced') – *karma* that has formed from mature seeds and is now active in our present life. It is this *karma* that we are most aware of, because of its effect on our lives from moment to moment, in the form of desires, aversion, insecurity, fear, anger, love, happiness, sadness, resentment, hatred, and so on. *Prārabdha karma* is destined to run its course. What has happened in the past cannot be changed, but with awareness one can reduce the development of dormant *karmas* that will reach the *prārabdha* state.
3. ***Āgāmi karma*** ('coming up') – the impressions of the current activities in our daily life, that are accumulating and will fructify in due course.
4. ***Kriyāmāṇa karma*** – *kriyāmāṇa* is interchangeable with *āgāmi karma* as both refer to that which is done in the present moment. But *kriyāmāṇa* is more to do with exercising our free will to make choices in the present.

KARMA – ANALOGY OF AN ARCHER

A classical example of how *karma* works is of an archer with a quiver full of arrows, which is cited to illustrate the archer's control over the three modes of *karma*. It is up to the archer how frequently he takes an arrow from his quiver and how and when he releases it against the target. This is his ability to perform actions with free will. But once the arrows have struck the target, their impact creates an effect. The archer is scored immediately according to the nature of the impact. This is equivalent to future consequences.

Once the arrow is released, the archer has no control over it. This the analogy of the fructifying *prārabdha karma*. The archer positions another arrow in his bow. He has the choice to shoot the arrow or throw it away. This represents the prospective *āgāmi karma*. The archer can also throw away the whole quiver of arrows if he chooses to do so. This represents our control over accumulated *sañcita karma* from the past that will fructify in a future life or lives.

6.8.3 THE *GUṆAS* – NATURE'S THREE FUNDAMENTAL FORCES

PURUṢA AND *PRAKṚITI*

The ancient school of Indian philosophy called *Sāṃkhya* (to have complete knowledge) – from *sam* ('union', 'completeness'), and *khyā* ('to be known', 'knowledge') – divides reality into two main principles: *puruṣa* (the Self; Spirit; the knower) and *prakṛiti* (primordial nature; matter; the known).

Puruṣa, the Self, is subjective and eternally separate. It is beyond *prakṛiti*, and so is not part of the Creation. *Puruṣa* is also without attributes; it is not the doer, it is pure consciousness – a Self-illumined, unchanging, uncaused, all-pervading, eternal Reality.

Unlike *prakṛiti*, there are as numerous *puruṣas* as there are conscious beings. Just as light from different candles can occupy the same space without any conflict, so there are numerous *puruṣas* occupying the same space.

All objects of the phenomenal world, including the mind, senses and intellect, are in themselves unconscious. They cannot function without guidance from an intelligent principle – the conscious Intelligence that guides the operation of *prakṛiti* and its manifestations is *puruṣa*, the Self.

Prakṛiti, the one all-pervading, unconscious primordial matter, is the material cause of the universe. Though it is conscious during its evolving stage, it can never be consciousness itself.

It is from the interaction of these two principles – *puruṣa* and *prakṛiti* – that evolution occurs. The entire universe evolves from their interaction. *Puruṣa* and *prakṛiti* act upon one another. *Puruṣa* gives the impetus and *prakṛiti* manifests. In an energy-packed state of tension, *prakṛiti* (primordial matter) undergoes transformation, but the *puruṣa* (Spirit; the Self) remains unaltered and unchanged.

At a very subtle stage of evolution, after *prakṛiti* arises from *puruṣa*, the three fundamental, creative forces of nature (*guṇas*) appear. These creative forces are called: *sattva*, *rajas* and *tamas*. These three *guṇas* are in equilibrium with each other. *Puruṣa* is without the *guṇas*.

Prakṛiti preserves a balanced tension between *sattva*, *rajas* and *tamas*. It is through the interplay of these three creative forces that *prakṛiti* manifests as the universe. Everything that is known in the world is a manifestation of these three *guṇas*.

The three *guṇas* are imperishable basic qualities of the matter principle (*prakṛiti*). They cannot be separated from each other and they cannot operate on their own; they are always together. As an analogy, the cooperation of the *guṇas* is likened to a lighted candle – without the cooperation of the wax, the wick and the fire, no candle flame is possible. Similarly, the world exists owing to the cooperation of the three *guṇas* – *sattva*, *rajas* and *tamas*.

Through awareness and understanding of how the *guṇas* operate, these three fundamental creative forces can help us in understanding our true nature – *puruṣa*, the Self.

THE THREE *GUṆAS*

The Sanskrit word *guṇa* literally means 'strand' or 'string'. The three *guṇas* are like the strands of a rope woven together to form the universe. *Prakṛiti* (subtle primordial nature) is like a rope made of three intertwined strands – *sattva*, *rajas* and *tamas*. Together they make up the rope of material existence that keeps us in bondage. These three inseparable forces of nature are also like the three sides of a triangle, they cannot operate individually – when one of the three forces becomes more prominent, the other two become correspondingly weaker. They function by balancing each other.

Sattva is the creative force of nature, *rajas* is the energetic and maintaining force, and *tamas* is the retarding or destructive force of nature. Although *sattva* is the purest and highest of the three *guṇas*, it is a part of *Māyā*, the delusive force inherent in creation. It is not inherent in the Self, and so is unable to give us freedom, or liberation from the ego.

The *guṇas'* cooperation and transformation can only occur when the *puruṣa* (pure consciousness; innermost conscious Self) is reflected in them. *Prakṛiti* and the *guṇas* exist to fulfil the dual purpose of *puruṣa*: experience and liberation. All objects (*prakṛiti*) exist to be experienced by *puruṣa*; without this ability to be known or experienced, Creation would have no meaning or purpose.

Prakṛiti borrows consciousness from *puruṣa* and begins to act as a conscious entity, causing the equilibrium of the three *guṇas* to be disturbed. This causes a conflict between the *guṇas* causing *prakṛiti* to undergo a gradual process of transformation. Through a progression of changes, evolution of the universe is finally manifested.

Characteristics of the three guṇas

> '*Sattva*, *rajas*, *tamas* – these qualities born of material Nature (*prakṛiti*) bind the imperishable soul to the body.'
>
> *Bhāgavad Gītā 14.5*

The *Bhāgavad Gītā* (chapter 14) gives us the knowledge of how we can measure our spiritual progress by understanding the mind through the knowledge of the three *guṇas*.

In Sanskrit, *guṇa* means 'quality' and refers to the three primary 'qualities' of nature (*prakṛiti*): *tamas* (the principle of inertia, darkness, ignorance), *rajas* (the principle of activity) and *sattva* (the principle of purity and illumination).

Tamas

Tamas or *tamoguṇa* is the quality of inertia, dullness, heaviness and darkness. Its source is impure, it brings ignorance and delusion to the mind, causing loss of awareness, deep-seated emotional blockages and attachments, resulting in misery. Its energy is negative and has a downward effect, drawing one's energy down the spine into the lower three *chakras* (*mūladhāra*, *svādhiṣṭhāna* and *maṇipūra*). Stagnation, lethargy and laziness are associated with *tamas*.

If you are under the influence of *tamas*, the dark quality that is controlled by negative and repressed emotions, you lose the sense of awareness and discrimination, and not being responsible for your life you remain in a state of ignorance, sleepiness, lethargy, carelessness and indolence. The mind in this state is full of misconceptions and errors. It is easily angered, and can become insensitive, confused, sad and depressed.

The *tamasic* person enjoys eating *tamasic* food that causes inertia, dullness and heaviness. These are foods that are impure, stale, left-over, unhealthy and non-nutritious. This includes meat, particularly pork and beef, and its derivatives. Such unhealthy and unwholesome food causes physical disease, mental dullness and no aspiration for spiritual development.

The predominance of *tamas* in the mind veils our true divine nature with thick dark clouds of ignorance. In this state one is not able to make spiritual progress at all.

For a *tamasic*-natured person to rise above this low level of consciousness, avoiding pain, suffering and unhappiness, they will need the influence, force and action of *rajas* to raise them to the next higher level of awareness.

Rajas

Rajas or *rajoguṇa* is the quality of activity, a force of passion, turbulence, uncontrolled desire, and change. It keeps our consciousness restless, distracted and disturbed.

If you are under the negative influence of *rajas*, you may become self-seeking, ego and habit driven, and continually active. Unawake to your spiritual purpose and dominated by your ego, you are never satisfied; with emotional excitement you restlessly pursue new sources of sense-pleasure, and become attached to enjoyments that eventually result in pain, distress and suffering. The mind in this state can be domineering, arrogant, critical, judgemental, envious, jealous, angry, and even hateful.

In the beginning, due to its stimulating action, *rajas* provides us with pleasure and happiness from the contact of the senses with their objects. But this is short-lived, followed almost inevitably by loss of control, frustrated desire, disappointment and sorrow, causing imbalance and dissipation of energy.

If you direct and use the active force of *rajas* in a positive way, it can lead you to be creative and constructive in ways that can help you to progress spiritually.

The *rajasic* person enjoys foods that stimulate and satisfy the senses – foods that are bitter, sour, salty, excessively hot and spicy. Onions, garlic, eggs, fish, fowl and lamb are all considered *rajasic*. Stimulating foods that are taken in excess can cause discomfort and disease in the body and make the mind agitated and restless.

For a *rajasic*-natured person to rise to the higher level of *sattvic* consciousness, the restless mind with its uncontrollable desires needs to be disciplined and the senses restrained. The *rajasic* person who is primarily centred in the emotions must become aware of their own spiritual nature, sincerely wanting inner peace and joy or bliss. Then with complete faith in finding the Truth within, and through persevering with the inner practice of meditation and other spiritual disciplines of Yoga, *rajoguṇa* can be subdued and *sattva guṇa* made predominant.

Sattva

Sattva guṇa has the qualities of purity, light, clarity, intelligence, peacefulness, serenity, calmness, selfless love, devotion. It is the basis for our higher awareness and experience of superconsciousness.

The *sattvic* person favours food that promotes optimum health, vitality and longevity. Such food that is vegetarian or vegan (non-dairy products), wholesome, nourishing and pure: fresh fruits, vegetables, whole grains, beans, pulses, nuts, seeds, honey, flax seed oil, olive oil, herbs, and food that is only mildly flavoured with spices. *Sattvic* food brings calmness, serenity and cheerfulness to the mind. For those who want to progress on the spiritual path of Yoga and meditation it is important to have a *sattvic* diet, not just for your health, but also for the spiritual upliftment and clarity of your mind, and spiritual aspiration. The *sattvic* person who follows the spiritual path also eats in silence in a quiet and peaceful atmosphere, and knowing that it is a manifestation of God, begins with a prayer to bless the food.

When *sattva* is predominant in your mind then it creates harmony, balance, stability, and purity of mind and heart. You have control over your senses. Your nature becomes harmonious, serene, and contented, and peaceful. You are compassionate and considerate and have respect towards others. There is a clarity in your awareness and your thoughts are positive and elevated, giving you mental and emotional equilibrium. In this state of *sattva* you experience calmness and joy. Its energy is positive and has an inward and upward motion in the spine, drawing your energy up the spine into the higher *chakras*, so that the consciousness is centred at the Spiritual Eye in the frontal lobe of the brain.

Transcending the guṇas

> 'When his own Self, endowed with the purest splendour, is hidden from view, a man through ignorance falsely identifies himself with this body, which is the non-Self. And then the great power of *rajas* called the projecting power sorely afflicts him through the binding fetters of lust, anger, etc.'
>
> *Madhavanda 2003, pp.52–53*

To find true and lasting joy beyond the happiness that is coloured by the *guṇas* – *tamas*, *rajas*, *sattva* – ultimately you need to experience and realise the pure bliss of the Self, which transcends them all. The blissful Self, pure Consciousness, is not coloured or tainted by the coloured filters of the three *guṇas*. The eternal light of the Self shines pure and clear. The yogi who has transcended even *sattvic* happiness abides in his own blissful Self.

The *rajasic* person, whose life is stimulated by activity, often ending in disappointment, may at some point in time feel that there is something missing from his or her life – this is when one begins to awake and seek that supreme and lasting joy that is found within. The *tamasic* person is less fortunate – they are totally unaware of their inner light and so remain in a dark and delusive state of ignorance, with no will for self-improvement.

For both the *tamasic* and the *rajasic* persons who have not reached the higher level of spiritual realisation and are attached to bodily enjoyments, the means for transcending them is through *action* and *discipline* of the body, mind, senses, thoughts, speech and actions; *satsang*, associating with spiritually-minded people; daily meditation; and by practising the spiritual disciplines of *Rāja Yoga*, the Eight Limbs of Yoga (*Aṣṭāṅga Yoga*), as outlined in Patañjali's *Yoga Sūtras*. In this way one can rise from the lower sensual natures of *tamas* and *rajas* to the *sattvic* nature of inner contentment and happiness.

> 'Remaining in solitude, with mind and body restrained, free from desires of the senses, and without avarice, the yogi should constantly concentrate on the inner Self.'
>
> *Bhāgavad Gītā 6.10*

To transcend the three *guṇas* of nature (*prakṛiti*) that create the body and this transitory world of delusion, you need to have one-pointed devotion and complete dedication to the supreme Self. Without purification of your mind, one-pointed devotion is not possible.

Such a spiritually elevated person who has transcended the *guṇas* becomes established in their true identity and divine nature, the inner Self, and remains ever calm and undisturbed by *tamas*, *rajas* and *sattva*, in all situations. Unaffected personally by joy or sorrow, praise or blame, pleasant and unpleasant, he or she maintains even-mindedness with undisturbed tranquillity. Having also transcended the ego, such a person is uninfluenced by honour or dishonour, and is free from personal aggrandisement or self-importance.

> 'Having transcended the three qualities of Nature, which bind the soul to the body, one is freed from the suffering of birth, old age, and death, and attains immortality.'
>
> *Bhāgavad Gītā 14.20*

One who is established in the supreme Self knows that the *guṇas*, the fundamental creative forces of nature (*prakṛiti*), are the agents of all actions that create the play of the universe, and that the Self is not the doer. Therefore, one who knows this and is free from identification with body consciousness, and is firmly established in the Self, does not become involved and enmeshed in the web of the *guṇas*.

6.8.4 WHAT IS CONSCIOUSNESS?

The mind is constantly fluctuating in thoughts, feelings, impressions, and states of waking, dreaming and sleeping. Behind these mental fluctuations is a constant awareness, an unbroken sense of Self or being that continually observes and witnesses the mind's activities. When we are not caught up in our mental activity, but are attentively aware, our Self-awareness can perceive and observe the mind. You cannot be your thoughts, feelings, sensations, or anything else of an objective nature, because when they subside, you are present and aware of them. These thoughts, feelings and sensations are transitory; they come and they go, but your real natural state or essential being – that single continuous consciousness in which the many and various aspects of objective experience come and go – is ever-present awareness that remains constant. It is all expansive without centre or periphery.

CONSCIOUSNESS-AWARENESS IS INDEPENDENT OF THE MIND

> 'Everyone knows that the drop is contained within the Ocean, but not everyone knows that the Ocean is contained in the drop.'
>
> *Kabir (1440–1518)*

Waves appear on the sea, but they have no independent reality, they are just appearances of the underlying water; the wave has no independent existence as something apart from its source. Similarly, the body, mind and objects of the phenomenal world do not exist as independent realities, like the waves of the sea, they are manifestations or appearances of consciousness. Just as waves consist of water, all things objective consist of consciousness.

The principle of awareness is independent of the mind and its activities, just as water is independent of its fleeting manifestation of bubbles, ripples and waves – these are nothing but water that rise and set. The water exists independently from the ripples and waves.

Without consciousness there is no world to witness or experience. Without the sense of 'I am' there can be no other experiences. That present awareness of 'I am' is your true nature.

To experience our thoughts and feelings requires the presence of consciousness. The phenomenal world, mind and body appear as objects within consciousness, within awareness. The fleeting objects of the world and the body and mind have no independent existence apart from being perceived in consciousness. Your body and mind are material objects that appear in consciousness, they do not exist as independent realities. The very nature of the mind is to express this awareness by means of name and form. You, the innermost Self, are the one to whom they appear. Consciousness is the eternal Reality alone that exists.

CONSCIOUSNESS IS ITSELF THE PROOF OF EVERYTHING ELSE

In reality there is only non-dual consciousness. Consciousness is a principle that does not have to be proved. It is itself the proof of everything else. Consciousness is self-existent. Those who experience consciousness in itself find that it is its own proof. Just as a light does not need the help of another light to show itself – its own light reveals it – so consciousness is its own proof. That Reality sees everything by its own light. It is Self-luminous.

THE MIND AND CONSCIOUSNESS ARE NOT IN THE BRAIN

Essentially, consciousness is not a mental state or mental process, but is awareness itself; the perceiver. If you were not aware you would not be able to take note of the mental and emotional states that you experience yourself in. So, therefore, awareness cannot be a mental function; if it was, it would disappear like all mental functions.

Consciousness or awareness does not disappear, it is continuous and always present. The states you experience are in awareness.

Thinking and perceiving are functional consciousness which is discontinuous, but Pure Consciousness is the continuous Presence beyond time and space. You are that Pure Consciousness, it is your true nature and is always awake, it does not sleep. It is unconditional Being and love.

Consciousness does not originate in the mind, nor the brain. The mind transmits the radiance of consciousness to the physical system. The brain, being material, is devoid of consciousness; it is only a medium or vehicle of consciousness, it is not its source. The mind is not in the brain. The brain is a physical organ, an instrument through which the mind works. This is why we say 'my mind' – we view the mind as an instrument. The mind only appears to be conscious to us because the light of pure awareness or Pure Consciousness is reflected onto the mind. The mind itself has no awareness and is not self-luminous. All cognitions and feelings are expressions of inner consciousness through different modes of the mind. Even our mental states are not conscious in themselves, but are illuminated by the light of the inner consciousness, the luminous Self, just as coal becomes aglow when permeated by fire.

Being of the nature of consciousness, the Self is awareness itself. Consciousness is the being of the Self, it is the Knower, the eternal constant Witness which is permanent and unborn. It is the subject and never the object. It is Self-existent. We cannot deny it any more than we can deny ourselves, and deny existence.

Consciousness is ever-present in us – in the waking, dream and sleep states. Waking consciousness and dream consciousness are but reflections of the light of the One Pure Consciousness in matter, in the form of the mind and the senses, in waking and dreaming.

Consciousness does not evolve, but the mind does. The mind can evolve from being gross to subtle; it has the potential to become refined and cultured. It can also become pure and illumined (*sattvic*) by the spiritual disciplines and practices of Yoga and meditation, which help to remove the subconscious tendencies and impressions of the mind that keep us in ignorance of our true nature and identity.

REGAINING YOUR TRUE BLISSFUL NATURE

To regain your true blissful nature, that divine and infinite Self, which is eternally yours but is veiled by the three fundamental forces (the *guṇas* – *sattva*, *rajas* and *tamas*), you have to reduce the *rajas-tamas* impurity, and increase the *sattvic* component of your nature. When consciousness functions through a predominantly *sattvic* mind, It expresses Itself as the God-principle.

When your mind has learned not to dwell on matter or the objects of the senses, then your spiritual life has begun – not until then.

Unless your mind becomes fine and subtle, and *sattvic* (pure), you will not be able to detach from the endless desires and urges of the senses and their objects. You have to learn the art of quieting and stilling the mind, to go within and feel and experience your own true essential nature as something different from the body, mind and senses. When you are able to go into stillness, and your mind becomes calm, then you begin to experience Pure Consciousness (*puruṣa*, the Self, *ātman*). When you discover your inner consciousness then you will find spiritual Truth.

6.8.5 THE PRACTICE OF *DHYĀNA* (MEDITATION)

> *'Tatra pratyayaika-tānata dhyānam.'*
> 'Meditation is a steady, uninterrupted flow of attention and awareness on the Divine reality within you.'
>
> *Yoga Sūtras 3:2*

Dhyāna is the seventh limb of *Aṣṭāṅga Yoga* (Eight Limbs of Yoga). The prolonged focus of concentration (*dhāraṇā*) without interruption becomes meditation (*dhyāna*). In this state the mind becomes fully one-pointed, opening the gateway though which the aspirant can enter the blissful, higher superconscious state of *samādhi*, the state in which one is established in one's true nature, and becomes one with the Supreme Consciousness.

WHY MEDITATE?

We have forgotten our true nature and need to be awakened to it. Our true essential nature, the divine inner Self, is ever one with the Divine, just as sparks are one with the fire, and waves are with the ocean, and rays of sunshine are with the sun. The Divine is the great Self of all – the Self of the entire universe. It has produced the multiplicity and manifestations of life as a kind of illusory projection from Itself. Therefore we are not really separate from the Divine, and never have been. When we awaken to our true divine nature then all feeling of separation, delusion and sorrow falls away, and we know that the spiritual core of our being – the inner Self – is one with the Divine. Yoga meditation is the method through which we spiritually awaken and realise our identity with that which is immortal and infinite within our own being.

Meditation is liberation of the mind from ego-consciousness – all disturbing thoughts, emotional reactions and restless desires – and becoming aware of your own true blissful nature. In meditation you turn your attention inwards, towards your own Self, where Bliss lies in its essential form.

The mind by its very nature wants to regain the stability, stillness, calmness and peace which is never attained without meditation.

In meditation the mind flows continuously in an unbroken stream towards the inner Divine Self. The identification with the body, ego, mind and senses is transcended. Meditation is not a technique, but a state of stillness. All movement has ended with *dhāraṇā* (concentration), and in *dhyāna* (meditation) you are at the inner source of your being. Yoga meditation leads you to the direct experience of your inner Self, your true nature and original identity. It is an inward journey; a return of consciousness from identification with the material body and mind to Supreme Consciousness, the ever-present Reality, that is always One and undivided.

When the Self is realised, all ideas about one's identity as a separate and limited being and ignorance are dispelled. Through meditation you come to realise that the infinite presence of the Divine is ever within you, which is *Sat-chit-ānanda* (Ever-Existing, Ever-Conscious, Ever-New Bliss), the true nature and reality of life.

WHY PRACTISE CONCENTRATION?

Without concentration the energy of the mind becomes scattered, diffused and unfocused. This causes the mind to be inattentive, distracted and disturbed, resulting in the mind being unable to fulfil its true potential. The more you can apply your attention and concentration in everyday life, the greater will be your success in meditation.

Meditation begins with concentration, for to enter the state of superconscious meditation the mind must become calm, steady and one-pointed. Concentration is the key that opens the door to meditation.

THE DIFFERENCE BETWEEN CONCENTRATION AND MEDITATION

There is a difference between concentration and meditation. In concentration (*dhāraṇā*), the attention is focused on a small limited area (the object of concentration). If at that time only one thought or idea functions in the mind, that is meditation (*dhyāna*). In meditation there is not even a suggestion of distraction. If there is awareness of distraction, you are only concentrating, not meditating.

The difference between concentration and meditation is that in concentration there is a peripheral awareness and distraction, whereas in meditation the attention is not disturbed, there are no distractions at all. In meditation the mind becomes one with its object, it is only conscious of itself and the object.

Yoga meditation is not ordinary concentration as in reading a book, watching a movie or listening to music. In ordinary concentration there is not the deliberate and conscious mental focus as in meditation, but a broken mixture of conscious and subconscious thoughts passing through the mind in quick succession. In meditation there is a continuous flow of the whole mind towards the spiritual object of concentration, like the continuous unbroken flow of oil being poured onto one spot.

Dhāraṇā (concentration) is like water dripping intermittently on a single spot; *dhyāna* (meditation) is like oil continuously flowing over the spot. The oil symbolises the mind and the spot the object of thought. If the mind flows uninterruptedly to its object of contemplation for a prolonged period of time, it is called meditation.

Another analogy is the unflickering candle flame burning steadily in a windless place. The mind is represented by the flame, and the disturbance and distraction by the wind.

> 'Just as a flame sheltered from the wind burns bright and steady, so shines the disciplined mind of a yogi practising concentration on the Self.'
>
> *Bhāgavad Gītā 6:19*

What is meditation?

'The purpose of meditation is to help you to enter the inner "kingdom of God".'

Walters 1996, p.17

'The secret of meditation lies not in affirming states that are foreign to us, but in reclaiming what we are. Meditation is a returning to our centre within.'

Walters 1996, p.186

Meditation is a practical, scientific and systematic technique for realising the truth of the essential nature of who you are – the inner experience of the blissful Self. It is an inner journey from the distracted state of mind to a state of inner stillness; a journey to discovering, realising and establishing yourself in your own essential spiritual nature – the divine Self. Meditation leads you to a state of inner joy and brings you contentment and inner peace. It makes you aware of the reality at the core of your being, revealing that your true nature is divine.

The word 'meditation' is misunderstood by some people, who understand it according to their own concepts. For instance, some people think meditation is sitting relaxed while thinking, reflecting, daydreaming or fantasising on a particular thought or idea. But even thinking about the Divine is not meditation, that is contemplation. The person contemplating can be compared to a bee buzzing around a flower, but a person in a state of meditation is like the bee who is seated on the flower absorbed in tasting the sweetness of the nectar.

In the process of meditation all mental activity is replaced with inner awareness and attention. The mind is brought into a sharp, one-pointed focus on spiritual aspects of reality – on a single internal focus of attention such as the breath or a *mantra*, such as *Oṁ* or *Hong Sau*, which is representative of the innermost source of consciousness.

Meditation is an art and science of realising the Ultimate Truth. It is not a religion, but it can be practised within a religion to help you to become conscious of your inner life, by understanding your mind. It also purifies the mind, preparing you to enter higher states of consciousness, in which the mind becomes calm and joyful, reflecting the inner Self. Everyone yearns to have everlasting joy. This longing is expressed outwardly through our desire for wealth, sense-pleasure, name, fame, power and position. It is through all of these desires or cravings that we are unconsciously trying to reach our Divine Self, the fountain of infinite joy within, which is *Sat-chit-ānanda* (Ever-Existing, Ever-Conscious, Ever-New Bliss). Finding lasting fulfilment through our worldly desires is impossible, because the joy derived from them is finite. Only Infinite Joy can give us the true fulfilment we are seeking. Eventually, through meditation we come to realise that searching for Infinite Joy through finite and external means will lead us nowhere.

Meditation is the highest form of worship. The divine inner Self is the true sacred shrine at which we worship when we meditate. You do not have to go on a devotional pilgrimage to the Himalayas or any other holy place to experience the grace and blessings of the Divine. The Divine is within you; your heart is your internal, portable sacred shrine that you carry with you every moment of your life. It is as close to you as your very breath; wherever you are, God is. Inner communion with your true Self in the direct experience of meditation is the highest form of worship.

There is also a distinction between prayer and meditation. In prayer there is a duality when it is offered to a divine personality or deity, perceived as being separate from us. Whereas in meditation, it may begin with concentration on a sacred sound, symbol or image, but it always ends in absorption, unity in oneness with the Divine. In prayer we commune with the Divine by talking to God, but in meditation we listen to the Divine sound of God (*Aum*) within us and achieve blissful union with it.

The goal of meditation

To understand the goal of meditation, the first question that needs to be asked is: 'What is the goal of our existence?' For a life devoid of meaning and purpose is of little value to you.

According to the ancient *Vedās* of India, there are four main human objectives or aims in life. They are called the four *puruṣārthas*: *dharma* (righteousness, virtue), *artha* (material wellbeing, prosperity), *kāma* (enjoyment, pleasure), and *mokṣa* (spiritual liberation). The first three serve one's wellbeing on the material plane, and also contribute to, and prepare the way to, the knowledge of Ultimate Truth and the attainment of the ultimate spiritual goal of Self-realisation and spiritual liberation. The fulfilment of human life is not in material progress, intellectual achievement, aesthetic pleasure, nor moral development, but in spiritual attainment – Self- and God-realisation. The fulfilment of life is to be free from delusion, suffering and sorrow. You have to realise the innate perfection of your divine inner Self.

Of these four objectives in life – *dharma, artha, kāma, mokṣa* – spiritual liberation/ Self-realisation (*mokṣa*) is the highest, because it is through Self-realisation that you can discover the essence of your true nature and spiritual identity. *Mokṣa* gives you freedom from ignorance (*avidyā*), which is responsible for your misidentification with the mind and body.

Meditation, the effort to perceive the presence of God, leads to the attainment of the highest goal of human life – Self- and God-realisation. God is omnipresent – within you and outside of you. To recognise this fact and, on the basis of it, to feel and later to perceive God's immediate presence – this is meditation. However, remember that meditation (*dhyāna*) is only the means. It is not the goal itself. The purpose of meditation and all spiritual practices is to fully manifest the inherent blissful Self, which only becomes fully manifest in the transcendent superconscious state of *samādhi* or Yoga.

Know your purpose in life

In this technological/digital age our culture is orientated towards action: an outward seeking, enjoying sense of fulfilment, that continually keeps us distracted and preoccupied. No time is made for inner reflection and meditation. We have become so separated from ourselves that we do not believe there can be anything particularly interesting or valuable within us. So, instead of meditating most people fill their free time with watching television or videos, or playing and socialising using their latest digital gadgets – iPad, tablet, laptop or mobile phone – keeping them in a constant state of restlessness, disturbing their inner balance.

The sense of fulfilment, completeness, balance and happiness that we are all seeking is experienced when we set aside the daily demands and distractions of the world that claim our attention, and go within in the stillness of deep meditation.

The three main purposes of finding true inner and outer fulfilment in life

1. To seek and find true lasting happiness.
2. To realise your full human potential.
3. To balance the material and spiritual aspects of your life.

When you have the right understanding that the purpose of all experiences are to stimulate and encourage your spiritual development, then you have the right attitude to life and to meditation.

If you do not know your higher purpose in life, meditation and inner reflection will help to reveal it. Then you will be able to unfold your innate qualities, and awaken your inner potential. Paramhansa Yogananda said, 'Focus your attention within. You will experience new power, new strength, and peace in body, mind and spirit. All limitations will be vanquished.'

PREPARING FOR MEDITATION

> 'Meditate daily, with earnestness and devotion. Love God without ceasing… Learn to love God as the joy felt in meditation.'
>
> *Yogananda 2010, p.133*

Beginning to meditate

Beginning to meditate can be likened to starting a long journey, a pilgrimage into the mind itself. It is a spiritual journey to the source of your Being. This journey begins when you start to become aware that there must be a higher Consciousness, a Truth to be realised, an inner spiritual goal as opposed to an outer material goal. The journey begins when the material world starts to lose its attraction for you. It is then that you start seeking, through philosophy, religion or spirituality, answer for the questions: 'Who am I?', 'What is the purpose of my life?', 'How can I be free of suffering?', 'Who or What is God?', 'What happens to me after death?'

We read books, and ponder on these philosophical questions. We seek out wise teachers or gurus who perhaps may be able to answer these profound questions. We may pray for the answers, or we may even doubt for a while that there is a Truth or God to be realised. But this is the beginning, generally where most of us start our spiritual journey of meditation. It is a process of emptying the mind of all that is of the non-Self, all the conditioning, ideas and wrong thinking, that is not our true divine nature. You have to empty yourself fully before the pure superconscious energies can freely flow through you. Having reached this state of emptiness and sincere searching, you soon start to realise the futile attempt to find Truth and happiness on the outside. Then you will begin to know that Reality, or the Self God, resides within you, and you must go within yourself to realise it.

Our spiritual journey is not always an easy one. Just by choosing to lead a spiritual life we are swimming against the current. The world around us is flowing in one direction but we have decided to go in another. Most people in the world are identified with their body, mind and personality characteristics, resulting in a false sense of separation from their true divine nature. By entering the spiritual path of meditation we have decided to remove this delusive error of perception by having direct knowledge of the Truth, Reality, or Self God; to experience directly in meditation what we are as pure existence-being.

In the early stages of your spiritual life it is quite likely that you will be faced with situations that show you what you need to work on – attachments you feel to desires of the world, strong inclinations of the ego, and dislikes towards certain things and certain people, that will test your ability to maintain right attitude. Your habits will probably be undisciplined and willpower ineffective. Old patterns of thoughts and emotions will surface which you will need to transform. You will have to mould the areas that are different into a new lifestyle so that there will be nothing in your subconscious mind that opposes what is in the conscious or superconscious mind. It is only when all three of these areas of consciousness act in harmony that meditation can be truly attained and sustained. In other words, you will have to reprogramme your subconscious mind to change through positive thinking, positive affirmations, and setting positive spiritual goals that will strengthen your will. As soon as strong initiative is taken to refine your personality, a new inner process will begin to take place within you.

Set the intention and resolve to meditate

To attain success in meditation you will need to cultivate dispassion and a strong aspiration or intense longing for Self-realisation. There are no short-cuts or instant success in meditation – it cannot be attained in a short while, it is a long and gradual process. It takes years of patient and steadfast effort to change the quality of the mind. A mind that has been conditioned through habit to seek enjoyment, pleasure and happiness outwardly for many years cannot be controlled, transcended and made pure overnight.

After setting the intention and making a resolve and commitment to meditating daily, you will then need to persevere with patience and vigilance over a long period of time.

To be successful in your spiritual practices and attain the greatest benefits from *Rāja Yoga* and *Kriyā Yoga* meditation, first set the intention to want to know the Absolute Truth. Whether we call the goal we are trying to reach Truth, Ultimate Reality, Absolute, *Brāhman*, *ātman*, *puruṣa*, Divine Self or God, know that it is the realisation of that highest and One Truth which liberates us from all illusion, ignorance, pain and suffering. Meditation is the key to unlock the secrets of life: it opens the doors of intuitive knowledge and leads us into realms of eternal Joy.

Decide now and positively resolve to make daily meditation part of your everyday life. Affirm that you will meditate on a regular daily basis with a clear sense of purpose for living, and for realising your true spiritual Divine nature; for becoming established in the awareness of your innermost Self, that is temporarily concealed, wrapped in the gross and subtle garments of the physical, astral and causal bodies.

Regular daily practice

Begin the habit of sitting for meditation at the same time, in the same place, and for the full length of time that you have set for yourself every day. Once you have developed this habit it will become easier to meditate. Then when you start to feel and experience the benefits of meditation – calmness, stillness, inner peace, inner joy, contentment, and feeling the energy – you will realise that meditation is actually your natural state of Being.

By practising regularly every day, you will reap the benefits that come from your sustained effort over a long period of time. When you establish stability in your meditation, you will create more freedom, balance, harmony, inner peace and joy in your life.

Train and discipline your mind to always put meditation first, by keeping it at the top of the list of your daily priorities, and remember to always practise with enthusiasm and joy! Meditation must never become a dull routine, with the thought that joy and freedom are a distant goal that you are trying to achieve. Your true eternal nature is Joy. So, always enter your meditation with the feeling that you are already free and are joy itself. Always remember, you are *Sat-chit-ānanda* (Ever-Existing, Ever-Conscious, Ever-New Bliss).

When to meditate

You can meditate at any time when it is convenient, but the most powerful times to meditate are at 6 am (sunrise), 12 noon, 6 pm (sunset) and 12 midnight. It is at these times that the gravitational pull of the sun works in harmony with the natural polarity of the human body.

In India, the yogis say that the most auspicious and peaceful time to meditate in the morning is between the early hours of 4 am and 6 am. This auspicious time is called *Brāhmamuhurta*. At this time there is the quality of peacefulness and goodness (*sattva*) predominant in the mind of the meditator and in the atmosphere. There is a natural peace and stillness in the atmosphere at this time which makes it particularly favourable for meditating. It is also at this time and at dusk that the energy in the *suṣumnā nāḍī* (main subtle energy channel) flows readily. You will know when the *suṣumnā nāḍī* is flowing, because your breath will be flowing equally through both nostrils. This is when the *prāṇa* is naturally balanced between the *iḍā* and *piṅgala nāḍīs*. Like the coastal tides, *prāṇa* flows back and forth, or rotates between predominance in the *iḍā* and *piṅgala nāḍīs*. During the daytime *prāṇa* is more active in *piṅgala nāḍī*, causing your consciousness to become more active and extroverted. While at night, *prāṇa* shifts to being more predominant in the *iḍā nāḍī*, causing you to become more introverted.

If you want to meditate early in the morning, then make sure you go to bed early enough. For example, if you are going to get up at 6am, you will probably need at least six or seven hours sleep to feel refreshed. So, you would need to be in bed by 10 or 11 pm. According to *Ā*yurvedic philosophy, *pitta* is most active in the middle of both the day and the night, so if you stay awake after 10 pm you will find it difficult to get to sleep properly as the vital force *pitta* ('to heat') has a fiery active nature. If you wish to live a healthy and balanced life then you will need to synchronise yourself actively with nature's rhythms.

Also, eat lightly at night. If you go to bed with a heavy meal in your stomach it will disturb your sleep, and you may not be able to get up early.

As you approach your evening meditation time and afterwards sleep, you need to prepare by relaxing your body, mind and nervous system. For the mind to be serene you should avoid reading the newspapers and watching television, as any stimulating or disturbing news or programmes may disturb or agitate your mind, causing you to become tense, restless or anxious. To keep your mind serene, be selective in what you watch, hear and read, and avoid arguments, heated debates and excessive talking, so that you may have a sound and restful sleep and rise refreshed early for meditation.

As soon as you awake at 6 am, get up immediately with the thought that you have an appointment with the Divine and that you are now going to meditate. You need to be careful that you do not procrastinate by allowing yourself to roll over and fall asleep again.

Length of meditation

If you are new to meditation, then sit for only 15 minutes in the beginning. It is more important to develop the constant habit of meditating regularly with alert attention than to sit for an hour feeling bored and restless, or to sit for half an hour one day and not meditate for the next few days.

Be consistent and regular in your practice. Begin with a daily 15-minute period of sitting for meditation, and try to sit for this period once in the morning and once in the evening, so that you have two meditations each day. If you can do this without creating any mental tension and can remain calmly centred without moving your body, then increase the length of your meditation to 20 minutes, and practise once or twice a day. As you progress and find it more comfortable and relaxed to sit, then you can gradually increase the amount of time you sit for your meditation. Longer meditations, practised with deep focus and devotion, will help you to meditate more deeply. Usually it takes at least 45 minutes to one hour to go deep in meditation. The active and restless mind that is outgoing needs this time to become calm before it can enter inward stillness. Until you are able to sit without effort for one hour, try a longer meditation once a week, perhaps at the weekend when you may have more time. You could also try sitting for a longer period of one and a half hours or more once a month. This could be your personal retreat into meditation.

As you progress, you will experience that the more you meditate, the more you want to meditate, because it will give you energy, joy, calmness, peace, contentment and creative inspiration. Rapid progress in meditation will depend on you being consistent and regular in your practice. It will require your aspiration, faith, sincerity, patience, perseverance, relaxed effort, interest and enthusiasm.

Where to meditate

For your daily sitting meditation, it is important to choose a private place, where you will not be disturbed, and which you will use regularly, and *only* for meditation. This will help to create a meditative vibration and a spiritual atmosphere in the place where you will sit. The place should be clean, comfortable, quiet and peaceful, with natural air-ventilation. Ideally, have a separate room in your home for meditation, otherwise you can use a corner or smaller space within a room. In this space, place a small cupboard or small table to make an altar with, and place on it candles, incense, sacred pictures of your guru, saints or deity, and fresh flowers as an inspirational focus. To keep the spiritual energy and vibrations of this sacred space pure do not allow anyone to eat, drink, smoke, sleep or socialise there.

If you can, try to have your altar positioned so that it faces east or north. This is because the polarity of the magnetic field of the Earth subtly influences us. Facing east or north will create a positive effect, while facing south will create a negative effect on the mind.

Meditation is a skill

If you find it difficult to go into meditative stillness, then set aside more time for each meditation session, and be willing to sit for a longer period of time to allow your thoughts to slow and settle down. As most experienced meditators will tell you, the meditative state of going into stillness usually occurs after between 45 minutes and one hour. So with a continued steady effort, you can reach this meditative state of inner stillness. Do not allow yourself to give up easily; if you feel a resistance to sitting longer, just remain seated and keep your awareness focused. Watch your resistance with detachment, and allow the resistant thoughts to dissolve with every exhalation of your breath as you mentally say, 'Let go.' The negative thought-energy will then dissolve.

If your body is uncomfortable and is causing your mind to be restless, then adjust your body position, stretch your legs slowly, and relax again into your sitting posture. Become aware of your breath and *mantra*. Stay aware and alert, and then you will gradually go deeper in your meditation and tap into your vital energy.

Maintain the right attitudes

The spiritual path of Yoga meditation is more than a technique, it is a way of life and requires the right attitude to life – to your relationship with others, your work, your study, and to God and Guru. Yoga is based on the classical teachings of Patañjali's *Yoga Sūtras*. In Patañjali's Eight Limbs of Yoga, the path of *Rāja Yoga* and *Kriyā Yoga*, he gives us the foundation stones on which to build our practice – *yamas* and *niyamas* – these are the right attitudes that we need to make our commitments.

No success can be attained on the path of Yoga without following the moral and ethical restraints (*yamas*), and observances, individual discipline (*niyamas*). These principles are an integral part of Yoga practice, and we cannot advance spiritually without practising them. They have to be continuously practised at all times.

GUIDELINES FOR PROGRESS IN MEDITATION

Vegetarian food is more sattvic than non-vegetarian

For a yogi, ideally a pure vegetarian or vegan diet is best for the practice of Yoga and meditation, as it has a more calming effect on the mind, and is more *sattvic*. There is more vital energy (*prāṇa*) in fresh, pure vegetarian foods to nourish your body and feed your mind. A vegetarian diet would include grains, beans and pulses, vegetables, nuts and fruits, and some dairy produce. A vegan diet (non-dairy) would mainly include grains, beans and pulses, vegetables, nuts and fruits.

According to the Yoga tradition, meat is considered impure, because its qualities are mainly composed of the *guṇas* of *tamas* (inertia) and *rajas* (dynamism, stimulation, activity), whereas the Yoga meditator seeks to increase the quality of *sattva* (illumination, lightness, purity) within their self, to dispel darkness. *Tamas* produces sluggishness, heaviness, dullness, and obstructs knowledge by ignorance; *rajas* generates aggressiveness, restlessness, pain and suffering. There is also the moral consideration. Eating meat involves harming the life of the animal, which goes against the Yoga principles of *yama* (moral and ethical restraints) of *ahiṃsā*, non-harming, non-violence. On all levels – ethical, physical, mental and spiritual – eating meat keeps one on a lower level of *rajasic* and *tamasic* consciousness. As humans our *dharma* (duty and responsibility) is to help, to protect and support, not to exploit and destroy. For a yogi or a true spiritual seeker of Truth, non-harming or non-violence is the highest principle.

Another reason for being vegetarian is that a vegetarian diet is the most energy-efficient and produces the lowest level of greenhouse gases. To produce one kilogram of meat requires seven kilograms of grain and 15 kilograms of pulses and 2500–6000 litres of water. To produce just one meat 'burger' requires the wasteful conversion of five square metres of rainforest into pasture or arable land. The amount of land required to feed just one meat-eater can feed 20 vegetarians. A cow can eat 50 kilos of grass a day and produce 500 litres of methane gas, releasing huge amounts into the atmosphere, and contributing to the pollution of the planet.

To nourish your mind and body and be soothing to your constitution, your food needs to be easily assimilated. As the *Bhāgavad Gītā* informs us, Yoga is not for those who eat too much or too little. Take everything in moderation.

Avoid all processed foods, and foods that are heavy and difficult to digest, such as meat and cheese, as these will be a drain on your energy.

Right attitude to eating

It is difficult and uncomfortable to meditate if you have a full stomach. A heavy meal impairs digestion, causing more blood to circulate to the stomach to assist in the digestive process. The after-effect of this makes it difficult to meditate; it will make you feel sleepy, as all the energy is directed into the digestion of the meal.

Eat only when your stomach is empty and avoid snacking between meals. Your stomach should be at least half-empty when you meditate. If you cup your hands together palm upwards and fill it with food, this would be about the right amount to eat at one meal, and would leave your stomach feeling comfortable.

Before a meal, always remember to wash your hands. Then try to put yourself into a calm, peaceful state of mind and remind yourself that you are about to receive elements that have been prepared for you in the laboratories of nature. Remember, God is in food in the form of life. God is life, and if food gives us life, it is because it contains God. That life needs to be raised to a higher spiritual level and stimulated and enhanced by our blessings, and above all by our gratitude. So, take a moment's silence, with your eyes closed and your hands joined in prayer give a blessing and thanks for the food you are about to eat:

> Receive Lord in Thy Light, the food we eat for it is Thine. Infuse it with Thy Love, Thy energy, Thy love divine. Aum, Amen.

Then, silently and in serenity, begin the process of nutrition. Proper digestion begins in the mouth where certain enzymes begin to break the food particles down, so chew your food for as long as possible – at least 30 times – until it turns to a liquid state, before you swallow it. By following this process you will train yourself to eat more mindfully with awareness. The subtlest processes are carried out in the mouth, for it is in the laboratory of the mouth that the etheric particles are absorbed and distributed to the mind and nervous system, whereas the denser elements are sent to the stomach.

Avoid sleeping too much or too little

The *Bhāgavad Gītā* tells us that Yoga is not for those who sleep too much or too little. Six or seven hours of restful sleep should be sufficient for most people, although children and persons who are ill may need more. Those who meditate regularly are able to sleep less hours than the average person, because both the body and mind are completely relaxed and rested in deep meditation. In fact, meditation revitalises the mind and body, giving them more rest than sleep.

It is also advised not to practise meditation if you are feeling very tired or lazy, if you are ill, or if your mind is in grief or extremely upset. The reason for this is that the mind will find it very difficult to concentrate.

Regulate your social life

For a meditator, too much socialising with worldly-minded people or people with secular interests can be distracting to the mind, and can lead to restlessness. Try to minimise any unnecessary or mundane talking as much as possible. Keep silence when you can and associate more with those people who are positive, optimistic and uplifting, who have a beneficial influence in your life, rather than those people who are negative, pessimistic and unsupportive.

Regulate your mental diet

When you have spare time, use it wisely. Do not waste your time and energy by sitting for hours in front of the television or playing video games, watching video films, and reading newspapers and novels. All the images and impressions from these things are distractions – they will sink into your subconscious mind and affect your conscious thinking and feelings. They will cause the mind to become restless and agitated, and then you will not be able to focus your concentration when you sit for meditation.

Read spiritually uplifting books that will inspire you to meditate. Study and understand the Yoga and meditation philosophy, such as Patañjali's *Yoga Sūtras* and the *Bhāgavad Gītā*, and know your true purpose in life. Develop your mental capacities to enable you to perceive accurately and improve your powers of creative imagination, will and positive intention.

OBSTACLES TO MEDITATION

In the *Yoga Sūtras* (1:30), Patañjali categorises nine obstacles (*antarāyas*) to one-pointed concentration that affect the activities of the mind, causing it to be distracted. These distractions of consciousness (*citta-vikṣepa*) that exist in the mind must be overcome if one is to enter one-pointed concentration (*ekāgratā*) and progress in meditation.

> *'Tat-pratiṣedhārtham eka-tattvābhyāsah.'*
> 'The persistent practice (*abhyāsa*) of one-pointed concentration on one single truth (*Īśvara*) is the best method to prevent the obstacles and their accompaniments (physical and mental disturbances).'
>
> *Yoga Sūtras 1:32*

It is by continuous, uninterrupted practice of *japa* of *Aum* (the Cosmic Vibratory Sound which indicates *Īśvara*, God) with one-pointed concentration at the Spiritual Eye, at the mid-point between the eyebrows, where the one truth, the absolute reality is experienced.

The nine obstacles (*antarāyas*) are:

1. **Disease (*vyādhi*).** The body and mind are intimately connected to each other. If the body becomes diseased or ill, causing pain and discomfort, the mind becomes affected and disturbed, making it very difficult for the mind to concentrate, meditate, and reach *samādhi*. That is why it is important for a meditator to remain fit and healthy, and to cultivate a spiritual awareness, so that one's thoughts and actions are positive and constructive in order to have a beneficial influence on the mind and body. To prevent disease and have total wellness you need to be committed to healthy living routines that support your spiritual practices, which means following a healthy lifestyle, eating a healthy diet, and taking sufficient exercise, sleep and rest. Take everything in moderation.
2. **Lack of interest (*styāna*).** Lack of interest is mental apathy and inertia. The mind becomes dull, which is a quality of *tamas guṇa*. The mind procrastinates

and makes excuses; there is an inability to put one's thoughts into action resulting in a lack of energy and focus. The mind becomes restless with distractions and is unable to constantly focus its attention for meditation. If it is not corrected there is the danger that the mind will return to worldly consciousness. It requires great willpower and energy to rise out of this mental inertia.

3. **Doubt (*samśaya*).** In the *Bhāgavad Gītā* (4:40) Sri Krishna informs us that doubt is one of the worst obstacles to higher consciousness: 'That person who is ignorant and without faith and of a doubting nature is lost. For the doubting self, there is no happiness nor success either in this world or the next.'

   The mind loses its steadiness if it hesitates and becomes uncertain by oscillating between two possibilities. The opposite of doubt (*saṃśaya*) is faith (*śraddha*). One needs to have faith in the true guru and the teachings he or she instructs. This faith develops when the disciple's interest and attraction towards spiritual knowledge increases. In the *Yoga Sūtras* (1:20), Patañjali tells us that *samādhi* (superconsciousness, absorption – the highest state of Yoga) is preceded by faith (*śraddha*), as well as energy, remembrance, awakening of wisdom, and meditation.

   The are many ways in which doubts can enter the mind, for example studying too many books of a varied nature written by different authors, each one contradicting the other, can cause confusion and doubt. When there is an absence of proper understanding of the guru and his teaching, it may cause one to keep changing one's guru and his teachings for another. Once you become convinced of the competency of your guru and the validity of his or her teachings and practice, what need is there for a change?

   It may take time and experience to develop faith and trust in the inner reality, but when it comes it brings clarity and calmness to the mind. When one has a genuine spiritual experience from meditation, it helps to strengthen one's faith by removing doubts, and inspiring one devotionally to attain the goal of oneness with the Divine Being.

4. **Carelessness (*pramadā*).** Carelessness or negligence is a lacking of interest in attending the object of concentration. It is lack of attention and mindfulness to the foundations such as *yamas* (restraints) and *niyamas* (observances), and *dhāraṇā* (concentration) that lead to *samādhi* (superconscious absorption). To progress spiritually one has to be self-disciplined, aware, and make a persistent effort.

5. **Lethargy (*alasya*).** *Styāna* is mental apathy, *alasya* is both mental and physical laziness. There is lack of effort and energy due to physical and mental heaviness (*tamas*). Lethargy paralyses the action of the mind to such an extent that the mind cannot even think properly in this state. Lethargy applies the brakes to onward progress. Such lethargy makes one unwilling to meditate; an indifference of attitude clouds over the seeker. Complacency sets in. The seeker may tell himself or herself: 'After all, I have made some progress. If today I don't sit for meditation, what does it matter? I'm too busy

today – I'll meditate tomorrow.' My guru, Paramhansa Yogananda, gives the appropriate answer to that: 'The most destructive shaft of *maya* delusion is unwillingness to meditate regularly and deeply, for by this attitude one prevents oneself from tuning in with God and Guru.' Those who do not meditate regularly usually become restless and give up after a short effort.

To overcome this obstacle of inertia and spiritual laziness, you need to change your consciousness, and not allow the narrow ego to obstruct or limit your full potential of attaining the Ultimate Reality. Willpower and energy are needed to make a sustained and determined effort. Cultivate positive mental attitudes and personal behaviours. If there is physical heaviness, then you may also need to change your diet and lifestyle, to make you feel more light-bodied and alert. Practise a vigorous *āsanas* sequence such as *Sūrya Namaskar* (Salutations to the Sun) daily, or some other stimulating exercise to awaken the energy in your body, and to get you out of the lethargic state. *Prāṇāyāma* will also help.

6. **Reluctance to give up sensuality (*avirati*).** Lethargy or torpidity is rather like a preparation for the contrary activity that is about to take place after some time. It is comparable to a dull, cloudy, silent sky, before the outbreak of thunder and lightning. Lethargy is a breeding ground for the mischief of the senses. They first paralyse the person by lethargy and then give him or her a blow by sensual excitement (*avirati*). The excited mind then jumps into various kinds of indulgence, and the fall into delusion from Yoga begins. Such mistaking of delusion for success is the subject of the next obstacle: false vision (*bhrānti-darśana*), by which one thinks one is progressing higher while falling down.

   Avirati is a lack of detachment and dispassion for indulgence and enjoyment of sensual attractions, which the mind gets attracted to and preoccupied with. To concentrate and meditate deeply with the mind calm and serene, one needs to withdraw the mind from sense cravings, sensual temptations and lustful desires, which pull one's energy downward in the spine to the lower centres of consciousness.

   This obstacle can be overcome by practising *vairāgya* (dispassion, detachment) and *abhyāsa* (repeated practice) by nurturing your spiritual growth. *Abhyāsa* is to know that all is One, that God is omnipresent, and to be constantly conscious that God is omnipresent. It is being established in Truth. *Vairāgya* is never to allow the idea of the world to arise in your mind. It simply means an absence of desires.

7. **False vision (*bhrānti-darśana*).** This is a state of false knowledge, and confused ideas, a distorted or deluded perception of what yogic attainment is. It is mistaking what is harmful to spiritual life as being beneficial and vice versa. It is taking truth as untruth, and distorting the teachings of the guru, or of Yoga scriptures. One needs to have a clear understanding and discernment at every stage of one's journey on the spiritual path.

8. **Losing the ground (*alabdha-bhūmikatvā*).** Even if by chance one recovers consciousness from deluded perception, it is not easy to regain ground that

has been once lost. Losing the ground (*alabdha-bhūmikatvā*) is a further obstacle in Yoga. One cannot start one's practice again with ease, due to the *saṁskāras* (past impressions stored in the subconscious mind) created by the impelling drive of the senses during the state of gratification.

This is the inability to know the real meaning and purpose of spiritual practice. As Patañjali states in his *Yoga Sūtras* (1.13): 'Practice is firmly grounded only after it has been cultivated properly and continuously for a long time.'

Without determined and completely unwavering self-effort one will not reach the higher levels of spiritual unfoldment.

9. **Instability (*anavasthitatvā*).** One may attain a certain state or level of Yoga, but due to ignorance, forgetfulness or carelessness one can become unstable and fail to maintain that state, lose interest in Yoga. and fall into worldly consciousness.

   When the mind is distracted it has the inability to maintain awareness and inner stability, thus it fails to attain the state of spiritual absorption, or if it is reached, to stay in that state of absorption (*samādhi*).

Kleśas – the five forces of ignorance

In addition to these nine obstacles Patañjali (*Yoga Sūtras* 2:3) recognises five more subtle and deeply rooted obstacles or psycho-physiological afflictions (*kleśas* – from the root *kliśh*, 'to cause pain') which disturb the equilibrium between the body, mind and self.

Ignorance of one's own real nature (*avidyā*)

Avidyā or ignorance is the root cause of the other four *kleśas*: egoism (*asmitā*), attachment (*raga*), aversion (*dveṣa*), and clinging to life or fear of death (*abhiniveṣa*). Ignorance exists in all four of these *kleśas*. It is a sequential chain action that causes suffering: ignorance breeds ego, the sense of self, which breeds attachment and aversion (likes and dislikes), which breeds clinging to this bodily individuality and a fear for the thought of the death of this body.

Ignorance is the belief that one knows, being all the while in error and misunderstanding. It is the root cause of all suffering. The ignorant, who lack awareness, confuse the temporary with the permanent, the pure with the impure, that which is painful with the pleasure, and that which is the ego-self with the true inner Self.

Egoism (*asmitā*)

First there is ignorance (*avidyā*). Then there comes the idea of the 'I', *asmitā* (ego-sense). Once the idea of 'I' is there it becomes the centre of the entire universe. *Asmitā* (I-am-ness) is not merely the ego, in the sense of vanity, but the essence of I-am-ness, the core of one's existence. It is this false identification of this sense of I-am-ness as being one's true nature, the Self (*ātman*). Through ignorance (*avidyā*) our sense of being becomes distorted and limited to the body and the mind. From one moment to the next we are constantly identifying with our physical and mental states; one moment we are happy, the next moment we are unhappy. It is the mind that experiences these changing states. Our true inner being or true nature is changeless, pure consciousness that is eternal, intelligent and Self-illuminated. The mind, which is an intermediary between the body and the Self, cannot be self-luminous, because it is an object of inner perception.

The true Self is the constant witness, ever present and ever aware of the appearance and disappearance of every mode, state, and function of the mind. It is only when we awaken to the true knowledge of our Divine nature that the veil of ignorance in the form of *asmitā* (I-am-ness) is removed.

Attachment (*rāga*)

From this 'I' comes *rāga* (attachment, attraction, approval, or liking).

As a result of our continued distorted self-understanding by identifying with the body-mind, we descend further into the affliction of *rāga* (attachment). Pleasure is based on attachment and desire. The more intense the desires, the more obstructions are experienced, bringing greater aversion. Desire brings pain in both the enjoyment of pleasure and in the obstruction of pleasure. We are all trying to avoid pain, but most of us pursue pleasure – and through our intense desires and attachment, which bring suffering, we experience pain. The mind clings to that which it identifies, thinking that its security comes from there. 'My security comes from there; without that I cannot live happily; without that I cannot live peacefully. My whole life is dependent upon that person, or that organisation or that group.' Being so thoroughly committed to this notion, you feel happy in that company. Once the feeling of happiness has arisen, the mind seeks that company more. It is a vicious circle – totally irrational – therefore no amount of reasoning is going to get us to an understanding of the truth concerning it.

Why is somebody's company pleasant to me? Because I have decided it is so – there is no other reason. In my own fear of loneliness I have chosen to identify myself with that person, calling that person my wife or husband, my son, or whatever it is. I have created this pleasure sensation within myself – it does not come from outside, it is in me. Unable to face self-ignorance, I have created the relationship and then I cling to it. Then I attribute pleasure to it. When I attribute pleasure to it, the mind flows towards it and the vicious circle is formed. Pleasure and pain and all the relationships based on that are totally irrational and therefore no amount of thinking concerning it can ever solve that.

Is there a way of looking at it without thinking? That is the problem of Yoga. Patañjali in his *Yoga Sūtras* (2:3) points out that these five *kleśas* (afflictions) – *avidyā*, *asmitā*, *rāga*, *dveṣa* and *abhiniveṣa* (ignorance, egoism, likes, dislikes and clinging to life) – are sources of psychological distress. Self-ignorance; identification (or the personality formation, which is the direct and immediate result of self-ignorance); 'I like this', 'I don't like this', and the fear of being a nobody (*abhiniveṣa*). When the identity is not known you feel frightened – you feel frightened to be a nobody. That is why we are all afraid to die – because then we are no*body*. Because this nobody frightens me, when I do not know who I am (what the identity is) I want to create an identity – 'I am Swāmi so and so.' That makes me sound solid strong and powerful! 'I am an American', 'I am a Christian.' That makes me part of an enormous beehive, a group, community, organisation, or even a religion, so that if you come against me, all of us will be against you.

To overcome this attachment one needs discriminative wisdom to not identify the activities of one's mind and body with the inner Self (*puruṣa*, *ātman*), the experiencer within.

Aversion (*dveṣa*)

Dveṣa is dislike, aversion or rejection. When you experience pleasure it creates a memory of happiness in your mind, and you want a repetition of it; and wanting the repetition sets up a craving, which is pain; and when you cannot have it when you want it, then it becomes painful. The very thought that this pleasure is going to end is painful. What makes it pleasure temporarily? Only your ignorance of its nature and your ignorance of your own true identity. When the attainment of a desire is thwarted, prevented or obstructed in any way, it gives rise to aversion (*dveṣa*), which causes delusion and suffering. It is a vicious circle because through aversion to pain we seek out and cling to that which is pleasurable. The aversion causes attachment and so creates an obstacle to experiencing the true ever-blissful inner Self.

Clinging to life/fear of death (*abhiniveṣa*)

Abhiniveṣa is often translated as 'blind clinging to life'. Why are we clinging to this life knowing that it will come to an end? We are clinging to this physical body even though it is bound to perish. Patañjali has concisely, precisely and scientifically expounded the facts of life and even says concerning this: *svārasavāhī viduṣo'pi* (*Yoga Sūtras* 2:9) – 'This blind clinging to life is there, it seems to be self-sustaining, and it is found even in wise persons.' Even very wise enlightened persons are irrationally unwilling to shed the body.

Abhiniveṣa is the instinctive yearning to live forever by perpetuating the existence of the physical body. It is the identification and attachment and clinging to the body and life that creates fear of death and an obstacle to experiencing the pure Self or pure Being that dwells in us all. This instinctive feeling of being immortal is not of the physical body, which is limited by the dimensions of time, space and causation, but of your very own Self, which is without form and has the quality of life *Sat-chit-ānanda* (Ever-Existing, Ever-Conscious, Ever-New Bliss). The divine Self is eternal Truth and Consciousness, and Bliss forever in Existence. Bliss is your true essence and nature; you are neither the body nor the mind. Ultimately, this clinging to life which is inherent within every individual mind can only be eliminated by transcending the identification with being the individual sense of 'I'.

This clinging to life that is known to be ephemeral, temporary, which is found even amongst the wisest, absurd though it seems, is a trend away from the centre, away from cosmic intelligence. Even though there is only this one single ocean of cosmic intelligence (which constitutes all the universe, including us), somehow or other there is this feeling 'I am', or rather 'I' is, the ripple, the wave, an individual entity.

The wave is not different from the ocean. The ocean is the entire volume of water, including what we call the current, the wave, the *vṛtti* (vortice of feeling). The diversity arises because you and I have created it. There is nothing called the Atlantic Ocean as distinct from the Pacific Ocean. It is one indivisible mass of water. To the ocean it is all ocean, it does not know anything about individual waves, parts. But somehow on account of that mysterious power we call *Māyā* (Illusion), *avidyā* or ignorance, the ocean limits itself, and that self-limited ocean is referred to as 'wave'. Why does this self-limitation occur? No answer. No one can answer these questions – Buddha remained serenely silent when asked such questions. He responded merely, 'When your house is on fire would you ask about the chemical composition of the fire or would you go and put the fire out?'

Even so, questions about God's reason for creating the world are irrelevant to us. One sees that in spite of one's intuitive perception or understanding, faith or belief that there is just the one indivisible cosmic being, and that the one being or ocean limits itself to the status of a wave, the wave immediately becomes as it were the centre of the ocean. From that wave's viewpoint, to the right is East and to the left is West. Otherwise these directions have no meaning whatsoever. The tragedy, the problem of our world, is that the human being, the individual, each 'I', becomes the centre of the universe as soon as the ego-sense arises. Why do two individuals fight? Because each one feels, assumes, that he or she is the centre and that everything must somehow be related to his or her pleasure, to his or her will.

This self-limited cosmic being which is the individual personality, *asmitā* or ego-sense, then goes on building relationships, assuming relationships. It is all ignorance! The child and the grandchild of ignorance can only be ignorance, just as all offspring of man can only be human. So everything which manifests in this cosmic being, Cosmic Consciousness, is born of ignorance. The self-limited ocean which is called the individual looks around, feels around, registers and reacts. Visualise a medium-sized wave in the ocean looking at a big wave with fear, anticipating, 'You are going to swallow me.' The medium-sized wave then looks at the little wave with superiority and contempt, and so it goes on. Fear, contempt, like, dislike, attraction, repulsion, approval, disapproval – all spring from the ignorant self-limitation that is called the ego. All these identifications, thoughts and feelings, pleasures and pains, likes and dislikes, are *vṛttis*. 'I' or ego is the central wave.

HOW TO OVERCOME THE OBSTACLES AND AFFLICTIONS

In the following *Yoga Sūtras* of Patañjali it is explained how to overcome the obstacles to Self-realisation.

> '*Īśvara* is the supreme Self, totally unaffected by afflictions of life (*kleśas*), actions and their consequent reactions (*karma*), or potential seed impressions (*saṁskāras*) of latent desires.'
>
> *Yoga Sūtras 1:24*

Īśvara, the inner ruler, the supreme principle of life, is *puruṣa-viśeṣaḥ* (a special or unique Conscious Being). This supreme and pure Consciousness that is omnipotent, omniscient and omnipresent is beyond duality; it is not conditioned by time, space nor causation. It expresses absolute Intelligence, and due to its intrinsic nature it transcends the totality of manifestation, making it both transcendent and immanent.

> 'The word that expresses *Īśvara* (the supreme Self) is the sacred syllable *Aum* (*Oṁ*). This is the *Praṇavaḥ* (primary Cosmic Sound Vibration of creation).'
>
> *Yoga Sūtras 1:27*

> 'Repetition of the sacred syllable (*Aum*), listening to it, and becoming absorbed in it (in deep meditation) with faith and devotion (*bhāvanam*) reveals its divine nature.'
>
> *Yoga Sūtras 1:28*

> 'From that practice (meditation on the inner sound of *Aum*), consciousness turns within, and realising its own true Self the obstacles cease to be.'
>
> *Yoga Sūtras 1:29*

The *Bhagavad Gītā* gives a similar method:

> 'Having closed all the gates (senses) of the body, and confining the mind in the heart centre, channeling the vital breath to the brain, established in Yoga (one-pointed) concentration, reciting the single-syllable *Aum* that signifies *Brāhman*, and meditating on Me, one who departs, renouncing the body, attains the supreme goal.'
>
> *Bhāgavad Gītā 8:12–13*

> *'Avidyā kṣetram uttareṣam prasupta-tanu-vicchinnodāraṇām.'*
> 'Ignorance is the field of growth of the other afflictions (*kleśas*), whether they are in a dormant, weak, alternated, or fully active state.'
>
> *Yoga Sūtras 2:4*

Ignorance (*avidyā*) is the root cause of all other afflictions (*kleśas*).

Just as a field of soil supports different plants, seeds, weeds and grass, so ignorance supports these five *kleśas* (afflictions) – *avidyā*, *asmitā*, *rāga*, *dveṣa* and *abhiniveṣa* (ignorance, egoism, likes, dislikes and clinging to life). And just as a fruit seed sown in the field of soil will germinate, and in time will grow into a tree and bear fruit, the seeds of afflictions (*kleśas*) germinate in the soil of ignorance (*avidyā*) and bear the fruit of suffering.

The *kleśas* manifest in four different states:

1. **Dormant (*prasupta*).** This is when the *kleśas* reside in the mind as potential seeds to become active in the future (except ignorance, *avidyā*, which is always manifest and never dormant, because it is their cause and support).

2. **Weak (*tanu*).** The afflictions and desires are gradually weakened, they become subtle, and are made dormant as one makes a persistent effort through the spiritual practices of Yoga and meditation. This is why self-discipline and regular practice is so important on the spiritual path. They can also be weakened by cultivating a state of mind that is the opposite of the *kleśas*.

3. **Alternating or counteracted (*vicchinna*).** The afflictions alternate between being active and inactive. For example, when the *kleśa* of attraction or

attachment (*rāga*) is present, anger and aversion (*dveṣa*) is not operative. This means that the power of aversion has been subdued and made latent by the intensity of attraction. Aversion may succeed attachment, but they cannot occur simultaneously. It is also interesting to note that, when attachment is seen with reference to one object, it is not non-existent in regard to another object or person. For example, if a person is attached to a particular woman, it does not mean that he is uninterested in another woman. His attachment has attained manifestation in regard to one, but he may become attracted to another woman in the future. These future *kleśas* of attachment are either in a dormant, weak or counteracted state.

The difference between dormant and counteracted *kleśas* is that dormant ones may take many lifetimes to appear and manifest, whereas the counteracted ones can be awakened and set in motion by the slightest stimulus.

4. **Fully active (*udāra*).** These are the afflictions that are functioning and are fully operative in the present.

A fifth state of *kleśas*

Although Patañjali only gives four different states in which the five *kleśas* manifest, there is also a fifth state according to the great sage Vyāsa. The fifth state is an inoperative state in which the *kleśas* (afflictions), that have a potential energy like seeds to germinate, are roasted or burnt and therefore made unproductive, completely losing their potential to germinate again. Just as seeds roasted by fire are made unproductive, so the Self (*ātman*, *puruṣa*) is no longer connected to the seeds of affliction (*kleśas*), which have been roasted by the knowledge of Truth.

According to the great sage Śaṅkāra, the most eminent philosopher of India, Patañjali did not include this fifth state because roasted seeds would not apply to everyone. It is not common in the ordinary person, but is only present in yogis who have reached the final liberation (*kaivalya*), through deep meditative absorption in *nirbija samādhi* (total absorption in which consciousness is established in itself, producing a permanent state of blissful, omniscient superconsciousness) – the state which very few persons achieve. In such a yogi, the mind (*citta*) remains active in order to keep the body functioning while living in the world, but it no longer responds to the stimuli that activate the *kleśas* in the presence of an object of the senses. The mind and the roasted seeds are resolved back into their original source (*prakṛiti* – matter principle), so that they have no potential to germinate again. As long as the mind (*citta*) exists, the afflictions will also exist.

> *'Te pratiprasava-heya sūkṣmāh.'*
> 'These inner afflictions (five *kleśas*) are subtle (*sūkshma*). They are eliminated by resolving them back into their original cause.'
>
> *Yoga Sūtras 2:10*

Patañjali teaches us that to overcome the five *kleśas* – the sources of psychological distress, disturbance or distraction that are subtle and can manifest in numerous forms of expression – then first they have to be weakened and reduced by the practices of

Kriyā Yoga (*tapas*, self-discipline; *svādhyāya*, self-study; and *Īśvara-praṇidhāna*, devotion to the Supreme Being), and then eradicated by the practice of meditation (*dhyāna*).

The *kleśas* can be likened to seeds lying dormant embedded in the soil, with their potency to germinate. Some of the seeds are active and can be recognised by their outer expression of a seedling beginning to sprout, while other seeds may be weak and will not germinate until the proper conditions are favourable. Still others may have no potency whatsoever to germinate.

The relation that exists between the five *kleśas* can also be likened to the interconnection between root, trunk, branches, leaves and fruit of a tree, each forming a connected series of causes and effects. The root (*mūla*) is the origin of the tree. In our analogy of the *kleśas* with the tree, the mind is like a field in which the root of the tree is the ultimate source of ignorance (*avidyā*). The root and trunk of the tree are the afflictions and the branches and leaves are the desires. As long as the root is present, it is going to generate action, and cause desires to grow, and therefore cause psychological distress, disturbance and distraction.

Ignorance is the fundamental cause of the *kleśas* (afflictions). It gives rise to ego-sense, which cannot be understood by the mind because it is born of the mind, and is part of the mind. Ignorance is known by its fruits. By cutting the root of ignorance with the axe of knowledge of Truth, the afflictions and desires are no more – they resolve back into their cause.

'Dhyāna-heyās tad-vṛttayah.'
'In the active state the *kleśas* (afflictions) are destroyed by meditation (*dhyāna*).'

Yoga Sūtras 2:11

In the above *sūtra* (2.11), Patañjali gives the words *tad-vṛttayah*, confirming that *vṛttis* (vortices of feeling) are produced by the *kleśas*.

The threefold process of eradicating these *kleśas* is illustrated by the analogy of a cloth that needs to be cleaned of impurities. First, the heavy dirt that is soiling the cloth is shaken away or washed off. Then, the finer, ingrained dirt is removed. But to completely remove the stains from the cloth it would have to be destroyed. Similarly, *Kriyā Yoga*, the Yoga of action, consisting of *tapas*, *svādhyāya* and *Īśvara-praṇidhāna*, weakens and eliminates the gross impurities, expressed as fully active *kleśas*. Then, the deeper subtle (*sūkshma*) *kleśas* or impurities are removed by further care and effort with meditation (*dhyāna*), which is synonymous with discriminating knowledge (*prasaṅkhyāna*). To completely remove all the subtle impressions there has to be a complete dissolution of the mind, which is attained in *asamprājñāta samādhi*, also known as *nirbija samādhi* or *nirvikalpa samādhi* – 'without support'. This is the highest and final state of total absorption, in which consciousness is established in itself.

SPIRITUAL PROGRESS

> 'A secret of progress lies in self-analysis. Introspection is a mirror in which to see portions of your mind which otherwise would remain hidden from you. Analyse what you are, what you wish to become, and what tendencies or shortcomings are impeding you. Decide what your deep and secret task is – your mission in life.'
>
> *Yogananda 2008b, p.21*

After engaging in spiritual practice for a short period of time, often the question arises, 'Have I made spiritual progress?' or 'How much spiritual progress have I made since I started meditation?'

Unfortunately these questions do not have straightforward answers. It is difficult to give a precise answer, because first we need to understand that the inner Self, our true identity, our essential Being, is pure, ever perfect and ever the same. It does not need improving, for the Self which is Pure Consciousness is complete, whole and perfect. It cannot progress or regress, and nothing needs to be added to it or taken away from it. The Self cannot be known by the intellect because the intellect is itself empowered by the Self. You perceive the activity of the mind by the light of the Self. You are the eternal Self – that consciousness with which you experience your very own existence – it is not something you have to attain.

So what is actually meant by the term 'spiritual progress'? What needs improving or changing? And how can we measure our progress?

Let us think of measuring our progress in terms of improving the quality not of our inner Self but of our mind. For a mind that is conditioned, restless, scattered, non-attentive and ruled by bad habits can never gather enough momentum to make spiritual progress.

Habits are your deadliest enemy

Every day our thoughts and actions are frequently repeated, forming habit patterns in our subconscious mind. From a positive point of view our habits free our conscious mind to concentrate on the necessary things that help us run our lives more efficiently, or to balance our lives. Without habit, we would be very limited in our freedom to accomplish anything. Paramhansa Yogananda used to say, 'It is not your passing thoughts or brilliant ideas but your everyday habits that control your life' and 'Habits are your deadliest enemy.'

To be free from the desires, bad habits, and negative or wrong attitudes formed from subconscious thoughts and actions, you need first to become aware of the habit patterns that are subconsciously controlling and directing your life. Once you have recognised them, then you can take the necessary action to change those patterns that are holding back your progress.

But beware, the mind will not easily abandon its old habits, even knowing that they cause you sorrow and suffering. The power of the suggestions from the subconscious mind is very strong!

The attention of the mind needs to be focused with awareness, and turned within, so that all the energies of the mind are brought under control. Your mind is an instrument of your inner Self; it is here to serve you, not to control you. If you are a slave to your mind and senses you cannot be happy or have inner peace, and you cannot experience the calmness and stillness of your inner Being, the image of God within you, whose divine eternal nature is *Sat-chit-ānanda* (Ever-Existing, Ever-Conscious, Ever-New Bliss).

Measuring your spiritual progress

> 'The four stages of spiritual progress are introspection, devotion, renunciation, illumination. Introspection is perception of the soul's qualities. Devotion is unconditional love for God. Renunciation is freedom from domination of the ego. Illumination is realisation of absolute oneness in God.'
>
> *Lahiri Mahasaya*

You can measure your own spiritual progress by improving the quality of your mind. This is not an easy or quick process by any means. For some people it can take years, and yet for others only months. Both patience and determination are required; you cannot expect quick results. If you sow a seed in the earth and pour water over it, and then the next day dig up the seed to find out how much it has grown, will you see any progress? Or if you were to plant a young sapling pear tree, and then every ten minutes measure how much it has grown, would you notice any progress in its growth? The answers are obvious. A much longer time would have to elapse before you had noticed how much growth or progress had occurred. And so it is with your spiritual progress. It takes place slowly and gradually over a long period of time, and it is almost impossible to perceive. It is no easy task to eradicate years of ingrained habits that enslave us – wrong attitudes and uncoordinated behaviour. Through sense indulgence and an undisciplined mind, we stubbornly hold on to and nurture these traits all our life.

In this technological age that we are now living in, everything seems to be moving fast. The irony of it is that although our latest mobile phones, tablets, iPads, laptops and other techno time-saving devices or gadgets have given us more freedom to communicate speedily, speed has not saved us time to truly relax for we tend to fill the time we save with more work and more tasks. The faster our lives become, the further we distance ourselves from our spiritual centre and Source – the inner Self. On our outward journey through our senses we forget the inward journey and the discovery of the God within us. Everything else in life seems to take on a greater importance than our divine mission to be Self-realised and united in God, the infinite goal. If your mind is only identified with your outward activities you cannot be consciously aware of the Divinity within you.

To grow and progress spiritually you will need to make a great and determined effort with patience to succeed. The dissipated forces of the mind will need to be gathered together until the mind becomes one-pointed through concentration. You should have one desire to fulfil your purpose in life – Self-realisation, to be united with the Absolute Truth. All your activities need to be directed towards that one goal. One-pointedness of mind through concentration and meditation is an important requisite to help you accomplish that. Without gathering together and concentrating the energy of the mind, the deeper state of meditation is not possible.

It takes willingness and willpower, and a strong, persistent effort, to overcome the habits that keep us enslaved to our desires, negative attitudes, negative thinking and wrong behaviour.

If your mind is scattered, restless and agitated, it becomes gross and limited in its function and power. And when that happens you lose awareness of that higher consciousness which is spiritual. As long as your mind has not realised its true nature, it will be restless and unsteady.

It is when your mind is quiet, calm and still, in unity in its subtlest state, that your own spiritual Self, your inner Divine Reality, becomes revealed to you. Deep meditation brings you to that higher state of consciousness.

Two types of restlessness

1. Restlessness arises due to desires. When you cannot satisfy your desire it turns into frustration, then anger, which leads to jealousy, envy, resentment and hatred.
2. When one advances spiritually and desires are eradicated from the mind, then a momentous longing compels the soul for the realisation of the Absolute, the Infinite Spirit.

The restless mind and the river of thoughts

> 'Whenever the fickle and unsteady mind wanders from its course, the yogi should restrain it, and bring it under the control of the Self.'
>
> *Bhāgavad Gītā 6.26*

The mind and its flow of restless thoughts can be compared to a river. If the water's flow is fast, the river flows fast. If the water is polluted then the river is polluted. Similarly, the mind is conditioned and defined by its thoughts. If the thoughts are restless, the mind is restless. If the thoughts are impure, the mind is impure. If the thoughts are positive, the mind is positive.

A river that is flooded and flowing its course with a tremendous momentum cannot be easily controlled; it sweeps away everything in its path. Similarly, as thoughts gather momentum they can take on a powerful force causing us to get swept away in uncontrollable emotions. Anger, for example, usually caused by the obstruction of one's desires, can be very powerful to the extent that it can cause sorrow and suffering to oneself and to others. To control the force of anger we have to first wait until the flood of angry thoughts have subsided. Like a quiet flowing river we need to maintain a steady flow on a single line of positive thought, or one idea, excluding all distracting, restless and agitated thoughts. This is concentration (*dharāna*). And if the flow is further reduced through deep focused concentration, the mind will become still like a calm and clear lake. This is meditation (*dhyāna*).

SIX QUALITIES OF GAINING CONTROL OF YOUR MIND

1. Calmness (*śama*)
2. Self-control (*dama*)
3. Self-withdrawal (*uparati*)
4. Forbearance (*titikṣa*)
5. Faith (*śraddha*)
6. Tranquillity (*samādhāna*).

1. Calmness (śama)

Calmness is one of the spiritual qualities of your true spiritual nature or Self within you. Paramhansa Yogananda eloquently stated that calmness is the living breath of God's immortality within you.

To have control of your mind you need to practise even-minded calmness, by remaining calm under all circumstances, so that nothing ruffles or disturbs you. This can be cultivated and maintained by regular deep meditation and awareness.

Calmness is the opposite of excitement, nervousness, restlessness, or being upset. Calmness is deeper than peace – it brings inner contentment and harmony.

The *Kriyā Yoga* meditation technique of Paramhansa Yogananda called *Hong Sau* deepens the concentration and brings deep calmness to the mind.

2. Self-control (dama)

> 'One who has perfect self-control acts in this world unaffected by it. Inwardly free from attraction and aversion, and under the control of the Self, one attains inner calmness.'
>
> *Bhāgavad Gītā 2.64*

Self-control, or self-mastery, is the ability and power to control one's emotions, speech and behaviour. It is also the discipline of restraining the sense-organs. The senses are so easily distracted and attracted to their objects, causing indulgence and attachment, ending in suffering and sorrow. It is the repetition of thoughts and actions that lead to the formation of bad habits. Control of the senses helps to control the mind, and through control of the mind egoism is eradicated, leading to Self-realisation. Self-control brings you a greater joy than the fleeting happiness indulged in the senses, because the consciousness returns to its own cause, its own Self that is motivated by this effort.

Self-control is not merely negation, but the channelling and redirecting of creative energies. True freedom means the power to act from the discrimination and guidance of the inner Self, not by instincts, impulses, whims, emotions and desires. True happiness is only gained when your will is guided by Self-discrimination.

You have to be vigilant and discipline your desires and impulses. To be free from the desires and impulses of the senses requires discrimination and willpower, and, as Yogananda said, 'Won't power!'

When your desires are not restrained or under your control the consequences can be very troublesome. For example, imagine a strawberry cheesecake. If your eyes see a delightful looking strawberry cheesecake, and your tongue tastes it, a message is communicated from your taste buds to your brain recording in your memory that this cake tastes absolutely delicious! It is so delicious that you want to repeat the experience, so you eat another slice of the cake, and perhaps another slice as well. Your desire for sensual delight continues until you can no longer eat another slice. Then, the suffering begins. You experience an uncomfortable feeling of having over-indulged in your senses. For those few moments of sensual indulgence it was as if the universe was not big enough to fill your passion. That tendency is what you have to be vigilant with. You have to very careful that your senses do not go out of control and create a habit. If you repeatedly do something, you will form a habit pattern. Habits are the results of your repeated actions that form your personality and your character.

The *niyamas* (personal observances/discipline) of Yoga are also helpful here. The second *niyama*, contentment (*santoṣa*), helps you to cultivate happiness in this present moment, and be content in not desiring or wanting more. It is not thinking, 'I shall be happy when I get everything I want.' But affirming, 'I have no lack or limitation. Centred in the oneness of Divine Consciousness as my spiritual Source, I am perfect and complete. As an expression of the Divine, I am infused with God's infinite wisdom and guided in wise and loving ways.'

The third *niyama* is *tapas* (austerity). Without austerity, it is so very easy to give into temptation and fall into sense indulgence. With the discipline of austerity you are able to establish boundaries for your senses.

Self-control educates the senses and gives you total freedom, allowing you to go beyond limitations, so that you may reach the Supreme goal of life. Expecting long-lasting joy from short-lived sense objects gives you only a momentary feeling of happiness. What you are really seeking is a sense of completeness.

In your will lies the greater, unlimited power of the Divine Will, that can help you to overcome all temptations, difficulties and obstacles that may trouble you. It is for you to utilise the divine gift of your dynamic willpower, so that you can direct your own destiny. You have tremendous power to improve your mind and personality; by using willpower to guide your thoughts, you can transform yourself. To progress spiritually and succeed it is important to know and train your mind in right ways. Give your mind the spiritual route to follow, then lead it in the right direction. Do not postpone your happiness – make the spiritual effort now, and make it your best effort!

If the ripples and waves of the river of thoughts that flow from the mind are not calmed, the true Self within cannot be experienced or realised. Be still and know that you are the God Self within. In that inner stillness you will experience your very existence of true joy and freedom.

3. Self-withdrawal (uparati)

> 'The result of dispassion is knowledge, that of knowledge is withdrawal from sense pleasures, which leads to the experience of the Bliss of the Self.'
>
> *Adi Shankaracharya, in Madhavananda 2003, p.159*

The absorption of the mind in the Supreme Consciousness by realising the Self in all objects is known as withdrawal of the mind.

In self-withdrawal a person's mental condition is not affected by the disturbance created by external objects, nor the internal attachment for egoism.

4. Forbearance, or silent endurance (titikṣa)

Silent endurance is an invaluable quality that gives you inner strength, helping you to overcome difficulties and obstacles along the spiritual path. This is also associated with *tapasya* or austerity, the second *niyama*. It includes accepting whatever happens as the best for your spiritual practice, and not being disturbed or ruffled by any discomfort that you may experience. It is accepting change calmly with equanimity and performing your duties in a spirit of inner freedom.

Whether in success or seeming failure you remain even-minded, knowing that the Divine Will is being accomplished. When you persevere with silent endurance, attuned to the Divine Will, you will have the inner power to conquer all difficulties.

True forbearance is a result of the mind being directed by an inner conviction that the divine goal of life is fulfilled through attaining Self-realisation. Knowing this to be true, the mind cooperates with the inner Self, facing all difficulties, challenges and obstacles – in joy and sorrow, success and seeming failures – to attain that Divine goal.

5. Faith (śraddha)

> 'One who possesses faith (*śraddha*) acquires knowledge.'
>
> *Bhāgavad Gītā 4.39*

Śraddha means implicit deep faith, which includes respect, trust, self-confidence and fearlessness. *Śraddha* is a natural inclination for those following the spiritual path with devotion. Deep faith is beyond mere belief; through deep faith you can conquer any doubts within yourself about the spiritual path, your guru and his teachings, and the goal of spiritual freedom or liberation. The spiritual path can be very challenging at times. Your patience, self-confidence and faith may be tested at any time as obstacles or difficulties arise. You will need implicit faith and inner strength to get you through those difficult times.

For the *tamasic* person whose mind is dulled, faith is inert. For a *rajasic* person, faith is active but with self-interest. In the *sattvic* person, faith is expressed with love and devotion, with intense spiritual enthusiasm.

Having firm faith in your spiritual ideal and belief in the existence of the Self is the first real step you take on the spiritual path. You begin your search with implicit faith in the possibility of knowing the Truth, knowing the Self within.

6. *Tranquillity (samādhāna)*

> 'For one aspiring to attain Yoga, action is said to be the means; for one who has already attained Yoga, tranquillity is said to be the means.'
>
> *Bhāgavad Gītā 6.3*

Tranquillity is the inner poise, perfect vibrationless peace, attained as a result of constant meditation, and contemplation of the Supreme Reality. It is to live every moment of one's life in the awareness and Presence of the Divine by inner attunement, devotion and dedication to that one principle.

SELF-DISCIPLINE – AN IMPORTANT KEY TO SPIRITUAL PROGRESS

> 'One who is regulated in eating and recreation, disciplined in actions, and moderate in sleep and wakefulness, attains Yoga, which destroys all suffering.'
>
> *Bhāgavad Gītā 6.17*

The word discipline comes from *discipulus*, the Latin word for 'instruction', 'knowledge'. Spiritual disciplines, known in Sanskrit as *sādhana*, are a means of self-instruction that we engage in for developing our inner spiritual awareness and one-pointedness towards Self-realisation. Self-discipline is a self-commitment to regulating yourself through disciplining your mind, speech and actions. It requires your zeal, enthusiasm, willingness, energy and determination; without these you will not succeed in your spiritual progress.

Discipline is divinely inherent in the universe, nature and humanity. Everything on our planet Earth is governed by physical laws of discipline and order. In the universe, the planets adhere to the discipline of staying in their own orbits. The universe could not exist harmoniously if there were not some established discipline and orderliness. Every living creature – human beings, mammals, birds, fish, insects and plants – acts according to its own disciplining law. In the insect world, ants are very self-disciplined. You will not find ants wandering around idly and aimlessly. They are self-disciplined in everything they do, and achieve incredible tasks. Such disciplines are necessary to bring order and harmony; without discipline there would be utter confusion and chaos in both the world and the universe.

Discipline is essential for success in all fields of life. At the social level we all practise the external discipline of following national or state laws, social norms and work ethics. At the individual level we have internal discipline, with which we choose to discipline ourselves. Discipline gives you the power to attain your goals in life. When you are disciplined you can be more productive and achieve more, because it creates space for your daily duties to be performed effortlessly. Being disciplined saves you both time and energy. So much time and energy is wasted in sense-indulgence – a joy that is short-lived – but the joy you attain through discipline is long-lasting.

Discipline is even more important when consciously following a spiritual path such as Yoga. To discipline yourself is absolutely essential for attaining success in your spiritual effort. Without discipline you will not be able to accomplish the purpose of life.

Guided by the spiritual wisdom of the great gurus and sages, and their holy texts, you can adopt a course of spiritual discipline that will give you the inner strength to overcome any obstacles that may arise. The greater the progress you wish to make on the spiritual path, the more self-discipline you will need to engage in. But never think of discipline as being a burden, a fearful punishment, a penitence, or restricting in any way; rather as an opportunity to end your delusion and give you success, fulfilment, joy and inner freedom. Without self-discipline an individual has no control over his or her own mind or senses, and so finds no lasting happiness or self-fulfilment.

A key point in Self-discipline is attention. Your consciousness needs to remain aware and give its full attention to all things and to whatever you are doing throughout the whole day. This will train your mind and lead to your concentration becoming effortless. Your mind will then become one-pointed instead of scattered aimlessly in all directions. If you do something with your full attention, you will increase your awareness and ability to perform what is right in your thoughts, speech and actions, so that you do not create unrest in your mind.

In the beginning self-discipline can be difficult to maintain, for the ego does not like to be limited, restricted or disciplined in any way whatsoever. The spiritual journey with its obstacles may seem formidable to a beginner starting out on the spiritual path of Yoga. The need for many changes in your diet, lifestyle, behaviour and attitudes soon becomes apparent, and can be discouraging for some people. But if you approach it carefully, and gradually make the changes, with perseverance, persistence and consistent practice, you will gain the inner strength to overcome each obstacle as it arises.

Make the effort now. Be very vigilant. Do not allow your sensory desires, habits and environment to control you. From today, determine that you will begin to discipline yourself. You do not need to be too rigid and strict with yourself, just start with changing the small things in your life and daily routines: 'I will go to bed at 10 pm and rise at 6 am.' Discipline yourself to those times, so it becomes a part of your daily routine every day. Once you have decided to do something, willingly persevere with fortitude and fervour, and do not give up. Be determined to succeed. In this way, gradually add more disciplines. Discipline your body, discipline your mind, and discipline your speech, so that the soul qualities and virtues hidden within you can be revealed. Be determined to break through the boundaries and limitations that hold you back from divine fulfilment.

If you find it difficult to remain resolute, firm, and steady on the path of Yoga and spirituality, re-dedicate and inspire yourself now to the yogic principles and apply self-discipline, with a willing, enthusiastic and aspiring seeking spirit. Then self-discipline will give you inner strength, confidence and satisfaction that will allow you to lead your life with purpose, awareness, love, respect and freedom. Then you will recognise the discipline as a source of inner joy and freedom.

NINE INDICATIONS OF SPIRITUAL PROGRESS IN MEDITATION

1. During meditation you experience a deep inner calmness. The mind becomes still with ineffable peace and inner joy.
2. Increased enthusiasm and love for meditation. The more you meditate the more you want to meditate. Your daily meditation becomes your most important engagement and an indispensable part of each day.
3. There is an absence of restlessness and agitation. The mind is attentive, has clarity, and is consciously aware.
4. A sense of oneness rather than separation from our divine Source. It is understanding that you are transcending duality, transcending the misunderstanding that you are separate from your own divine Source – the Blissful Self.
5. Spiritual progress is authenticated by your character and behaviour as you begin to perceive and develop noble and divine qualities – truthfulness, love, inner peace and care for all beings.
6. Increased one-pointed awareness and unwavering commitment to living in Truth. There is a sense of dedication and devotion towards the spiritual ideal you are following.
7. An expansion of consciousness, experiencing a oneness of unconditional love and harmony towards all beings and all life.
8. Every moment in life is utilised for meditation. The inner subjective state becomes important, not the outer circumstances. One has a strong conviction to act on a calm intuitive state of inner perception.
9. The mind becomes calm and steady as you have control over your thoughts, emotions, speech and actions. A meditator knows success when he transforms his character and reduces his desires, bad habits and sense-attachments to bring balance and harmony to his daily life.

DISCOVER YOUR SPIRITUAL IDENTITY, AND KNOW YOUR TRUE PURPOSE IN LIFE

1. For as long as the mind and senses are restless you can never make spiritual progress. It is through diligent practice (*abhyāsa*), higher awareness, and sincere pursuit of the higher values of life that you will make spiritual progress.
2. Be sincere and regular in practising daily meditation; make consistent efforts to know and realise your real Self that is within you.
3. At all times practise the presence of being in Divine Consciousness, your Eternal Being.

4. Never forget your true identity, your essential Divine Nature, as *Sat-chit-ānanda* (Ever-Existing, Ever-Conscious, Ever-New Bliss).
5. Remember your important mission in life and the ultimate spiritual goal of perfection you want to achieve.
6. All spiritual practices (*sādhana*) are for training your mind, and to remove the obstacles that prevent you from realising your true essential nature of Pure Existence, Pure Awareness and Pure Joy, and freedom – the immortal divine Self within you. When the clouds of ignorance are removed, the light of the inner Self is illumined in all its glory.
7. To know the subtle Pure Self within is to realise it directly. It cannot be perceived through the limited senses or the mind, intellect or ego. The Self becomes aware that the knower, knowledge and the object of knowledge (the known), and the seer, the seeing and that which is seen, are all One. This pure, unseen Self, the inner Witness of our experiences, is always within; it is never outside. This is why we meditate. Be still and look within. The Self or God can never be found outside of you.

GURU–DISCIPLE RELATIONSHIP

> 'Self-redemption must come ultimately from ourselves. The external props such as temples, idols and gurus are all encouragements and aids. They must be intelligently used to help build up inner perfection.'
>
> *Thapan 2005, p.149*

> 'The true gurus only show you the way and encourage you.'
>
> *Thapan 2005, p.158*

In our modern times the word 'guru' has become fashionable and commonly used to refer simply to an influential teacher or an expert in whatever field they are teaching. But a true guru (*satguru*) is one who is Self- and God-realised. The Sanskrit word *guru* is composed of two syllables: *gu* (darkness) and *ru* (that which dispels). The *satguru* leads the disciple from darkness into the Light. The *satguru* is the disciple's spiritual guide and preceptor, friend and companion on the spiritual path. The Self-realised guru who has attained self-mastery and has purified his or her ego is the dispeller of spiritual darkness (ignorance). He or she illumines our way along the spiritual path. Such a spiritual master who has attained Infinite consciousness is no longer bound by the limiting ego. Instead he or she abides serene and calm in the uninterrupted stillness of superconsciousness.

The need for a guru

Many of you may have started your journey on the spiritual path by being inspired through reading books on Yoga, meditation and philosophy, which is useful and needed in the beginning to help you find your way. But sooner or later you will need to find a true and competent spiritual teacher or guru, who can give you personal guidance and wise counsel in the art and practice of *Rāja* and *Kriyā Yoga*. The personal guidance of such a wise, experienced and competent guru can give more subtle details than a book can give.

The *satguru* can help you to transcend your mind and reach the ultimate Truth. He or she can point out your weaknesses, defects and shortcomings, and help you to avoid the pitfalls and snares that may arise on your spiritual journey. The enlightened guru can help you to purify your ego-personality, helping you to overcome the many obstacles and difficulties that you may encounter on your journey along the spiritual path. The Self- and God-realised guru can shower God's grace upon you and can enlighten you. He or she (yes, there are female gurus too) is the visible representative of the Supreme Lord.

How do we find a guru?

In the beginning God sends us indirect guidance through books and other teachers. It is only when you start to develop a sincere yearning to know the Truth, Supreme Reality, or God, when you truly feel that there is something missing in your life, that God answers you by sending you a Self-realised guru. It is not that you have to go to India, or anywhere else, to search for a guru. Although if your true guru really is in India, you may be called there to meet him or her. In India it is said, 'When the disciple is ready the guru appears.' By God's grace, you are sent a guru when you are spiritually ready and the time is right. The guru may not even come in his physical form, but may appear to you in a superconscious dream, in which he or she will affirm that you are his or her disciple and initiate you.

This is exactly what happened in my own life in 1982. After many years of Yoga purification, through practising different forms of Yoga – *Haṭha*, *Karma*, *Bhakti*, *Gyana*, *Kuṇḍalinī* and *Rāja*, and meeting many eminent gurus over a period of ten years, I finally met Swāmi Kriyananda (1926–2013), an American direct disciple of Paramhansa Yogananda. He was doing a tour of Europe and stopped over in England to give an afternoon *Kriyā Yoga* workshop at the Mind-Body-Spirit Festival at Olympia in London, which I attended. I had already heard of Paramhansa Yogananda through reading his *Autobiography of a Yogi* ten years previous to meeting Swāmi Kriyananda, but had never met a disciple or follower of him.

Swāmi Kriyananda instantly inspired me with his warm, friendly and exuberant joy! In his presence I felt at peace. By the end of the three-hour workshop I felt I had become part of a new spiritual family, and had formed a wonderful spiritual relationship with *swāmiji*, who was to be my *Kriyā Yoga* teacher, and introducer to my guru-to-be, Paramhansa Yogananda.

That night after meeting Swāmi Kriyananda I had a superconscious dream in which Paramhansa Yogananda appeared to me very clearly. Yogananda stood close and, facing me directly, he looked into my eyes and said: '*Kriyā Yoga* is the path you shall follow, I am your guru, Paramhansa Yogananda.' I awoke the next morning feeling very refreshed and joyful with the clarity of that dream imprinted on my mind. All day long I was thinking of Yogananda, and feeling very happy and humbled that this great spiritual master had chosen and accepted me to be his disciple.

> 'God sends the seeker indirect guidance at first, through books and lesser teachers. Only when the desire for Him is very strong does He send help in the form of a Self-realised guru.'
>
> *Kriyananda 1990, p.127*

The guru does not have to be with you in his physical form, because the relationship between guru and disciple is an inner relationship.

Yogananda himself said, 'The friendship that exists between guru and disciple is eternal.' It is our loyalty and devotion to God and Guru that keeps us in attunement to them. Our loyalty attracts attention of the Divine. When we meditate deeply every day and sincerely pray from our hearts with devotion, we enter an inner communion with the awareness and presence of God and Guru. The divine power and potential within you – the inner Self, or the God within you – is ultimately the guru.

What are the characteristics of a true guru (satguru)?

Yogananda said, 'One may have many teachers, but only one guru, who remains as one's guru throughout many different lives until the disciple attains the final goal of liberation in God.'

A true guru, in Sanskrit known as *satguru* or *sadguru*, has to be Self- and God-realised. He or she has attained the highest realisation of the Absolute Truth, full knowledge of the Self. A teacher has some knowledge and experience, but has not yet achieved complete realisation.

A true guru has a genuine spiritual lineage (*guru-parampara*), in which the spiritual teachings are passed down in succession from guru to disciple. The teachings of *Kriyā Yoga* were passed down in spiritual succession from Mahavatar Babaji to Lahiri Mahasaya to Swāmi Sri Yukteswar, who imparted the knowledge to Paramhansa Yogananda.

Ultimately, the *satguru* is God Himself manifesting in a personal form to guide the disciple. The grace of God takes the form of the *satguru*. Such an enlightened guru inspires love and devotion in others and his or her presence purifies all. The *satguru* is the embodiment of wisdom which is the basis for all types of knowledge.

All great spiritual gurus and saints have humility, which is the manifestation of an understanding heart. A true guru is free from egoism, anger, lust, greed, envy, pride, jealousy, selfishness, and other negative qualities. He or she not only speaks the truth, but also lives by it. The genuine guru's character is perfect and his or her behaviour exemplary. A true guru lives the *yamas* and *niyamas*.

True gurus transcend the pair of opposites (such as happiness and sorrow, gain and loss); they do not desire or crave praise, honour, fame or wealth. They have no ulterior selfish motives, and they never charge money for giving spiritual instructions.

Attunement with the guru

> 'Everything in future will improve if you are making a spiritual effort now.'
>
> *Swāmi Sri Yukteswar, in Yogananda 1946, p.119*

The relationship between the guru and the disciple is based on mutual faith and trust. If the disciple has no faith in the guru, he or she will not follow the guru's guidance and instructions. And if the guru has faith in the disciple it will help the disciple's yearning to learn more. The guru selflessly inspires and uplifts the disciple.

Along with faith and trust, the disciple also needs to be loyal to his or her guru and to God. The true guru who gives unconditional love is your true friend, counsellor and spiritual guide. So it is only natural to reciprocate with loyalty to such a guru. It is through your loyalty that you can establish your oneness with both God and Guru.

The disciple also needs to make a strong, persistent and repetitive effort to progress spiritually. The guru cannot do everything for you – he or she can only inspire you and give you spiritual counsel, guidance and instruction. There are no short-cuts; you have to make an intense spiritual effort if you want to succeed along the spiritual path, just as you would have to make an intense effort to study for an educational degree at university. The teacher is there to guide and instruct you, but you have to make the effort by working hard to attain success.

The guru will not effortlessly remove all your problems and difficulties. The guru wants you to develop your own inner strength so that you can stand independently and wisely on your own two feet. But the guru will make you aware of any negative attitudes, selfishness, negative emotions and misgivings that you have limited yourself by. Like a sculptor, the guru will chip away all the flaws that are not your true Self to reveal the true image of God within you. God and the guru's grace and power will help you and guide you, but it is you who will have to make a great self-effort. The deep truths that the guru imparts to you have to become part of your life and being, then they will help you by giving you tremendous strength and understanding to overcome your difficulties. Every situation you face in life offers you a means to cultivate the right attitudes and qualities needed to help you succeed on the spiritual path to the God.

For your part, cultivating right attitudes (*yamas* and *niyamas*) – selflessness, devotion, receptivity, cooperation and loyalty to God and Guru – is needed to attain divine freedom; it is not attained by *Kriyā Yoga* techniques alone. Paramhansa Yogananda gave the formula that to attain divine freedom requires 25 per cent of devoted practice of meditation techniques, 25 per cent blessings of the guru, and 50 per cent grace of God. This is why many seekers do not attain Self- and God-realisation, because they do not persevere with their effort to succeed in meditation and their attunement to God and Guru. As Yogananda said, 'Those who don't meditate regularly and deeply are restless whenever they do meditate, and give up after a short effort.'

Attunement with the guru and the Divine is not achieved merely by thinking of them for a short while, but by practising the Presence of God and Guru throughout the day and by meditating every day on them. By remaining as much as possible in the inner silence and peace gained from deep meditation you can align your consciousness and heart with the guru, so that your life becomes naturally directed by his or her wisdom. Then you will be able to remain steadily in tune with the will, guidance and blessings of God and Guru.

Ways of cultivating your attunement with the guru

- Practise *japa* (mental repetition) of your guru's name throughout the day and evening. For example, when I walk to the station from my house I mentally chant, '*Jai guru, jai guru, jai guru jai, Paramhansa Yogananda jai guru jai*' (*jai* means victory). Or sometimes I repeatedly chant, '*Aum Guru*'. Chanting the *mantra* '*Aum Guru*' is like a prayer to the guru asking for God's grace to flow through *Aum* to you. As you chant *Aum*, attune yourself to its divine consciousness. Paramhansa Yogananda said that *Aum* is the Great Comforter – when you are in that omnipresent consciousness of *Aum*, nothing can touch you.
- Read your guru's words from the books that he or she has written. Make a habit of reading a few paragraphs each day, and absorb into your consciousness some truth that your guru has given.
- Find ways to serve your guru – help to promote his or her teachings.
- Meditate on a picture of your guru. Feel that you are meditating with him or her. Gaze into his/her eyes and focus your attention at your guru's Spiritual Eye, at the midpoint between the eyebrows. Try to see beyond the physical form and personality of your guru into his or her expanded consciousness. Feel a divine attunement and divine love connecting your heart with the Divine through your guru. Feel that your guru and God are One.
- Practise *Kriyā* meditation with devotional self-offering to God and Guru. Paramhansa Yogananda said, 'To those who think me near I will be near.'

6.9

SAMĀDHI (TOTAL ABSORPTION)

> 'When the consciousness of the duality of subject and object disappears and only the true nature of the object contemplated remains, that is absorption (*samādhi*).'
>
> *Yoga Sūtras 3:3*

In the beginning, in our true original state, there is only one infinite Being, which you are, or God is. There is no sense of separation or otherness. In Reality there cannot be anything other than the Infinite. The Infinite has no boundaries. If the consciousness within you was separate from the Infinite Consciousness then the Infinite could not be infinite. There is no separation in that One Supreme Consciousness that lives and expresses through all. The Infinite Consciousness has not divided Itself but has individualised Itself. It is individuality in unity. You live in God and God lives in you. Realising this we can affirm, 'I and the Father are One', 'Wherever I am, God Is', 'I exist because God Is.' It is important to realise the Divine Consciousness within yourself, because it is through that alone that you have come into being and exist. The only way God can express Itself in all Its manifestations is through Its Consciousness, becoming aware of Its manifestation, and Its awareness in Its manifestation becomes the Consciousness in you and me.

Due to having forgotten the consciousness of our own true and essential nature, we are experiencing ourselves as limited, mortal, finite beings. We feel separated from God, separated from one another, and we falsely identify ourselves with our minds and bodies.

Actually, the soul, or Self, has no lack or limitation, it is of the very nature of perfection. Your true spiritual Self has never been lost, it has always been present here and now. All that you are seeking is already within you. The Self is eternally fulfilled and eternally established; that is its divine nature. The division and separation that you feel is only an appearance, it is not real. You have forgotten because your attention and identification is outward looking. Therefore, the spotlight of your awareness and attention has to be turned inwards, towards your own inner divine Self, a Reality which is the real you where bliss lies in its essential form.

It is the inner Self that you have to meditate upon; then you will come to realise that the joy you are seeking in outer objects, persons and things is not in them, but actually contained within your very Self – the Source of all Joy or Bliss! When you truly connect with your essential nature, then you will experience a true and fulfilling joy.

Rāja Yoga, the supreme path to Self-realisation, which is also known as *Kriyā Yoga*, and was first brought to the Western world by Paramhansa Yogananda, gives us the way to attain and realise that blissful superconscious state of absorption known as *samādhi*.

Kriyā Yoga reverses the outward flowing energy of the senses and the body that keeps the soul bound to matter. The *prāṇāyāma* technique of *Kriyā Yoga* directs the energy inward and upward through the centres of consciousness (*chakras*) in the astral spine to the *sahasrāra*, the thousand-rayed petalled lotus at the crown of the head, the centre of Cosmic Consciousness. It is through this astral spinal pathway that the soul first makes its descent from the subtle causal state into gross matter, into the physical form or body, and becoming engrossed in it, forgets its original nature and its eternal relationship with the Infinite Divinity. As the soul descends through each *chakra* the consciousness becomes less aware of its divinity and more identified with the physical form and mind. When the soul reaches the three lowest *chakras* or centres of consciousness (*maṇipūra*, *svādhiṣṭhāna* and *mūladhāra*), it has reached its lowest point in its descending journey through the *chakras*. At this stage the soul is conscious but feels separate from God, and separate from other souls, because it has forgotten its true essential spiritual nature. Here the soul's Divine awareness is obscured; the individual soul perceives everything in terms of the mind and physical body.

At the base of the spine lies the Divine Energy known as *kuṇḍalinī śakti*, which is lying there waiting for the soul to awaken it, so that it can rise to higher Consciousness to be established again in that ever-awareness of the presence of God.

THERE IS NO SHORT-CUT TO *SAMĀDHI*

> '*Samādhi* alone can reveal the Truth. Thoughts cast a veil over Reality, and so It is not realised as such in states other than *samādhi*. In *samādhi* there is only the feeling of "I am" and no thoughts. The experience "I am" is being still.'
>
> *Maharshi 1972*

The spiritual practice of *Kriyā Yoga* is an art based on science that a spiritual aspirant needs to be guided in to attain the higher states of Divine Awareness. The mind, body and breath have to be purified and prepared for the return ascent of the soul in the spinal pathway to God.

The spiritual aspirant's self-effort, with loyal commitment to practicing *Kriyā Yoga*, with devotion, and with God's grace and the guru's blessings, can attain the state of *samādhi*. Over many years of such devoted practice the *Kriyā* yogi is able to strongly magnetise his or her spine with energy and interiorise his or her consciousness in Divine Consciousness. In that state of Divine Unity or Oneness the yogi rises above ignorance (*avidyā*) and delusion (*moha*) and regains his or her blissful, immortal divine nature that is inseparable from God. Now transformed into the divine state of Consciousness, the mind no longer has its former characteristics of weakness, limitation, and the sense of duality.

That infinite state of Divine Awareness is the realisation of true freedom and oneness in the Supreme Consciousness, the One Eternal Reality, and is attained through the state of *samādhi* (total absorption, superconsciousness).

THE DIFFERENCE BETWEEN MEDITATION (*DHYĀNA*) AND *SAMĀDHI*

The word *samādhi* comes from the Sanskrit root *sam*, which means 'perfect' or 'complete', and *dhi*, which means 'consciousness'. The goal of Yoga culminates in the highest state of *samādhi*.

In the state of *samādhi* the mind is so totally absorbed in the Divine Self that the mind is no longer aware of itself meditating. All distinctions between the person who is the subjective meditator, the act of meditation, and the object of meditation merge into oneness. There is no sense of a separate subjective experience.

In meditation (*dhyāna*) there is a *continuous* and *uninterrupted* flow of attention towards the object of meditation, whereas in *samādhi* there is a dissolution of the subjective/objective duality of consciousness of observer and observed. The mind is no longer conscious of itself as it merges with the object of meditation. Body consciousness also vanishes. When the mind becomes one with absolute bliss in *samādhi*, it is totally transformed, just as a snowflake melts and changes into water. Then it knows that it has always been water. Similarly, the mind being transformed into the *Sat-chit-ānanda* (Ever-Existing, Ever-Conscious, Ever-New Bliss) state begins to know that its own true spiritual nature is Divine.

In meditation there is a succession of identical thought waves towards the object of meditation, but when meditation culminates in the enlightened state of *samādhi*, the meditator loses his or her individuality (ego-consciousness); expansion of consciousness and absorption begins. Beyond the mind, time and space, the individual consciousness of the meditator becomes totally absorbed and completely identified with the Absolute, the all-pervading, nameless, formless Cosmic Consciousness, in which all sense of duality completely disappears.

Here is a simplified analogy. When the attention is limited to a particular focal point, that is concentration (*dhāraṇā*); when it is continually flowing there, it is meditation (*dhyāna*). For example, if I keep looking at you, it is concentration. When I am completely absorbed in looking at you, it is meditation. If I go deeper, these three (I – looking – you) become one, so that it is as though you alone are the reality and 'I' is non-existent; that is *samādhi*.

Since my whole consciousness is filled with this object to such an extent that I do not exist, that object alone exists fully and truly, I *know* that object intimately, immediately, in its complete essence.

THE DIFFERENCE BETWEEN SLEEP AND *SAMĀDHI*

Samādhi is the complete merging of the mind in God-Consciousness. It should not be confused with a state of unconsciousness, coma, trance or sleep. There is some similarity between the transcendental experience and what we call trance, coma or sleep, because in both the sleep state and the *samādhi* state the mind and senses are disconnected from the objective world. But there is a vast difference between these two states.

In the dream state, the mind operates in the subconscious level. In the dreamless deep sleep state, the mind enters into a causal state in which cognition and all its functions lie dormant and suspended. Even the ego disappears (it only arises when the person awakes from deep sleep and says, 'I had a beautiful sleep and did not know anything about it'). There is no experience of memory, fear, pain, pleasure or imagination, because the ego becomes submerged and all mental operations cease, due to consciousness receding from the mind altogether. But in *samādhi* the mind does not become submerged in darkness, it goes beyond and above ego-consciousness. This superconscious experience is called the fourth kind of experience as distinct from waking, dream and deep sleep.

So the difference between *samādhi* and sleep is that in the deep sleep state a person's mind is completely in darkness and ignorance, and ego consciousness does not exist. Whereas in the transcendental state of *samādhi*, the mind goes into the Divine Light. The mind enters that Light and becomes illumined and all trace of ignorance is removed. *Samādhi* spiritually transforms the person, whereas sleep does not. A person awakes from sleep without any change to his or her consciousness, and therefore he or she still continues to identify with their body. The yogi who has attained the highest *samādhi* becomes enlightened, one with the Supreme Reality, and so is ever free from the bondage of this life completely.

THE STAGES OF *SAMĀDHI*: THE BLISSFUL STATES

Rajā Yoga divides *samādhi* into two main categories: *samprajñāta samādhi* and *asamprajñāta samādhi.*

Samprājñāta samādhi – *samādhi* with complete consciousness; with wisdom or perfect knowledge (*prājñā*). Also known as *sabīja samādhi* – superconsciousness 'with support' or 'with seed'. In this first stage of superconsciousness, the meditator's consciousness is expanded and he realises that he is *Sat-chit-ānanda* (Ever-Existing, Ever-Conscious, Ever-New Bliss), but he retains a sense of individuality; some duality of subject and object still remains in his consciousness.

Samprājñāta samādhi is the first category of *samādhi* in which the mind needs an object (gross or subtle) or supportive factor (*ālambana*) in concentration until *dharma-megha samādhi* is reached. *Dharma-megha samādhi* ('raincloud of virtues') is the supportless *samādhi*, the higher stage of the *asmitā*-accompanied *samādhi* in which the mind dwells in itself by itself, and it is the initial stage of the acognitive *samprājñāta samādhi*. *Dharma-megha samādhi* acts as a bridge between *samprājñāta samādhi* and *asamprājñāta samādhi*.

Asamprājñāta samādhi – superconsciousness beyond perfect knowledge. Also known as *nirbīja samādhi*, superconsciousness 'without support' or 'without seed', and *nirodha samādhi,* total control and final cessation of mental fluctuations (*vṛttis*). This is the highest and final state of total absorption, in which consciousness is established in itself. Just as salt dissolves into oneness with water, the yogi's mind becomes blissfully dissolved in the infinite ocean of Divine Consciousness.

This is the state where the awareness of *puruṣa* is no longer aware of any external object. The mind is not supported by any active thought, there is a cessation of *vṛttis* (thought waves); this includes all mental activities that arise in the *citta* (mind-field) including the object of meditation. There is no mind-field, only Self-awareness. The Seer abides in the Self.

To attain liberation (*kaivalya*) the yogi first has to bring the *rajasic* and *tamasic vṛttis* under control (*nirodha*) by means of practice (*abhyāsa*) and dispassion (*vairāgya*). Then the yogi has to gradually progress through each of the different refined and subtle *samprajñāta samādhi* levels from *savitarka* to *sāsmitā*, until Self-realisation is attained, in which there is true and direct realised knowledge of the 'real' and dispassion for the 'unreal'. Complete cessation of fluctuations of the mind emanates from the constant practice of *paravairāgya* (supreme detachment) which is free from any material cogitation. Both the knowledge of non-self and the knower of non-self (the 'I-sense') disappears. *Paravairāgya* (supreme dispassion; supreme non-attachment) produces no *saṁskāras* (latent impressions) in the mind-field other than its own latent impressions of dispassion. And no other *saṁskāras* can replace these because there is no higher stage. Without the seeds of *saṁskāras*, there cannot be *kleśas* (afflictions), *karma* (action) and *vipāka* (fruition of action).

THE PROGRESSIVE STAGES IN THE PROCESS OF ACHIEVING ABSORPTION IN MEDITATION

> *'Vitarka-vicārānandāsmitā-rupānugamāt samprajñātaḥ.'*
> '*Samprājñāta samādhi* is that deep absorption which is accompanied by reasoning, reflection, bliss and pure sense of "I-am-ness".'
>
> *Yoga Sūtras 1:17*

The act of meditation leads to the attainments known as *samāpattis* (a synonym for *samādhi*: 'absorption', 'engrossment'). Patañjali gives us an important *sūtra* (1:41) explaining that when the mind is freed from all distractions in the form of *vṛttis*, it becomes like a pure, transparent crystal. In this state with the mind in its one-pointed (*ekāgra*) concentration, released from the effects of *rajas* and *tamas*, it can reflect reality as it is, and thus gain a deep insight into its nature. In the highest *samāpatti* when the mind is pure, calm and steady it can reflect *puruṣa* (Self) to itself. The Self becomes aware of itself. There is a complete identification of the mind with that which is being meditated upon.

Patañjali in his *Yoga Sūtras* speaks of *vitarka*, *vicāra*, *ānanda* and *asmitā* stages in these attainments, which are again subdivided into the stages known as *savitarka*, *nirvitarka*, *savicāra*, *nirvicāra*, *sānanda* and *asmitā*. These attainments (*samāpattis*) are the graduated attunements and refinements of the meditating consciousness with the cosmological categories enumerated in the *Sāṃkhya* (*Sāṅkhya*) philosophy.

As each stage becomes complete, the subtle aspect of the object of concentration becomes the supportive factor for the next level of concentration. When these four levels are achieved in gradual succession, wisdom and knowledge is attained in its perfect expansion (*samprājñāta* – complete higher consciousness). Each level attained is purer and more refined than the previous level because of the increased *sattva guṇa* (pure illumined quality of consciousness).

The following is a summary of Patañjali's *Yoga Sūtras* 42 to 51: the four stages of meditation known as *samāpatti*, and the final stage called *asamprajñāta samādhi* (superconsciousness beyond perfect knowledge).

Savitarka samādhi (absorption with physical awareness, with question). There is an absorption of consciousness upon the contemplated object as involved in its name, memory, meaning and idea, which relies on gross thoughts and objects knowable through the senses. The subconscious *saṁskāras* of memory and recognition are still not fully inactive in this *samādhi*. According to the *Sāṃkhya* philosophy the entire Cosmos is composed of five external gross elements called *mahābhūtas*. Here the mind is concentrated inquiringly on the five *mahābhūtas*, the lowest forms of the manifestations of *prakṛiti* (primordial nature).

Nirvitarka samādhi (absorption without conceptualisation, without question). Based on *direct perception*, beyond words, meaning and ideas, the objects of contemplation (the five *mahābhūtas*) are taken out of time and space and completely known as they are in their true essential nature or reality. The mind being totally focused is unaware of anything else but the object; it has completely transformed itself into the object being contemplated.

Savicāra samādhi (absorption with subtle awareness, insight, reflection). Here the intense focus on the object of concentration deepens and the gross thoughts have turned towards *subtle* aspects of the physical object, but still with some awareness of space and time in the present. There is a movement of the mind's concentration from gross to subtle aspects of the object focused on. This is the subtle energy that gives rise to the five subtle elements (*tanmātras*) in the subtle body: sound (*śabda*), touch (*sparśa*), colour/form (*rūpa*), taste (*rasa*) and smell (*gandha*). These are the subtle components of the ultra-atomic particles that form the nuclei of our physical world.

Nirvicāra samādhi (absorption super-reflective, beyond insight). There is no awareness of time or space in this higher level of absorption on the *tanmātras*. The form of the object, space and time dissolves from the meditator's mind, and then there is only the experience of omnipresent subtle energy pervading reality. There is complete knowledge of the object of contemplation, from gross to subtle.

Sānanda samādhi (absorption with bliss). This relies on a more subtle support accompanied by bliss or joy, the pleasure of sattva (serenity, illumination), with no qualities of activity (rajas) and dullness (*tamas*). Here the mind itself is used as the object of meditation.

Sāsmitā samādhi (absorption with the subjective pure 'I-sense'). In this *samādhi* there is only Self-awareness (awareness of the 'I-existence'). The Self dwells in the Self.

The final or seventh stage is ***asamprajñāta samādhi*** (superconsciousness beyond perfect knowledge), or ***nirbīja samādhi*** (superconsciousness 'without seed').

Another way of understanding it is using the analogy of the Sun as an object of concentration or the seed of meditation:

> ***Savitarka samādhi*** corresponds to focusing on the Sun without distraction, but *with* awareness of its name, function, size, shape, distance, composition, etc.
>
> ***Nirvitarka samādhi*** corresponds to seeing the Sun as a luminous object but *without* awareness of its name, function, size, shape, distance, composition, etc.

Savicāra samādhi corresponds to perceiving that the fire element of the Sun is a subtle element (*tanmātra*) of light in the present, not the past or future.

Nirvicāra samādhi. All awareness of space and time dissolves. The meditating yogi just perceives the omnipresent pure light of the Sun pervading all things.

Nirbīja samādhi. The yogi's mind becomes free from all seeds of potential thought. In this state there is no perception or cognitive functioning of the *citta*, because the yogi's mind becomes completely inactive, all *vṛttis* cease. Space and time dissolve and the individual consciousness merges into oneness with the Self, the Universal Consciousness. The final and ultimate goal of Yoga has been attained.

AN EXEMPLARY YOGI AND A SAINT OF INDIA WHO ATTAINED *SAMĀDHI*

The following yogi and saint appear in Paramhansa Yogananda's *Autobiography of a Yogi* (First edition 1946).

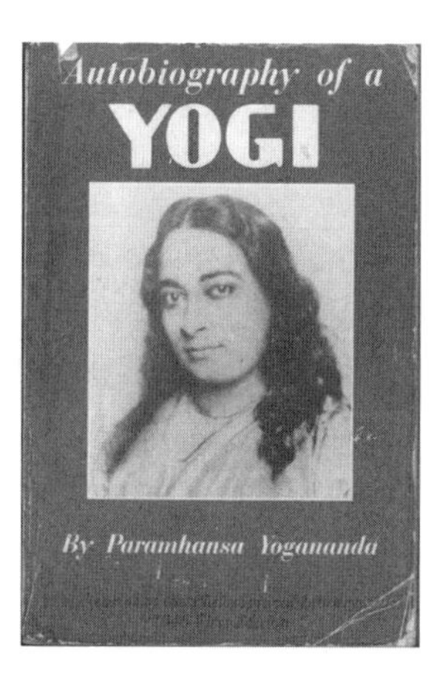

Trailanga swāmi (1607–1887)

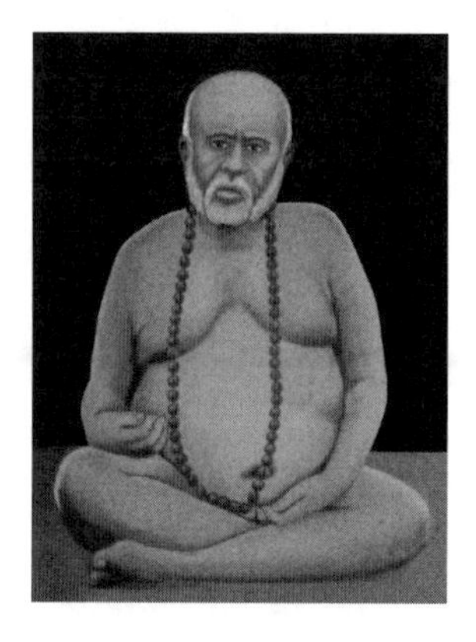

A remarkable and famous yogi named Trailanga *swāmi*, famed for his spiritual powers and longevity, was said to have lived for 150 years in the holy city of Benares, also known as Kashi (now called Vārānasī). Some reputed that Trailanga *swāmi* was over 300 years old when he died. The word Trailanga, used mostly in Benares, is derived from the area where Telugu language is spoken. Trailanga *swāmi* was born to a Brahmin family in a small village near Vizianagaram (now the modern Andhra Pradesh). His name at birth was Śivaram, then Swāmi Ganapati Saraswati, and finally he was known as Trailanga *swāmi*.

When Trailanga was 40 years of age, his parents (followers of Lord Śiva) died. He renounced the worldly life and lived as a recluse for 20 years. Then in 1679 he met his spiritual guru, Swāmi Bhagiratananda Saraswati, a yogi with whom he stayed for many years. Six years passed, then in 1685 Swāmi Bhagiratananda initiated him with the name Swāmi Ganapati Saraswati into *sannyasa* (monastic vows). After living many years of austerity (*tapasya*), Swāmi Ganapati Saraswati went to Prayag on a spiritual pilgrimage, and finally in 1737 settled in Benares (now Vārānasī).

Trailanga *swāmi* was a friend of the *Kriyā* yogi, Lahiri Mahasaya, and they often sat together in deep meditation. It is also said that Sri Ramakrishna Paramhansa, a contemporary Bengali saint, was greatly attracted towards Trailanga *swāmi*, who referred to him as 'the walking Śiva of Benares'. Trailanga was regarded by his disciples as an incarnation of Lord Śiva. Ramakrishna once asked Trailanga *swāmi*, 'Is God one or many?' Trailanga answered, 'In *samādhi* you will know that God is one. And when you have a taste for the world, God is many.'

Trailanga *swāmi*'s body, which exceeded 300 pounds (about 140 kg) in weight, always remained completely nude. As he ate very seldom, the mystery is increased. On many occasions the *swāmi* was seen to drink, with no ill effect, the most deadly poisons. Thousands of people observed Trailanga *swāmi* floating on the Ganges. For days he would sit on top of the water, or remain hidden for very long periods under the waves. A common sight at the bathing *ghats* on the banks of the Ganges at Benares was the *swāmi*'s motionless body on the blistering stone slabs, wholly exposed to the merciless scorching rays of the sun. By these feats Trailanga sought to teach us that a yogi's life does not depend upon oxygen or ordinary conditions and precautions. Whether he was above water or under it, and whether or not his body lay exposed to the fierce solar rays of the sun, the master proved that he lived by divine consciousness: death could not touch him. In the later part of his life the *swāmi* remained almost entirely absorbed in *samādhi*; with no sense of individuality, he had become identified with God.

Sri Anandamayi Ma (1896–1982)

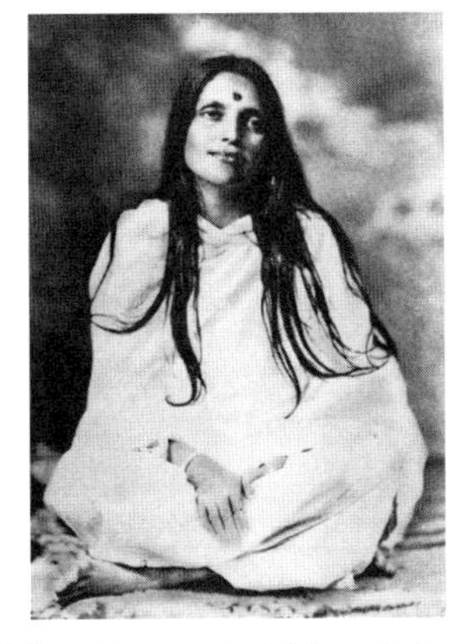

Sri Anandamayi Ma was born on 30 April 1896 in Kheora, a tiny village in East Bengal (now Bangladesh), surrounded by Muslim dwellings. She was the second child, born three years after the first. Four brothers and two sisters were born after her. At birth her mother named her Nirmala Sundari ('Immaculate Beauty'); she later came to be popularly known as Anandamayi Ma ('the bliss permeated mother') and simply as Mataji or Ma. Nirmala's parents were from Brahmin families (the Hindu priest caste), devout Vaisnavas (devotees of Krishna) who loved to chant devotional songs, and were also strict followers of caste regulations. Her mother, Mokshadasundari Devi (popularly known as Didima), married Nirmala's father, Bipin Bihari Bhattacharya, at the very young age of 12. The family were living quite poorly on a slender budget, which affected Nirmala's education, and so she was only able to attend school for less than two years.

While Nirmala was still a child, it was customary at the time for her parents to find a husband of Brahmin caste for her to marry. After a careful search her parents arranged for the marriage of Nirmala. So on 7 February 1909, when Nirmala was almost 13, she was married to Ramani Mohan Cakravarti, later referred to as Bholanath (a name for Śiva), he was considerably older than her. For the first five years of their marriage they did not live together; instead, she lived with her parents. It was not until 1914 that they actually began their married life together, in Aṣṭagrāma in East Bengal. But this was quite an extraordinary marriage, for at the beginning Bholanath had no idea that Nirmala was a saint – he had thought he had married an ordinary village girl. Their marriage was never physically consummated. It is said that when he first tried to approach her with physical desire he received such a violent electric shock from her inner being that all thought of a physical relationship went out of his mind. This was most unusual because at that time a wife was expected to be submissive to her husband and to worship him as a guru or god.

By virtue of Nirmala's spiritual power she helped Bholanath to live a celibate life with her. Recognising her exalted spirituality he accepted this most unconventional marriage and became her disciple, leading a life of self-denial and asceticism.

Paramhansa Yogananda speaks lovingly with reverence of Anandamayi Ma. In his first meeting with her in Calcutta when she was blessing a throng of about one hundred disciples from an open-topped car, she referred to Yogananda as Father: 'Father, I am meeting you for the first time in this life, after ages! Please do not leave yet.'

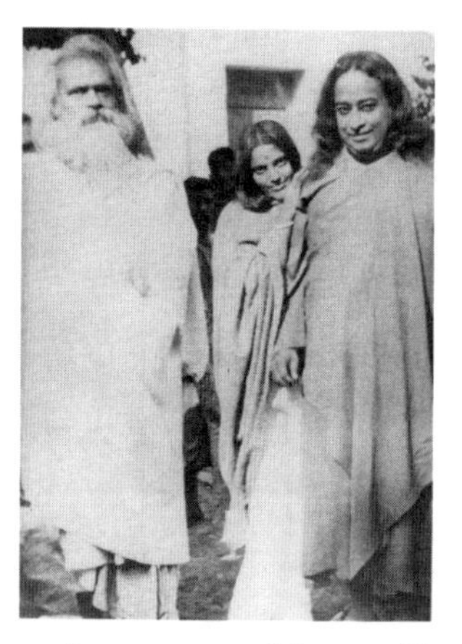

BHOLANATH, ANANDAMAYI MA AND YOGANANDA

They sat together in the rear seats of the car. The Blissful Mother soon entered the immobile ecstatic state. Her beautiful eyes glanced heavenward and, half-opened, became stilled, gazing into the near-far inner Elysium. The disciples chanted gently, 'Victory to Mother Divine!'

Yogananda said, 'I had found men of God-realisation in India, but never before had I met such an exalted woman saint. Her gentle face was burnished with ineffable joy that had given her the name of Blissful Mother. Long black tresses lay loosely behind her unveiled head. A red dot of sandalwood paste on her forehead symbolised the Spiritual Eye, ever open within her. Tiny face, tiny hands, tiny feet – a contrast to her spiritual magnitude!

'Anandamayi Ma sank into a deep meditative state. Her form was statue-still; she had fled into her ever-calling kingdom. The dark pools of her eyes appeared lifeless and glassy. This expression is often present when saints remove their consciousness from the physical body, which is then hardly more than a piece of soulless clay. We sat together for an hour in the ecstatic trance. She returned to this world with a gay little laugh.'

Paramhansa Yogananda asked Anandamoyi Ma to tell him something of her life. Ma replied, 'Father, there is little to tell. My consciousness has never associated itself with this temporary body. Before I came on this earth, Father, "I was the same". I grew into womanhood, but still "I was the same". When the family in which I had been born made arrangements to have this body married, "I was still the same". And, Father, in front of you now, "I am the same". Even afterwards, though the dance of creation changes around me in the hall of eternity, "I shall be the same".'

Anandamayi Ma's followers often claimed that she was continuously in the highest state of *samādhi*. They said that even as she looked at you, you would be aware of the fact that she is with you and yet far beyond you; that she had that dual vision encompassing the manifest and the transcendent. Her days were not divided into mornings, evenings and nights, but there was only one prolonged period of indescribable bliss. Once she stayed in *samādhi* for five days without any response to outside stimuli. When she was asked what her experience of *samādhi* was like, she would only reply, 'It is a state beyond all conscious and supra-conscious planes – a state of complete immobilisation of all thoughts, emotions and activities, both physical and mental – a state that transcends all the phases of life here below.'

When she was asked 'What is the nature of your *samādhi*? Is it *savikalpa* or *nirvikalpa*? Does mind then persist?' Ma answered, 'Well, it is for you to decide this question. All that I can say is that in the midst of all apparent changes of state in body and mind, I feel, I am aware, that I am always the same. I feel that in me there is no change of states. Call it by any name you like. Is it *samādhi*?'

PART 7

KRIYĀ YOGA

7.1

AN ADVANCED SPIRITUAL ACCELERATOR

'This *Kriyā* can be called "*Kevali*" inner *prāṇāyama*, as mentioned in the scriptures. This technique does not use the difficult breath-holding methods of the usual types of *pranayam*, and as such, one does not have to fall into the dangers caused by those practices. This method uses a special technique by which the scattered currents of the nervous system are gathered, decay is prevented and the need of breath is dispensed; as in the gap of inhalation and exhalation, the restless breath within becomes still.'

Swāmi Satyananda Giri, in Niketan 2004, p.41

Kriyā Yoga is the essence and synthesis of all Yogas and religions, which includes the highest Yoga and meditation techniques from *Haṭha Yoga*, *Rāja Yoga*, *Laya Yoga* and *Mantra Yoga*.

The Sanskrit word *kriyā* means 'to do', 'action'; and *Yoga* means 'union'. *Kriyā Yoga* therefore means the 'activating power (*prāṇa*) of the divine Spirit manifested in creation', or the active process to achieve the science of uniting the soul with God. *Kriyā* is a scientific technique based on the vital life force (*prāṇa*).

The ancient spiritual art and science of *Kriyā Yoga* awakens the divine memory of the soul, of which it has forgotten its real nature due to identification and attachment to the body, mind and ego-self.

We have forgotten that our soul or inner Self and God are one, so we must learn to manifest our Divinity. When we realise this, then we will discover that we are Divine, everything is God, and nothing exists but God.

Kriyā Yoga is the quickest means of attaining spiritual success. By practising *Kriyā Yoga* a person transcends human consciousness and attains Divine Consciousness.

It is through the divine dispensation, through a great line of Spiritual Masters – Christ, Krishna, Mahavatar Babaji, Lahiri Mahasaya and Swāmi Sri Yukteswar – that Paramhansa Yogananda was selected and blessed to impart the supreme science of *Kriyā Yoga* worldwide.

The practical science of *Kriyā* is based on the inner Yoga science of advanced yogis, who since ancient times and through their own direct experience realised the God Self within. These great *Kriyā* yogis evolved a system of Yoga techniques from *Haṭha Yoga*, *Rāja Yoga*, *Laya Yoga* and *Mantra Yoga* that became known as *Kriyā Yoga*.

The *Kriyā* techniques work directly with the *prāṇic* life force in the subtle astral spine. *Kriyā Yoga* helps you to withdraw the consciousness and *prāṇic* energy from the *iḍā* and *piṅgala nāḍīs* (the two outer *prāṇic* subtle channels), into the *suṣumnā* (central subtle channel).

> 'The *Kriyā* yogi mentally directs his life energy to revolve, upward and downward, around the six spinal centres (medullary, cervical, dorsal, lumbar, sacral, and coccygeal plexuses) which correspond to the twelve astral signs of the zodiac, the symbolic cosmic man. One half minute of revolution of energy around the sensitive spinal cord of man effects subtle progress in his evolution; that half minute of *Kriyā* equals one year of natural spiritual unfoldment.'
>
> *Paramhansa Yogananda*

The science of *Kriyā Yoga* is the means and inner highway for attaining the direct experience and the highest spiritual realisation of uniting the individual soul-consciousness with the Supreme Consciousness; that Eternal Reality we call God.

The *Kriyā* yogi, through his or her own self-effort, using the Yoga techniques of *prāṇāyāma*, *mudrā*, *mantra* and meditation to magnetise the spine and reverse the downward and outward-flowing life force that keeps his or her consciousness habitually externalised (the actions of the breath, heart, mind and senses) with attachment to the objective world by identification with the body, redirects that life energy inward and upward through the deep inner spinal pathway, from which it had descended, to the higher centres in the brain.

The soul has descended from its original divine awareness of oneness with the Eternal Reality, God, from the causal to the gross physical plane in which we have forgotten our original spiritual, blissful and immortal nature, and have become more identified with this physical form in which we feel separate from the Divine and one another. The further we descend down through the spinal centres of consciousness (*chakras*) the more we become identified with matter and more enmeshed in bondage and delusion. Divine energy, which has brought the individual soul in the descent through the *chakras* to the lowest point of the spine (the three lowest *chakras*) is as if it were lying coiled asleep there. The goal of *Kriyā Yoga* is to reawaken the sleeping Divinity within you; to turn your attention inwards, towards your own God Self, where bliss lies in its essential form, and to realise it.

KRIYĀ YOGA IS MORE THAN JUST TECHNIQUES

Kriyā Yoga techniques prepare the body and mind to know God by helping to remove the obstacles, so that subtle currents are awakened in the spine, and the consciousness is interiorised and expanded.

Kriyā Yoga is not just about doing techniques, it is a way of being and living, thinking and behaving with right attitudes, and being established in God-awareness, living skilfully with conscious intention. It is no less than a complete transformation of your consciousness and personality from the lower nature to divinity. Transformed into that divinity, the mind never again becomes ignorant of its own true nature. The realisation of your true nature which comes through deep *Kriyā Yoga* meditation results in the perfect knowledge that your real Self is immortal, undying and unchanging, while your body and ego-personality that you identify with is always subject to change.

7.2

THE FOUR YUGAS

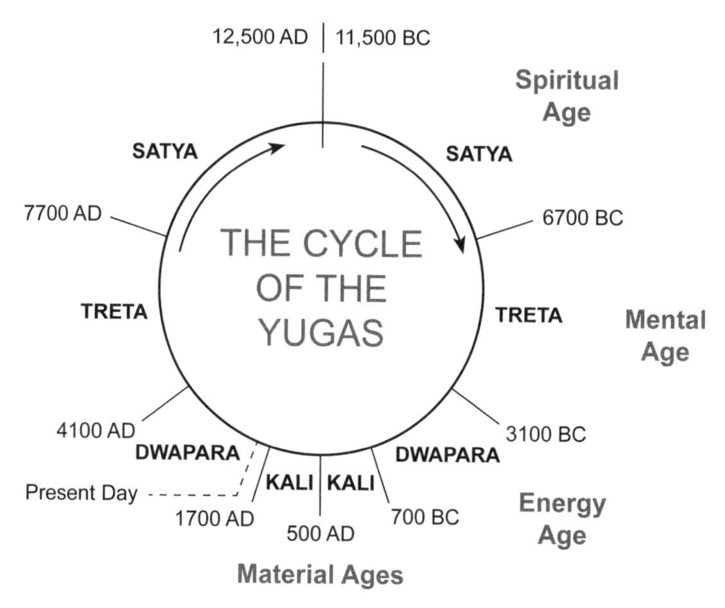

THE CYCLE OF THE YUGAS

In the *Bhagavad Gītā*, the Lord said to Arjuna:

> 'I gave this imperishable Yoga to Vivasvat (the sun-god); Vivasvat passed on the knowledge to Manu (the Hindu lawgiver); Manu taught it to Ikshvaku (founder of the solar dynasty of the Kshatriyas). Handed down in orderly succession, the Rajarishis (royal sages) knew it.
>
> With the long passage of time, however, O Scorcher of Foes (Arjuna), this knowledge of Yoga has become greatly diminished on Earth.'
>
> *Bhāgavad Gītā 4:1–2 (Author's translation)*

These two verses from the *Bhagavad Gītā* are referring to the decrease and decline in spiritual knowledge and the supreme science of *Kriyā Yoga*, during a long cycle of time, when our planet Earth was descending from a higher Spiritual Age of consciousness and wisdom (*Satya Yuga*), that was gradually diminishing through the successive ages of *Treta Yuga* (age of discrimination), *Dwapara Yuga* (age of energy), and then entering into a darker age of consciousness known as *Kali Yuga* (in 700 BCE). This decline in knowledge, awareness, perception and understanding only reached its lowest point as the Earth entered the ascending cycle of *Kali Yuga* in 500 CE.

Then the upward arc of the cycle began. In 1700 CE it entered the ascending cycle, a transition period (called a *sandhi,* which is one tenth of each *Yuga*'s length), into ascending *Dwapara Yuga*, the age of energy. We are now in the proper *Dwapara* age that started in 1900 CE, in which there is a rapid expansion in electronic, digital and medical technologies and other advanced technologies in which energy has revolutionised our lives. This present cycle will last until 4100 CE, before entering the next cycle of *Treta Yuga*.

These great cycles of evolution and devolution (four *Yugas* or Ages) are recorded in the ancient scriptures of India to last as follows: *Kali Yuga* (1200 years), *Dwapara Yuga* (2400 years), *Treta Yuga* (3600 years) and the Golden Age *Satya Yuga* (4800 years). This amounts to 24,000 years – 12,000 years of upward evolution followed by 12,000 years of gradual degeneration – that occurs continually over incomprehensible eons of time.

7.3

THE KRIYĀ YOGA MASTERS

The imperishable science of Yoga that had been lost down through the ages was revived again by the great householder yogi, Lahiri Mahasaya (1828–1895), a young Bengali accountant of Vārānasī, India, who received it from his guru, Mahavatar Babaji, in the foothills of the Himalayas near Ranikhet, when he was aged 33 in the autumn of 1861. Babaji had rediscovered the lost science of Yoga and gave it the name *Kriyā Yoga*. Babaji initiated Lahiri Mahasaya into the ancient art and science of *Kriyā Yoga* and instructed him to serve humanity as an ideal guide to follow, by being both a married householder and a yogi: 'The millions who are encumbered by family ties and heavy worldly duties will take new heart from you, a householder like themselves. You should guide them to understand that the highest yogic attainments are not barred to the family man.' When Babaji gave Lahiri Mahasaya permission to initiate others into *Kriyā Yoga* he also told him to advise each new initiate in the words of Krishna (*Bhagavad Gītā*, 2:40): 'Even a little of the practice of this *dharma* will save you from great fear.'

LAHIRI MAHASAYA (1828–1895) AND MAHAVATAR BABAJI

Lahiri was the family name of Shyama Charan Lahiri, and Mahasaya means 'great-minded'. Lahiri Mahasaya is well-known as being the disciple of Mahavatar Babaji, and the guru of Swāmi Sri Yukteswar, who initiated Paramhansa Yogananda into this great line of *Kriyā Yoga* Masters. It was Lahiri Mahasaya to whom the ancient art and science of *Kriyā Yoga* was revealed after having been lost for centuries.

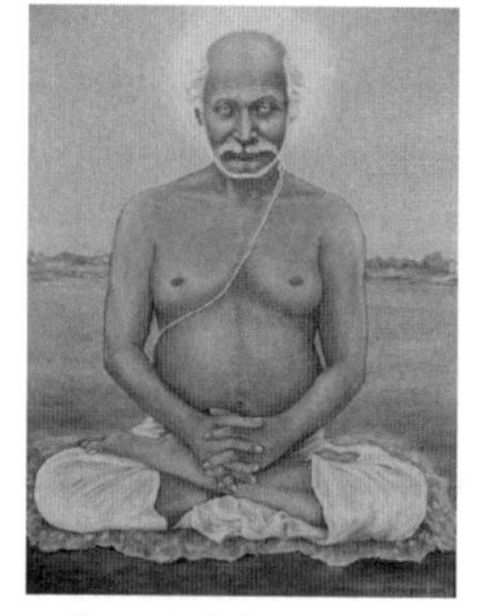

LAHIRI MAHASAYA BY STEPHEN STURGESS

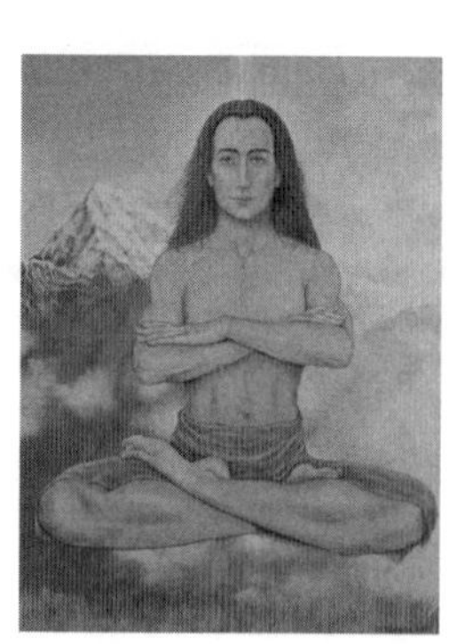

MAHAVATAR BABAJI BY STEPHEN STURGESS

In Yogananda's *Autobiography of a Yogi* (chapter 34), Lahiri Mahasaya's first meeting with Mahavatar Babaji is recounted. In the autumn of 1861 during a ramble one early afternoon at the Himalayan site of Raniket in the Almora district, Lahiri was astounded to hear a distant voice calling him. So he continued his vigorous upward climb on the Dronagiri Mountain. After some time he finally reached a small clearing in the forest whose sides were dotted with caves. It was here that he first met the young Babaji with his long copper-coloured hair, who struck Lahiri gently on the forehead, releasing the seed-memories of his previous life. In that instant, Lahiri remembered that Babaji was his guru, who had belonged to him always. The recollection of the many years of his last incarnation came back to him in the cave where they sat together. 'Here in this cave I spent many years of my last incarnation!' said Lahiri.

At midnight, Babaji miraculously materialised a magnificient and enchanting golden palace studded with jewels, set amidst landscaped gardens. In the grand hall of this palace Babaji sat in the lotus posture on a golden throne. Lahiri knelt before him and Babaji initiated him into the liberating Yoga technique of *Kriyā*. By early dawn the *Kriyā* rites were completed. Lahiri was in such an ecstatic blissful state that he felt no need for sleep. Later that afternoon as he sat on his blanket, hallowed by associations of past life realisations, Babaji approached him and passed his hand over Lahiri's head, causing him to enter the superconscious state of *nirbvikalpa samādhi*. Lahiri remained in this unbroken state of bliss for seven days. Then on the eighth day he prostrated at Babaji's feet and implored him to keep him always near him. Babaji embraced him and replied, 'My son, your role in this incarnation must be played on an outward stage. Prenatally blessed by many lives of lonely meditation, you must now mingle in the world of men. A deep purpose underlay the fact that you did not meet me this time until you were already a married man, with modest business responsibilities. You must put aside your thoughts of joining our secret band in the Himalayas; your life lies in the crowded marts, serving as an example of the ideal householder… You have been chosen to bring spiritual solace through *Kriyā Yoga* to numerous earnest seekers.'

SWĀMI SRI YUKTESWAR GIRI (1855–1936)

Swāmi Sri Yukteswar Giri was born on 10 May 1855 in Serampore, situated on the banks of the river Ganges. At birth he was given the name Priyanath Karar (Priyanath means 'beloved to God', and Karar was his family name. His father Kshetranath Karar and his mother Kadambini Devi were both from the well-known and honoured family of Karar.

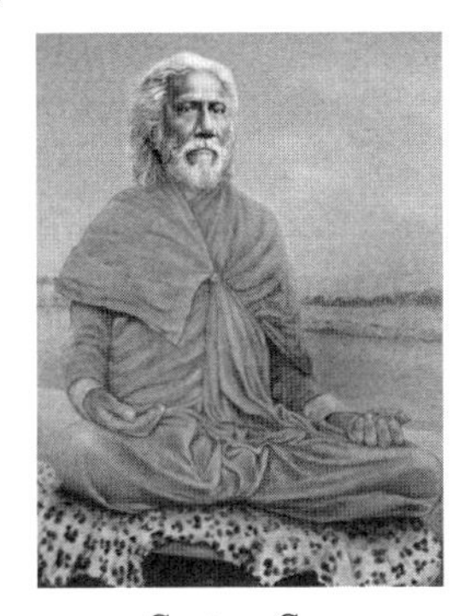

Swāmi Sri Yukteswar Giri by Stephen Sturgess

While Priyanath was still a young student, his father died, and so his loving mother became his sole guidance and inspiration. Priyanath continued his studies and helped his dear mother in looking after their family business.

When he finished university, Priyanath was persuaded by his mother to look after the ancestral land, properties and business. Honouring the wish of his mother, he became married and developed a sense of responsibility, and worked to maintain his family.

From the marriage he had only one child, a daughter. After some years of married life his wife died and later his daughter died due to an illness. She was married and left a granddaughter, who was taken care of by her father. Now at the age of 28 years Priyanath, with only himself and his mother left, started to become interested and attracted to the great *Kriyā* yogi, Shyama Charan Lahiri Mahasaya, indirectly through some of his disciples living in Serampore. These disciples were of wealthy and noble families such as the Goswāmi family, who were well known in Serampore as a humble spiritual family who had high morals, and who were known to him. Because these initiated disciples of Lahiri Mahasaya were practising *Kriyā Yoga* in secret, Priyanath had no way of knowing the technique they were practising. This made him restless and eager in his interest and desire to meet Lahiri Mahasaya. He started to enquire more intensely, by questioning the disciples on the whereabouts of the great *Kriyā* yogi. It was not long before he succeeded in locating the city where Lahiri Mahasaya was, and without informing anyone he immediately set out towards Kashi (Benares, now Vārānasī), determined to find the holy residence of Lahiri Mahasaya. On arrival in Kashi he had to search the labyrinth of streets until he found the right house. After some time he found it and entered. There in front of him seated in a meditative Yoga posture was the great yogi, Lahiri Mahasaya, absorbed in the stillness of deep meditation, with many devotees around him.

Priyanath in his delighted state felt great joy at seeing the Master, and with great respect and reverence of love and devotion he prostrated before him and then sat quietly meditating among the other devotees. In the evening when all the devotees had left, Priyanath devotionally approached Lahiri Mahasaya and expressed his sincere desire to be initiated by him into *Kriyā Yoga*.

Recognising his disciple-to-be, Lahiri joyfully accepted him, and on the auspicious day of 19 August 1883, Priyanath was initiated into the ancient art and science of *Kriyā Yoga*. He stayed with his guru in Benares for many days learning and practising *Kriyā*, before returning to Serampore. Because Priyanath had been a seeker of Truth and wisdom from his early childhood, Lahiri Mahasaya gave him the title of '*Jñānāvatāra*' ('Incarnation of wisdom or divine knowledge').

Around February or March 1894, 11 years after Priyanath had been initiated into *Kriyā*, He went on a pilgrimage to Allahabad in India, where a great spiritual fair called the *Kumbha Melā* (the largest religious festival in the world of several million people who make the pilgrimage every 12 years to Allahabad, when the alignment of the stars is particularly auspicious) was taking place at the confluence of three spiritual rivers – Ganges, Jamuna, and a subterranean river called Saraswati. A huge assembly of thousands of spiritual pilgrims, sages, yogis, ascetics and saints gathered there to bathe in the spiritual atmosphere and be blessed.

Priyanath set up his temporary residence on the Allahabad side of the river Jumuna. One day during his visit to the *Kumbha Melā* he crossed over to the other side of the river Jumuna in a small boat. On reaching the opposite bank he continued walking along by the river, musing over the similarities of the Gospel teachings of Christ with those of Krishna's teachings in the *Bhāgavad Gītā*. While absorbed in these deep thoughts as he continued walking, he suddenly heard a voice calling out from somewhere behind him, '*Swāmiji! Swāmiji!*'

Priyanath was bewildered by this, and thought: 'Is he calling me? But how can that be? I'm not a *swāmi*.' And so he did not respond and continued walking. Then, as Priyanath turned and looked around, he saw a young *swāmi* monk approaching him and pointing to a tent nearby, saying, '*Swāmiji*, follow me, there is a saint who wants to see you.' So the surprised Priyanath followed the monk to the temporary hermitage of tents, and as he arrived at one of the tents he was divinely greeted by a beautiful young yogi with a radiant aura, who looked about 25 years of age. His long reddish-brown hair fell around his shoulders, and his perfectly proportioned toned body stood gracefully upright. The yogi's face broke into a radiant and joyful smile, and he said to Priyanath, '*Swāmiji*, please sit here. I have something to share with you.'

Priyanath seemed perplexed, and replied, 'Why are you addressing me as *swāmiji*? I'm not a renunciate.' The saintly yogi replied, '*Swāmiji*, why are you disagreeing with me? Nobody contradicts my words. Those who are of a higher consciousness speak in their own language. I address you in such a language, so do not be upset.'

This was the time now for Priyanath to renounce the worldly life, for he had no attachments, his wife had recently died and his daughter had got married. It was only his elderly mother that was living with him.

Priyanath felt a strong attraction to this mysterious yogi, who resembled his beloved *Kriyā* guru, Lahiri Mahasaya, with the same spiritual magnetism. He recognised the same divine qualities in his being of compassion, and love and devotion for God. With deep respect and devotion Priyanath joyfully prostrated at the holy feet of Mahavatar Babaji, the great immortal Himalayan yogi.

Babaji then gave him his blessing and said, 'At the request of your guru, you wrote a commentary on the *Bhāgavad Gītā*, now I request you to write something for me.'

Priyanath then recognised that this yogi saint was the great guru of Lahiri Mahasaya, the immortal Himalayan yogi, Mahavatar Babaji. With feelings of great joy and devotion he prostrated at the holy feet of Babaji. As he rose from the floor he humbly asked Babaji, 'What would you like me to write?'

Babaji replied, 'Write a book about the spiritual philosophies of East and West, to give an understanding and unity of Truth to those living in the Western countries.'

On hearing these instructions from Babaji, Priyanath, feeling unqualified for the task, said, 'Gurudeva, my apologies, but my knowledge is limited, how can I write such a spiritual book?'

This caused Babaji to laugh out aloud, and raising his right hand in giving a blessing, replied, 'The thought of this divine work is of a higher inspiration that has been expressed through divine intuition through me. You have heard these words from my mouth and so the work will be done. It is the work of the Divine that He will do.'

With great respect and devotion Priyanath gladly accepted his Master's wish, and said, 'Gurudeva, when I complete the holy book I will need to see you again so that you can check it. How will I see you?'

Babaji smiled lovingly at his disciple, 'Don't worry, we will meet again!'

It was now time for Priyanath to leave the *Kumbha Melā* at Allahabad. As he gave his last respects and farewell to Babaji and turned to depart, Babaji expressed some last words to him. Priyanath, looking puzzled, could not understand the meaning of the mystical words, but as he left he made a mental note of them.

Divinely blessed by the grace of Babaji, Priyanath returned to see his divine guru, Lahiri Mahasaya, in Benares. On his return he saw Lahiri sitting in a meditation posture surrounded by his *Kriyā* disciples. Priyanatha bowed before him and began to give him an account of his blessed experience of meeting Babaji at the *Kumbha Melā*, and related to Lahiri the holy words of Babaji that were spoken to him.

For a few moments there was a solemn silence. Hearing the words of Babaji related to him by Priyanath caused Lahiri great concern. His feeling of joy and countenance turned gravely serious, so much so that he turned pale and became very quiet. Lahiri remained in silence for three hours. This caused some anxiety in his disciples, and Priyanath began to feel responsible for causing this situation of sorrow.

When the three hours had passed, Lahiri Mahasaya returned to his normal joyful self, which brought great relief to both Priyanath and the disciples.

Priyanath now realised that he had been entrusted with a necessary task that must be carried out, and so on his return to Serampore he began to plan out the writing of the book. And by the end of the year he had completed the book, which was titled *Kalvalya Darshanam* (*The Holy Science*).

It was known later that Lahiri Mahasaya had understood from Babaji's words that he was going to die soon. His mission to establish *Kriyā Yoga* was almost fulfilled and his sojourn on Earth was close to coming to an end.

PARAMHANSA YOGANANDA (1893–1952)

Paramhansa Yogananda was born in Gorakhpur, northern India, on 5 January 1893 to his Bengali parents, who were of the *Kshatriya* caste (caste of warriors and rulers). His birth name was Mukunda Lal Ghosh. He was the second son and the fourth child of eight. His father, Bhagabati Charan Ghosh, was a direct disciple of the great *Kriyā* Master, Lahiri Mahasaya. Lahiri had left his body in *mahāsamādhi* two years after Mukunda was born. When Mukunda was a baby, his parents took him to Lahiri Mahasaya to receive spiritual blessings. Lahiri foretold his future by saying, 'This baby when he grows up will enlighten the whole universe with his divine wisdom and will guide many spiritual aspirants on the path of *Kriyā Yoga*.'

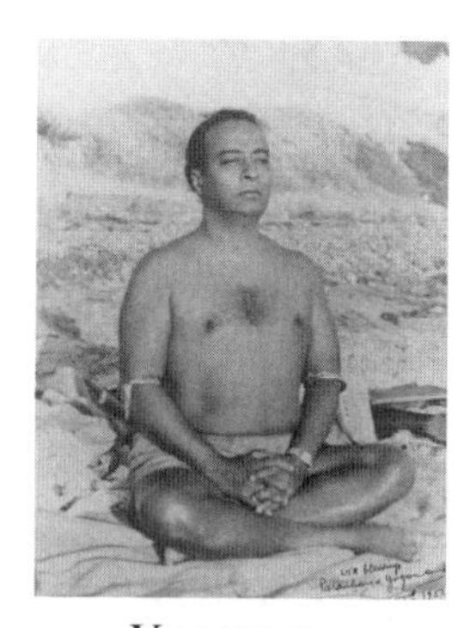

YOGANANDA MEDITATING IN THE DESERT

Yogananda is revered worldwide and known mainly through his successful book *Autobiography of a Yogi*. Yogananda is a great spiritual master of *Kriyā Yoga*, and was the last *Kriyā* Master in a particular line of gurus going back to Mahavatar Babaji.

Soon after graduating from Calcutta University in 1915, Mukunda Lal Ghosh took the formal vows of the monastic Swāmi Order and was given the name of Swāmi Yogananda Giri by his beloved guru, Swāmi Sri Yukteswar Giri (whose family name was Priya Nath Karar). His main hermitage was in Serampore, near Calcutta, an ancestral mansion that he inherited from his father.

In his *Autobiography of a Yogi*, Yogananda tells us of his experience of being initiated into *Kriyā Yoga* by his guru, Yukteswar: 'The technique I had already received from two disciples of Lahiri Mahasaya – Father and my tutor, Swāmi Kebalananda – but in Master's presence (Sri Yukteswar) I felt transforming power. At his touch, a great light broke upon my being, like glory of countless suns blazing together. A flood of ineffable bliss, overwhelming my heart to an innermost core, continued during the following day. It was late that afternoon before I could bring myself to leave the hermitage.'

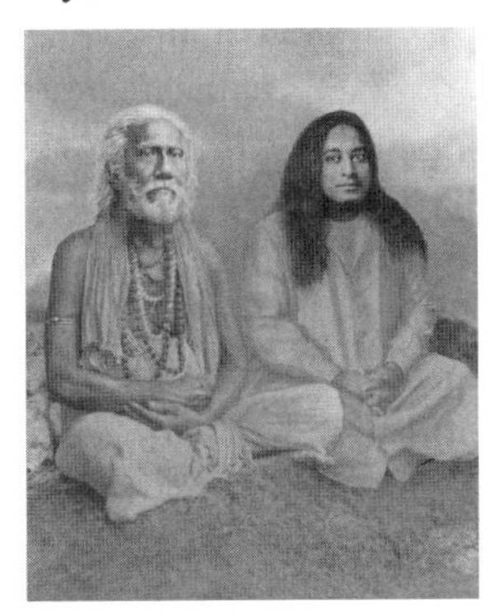

In 1920, after ten years of intensive Yoga training with Swāmi Sri Yukteswar, Yogananda was invited to visit America to attend a seminar of world religions in Boston organised by the Congress of Religious Liberals, as a representative of India. Sri Yukteswar told him, 'If you go now, all doors will be open to you.' Yogananda accepted the invitation and travelled by ship to America, spoke at the Congress and remained in Boston for three years teaching *Kriyā Yoga*. This was an immediate success, and afterwards thousands of spiritually inspired Americans were blessed to take *Kriyā* Initiation from him. After this, Yogananda did an extensive lecture tour of the USA, travelling to many of the major cities, paid for from funds donated by his Boston disciples.

During Yogananda's first visit to Los Angeles in 1925, more than 3,000 people attended his lectures. Following this great interest in *Kriyā Yoga*, Yogananda soon established the organisation Self-Realization Fellowship (SRF) in Los Angeles, California. A hotel building and several acres of land was purchased for the ashram site. There, accommodation was provided for disciples, both male and female, who wanted to live the renunciant life as *Kriyā* yogis.

Yogananda had much to do in completing his mission of disseminating the teachings of *Kriyā Yoga* in America and so he had not seen his master, Swāmi Sri Yukteswar, for 15 years. But in 1935, after Sri Yukteswar's many requests over the years for Yogananda to return, he sent a final message to him, 'You must come back to India with a return ticket at least for a few days, leaving your activities there however important they may be.'

Realising the importance of his master's urgent message, Yogananda, now 42 years of age, returned for the first and last time to Sri Yukteswar's hermitage in Serampore. On arrival at the hermitage, and filled with great anticipation, Yogananda once again met his beloved guru in the peaceful courtyard of the two-storeyed hermitage. Swāmi Sri Yukteswar, the 80-year-old *Kriyā* guru stood clothed simply in a faded orange-coloured *dhoti* and shirt, calmly and nobly in front of him. Yogananda lowered himself to his knees and with bowed head offered with great respect and humility his soul's gratitude and greeting, touching with his hand his guru's holy feet and then, in humble obeisance, his own head. He then rose and was lovingly embraced on both sides of his chest by Sri Yukteswar. They were both so filled with intense joy, with the warmth of renewed soul-union, that at first no words were expressed between them.

After this heart-filled reunion with his master in Serampore, Yogananda visited Ranchi and then Mysore in southern India, and to other parts of India. One of the ashrams he visited was that of Sri Ramana Maharshi (1879–1950) in Tiruvannāmalai. Ramana Maharshi was one of the greatest spiritual gurus of modern-day India. At the age of 17 he attained a profound experience of the true Self without the guidance of a guru and thereafter remained conscious of his identity with the Absolute at all times, until his passing in *mahāsamādhi* in 1950.

This sacred pilgrimage site in Tiruvannāmalai and his meeting with an adept disciple of Ramana Maharshi, named Yogi Ramiah, had a spiritually inspiring influence on Yogananda. Later, after returning to Calcutta, Yogananda quietly told Richard Wright, the young American writer companion travelling with him, 'It seems like Yogi Ramaih is even more advanced than his guru!'

Yogananda then returned to his guru's hermitage, and after a few days he gave a talk before a large audience at Albert Hall in Calcutta, with Swāmi Sri Yukteswar seated beside him on the platform.

He then gave a talk before the alumni of Serampore College, where Yogananda had once been a student.

At the end of December 1935, a Winter Solstice Festival was celebrated at Yukteswar's Serampore hermitage. Many of Sri Yukteswar's disciples gathered there from far and near, and joined in devotional chanting and a feast served by young disciples. In the courtyard under the starry night sky, Swāmi Sri Yukteswar requested Yogananda to give a talk in English about his journey to America to the disciples. He concluded his talk with a fervent tribute to his beloved master, Yukteswar: 'His omnipresent guidance was with me not alone on the ocean steamer, but daily throughout my 15 years in the vast and hospitable land of America.'

When the guests had departed, Sri Yukteswar called Yogananda to his bedroom where once he permitted him to sleep on his wooden bed. Sri Yukteswar sat quietly on the bed, surrounded by his disciples seated at his blessed feet. As Yogananda quickly entered the room, Sri Yukteswar smiled and said to him, 'Yogananda, are you leaving now for Calcutta? Please return here tomorrow. I have certain things to tell you.'

The next afternoon Yogananda returned to the hermitage to see his guru. Sri Yukteswar said a few simple words of blessing and bestowed Yogananda with the further monastic title of *Paramhansa*. From then onwards Swāmi Yogananda came to be known as Paramhansa Yogananda.

Sri Yukteswar become quiet for a moment. Then with gentleness he calmly looked at Yogananda, and speaking quietly said, 'My task on earth is now finished; you must carry on. Please send someone to take charge of our ashram at Puri (near the bay of Bengal). I leave everything in your hands. You will be able to successfully sail the boat of your life and that of the organisation to the divine shores.'

Hearing these words from his guru caused Yogananda's heart to palpitate in fear, and with tear-filled eyes he lovingly embraced Sri Yukteswar's feet. With compassion for his disciple, Sri Yukteswar stood up and blessed him endearingly.

The following day Yogananda carried out his guru's wishes by summoning Swāmi Sebananda, a *Kriyā Yoga* disciple from Ranchi, and sent him to Sri Yukteswar's Karar ashram in Puri to assume the ashram duties there.

Sri Yukteswar, now nearing his eighty-first birthday, knew that his bodily departure from earth was approaching. He was prepared for it, but it was difficult for Yogananda to accept the hints he had been given, that his beloved guru would soon be departing this world.

One day while at his guru's ashram in 1936, Yogananda said to Sri Yukteswar, 'Sir, the *Kumbha Melā* is convening this month at Allahabad.'

Reluctantly, Sri Yukteswar replied, 'Do you really want to go?'

Not sensing his guru's reluctance to let him go, he replied, 'Once you beheld the blessed sight of Babaji at an Allahabad *Kumbha*. Perhaps this time I shall be fortunate enough to see him.'

Sri Yukteswar replied, 'I do not think you will meet him there.' He then became silent, not wishing to obstruct Yogananda's enthusiastic plans.

And so the next day as Yogananda set out for Allahabad with a small group, Sri Yukteswar quietly blessed him. Yogananda and his group arrived at the *Kumbha Melā* on 23 January 1936, to an overwhelming and impressive sight of a surging crowd of nearly two million persons. Holy sadhus, yogis, and shaven-headed *swāmis* wearing ochre or orange-coloured robes appeared by the thousands, their faces beaming with enthusiasm and joy.

Yogananda, fascinated and inspired by the spiritual ardour of these devotees, spent his first day there just observing them. On the second day at the *Kumbha Melā* he visited various ashrams and temporary huts, receiving blessings from saintly persons who were staying there.

Driving in a Ford car, Yogananda and his American companion Richard Wright crossed a creaky pontoon bridge spanning the very low water of the Ganges river. The car crawled slowly like a snake through the crowds of pilgrims, and along narrow twisting lanes, passing the site on the river bank where Babaji and Sri Yukteswar had once met at a *Kumbha Melā*.

After having two more days at the *Kumbha Melā*, Yogananda and his group headed north-west along the banks of the holy river Jumuna to Agra to see the Taj *mahā*l, and then onwards to Brindaban to the Katayani Peith Ashram of Swāmi Keshabananda, a direct disciple of Lahiri Mahasaya.

Yogananda and his group were warmly welcomed by Swāmi Keshabananda, a yogi nearly 90 years of age, with long hair, a snow-white beard, joyful twinkling eyes, and a surprisingly muscular body that radiated strength and health.

Yogananda informed Keshabananda that he wanted to include him in his forthcoming book (*Autobiography of a Yogi*). Swāmi Keshabananda agreed and began telling Yogananda some stories about his life. He told Yogananda that practically his whole life had been spent in Himalayan caves that he travelled to on foot, and for a short time he had maintained a small ashram outside Hardwar, but later the Ganges river flooded and swept it away.

After two hours of listening to Swāmi Keshabananda's interesting stories they sat together on the dining patio for a banquet dinner that had been prepared in Yogananda's honour.

When they had finished dinner, Keshabananda quietly led Yogananda to a secluded spot outside the ashram where they could talk. He looked at Yogananda and said, 'Your arrival is not unexpected, I have a message for you.'

Yogananda was completely taken by surprise at Keshabananda's words, for no one had known of his plan to visit him.

Keshabananda continued, 'While roaming last year in the northern Himalayas near Badrinarayan, I lost my way. Shelter appeared in a spacious cave, which was empty, though the embers of a fire glowed in a hole in the rocky floor. Wondering about the occupant of this lonely retreat, I sat near the fire, my gaze fixed on the sunlit entrance to the cave. Then, suddenly from behind me I heard the words, "Keshabananda, I am glad you are here." I turned, startled, and was dazzled to behold Babaji! The great guru had materialised himself in a recess of the cave. Overjoyed to see him again after many years, I prostrated myself at his holy feet.

'Babaji continued, "I called you here. That is why you lost your way and were led to my temporary abode in this cave. It is a long time since our last meeting; I am pleased to greet you once again."

'The deathless master blessed me with some words of spiritual help, then added: "I give you a message for Yogananda. He will pay you a visit on his return to India. Many matters connected with his guru and with the surviving disciples of Lahiri will keep Yogananda fully occupied. Tell him, then, that I won't see him this time, as he is eagerly hoping; but I shall see him on some another occasion."'

This message of consoling promise from Babaji deeply touched Yogananda's heart.

Yogananda and his party stayed one night as guests of Keshabananda's ashram and the following afternoon continued their tour to Calcutta.

Yogananda was eager to see Swāmi Sri Yukteswar, but on arrival in Calcutta was disappointed to hear that his beloved guru had left Serampore and was now in Puri, about 300 miles to the south.

A telegraph message had been sent to one of Sri Yukteswar's disciples (Atul Chandra Roy Choudhury) in Calcutta, informing him to come immediately to Puri. News of this message reached Yogananda, and, anguished at its implications, he dropped to his knees and implored God to spare his guru's life. As he was about to leave his father's home for the train to Puri, a divine voice spoke within him, 'Do not go to Puri tonight. Your prayer cannot be granted.'

Overcome with grief, Yogananda obeyed the divine inward command and remained in Calcutta until the following evening when he took a train to Puri. Later when the train entered Puri, Yogananda had a vision of Sri Yukteswar, who was sitting with a very grave countenance, and with a light on each side of him.

Yogananda asked, 'Is it all over?'

His guru nodded, then slowly vanished.

The following morning at Puri, Yogananda stepped down from the train, and still hoping against hope, stood on the platform. An unknown man approached him and said, 'Have you heard that your Master is gone?' The man then left without uttering another word.

Yogananda was stunned, but soon realised that in diverse ways his guru was trying to communicate to him the devastating news.

Swāmi Sri Yukteswar Giri (81 years old) had passed away in *mahāsamādhi* at 7.00 pm, 9 March 1936.

On finally reaching his guru's Puri ashram, Yogananda entered the room where his guru's body was sitting in the lotus posture, with a beatific expression of tranquillity on his face. A short time before his passing, Sri Yukteswar had been slightly ill with fever, but before the day of his ascension into the Infinite, his body had become completely well. He had relinquished his body at the hour of mystic summoning.

The next day Yogananda prostrated at his Master's holy feet, then after carrying out the ancient rituals of the *swāmis* he buried Sri Yukteswar's body in the garden of his Puri ashram. Afterwards a thatched hut was built over that place.

Yogananda remained for some time at the Puri Ashram, but this was to be his last time in India. He never returned. His divine mission was now to take place in America, to spread the teachings of *Kriyā Yoga*.

Three months later, before leaving India, in the afternoon of 9 June 1936, Yogananda was sitting on his bed in a Bombay hotel in deep meditation. Suddenly, before his opened eyes he was astonished to see the whole room transform into another world of bright illumination and splendour. Waves of rapturous delight engulfed him, for there before him stood the resurrected body of his beloved Master, Sri Yukteswar, that he had missed so much. Yogananda was astounded; he could not believe what his eyes were seeing.

'But is it you, Master, the same Lion of God? Are you wearing a body like the one I buried beneath the cruel Puri sands?'

'Yes, my child, I am the same. This is a flesh and blood body. Though I see it as ethereal, to your sight it is physical. From the cosmic atoms I created an entirely new body, exactly like that cosmic dream physical body which you laid beneath the dream sands at Puri in your dream world. I am in truth resurrected – not on earth but on an astral planet.'

Sri Yukteswar then proceeded to give Yogananda a wonderful exposition on the astral Cosmos. Then after some time of listening with great interest and devotion, Yogananda said, 'Angelic guru, your body looks exactly as it did when I last wept over it in the Puri ashram.'

Sri Yukteswar replied, 'O yes, my new body is a perfect copy of the old one. I materialise or dematerialise this form any time at will more frequently than I did while on Earth. By quick dematerialisation, I now travel instantly by light express from planet to planet or, indeed, from astral to causal or to the physical Cosmos.' Sri Yukteswar smiled. 'Though you move about so fast these days, I had no difficulty in finding you in Bombay!'

In 1946 Yogananda's *Autobiography of a Yogi* was published (now available in 32 languages, and truly a spiritual classic). A few years later, when Yogananda was asked why so many people declared that reading it had transformed their lives, he quietly said, 'Because my spirit is in it.'

As well as spreading the teachings of *Kriyā Yoga*, Yogananda also demonstrated the underlying unity between the spiritual teachings of India, as expressed in the *Bhagavad Gītā*, and the original teachings of Christ as given in the Gospels of the Bible. Yogananda showed that all religions, whatever their outward forms, are rooted in the same essential Truth.

The last two years of Yogananda's life were spent mostly in seclusion at his retreat house near Twentynine Palms, California, writing commentaries on the *Bhāgavad*

Gītā. He consciously left his physical body in *mahāsamādhi* (superconscious exit from the body) on 7 March 1952 while giving a banquet and talk welcoming the newly independent India's first ambassador, Binay Ranjan Sen, and his wife Srimati Sen, to California. Yogananda was giving his final speech and at the end of his talk, with love and devotion, he recited his poem 'My India', which praised the spiritual wealth of India. The poem touched the audience's hearts and they responded with ecstatic applause, but as Yogananda went to take his seat, suddenly his body collapsed on the stage. The last of this great line of enlightened *Kriyā* Masters had expired his last breath.

7.4

KRIYĀ YOGA PLUS DEVOTION

> 'Win conviction of God's presence through your own joyous contact in meditation…I myself consider *Kriyā* the most effective device of salvation through self-effort ever to be evolved in man's search for the Infinite.'
>
> *Swāmi Kebalananda Giri, in Yogananda 1946, p.40*

Yogananda also said, 'Without devotion, you can't touch God; you keep Him at a distance.' And Jesus Christ also reminds us that devotion is needed: 'Love the Lord thy God with all thy heart, and with all thy soul, and with all thy mind, and with all thy strength..' (Luke 10:27). With devotion in the heart, sincere effort, and consistent regular practice of the techniques of *Kriyā Yoga* over a long period of time, a devotee attains an inner awakening more fulfilling than any experience that the mind, senses or feelings can give. It is only when the soul becomes conscious that the sense of self-division, the sense of finitude and limitation, is part of an illusion and that everything is already within itself, that its desire for experience will stop. Freed from the mind's restless nature, and the obstacles of distraction, the devotee's attention is concentrated and interiorised with love and devotion on the God Self within.

The *Kriyā Yoga* techniques should never be practised in an unaware, dry and mechanical way. One has to have the right attitude, and practise with awareness and devotion, in an attitude of self-offering to the Divine.

Without the natural love of the heart, spiritual progress is ineffectual and the mind becomes dry like an arid desert; the sweet water of love is not present. Without devotion, knowledge and wisdom becomes dry intellectualisation.

The *Kātha Upaniṣad* informs us:

> 'The Self cannot be known through study or learning, nor through the intellect, nor through hearing or memorising the sacred scriptures. The Self is known and realised by those whose heart and mind is pure, and who by being able to concentrate deeply upon the Self, abide in their own true nature.'
>
> *Kātha Upaniṣad 2:23–24 (Author's translation)*

When the heart's feelings are awakened they need to be directed upward in the spine in devotional calm meditation, otherwise, if they are not directed these feelings will feed the emotions, causing the heart's feelings to become unsettled and turn outward in the form of restless desires, in seeking fulfilment outside. The practice of meditation is directed towards calming and neutralising the *vṛttis*, vortices of ego-feeling – waves of desire, likes, dislikes – which cause mental ripples to rotate around the ego. Meditation is the process of neautralising these waves of feeling, by releasing the ego's involvement with them. How? By calmly observing with awareness the waves of feeling as they arise without becoming involved or identified with them. In this way the waves gradually subside into calmness.

CHARACTERISTICS OF A TRUE DEVOTEE

To develop spiritually and to progress to higher meditation one must have a totally integrated inner personality. The following noble disciplines and characteristics nurture, nourish and strengthen the inner spiritual seeker, the devotee who seeks to realise his or her own Infinite and Divine Nature.

Never harbours malice or hatred towards anyone. Does not restrict the blessings that are unfolding in his or her life by harbouring malice or animosity towards others.

Always kind, friendly, and compassionate towards all. Kindness teaches one to be merciful and compassionate. In kindness the devotee expresses love to all, always seeing the Divine in them, knowing that Spirit in All is his own Self.

Free from attachment, egoism and pride. Free from the sense of 'I', 'me' and 'mine' (ego attachment), the devotee knows that whatever pleasures arise from the sense objects are only a source of attachment ending in suffering.

Even-minded in pleasure and pain. The devotee is even-minded under all conditions – in pleasure and pain, respect and disrespect, criticism or praise. The devotee does not seek fame or recognition and is not flattered by praise nor vexed by envy, nor angered or grieved at nonfulfilment of desires. Having attained the true joy of the inner blissful Self, the devotee has such a complete sense of fulfilment that there is no desire for attaining anything.

Always forgiving towards all. Does not hold hurt, wronged feeling, grudges, resentment, blame, harsh judgement or malice towards anyone. Peace comes not through logic or reason, but through spiritual understanding. By choosing forgiveness, the heart and mind are at peace. Forgiveness creates understanding and harmony. The devotee affirms: 'I am ready to forgive, ready to release what was or could have been, and accept what is.'

Inwardly content and balanced in mind. There is no room for mundane desires in the heart of the devotee, who is fulfilled. The devotee finds joy and heart satisfaction inwardly in the divine Self, and so does not wish for any material desires to be fulfilled.

Steadfast in meditation. Established in regular daily meditation practice, with thoughts and senses controlled, the devotee's mind, intellect and heart are focused inwardly on the Divine Self.

Self-disciplined and self-controlled. Self-discipline and self-control are essential for concentrating the mind and making it one-pointed, so that one's energies can be focused, channelled and directed towards the Divine.

Firm in conviction. Steady-minded with a determined resolution and firm faith, the devotee lives joyfully with mind and intellect centred in the Divine. Determination builds willpower and courage, leading to success in all fields of life. Firmness leads to self-reliance and fearlessness.

Heart and mind dedicated to the supreme Reality. The spiritual life requires a continual spiritual awareness. With self-discipline, the mind, heart and intellect of a devotee is one-pointed in dedication towards the supreme Self, the absolute Existence, Consciousness, Bliss, Eternity and Purity.

Free from agitation. The devotee does not agitate others, nor is agitated by others. Since the devotee is not entangled in the world of attachments and superficial conditions, he or she is not disturbed by such emotions as envy, jealousy, fear and anxiety, and intolerance. The devotee remains inwardly calm, serene, undisturbed and undissipated. A mind that is calm is undisturbed in all situations whether they be favourable or unfavourable.

Free from dependence. Free from material desires, attachment, and from dependence, not identifying oneself with the body, mind and the objects of the senses, the devotee always draws inspiration, equanimity and joy from the true source of supreme Bliss – from the inner Self.

Pure in body, mind and heart. Cleanliness in body means outer bodily cleanliness and eating pure *sattvic* vegetarian food. Being pure of heart and mind is the cleanliness of the inner Self. The devotee follows the ten attitudes (*yamas* and *niyamas*) that help to create the necessary basis for the higher practices of *Kriyā Yoga* meditation to realise one's true spiritual nature, the inner blissful Self.

Enthusiastic. The devotee is clear about the spiritual goal and the path, method and techniques by which to attain it. The devotee is positive, energetic and enthusiastic, and seeks the Divine with their entire personality and wholehearted devotion.

Cheerful and optimistic. Being cheerful and optimistic enables one to avoid thoughts or feelings of fear, limitation or incompetence.

Love and devotion. Of all spiritual practices, the highest is the constant remembrance of the Supreme Lord with a heart overflowing with love and devotion. Whether you relate to that Supreme Reality with love and devotion as God or Self, it is the same eternal Consciousness, that is One. God is within you as you (the Self). For one who has realised the absolute Truth, everything that exists is God, the supreme Self, who exists in every perceivable form. God, the Self, is simultaneously both the subject and the object. The highest form of prayer is the mental repetition (*japa*) with aspiration and love of the name of God, which is a concentrated focus upon itself.

NINE QUALITIES OF A *KRIYĀ* YOGI

Loyalty and dedication

Loyalty is acceptance of God and guru with open heart and mind. It is being devoted, receptive and cooperative with your guru.

The disciple remains steadfast, dedicated and devoted to both the enlightened guru and his teachings to find inner freedom in God.

Kriyā Yoga is a full-time pursuit. It requires commitment to achieving the goal of realisation, of seeing divinity at all times and in all places. Self-transformation requires constant dedicated practice with zest and enthusiasm. Those who have a high level of loyalty, commitment, enthusiasm and devotion, who persevere without giving up easily, and who are constant in their spiritual practices and meditation, achieve successful results.

Faith

In Sanskrit the word for faith is *śraddha*, meaning respect, implicit faith and self-confidence. This means you must have great respect, implicit faith and trust your guru and his teachings. You must also have self-confidence that God's grace and your guru will guide you through the obstacles and difficulties that you may encounter on the spiritual path.

By regularly meditating deeply, and feeling and experiencing that deep inner calmness, bliss, love, peace and energy – divine qualities of God – we attain deep faith.

Devotion

> 'The nature of spiritual devotion is the supreme love. And its essence is the nectar of immortality.'
>
> *Narada Bhakta Sūtras, verses 2–3, in Prakash 1998, pp.8–9*

Devotion is the state of mind in which one has no separate existence apart from God. To be devoted is to engage with love. All expressions of love are manifestations of that supreme Love which is the love of God, the highest state, and ultimate goal. Complete devotion is love for both the formless, transcendent God and the immanent God. Within you is the Divine Love that is God, and it is revealed to you when your heart is pure enough to receive it.

Devotion is cultivated by slow, constant and steady effort. Devotion promotes humility, love for the Divine, and love towards all beings. When we no longer seek return for love given, we can love all beings as expressions of God's omnipresence, for God resides in all beings.

Study alone cannot give us God-realisation: our knowledge must be balanced with meditation and devotion to receive God's grace. Similarly, devotion without study, service, and meditation limits our realisation of our full spiritual potential.

> 'Love is patient, love is kind. It does not envy, it does not boast, it is not proud. It is not rude, it is not self-seeking, it is not easily angered, it keeps no records of wrongs.'
>
> *I Corinthians 4–5*

Without devotion, the Yoga of knowledge of the Self (*Jñanā Yoga*) becomes dry intellectualisation. There must be a balance of the heart and mind to attain the highest perfection – knowledge of the Self and love of God. Devotional love without discrimination falls into sentimentality and sensuality, whereas intellect without the sweetness of the heart's love is unable to radiate any joy or bliss.

Humility

The disciple has an understanding heart. Not seeking fame, flattery or admiration, he or she is free from the sense of self-importance. The disciple's will is attuned to God's Will, whatever action or work is performed is done selflessly, guided by the creative power of Divine Spirit.

Humility is not humiliation. To have humility is not the same as being diminished or degraded, which is what humiliation is. Humility reminds you to receive others with kindness, understanding and compassion; aware of your own limitations, you can accept theirs.

Right attitude

Having right attitude is essential on the spiritual path to break free from the conditioning of limiting and negative beliefs of the ego-self, so that you can express your true divine nature. In your attitude lies either your greatest obstacles or your transformation to higher consciousness. Your opinions are the root cause of your negative attitudes. When these opinions are reinforced by your feelings and emotions, your attitudes arise. These attitudes can be positive or negative, and can be divided into those that you have towards life, towards yourself, and towards others. Accepting a spiritual perspective to life and adopting attitudes that are aligned with love and understanding will guide you towards a more fulfilling and joyful life.

A *Kriyā* yogi cannot attain spiritual realisation with *Kriyā* technique alone. Practising the *yamas* and *niyamas* are important and necessary for the *Kriyā* yogi in cultivating right attitudes, devotion and selflessness.

Right attitude is having the right mental attitude towards God and guru; towards life; towards work and service; towards your family, relationships and all others. It is having a cheerful disposition, and a positive and optimistic outlook on life, not dwelling upon the negative aspects. The wrong and negative attitudes of finding fault with or criticising others, or being moody, irritable, holding grudges and resentments, are all obstacles to spiritual progress.

Sincerity

Spirituality and sincerity are inseparable. Spiritual sincerity leaves no room for doubt or falsehood. It is to be true to the Spirit, to the will of the Divine. Sincerity elevates us from the falsehood of ego into the higher vibration of Truth. Loyalty to a spiritual guru and his tradition and teaching without sincerity and conviction is hypocrisy. If you are sincere you will truly follow your deepest spiritual aspirations by being constant and faithful in practising *Kriyā Yoga* disciplines and meditating regularly, to raise your consciousness.

Sincerity is also practising what you preach. It is being true to yourself. A sincere attitude is one in which your expressions of friendship towards others is sincere, and the promises you make are kept and honoured. Being truthful, genuine, honest and having integrity are also related to sincerity. A person whose thoughts, words and deeds are consistent has integrity. To tell a lie to someone is the ego's attempt to establish its apparent separation, for lying is a means of avoiding respect and love for another person.

To disguise, hide under a false appearance, conceal facts, intentions, thoughts and feelings under some false pretence, is dissimulation or insincerity.

Self-discipline

Discipline is required in every field of endeavour, but is particularly essential for success in spiritual effort. The disciple must have a steady, unceasing zeal to progress spiritually. In the beginning there will be need for many changes in your lifestyle and your attitudes.

Spiritual disciplines are means of self-instruction that we engage in for the growth of our higher awareness. To be successful spiritually – to realise our identity with the Ultimate Reality – requires a high degree of inner discipline.

By practising the *yamas* you can restrain harmful physical urges, and unwholesome thoughts and impulses. And by cultivating the *niyamas* you can improve the quality of your mind and make it stronger.

Willingness

> 'Never relax your efforts until there is Enlightenment. Let no gaps interrupt your attempt, for a gap will produce An eddy, whereas your striving must be continuous like the flowing of oil; it must be sustained, constant, an unbroken stream.'
>
> *Anandamayi Ma, in Atmananda 1982, p.20*

Few are willing to work hard to achieve spiritual progress. Those who are willing to make an intense spiritual effort over and over again to achieve the spiritual goal of life have success. Lethargy (*alasya*) makes one unwilling to meditate.

One of the first things you can do to help yourself along the spiritual path is to develop greater willpower. Yogananda said, 'The stronger the will, the stronger the flow of energy.' A strong willpower gives sustained and determined effort to succeed.

Selfless service

Selfless service is a natural expression of love, given joyfully and spontaneously, and is an integral aspect of spiritual life. It purifies the heart and mind. Service means carrying out all your duties conscientiously with dedication of purpose, and doing them well. Faith, humility, devotion, service and love towards all are the primary requisites. Our highest duty is to realise our divinity – the inner Self as *Sat-chit-ānanda* (Ever-Existing, Ever-Conscious, Ever-New Bliss), which is the same nature as God.

Serving others selflessly, without expectation of reward or recognition, is a devotional practice of a high order, and it provides a field for reducing the ego.

WAYS OF CULTIVATING LOVE AND DEVOTION FOR THE DIVINE

Some of the ways of cultivating love and devotion for God are:

Practising the Presence of God.

Chanting devotionally. Remember, though, that devotion is not merely an outward show of emotion and continuous loud chanting, but an inward awareness of the consciousness of God.

Prayer.

Reading and contemplating such devotional works as the *Bhāgavad Gītā* and *Narada Sūtras*.

Practising *japa*, mental repetition of a Divine Name, such as *Sri Rāṁ*, *Oṁ Namah Śivaya*, *Oṁ Namo Bhagavate*, *Aum Guru*, or just *Aum*. There are infinite names we can call God. The practice of *japa* neutralises vibrations of material consciousness. All that is needed is a true and sincere love for the Divine whom that name signifies, who is enthroned within the hearts of each and every one of us. When the mind is focused on a *mantra* of the Divine Name, the mind's normally scattered flow of worldly thoughts becomes one-pointed in its concentration. Calmly focused in awareness and devotion, the mind and heart become full of peace and inner joy.

Satsang or associating with others who are of a devotional nature.

PRACTISING THE PRESENCE OF GOD

Yogananda said, 'When you learn to practise the Presence of God in every moment that you are free to think of Him, then even in the midst of work you will be aware of divine communion.' Yogananda's words bring to mind the seventeenth century monk, Brother Lawrence (1611–1691), who was a lowly, unlearned man who served as a lay brother in a Carmelite monastery in Paris. Today he is most commonly remembered for the classic Christian text, *The Practice of the Presence of God.* Much of his life was spent within the walls of the priory, working in the kitchen. He was known for his profound peace and many came to seek spiritual guidance from him.

Brother Lawrence discovered how to live in the presence of God in continual joy every waking moment. To live a life in which every single thought, word and deed is pure and loving enough to be a continual prayer to God every single minute of every single day. The most effective way for Brother Lawrence to commune with God was to simply do his ordinary work out of a pure love for God. He believed it was a serious mistake to think of our prayer time as being different from any other, and that our actions should unite us with God when we are involved in our daily activities, just as our prayer unites us with God in our quiet time.

This is a practice in loving awareness of the Divine that we can all try to make a part of our everyday living. Whatever your activities or duties are, spiritualise them by repeatedly chanting a devotional thought from your heart, the centre of feeling in you. Be fully aware and present in those moments as you chant or pray from your heart. Whatever you are doing, try to keep your consciousness established in the Divine as much as possible; then in time you will experience the Divine's response through your feeling of inner peace, joy and love.

True devotion is seeking to know God, by contacting that Divine Presence within your own heart. Wherever you are, God is – there is no separation except in the thought that creates it. The true meaning of total love of God is not to love God to the exclusion of everything and everyone else, but to love God and to love *all* in God. Love is the ultimate and highest goal to which we can aspire. Every relationship with life should be ultimately a relationship with God, because God is the very ground of our being. God's absolute love is universal, unconditional and unlimited, and is constant, not subject to change. The very desire for love proves the existence of God; love is the doorway to God. God is that very love that we feel deep within us. Be still and know that you are one in God.

DEVOTIONAL CHANTING

> 'Learn to love God as the joy felt in meditation.'
>
> *Yogananda 2003, p.7*

> 'Hear in all songs the heart-stirring ecstasy of God's song. Tune in – hear God's radio programme of celestial inspirations.'
>
> *Yogananda 2003, p.11*

Chanting or singing and listening to devotional chants opens the heart. The sweet attraction of chanting is that it gives you energy and joy. It draws your attention away from the ordinary sense attractions of the outer world, and draws you towards the Divine Consciousness within your own heart. Yogananda said, 'Chanting is half the battle!' This means that chanting can give great effect in helping us to overcome our egoic tendencies on the battlefield of life, so that we may have a perception of God.

Chanting with an intense aspiration can lift the individual soul to the awareness of God. The way to chant is joyfully with focused devotion and meditative concentration. When you chant, listen to the words and feel what they are expressing, and focus on attuning yourself to the aspects of Divine consciousness within each chant. The purpose of chanting is to interiorise the mind, heart and soul into calm stillness.

Begin by chanting softly and gradually increase the energy of chanting to a louder voice. Then gradually decrease your voice so that you are chanting softly, then into a whisper, and finally, feeling the melody, words and spiritual vibration of the chant mentally. The mental chanting will naturally interiorise your mind and heart, bringing you into a state of meditative stillness in which you perceive the Presence of the Divine as joy and bliss permeating through you. As you chant, keep your attention at the Spiritual Eye, at the midpoint between the eyebrows.

Traditionally, the Indian harmonium is used to play the chants, but an electronic keyboard or other instrument such as a guitar can be used. To maintain the rhythm on some chants you can also have someone join you playing an Indian drum such as a *dholak*, *mridaṅga* or *tablas*.

Here are two of my own chants that I composed for guitar: *Jai Guru* and *Oṁ Guru Yogananda*. Both chants are praising my guru, Paramhansa Yogananga.

Jai Guru Yogananda

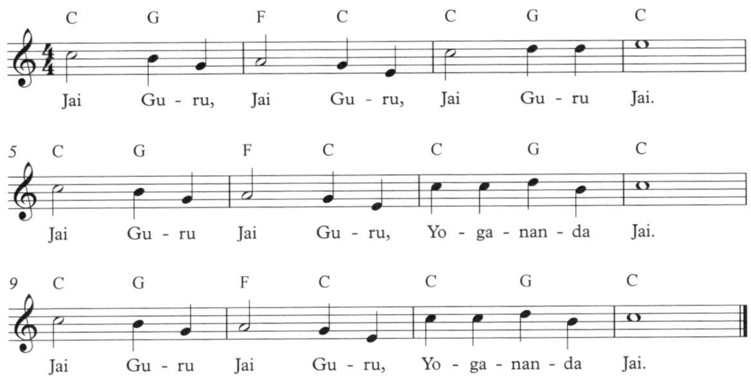

Om Guru Yogananda

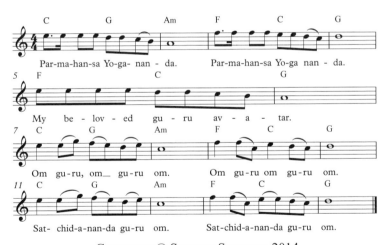

PRAYER

'If we neglect prayer and if the branch is not connected to the vine, it will die. That connecting of the branch to the vine is prayer. If that connection is there then love is there, then joy is there, and we will be the sunshine of God's love, the hope of eternal happiness, the flame of burning love.'

Mother Theresa 1998, p.113

The process of prayer is another way of focusing the mind on the Divine. Through prayer the scattered rays of the mind concentrate upon the object of prayer. It helps you to turn your attention inward to connect consciously with the Divine, so that your thoughts, feelings, beliefs and attitudes are in harmony with the flow of the cosmic process. Prayer opens and enlarges the heart; it opens the door to deeper levels of consciousness, and to God's omnipresent grace.

More than merely an outer posture or position, true prayer is an inner attitude. When we pray in the silence of our hearts, with the heart's intention to feel the presence of God, we enter inner communion with the Divine, a presence, power and activity that helps us to release our outer concerns and open the door of our hearts to God's love, wisdom and guidance.

> 'If we really want to pray, we must first learn to listen: for in the silence of the heart God speaks.'
>
> *Mother Theresa 1998, p.22*

Prayer is the conscious intention to experience the presence of God, seeking to recognise our awareness of God, and of opening ourselves to God's omnipresent power that flows through us. When we pray in this way, we are not praying to God or for God, as something separate from us, but from that divine presence which is our essential Being or Self. Pray with the realisation that you are one with God, and God's Will is done in you. When you pray, do not think of God as being outside of you, for God is within you in the Eternal Now, the prayer and the answer are as one. God the Ultimate Reality is always the only Life expressing in and through all. Your consciousness is the point through which God expresses Itself. And it is also through your consciousness that you express the living Presence of God the Christ within you.

As a drop of ocean water that has been separated from its source eventually makes its way back to the ocean, we are inevitably drawn back into the awareness of our oneness with God. The drop of water may evaporate high up into the clouds then, blown by the wind, fall as snow on a mountain. Eventually the snow will melt and the drop will become part of a small trickle of water, that flows into a brook, and into a stream, then into a river, until it finally returns to the sea and the ocean.

Like the drop of water that cannot be forever separated from its source, the ocean, so our prayers, which are for the purpose of knowing God, return us to the awareness of our oneness in God.

> 'Fix a definite time everyday for praying to God and let that period be dedicated to Him for the rest of your life.'
>
> *Sri Anandamayi Ma, in Ganguli 1995, p.192*

Prayer is allowing ourselves to enter into the Presence of the Divine Being, and that Presence is not sitting on a golden throne in some undefined quarter of a celestial city. If we think that, we have definitely got our geography wrong. The Presence is with us all the time. We have but to allow it to move within us. In the silence of our hearts the Divine speaks to our soul and listens to us.

> 'Regular and ardent prayer, ending with deep and steady meditation, alone can unfold enthusiasm, patience, and the inner sharpness to detect and avoid false

tones in thought, word and action. Through prayer and meditation let us come to feel our oneness with the Infinite Lord.'

Swāmi Chinmayananda, in Thapan 2005, p.223

In prayer you need not request anything at all, because we already have access to all that God is. Many times the things for which we pray are obstacles to our spiritual progress. It is best to pray for results which reduce your desires and promote peace, love and understanding in you. Prayer without any material motive is a powerful means for attaining spiritual fulfilment. We do not pray to God or for God, but from an awareness of the Divine presence within us. In prayer we can affirm what already exists in Truth. By praying affirmatively we assert that we are being guided to our highest good, irrespective of any outer circumstances or temporary appearances. Through affirmative prayer we faithfully pray, giving gratitude in advance that the Divine is blessing our lives with unlimited possibilities and meeting our needs. Below is the well-known prayer associated with saint Francis of Assisi (1182–1226 CE): 'Make me an Instrument of Thy peace.' The prayer has been slightly adjusted to make it an 'affirmative prayer'.

Lord, I am an instrument of Your peace.
Where there is hatred I sow love;
where there is injury, pardon;
where there is doubt, faith;
where there is despair, hope;
and where there is sadness, joy.

O Heavenly Father, I do not so much seek
to be consoled as to console;
to be understood as to understand;
to be loved as to love.

For it is in giving that we receive;
it is in forgiving that we are forgiven;
and it is in dying to ego-consciousness
that we are born into eternal Divine Consciousness.

The best type of prayer is that which asks for the highest things: awareness and Presence of the Divine. The highest prayer of all is for the love of the Supreme Being, the Source of lasting happiness and true security. It is not praying *to* God, but praying from a consciousness of God, so that you become a radiating centre of God-consciousness and immersed in this energy, power, love and light to draw to you whatever you need for your health and wellbeing, abundance, prosperity and success here and now.

Prayer begins with words and thoughts but ends deep inside ourselves in silence, in absolute stillness in the presence of God. It is in this still silence that we find inner peace, contentment, strength, healing and joy. 'Be still and know that I am God' (Psalm 46:10). In other words: Be still and know your Self. In stillness, there is no movement because you are beyond space and time. The moment you are still, you will know the 'I Am' within you; there is just the awareness of the oneness of Being.

The Sanskrit *mantra so'ham*, which is the sound of the inhalation and the exhalation, is really an echo of 'I Am'.

You can pray at any time and in any place, but it works particularly well when you meditate first and enter into the stillness of your heart, the realm of soul intuition within the essence of your being. It is in that inner silent peace and joy of deep meditation that you have made the Divine connection.

Every day, begin and end your meditation with a prayer. Sit quietly, and with a calm mind and an open heart, pray deeply in the spontaneous language of your heart with faith, love and devotion – '*Infinite Spirit, Heavenly Father, Divine Mother, Friend, Beloved God, bless me, guide me, and protect me, show me the true path to Self-realisation.*' Pray using the words that come to you naturally and in the consciousness that the Divine is with you. Then in the inner silence of your Self, the Divine will communicate to you through the silence of intuition. Prayer begins with words, flows into a silent aspiration in the heart, and transforms itself naturally and spontaneously into meditation – the ultimate goal of prayer.

Prayer becomes effective only when it has the total support of your faith, a spirit of self-surrender of ego, devotion and intense aspiration with divine will-force as a continual spiritual discipline. First you attain divine attunement with the Divine in the stillness of meditation, immersing yourself in calmness and inner peace. In this way, prayer detaches the will from desires and objects and spiritually focuses the mind, lifting it upward to a higher reality.

Before you pray it is good to have a concept of God, which can be with form or without form. In the formless aspect God, the Supreme Reality, which has the Divine aspects of infinite Love, Joy or Bliss, is Infinite, Omnipresent, so wherever you are, God is. You can establish your connection with God in meditation and prayer by feeling God's formless Presence in any of God's qualities – love, peace, calmness, wisdom and joy – within you, as you pray *in* God. When your mind is calm and still through deep meditation, then pray for the awareness of God's Presence to be felt within you. In meditative silence with your consciousness inwardly calm and focused, intuitively listen to hear God's silence. Enter an inner communion with the Divine, dissolving all sense of individuality and separation until you experience a oneness with that great Love, Bliss, Wisdom, Calmness, Peace, and Light of God. You can end your prayer for those close to you, your family and friends, and for world peace.

Sanskrit prayers

The following Sanskrit prayers are traditionally used in India, and are commonly chanted before or after meditation.

Sarveśām svastir bhavatu
Sarveśām shāntir bhavatu
Sarveśām pūrnam bhavatu
Sarveśām mangalam bhavatu
Oṁ śhānti, śhānti, śhānti.

May there be happiness for all
May there be peace for all
May there be completeness in all
May there be success for all
Oṁ peace, peace, peace.

Oṁ, Sarve Bhavantu sukhinah
Sarve santu nirāmayāh
Sarve bhadrani paśyantu
Mā kashchit dukha bhāgbhavet
Oṁ śhānti, śhānti, śhānti.
May all be prosperous and happy
May all be free from disease
May all see what is spiritually uplifting
May no one suffer.
Oṁ peace, peace, peace.

Asato mā sadgamaya
Tamaso mā jyotir-gamaya
Mrityor-mā āmritam gamaya
Oṁ śhānti, śhānti, śhānti.
From the unreal (of transitory existence) lead me to the Real (of the eternal Self)
From darkness (of ignorance) lead me to Light (of Spiritual knowledge)
From (the fear of) death lead me to (the Knowledge of) immortality
Oṁ peace, peace, peace.

Praying for others and sending them healing

When praying for others for their wellbeing and to help them overcome their difficulties, it is always good to pray first that they be receptive to God's blessings. This helps by opening the channels so they can be open to receiving God's blessings and grace.

Healing prayer technique

> 'Convert yourself into a divine battery, sending out through your hands divine healing rays whenever and wherever they may be needed. Then your hands, charged with Divine Power, will throw healing rays into your patient's heart and brain. Thus his or her seeds of ignorance will be destroyed, and he or she will smile with the health of God-love.'
>
> *Yogananda 2003, p.10*

To send healing to others through your prayers, first bring your focused attention to your Spiritual Eye, at the midpoint between your eyebrows, and with your consciousness calmly focused visualise the Vibratory Light of God there. Visualise Cosmic Energy surrounding and entering your body through your medulla oblongata at the base of your brain stem, and flowing into your spine. Feel that it is the powerful vibrations of God's Love, Light and Cosmic Energy flowing through you.

By the power of your will at the Spiritual Eye, feel this Cosmic Energy flowing down through your arms into your hands. Energy follows thought and Yogananda said, 'The stronger the will, the stronger the flow of energy' and 'Strong will pulls energy from the Conscious Cosmic Rays surrounding the body through the door of the medulla oblongata.'

First, pray: '*Dear Heavenly Father (or Divine Mother) Thou art omnipresent. Thou art in all Thy children. Thou art in (name). Manifest Thy healing presence in his (or her) body, mind and soul.*'

Then firmly rub up and down your left arm with your right palm, followed by your right arm with your left palm, to stimulate energy in them. Then relax, continuously visualising and willing Cosmic Energy to descend from your medulla through your arms into your hands. Next, with your eyes closed, rub your palms together vigourously until they feel warm and are charged with a tingling sensation of energy. Then, separating your hands magnetised with energy, raise them shoulder-width apart above your head with the palms facing away from you. Feel the life current of energy flowing from your medulla into your Spiritual Eye, arms and hands, and chant the Vibratory Sound *Aum* (*Oṁ*) aloud three times. Feel this Cosmic Energy flowing out though your hands and flowing into the person you are sending healing to, and visualise him or her bathed in God's healing Light and Love, penetrating every cell and atom in their body, dispelling all illness and imperfection. Affirm: '*You are well and whole for God's healing light is within you.*'

Healing prayer for disharmony with others

If you are having challenges with another person over something and you want to lift your own consciousness out of negative thought patterns towards that person, visualise that person bathed in God's Light and for one minute pray: '*Lord, fill him or her with peace and harmony.*' Then visualise yourself bathed in God's Light and pray for 30 seconds: '*Lord, fill me with peace and harmony.*' Practise this five or six times a day.

This simple and clear focused prayer directs the mind towards attunement with God, giving you a practical way to draw God's grace in important aspects of your life.

Satsang

The coarser the object of pleasure, the more short-lived and less elevating is the pleasure arising out of it. Gambling, drinking alcohol, smoking and taking narcotic drugs are all examples of very unrefined pleasures. They do not satisfy or fulfil our soul except for a brief while, and they degrade the mind, making it impure and worldly. The short-lived excitement they cause is a waste of time and energy, and they cause suffering and pain, both mentally and physically. For example, smoking is recognised as the single biggest cause of preventable disease and early death in the United Kingdom, claiming more than 102,000 lives a year.

All these useless distractions cause us to become restless, pulling us away from our Divine Source, causing us to forget our true essential nature – the blissful Self within.

The mind can also become impure by indiscriminately associating and mixing with others who are selfishly self-centred, emotionally negative, weak-willed with bad habits, pleasure seeking and greedy, lustful and hateful. It is like mixing clear, pure water with mud.

Satsang is a Sanskrit word, meaning 'fellowship of Truth'. In other words, keeping company or associating with those who are spiritually minded, those who are wise and virtuous, and who live in Divine Truth. It is sharing your time with those who spiritually inspire, uplift, encourage, and remind you of the spiritual goal: Self- and God-realisation. Good company is essential on the spiritual path, for the company you keep determines whether your energy will move inward towards the Divine, or outward towards the world. By cultivating the right company, *satsang* helps to strengthen and protect you from the temptations and lures of lower goals. When we meditate with others, a beautiful spiritual atmosphere of devotion is created, in which each person meditating is reinforced and supported by the enthusiasm and deep concentration of the other meditators in the group. Meditating regularly and deeply together also helps us to form bonds of spiritual friendship and harmony in Truth.

> 'Environment and the company you keep are of paramount importance. Your outer environment, in conjunction with your inner environment, through your habits, controls your life and molds your tastes and habits.'
>
> *Yogananda 2007a, p.46*

> 'For the beginner, especially, association with others who are firmly on the path is essential. He needs their spiritual magnetism to help him to develop the power to rise above vitiating influences in the world around him, and in himself.'
>
> *Kriyananda 2003, p.324*

7.5

CONSCIOUSNESS AND COSMIC ENERGY

> 'The conscious cosmic energy first enters through the medulla oblongata (in the brain stem) and remains concentrated in the brain as the thousand-petalled lotus. Then it descends into the body through the spinal cord and sympathetic nervous system.'
>
> *Yogananda 2003, p.17*

All of life is Consciousness and Energy, which are two aspects of the same Ultimate Reality. Cosmic Consciousness and Cosmic Energy pervades the universe and is beyond the universe. This Consciousness and Energy is in all things visible or invisible, conceivable or inconceivable, animate or inanimate. It is in every tree, rock, grain of sand, blade of grass, drop of water, insect, fish, bird, animal and human; all are vibrating with timeless All-Pervasive Consciousness and Cosmic Energy. Every part of Consciousness holds within it the whole of creation.

To see a World in a grain of sand,
And Heaven in a Wild Flower,
Hold Infinity in the palm of your hand,
and Eternity in an hour.

William Blake, Auguries of Innocence

Scientifically this can be understood according to Einstein's famous equation $E=mc^2$, c being the speed of light (300,000 km per second, which is a universal constant of nature, absolute and not relative) and m being mass. This shows that mass and energy, being mutually convertible, are intrinsically the same. There is no separation between matter and energy, or matter and mind. They are aspects of one energy. In other words, there is a basic oneness and unity of life. It is the Ultimate Reality that underlies and unifies the multiplicity of everything. This equation $E=mc^2$ not only gives a clue to the production of energy which can be generated from a small amount of mass but its corollary gives an equation for mass that is $m=E/c^2$; and that a beam of light is pure energy ($c^2=E/m$). It gives also a clue to the power and potential of a human being

Ultimately, our bodies are nothing but energy. As Paramhansa Yogananda said, 'Behind the light in every bulb is a great dynamic current; beneath every little wave is the vast ocean, which has become the wave.' Our *chakras* act as dynamos of Cosmic Energy, allowing our subtle bodies to plug in to the universal power source. They serve as transformers and regulators to receive, assimilate and distribute *prāṇa* to the astral body, which then distributes it to the spinal nerve plexuses, where it is, in turn, transferred to the blood and organs of the physical body.

The *prāṇa* enters the body at the base of the brain in the brain stem (an area known as the medulla oblongata; Yogananda referred to it as the 'mouth of God', the finite opening in the body through which God breathes His Cosmic Energy or Life into physical flesh) and flows to the higher brain centres. It then filters downward through the six major centres of consciousness (*chakras*) below that, starting at *ājñā chakra* (at the eyebrow centre) and working its way down to the base of the spine to *mūladhāra chakra.*

Sahasrāra (also known as *Brāhmarandhra*, 'the door of God'), the main generator of the energies that power these six *chakras*, is located at the crown, above the medulla oblongata, and operates on a higher plane of consciousness.

As this energy spirals down through each *chakra*, it becomes increasingly dense, until it forms what are known as the 'five great elements' (*panchamahabhuta*). These are essential 'states' of matter, not to be confused with the periodic elements of modern chemistry, and they represent the stages of creation from Spirit to matter.

When these seven centres of consciousness and *prāṇic* energy are withdrawn from the body at death, the body disintegrates – the cosmic energy is switched off, and the soul has to leave the physical, astral and spiritual bodies through the seven astral doors or *chakras* in order to reach, and merge into, the Spirit.

> 'The spinal cord may be likened to a wire. In it are located these seven centres of light which are the subcentres for the conduction and distribution of life current throughout the body. The body is nothing but a condensation of this spinal energy. Just as invisible hydrogen and oxygen atoms can be condensed into visible vapour, water and ice, so light can be transformed into body which is nothing but frozen energy.'
>
> *Yogananda 2003, p.11*

Cosmic Energy projects the galaxies and governs the movement of the stars and planets. It is this same energy that is vibrating in our bodies and minds. We live, move and have our being in Consciousness that is whole, complete, self-contained and self-evolving. Consciousness is the field and the Source of all, and creation is the manifestation that happens from the Cosmic Energy within that.

Due to ignorance and the power of delusion we have forgotten the source of our being and the power of Supreme Consciousness and Cosmic Energy that permeates every particle of our being, and that is an inherent part of each of us. We are like a wave that gets separated from the ocean; it forgets it is a part of the ocean. Beneath the wave of your consciousness is the infinite ocean of Divine Consciousness. That potential of energy is so great within you that Yogananda said, 'There is enough energy in a gram of flesh to run the city of Chicago for two days!'

ENERGY AND WILLPOWER

Energy is a manifestation of Consciousness, and matter is a manifestation of that Cosmic Energy. This energy is available and accessible to us at all times – all we have to do is consciously plug into or tune into it. Using the power of your will you can directly access and draw on the energy of the universe, which has an unlimited supply. My guru, Paramhansa Yogananda said, 'The stronger the will, the greater the flow of energy!' The centre of positive will in the human body is the Spiritual Eye located at the eyebrow centre, the positive pole of the sixth centre of consciousness (*ājñā chakra*), and the seat of spiritual perception and intuition.

If you concentrate strongly with determination at that point between the eyebrows, you can draw on the limitless flow of Cosmic Energy through your medulla oblongata, the negative pole of the *ājñā chakra* and the seat of the ego, located in the brain stem at the base of the brain. Paramhansa Yogananda referred to the medulla oblongata as the 'mouth of God' and the 'door of God', meaning that it is the portal through which the body receives its energy from the universe and God.

> 'The astral body, in appearance like a vast nebula or the tail of a comet, charges the physical body with Cosmic Energy through the medulla oblongata.'
>
> *Yogananda 2003, p.8*

FEELING AND DIRECTING THE ENERGY

Yogananda said that the medulla oblongata is fed by conscious Cosmic Energy which surrounds the body and which is drawn into the body by the power of the will. Therefore, you should never say or think you are tired, for by doing so you become even more tired. Your will becomes paralysed with thoughts of tiredness and fatigue and cuts off the supply of energy. The will must be active in order to draw Cosmic Energy into the body.

We all have willpower, but not all of us use it in a conscious way to draw energy into the body. Yogananda pointed out that many people die mentally long before they die physically: 'When one ceases to have ambitions and to be interested in life, the will becomes paralysed. When this will-radio is untuned or destroyed, Cosmic Energy ceases to supply the reserve dynamo of the medulla, and physical health slowly fails from want of life-force. This is the principal cause for the symptoms of old age. *The stronger the will, the greater the flow of energy into the tissues and body parts.*'

A simple test for you to feel and experience energy being directed by your will is to look at your right hand, palm upwards. First, let it relax; as it relaxes, the fingers naturally curl inward towards the palm. Now, stimulate an inward awareness of energy in your hand by slowly clenching your fist, and remembering what Yogananda said, '*The stronger the will, the greater the flow of energy into the tissues and body parts.*' Using your concentrated willpower, slowly tense your fist tighter and tighter, feeling the energy building up in the muscles of your fisted hand, until it is vibrating with energy (tension with will produces more energy than concentration alone). Then, with awareness, slowly and gradually release the tension in the muscles of your hand to complete relaxation. Now relax and feel the energy. Compare the feeling in your right hand to the feeling in your left. You should notice a marked difference in energy.

These principles of energy to recharge the body at will were innovated by Paramhansa Yogananda in 1916 in India for his students, and were developed into the Energisation Exercises, a system of 39 exercises which teach one how to recharge the body with energy through the conscious power of will.

> 'The Energisation Exercises teach how to recharge the body battery with fresh life current by increasing the power of will. They strengthen and recharge the muscles with vital force, not only collectively but individually, and teach how to surround each body cell with a ring of super-charged electrical vital-energy and thus keep them free from decay or bacterial invasion. They keep not only the muscles, but all the tissues of the body, bones, marrow, brain, and cells in perfect health, and cause the resurrection of dying tissue cells and worn out faculties, and the formation of billions of new cells.'
>
> *Paramhansa Yogananda*

USING 'WILL' AND 'ENERGY' TO HEAL

The following technique of using energy for healing is a method that Paramhansa Yogananda taught:

1. Sit upright in a comfortable position. As you inhale deeply, slowly and gently tense all the muscles in your body. While tensing your body muscles hold your breath in for a few seconds, then exhale with a double breath (ha-haaa) through your mouth. Then relax and feel the energy flow into your body.
2. Now remain relaxed and calm. Touch your medulla oblongata at the base of the brain (the indentation at the back of the head, where the neck meets the skull) in order to make it easier to concentrate on it. Then visualise Cosmic Energy surrounding and entering your body through the medulla and at the midpoint between your eyebrows, and flowing down into your spine.
3. Feel the energy flowing down the whole length of your arms into your hands. Continue tensing and relaxing your body and feeling the life force flow from the medulla and the midpoint between your eyebrows through the spine to your hands.
4. Then stop tensing and relaxing, and by using your right palm, firmly rub your entire bare left arm up and down several times. Do the same to your right arm with your left palm. Then relax, continuously visualising and willing Cosmic Energy to descend from the medulla through your arms into your hands.
5. Now, with closed eyes and, with your attention at the eyebrow centre, rapidly but gently rub your palms together about 20 times. Then separate your hands and raise them upward. You will feel the life current of energy flowing from the medulla into your spine, especially through both arms and hands, with a warm, tingling sensation.

Now that your hands are magnetised with energy, they can be used either for healing any diseased part of your own body or some other person's. If it is for another person they need not be present; they can even be on the other side of the world. This Cosmic Energy or *prāṇic* energy passing through your hands has infinite power of projection. Energy follows thought. However, Yogananda said to visualise the person you are sending healing to. In other words, hold that person in God's healing Light, Love and Wholeness. Send that person healing on all three levels of their being – physical, mental and spiritual. And with unquestioning faith know that healing energy is working on all those levels, pouring strength, energy, power, love, light and happiness into that person. Let there be no suggestion in your mind of limitation. Be like Jesus, who saw a person's wholeness, not their illness. See them with renewed life, vitality and strength.

To send that healing force of energy through the ether or space after following the above steps, you can then raise your energy-charged hands above your head with the palms facing forward. With your eyes closed, and with your concentration at the eyebrow centre, send out through the palms of your hands divine currents of healing rays to the person who is unwell or diseased. As you do this, chant *Aum* aloud or mentally three times. Visualise and hold that person in the divine light for as long as you feel the need to do so.

It is best to prepare yourself for sending distant healing by meditating first until you are calm and still, then to offer a prayer to the Divine, so that you feel God's presence as the Divine Source of the healing you are sending.

You can use this prayer just before rubbing your hands together to magnetise and charge them with energy, then raising them to send the divine healing rays as you chant *Aum* three times: '*Divine Mother, Thou art omnipresent. Thy art in all Thy children. Thou art in (name of person you are sending healing to). Manifest Thy healing presence, love, peace, light and joy in his/her body.*'

SENDING HEALING PRAYERS FOR WORLD PEACE

After praying for individual persons you can send healing blessings out to the world to bring harmony and peace to all people.

From the stillness of your meditation, visualise peace radiating out from you like ripples on a lake, in ever-expanding circles. Feel that your peace is touching everything and everyone. Feel that you are expanding that feeling of peace farther and farther, beyond all limitations of your body and personality. See the whole planet with its blue aura floating in space, bathed in God's universal peace. See the Earth's surrounding aura filled with light, harmony, love, peace.

Then pray affirmatively: '*As I radiate God's peace, light, love and goodwill to others, I open the channel for God's love to flow through me.*'

Visualise and feel that Cosmic Energy is surrounding and entering your body through the medulla at the back of your head and at your Spiritual Eye, flowing into your spine, and down your arms into your hands. Then rapidly but gently rub your palms together until they feel warm and tingling with energy.

Raise your arms to the level of your head or above with your palms facing forward, inhale deeply and then chant *Aum* as you exhale. You can chant *Aum* three times. Then say '*Aum Shanti, Peace, Amen*' to end your prayer session. Take the divine qualities within you of calmness, peace, love, and joy into your everyday-life activities, and keep your connection to the Divine Presence.

7.6

KRIYĀ YOGA PRACTICE

THE ART AND PRACTICE OF *KRIYĀ YOGA*

> 'Meditate unceasingly, that you may quickly behold yourself as the Infinite Essence, free from every form of misery. Cease being a prisoner of the body; using the secret of *kriyā*, learn to escape into Spirit.'
>
> *Lahiri Mahasaya, in Yogananda 1946, p.315*

Through the grace of the great line of *Kriyā* Masters, Mahavatar Babaji, Lahiri Mahasaya, Swāmi Sri Yukteswar and Paramhansa Yogananda, *Rāja Yoga* has been revived as *Kriyā Yoga*, the scientific technique of God-realisation.

Your spiritual practice (*sādhana*) is important if you want to make progress on the spiritual path towards awakening and realisation in God Consciousness. Remember that the goal of Yoga science is to calm the mind so that it may hear the still inner voice of the divine Self within. The *Kriyā Yoga* techniques are not an end in themselves, they are not meditation itself, they are instruments or vehicles to be used to take you into the inner stillness of meditation. When practised as a regular daily discipline, the *Kriyā* techniques can stimulate, energise, and magnetise the *prāṇic* life force in the seven spiritual centres of consciousness (*chakras*) located in the subtle astral spine and brain. Then, with the spine and brain magnetised, the current of life force that is normally uncontrolled and flowing out through the mind, body and senses can be turned inward towards the consciousness of Self, which is *Sat-chit-ānanda* (Ever-Existing, Ever-Conscious, Ever-New Bliss), beyond the mind, body and senses to the Source of wisdom, bliss and divine love.

Practise the following *Kriyā* techniques regularly every day with willingness, enthusiasm, faith, and above all love and devotion, you will transform your consciousness and you will attain that ineffable peace, freedom and joy that you seek. So be patient, persevere and never give up, then, eventually you will experience the joy of pure Bliss-consciousness.

In addition to practising the *Kriyā* techniques, devotion and meditation are important. Practise the Presence of God – think of God, the Supreme Consciousness, and Guru. Bring them more and more into your everyday life, into your thinking and activities – that is practising the Presence. And in that Presence you will enjoy the ineffable peace of the Divine in the stillness within you. When you have the perception of the Divine, your life will become more harmonious, purposeful and meaningful. You will feel that you are not separated from the Divine Consciousness, but are one with It. And you will know that it is your natural state of being.

Remember these words from the Bible: 'Be still and know that I am God' (Psalm 6:10). That stillness is ever present within you, you simply have to discover it. 'I and my Father are one' (John 10:30). There is no separation except in your mind, you are eternally in God. Affirm these words regularly to yourself and meditate on these words, then you will feel peace and joy enter your heart.

7.6.1 *HONG SAU* TECHNIQUE OF CONCENTRATION

An excellent technique for deepening the concentration, and calming the mind in preparation for deep meditation, is a technique in which you focus on the inhalation and exhalation with the two seed-syllable (*bīja*) *mantra*, *Hong Sau*. This *mantra* works on a pure vibrational level by stilling the mental energy in the form of restless thoughts and purifying the ego. *Hong Sau* is the inner sound of the inhaling and exhaling breath. It also calms and interiorises the *prāṇa* in the body.

Hong Sau corresponds with the two *prāṇic* currents: *iḍā* and *piṅgala nāḍīs* (subtle *prāṇic* channels) either side of the central *prāṇic* channel (*suṣumnā*) in the astral spine. During the inhalation there is a rising of energy in the spine that corresponds to a mental attitude of going outward. During the exhalation there is a downward movement in the spine that corresponds to an inwardness of the energy in the body and consciousness.

The mind can never be focused without a mental object. Therefore you must give your mind an object that is readily available in every present moment. Your breath is the closest object. Every moment, the breath is flowing in and flowing out through your nostrils. The concentration technique of *Hong Sau*, practised by concentrating intently on the breath with total attention, trains the mind to stay focused like a 'one-pointed' laser beam. By training your mind to maintain a concentrated focus on a single point on the breath, while following it with the *mantra*, the other techniques and meditations that you practise will become increasingly deeper.

Hong Sau means 'I am He', 'I, the manifested Self, am He, the Unmanifested Spirit (the Absolute)'. By consciously repeating mentally the seed-syllable *mantra Hong Sau*, in conjunction with the concentration on the breath we affirm that the ego-self is one with the Infinite Spirit. *Hong* as the inhaling breath represents the contraction of consciousness into finitude. *Sau* as the exhaling breath represents the expansion of consciousness and the reabsorption of differentiation and separation into pure Unity.

Hong Sau possesses a vibratory connection with the breath. It is the natural, subtle sound of the breath – *Hong* vibrates with the inhalation, corresponding to the ascending current in the *iḍā nāḍī* (see *Nāḍīs*, Chapter 4.4). *Sau* vibrates with the exhalation, corresponding to the descending current in the *piṅgala nāḍī*. Throughout the 24 hours of the day and night the breath flows in and out 21,600 times in a continuous *mantra* of *Hong Sau*. Unknowingly, we are all repeating this *mantra* in a process of automatic and continuous recitation. In Yoga, continuous recitation of a *mantra* is called *ajapā japa*. The *japa* becomes *ajapā* when the *mantra* gets repeated in the mind on its own. The difference between *ajapā japa* and *japa* is that *ajapā japa* goes on subconsciously all the time, while *japa* is done consciously.

Paramhansa Yogananda, as a young boy named Mukunda, would sit in meditation and practise *Hong Sau* meditation technique for seven hours at a time, until he became breathless. He called *Hong Sau* 'the Baby *Kriyā*'. In the actual *Kriyā* meditation technique that has been passed down through a succession of enlightened *Kriyā* Masters from Mahavatar Babaji to Paramhansa Yogananda, the *kuṇḍalinī* life force flows in the spine and rises up through the *chakras* to the pituitary gland at the *ājñā chakra*, and then it is offered to the Divine at the crown centre (*sahasrāra*) above the head.

> 'The purpose of the *Hong Sau* technique is to help you to free your attention from outwardness, and to withdraw it from the senses, for breath is the cord that keeps the soul tied to the body... By dispassionately watching the breath coming in and going out, one's breathing naturally slows, calming at last the peace-disturbing activity of the heart, lungs, and diaphragm.'
>
> *Yogananda 2010, pp.110–111*

PREPARING FOR THE PRACTICE OF *HONG SAU*

To prepare for the practice of *Hong Sau*, follow this procedure:

1. **Tensing and relaxing.** Sit in a comfortable and steady meditation posture with your head, neck and spine aligned. To relax your mind and body, inhale deeply, hold the breath, and tense all the muscles in your body. Hold both the breath and the tension in your muscles for a few seconds, then simultaneously release the breath and the tension and relax. Repeat the process of tensing and relaxing three times, then finish by completely relaxing, and feel the relaxation and the flow of energy into your body.

2. ***Loma prāṇāyama.*** Continue to remain relaxed as you practise a minimum of nine rounds of *Loma* ('Natural Force') *prāṇāyama*. This is a three-part equal breath ratio, breathing through both nostrils. Inhale for a count of 12, hold your breath for a count of 12, exhale for a count of 12 (12:12:12). If this is not within your lung capacity then, keeping the same ratio, halve it to 6:6:6. The number of rounds can be gradually increased over a period of time to 27 rounds.

3. **Sit calmly for meditation.** Remain sitting still and concentrate your relaxed attention at the midpoint between the eyebrows (Spiritual Eye). Let go of all thoughts and be totally centred in the present here and now moment. Place your hands palms upward on the knees in *chin mudrā* (gesture of consciousness). Close your eyes and relax, with your awareness on the natural breath. Keep the body still and bring your attention and awareness to the frontal part of the brain at the midpoint between the eyebrows (the Spiritual Eye, the seat of spiritual consciousness). If your mind wanders, gently bring it back to the practice of watching the breath with awareness.

Watching the breath is a present-moment experience. Focus and interiorise your mind by deepening your attentive awareness and concentration.

PRACTISING *HONG SAU*

1. With your body and mind still, uniting your mind with the present moment, begin the practice of *Hong Sau*. With closed eyes and without straining, gently lift your gaze upward to the midpoint between the eyebrows, and with steady concentration and inner calmness look into the Spiritual Eye, the seat of intuition and omnipresent perception.
2. Feel the natural breath flow in and out of your nostrils. Feel the tactile sensation of the breath, and try to feel where the flow of breath is strongest in your nostrils. The sensation of breath is subtle, and yet it is quite distinct when you learn to tune into it. Once you have found the point where the breath is strongest in your nostrils (usually just inside the tip of the nose), then concentrate on the breath at that point. It is from this point that you will follow the whole passage of your breath.
3. Use this single-point sensation inside the nose to keep your attention fixed. Observe each breath with attention and precision in present-moment awareness, taking it one split second on top of another. In this way, continuous and unbroken awareness will eventually result.
4. Then begin to feel the sensation of the air that passes in and out of your nostrils higher up in the nasal passages by the midpoint between your eyebrows; concentrate at this point. As your concentration deepens, your breathing will begin to slow down, and you will be able to focus on it more clearly, with fewer and fewer interruptions.
5. As you concentrate on your breath, make no attempt to control it. This is not a Yoga breathing exercise. With focused awareness just let go, and allow this natural process of subtle breathing to move in its own rhythm.
6. Inhale deeply, then slowly exhale. As the next inhalation naturally arises and flows into your nostrils, feel the breath where it enters the nostrils, and with your inner focus, simultaneously repeat mentally the *bīja* (seed-syllable) *mantra Hong* (rhymes with 'song'). Imagine that the breath itself is making this sound.
7. And as your breath flows out naturally, simultaneously mentally repeat the seed *mantra Sau* (rhymes with 'saw'). Remember, make no attempt to control your breath, just allow its flow to be completely natural. The process of *Hong Sau* is not a breathing technique, it is simply being consciously aware, with your concentration on the *Hong Sau mantra* as the breath flows. Feel that your subtle breathing is silently making the sounds of *Hong Sau*.

8. Continue focusing on your Spiritual Eye, at the midpoint between your eyebrows, and as the breath naturally flows in, simultaneously repeat mentally the seed *mantra Hong*. As the breath flows out, simultaneously repeat mentally the seed *mantra Sau*. By concentration on the breath, the breath gradually diminishes. This gradual subtle refinement leads naturally to an interiorised meditative state. When the mind is united with the breath flowing all the time, you will be able to focus your mind in the present moment.
9. If your mind begins to wander on to other thoughts, gently bring it back to the awareness of watching the breath in unison with *Hong Sau*.
10. As you go deeper into the practice of watching your breath in unison with *Hong Sau*, the breathing becomes more subtle and the mind becomes very calm and still. You may notice that, between each inhalation and exhalation, there is a natural space or pause, a point of complete stillness, where the form of the breath is briefly suspended. This is the space of the innermost Self. Softly focus your attentive awareness on those pauses, where the inhalation subsides and the exhalation arises. And as your mind becomes more calmly interiorised, notice the spaces extending between your breaths, into a breathless state, and enjoy that experience of expansion into the freedom of infinite spaciousness while inwardly gazing into your Spiritual Eye. Then, when the breath naturally returns, continue with the practice of *Hong Sau*.

During and after practising *Hong Sau*, remain in the inner calmness and stillness for as long as possible. Remember to feel that inner calmness from your meditation, and remain calmly centred within your Self, allowing the calmness to permeate your everyday consciousness.

If the technique of *Hong Sau* is practised correctly and regularly, it will eventually bring you to a state of mental calmness, drawing your energy inward, and leading you naturally into breathlessness as the pauses between your breaths naturally lengthen. By entering the space between one breath and another, consciousness can fully expand. These natural pauses between the breaths arise at the beginning of every inhalation and at the end of every inhalation, and at the beginning of every exhalation and at the end of every exhalation.

When you are attentive to these pauses or moments between the breaths, the awareness behind your breath and mind will merge and expand, taking you into the 'breathless state', and in that inner fullness in which the breath expands, the twofold vibration of *Hong* and *Sau* merges into the single omnipresent vibration of *Aum*. In other words, you enter into the fullness and spaciousness of the inner kingdom of the Absolute, the Supreme Self. This *mantra Hong Sau* reminds us that we are not separate from the Source of Life.

7.6.2 THE ENERGISATION EXERCISES

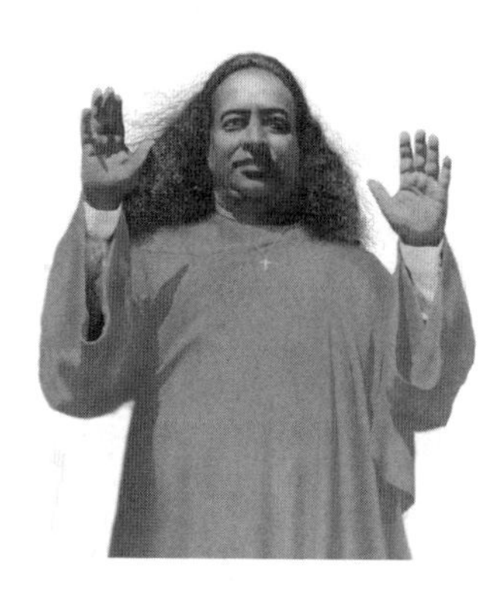

The following 39 Energisation Exercises, a unique system devised by Paramhansa Yogananda for consciously drawing Cosmic Energy into the body, are best learned from a teacher who can guide you through them correctly. It will be much quicker to learn the exercises from a teacher than trying to follow them from a book. If you cannot find a teacher then the next best way is to obtain a guided video or a guided audio CD, which can be obtained online (see 'Kriyā Yoga Resources' at the back of this book).

The two most important things for bringing the energy in the mind and body under control are: *awareness* and *willpower*. These energisation exercises are a means of using conscious willpower with awareness, to consciously draw this cosmic energy or life force, the infinite potential of God within you, into the body cells and, afterward, to withdraw it again from the body in meditation. The mind cannot act directly upon the body. It must act through a medium of energy. The will first acts upon the energy, then the energy acts upon the body. Developing a deep inner flow of energy is important to our experience of spiritual awakening because like a flowing river it washes away all the debris – the obstacles and blockages that keep us bound to body consciousness, and our separation from the Divine Consciousness. By expanding the flow of energy within, you have greater access to freedom and inner joy.

The Energisation Exercises give awareness of the energy, and that awareness gives the ability to manipulate its flow in the body at will. We incorporate that awareness into our disciplined inner practice by establishing a flow of energy within. This is how we come to experience spiritual energy moving through our body. It is this divine Cosmic Energy, which is a communicating link between the mind and body, that truly sustains those who serve with willingness and awareness of Divine Presence. It flows from the medulla oblongata, located at the base of the brain in the brain stem at the back of the head, and from there flows to the rest of the body throughout the network of *prāṇic* subtle channels or *nāḍīs*.

When you practise these Energisation Exercises, do them with the will, the power of God within you. Usually when we use the word will, we think of tension in an effortful way, so use the word 'willingness'. The greater the willingness, the greater the flow of energy. Yogananda defined will as desire plus energy, directed towards fulfilment. In other words, it is something you should enthusiastically want to do. In that way, practise these energisation exercises with willingness, with the desire that your body be filled with energy and joy. The positive 'will centre' in the body is the Spiritual Eye, at the midpoint between the eyebrows. By strong concentration at this point, willpower can be exerted to draw a limitless flow of energy through the medulla oblongata.

CONCENTRATE ON THE FLOW OF ENERGY

As you do the movements with a calm inward awareness, be conscious of the energy flowing through a subtle portal located at the medulla oblongata, inside the brain stem at the base of the skull. Then by using your willpower concentrate on the flow of energy to the specific body part or centre of the particular muscle group, and consciously direct the flow of energy to it. You can try visualising the flow of limitless energy as a stream of light, coursing through your body to the various parts you are directing it to.

From a gradually increasing flowing rhythm – low, to medium, to high tension – to the point where it vibrates, hold the tension for a few moments, consciously filling that body part with energy. Then exhale and slowly relax in the reverse order, in a decreasing flowing rhythm from high, to medium, to low, and completely relax, feeling the energy as it withdraws from the body part. Be consciously aware of the energy inwardly behind that tension and vibration. The more aware you are of the energy, the greater will be your control over it. Always tense with will, relax and feel.

At first, what you will feel is just the physical tension inside the muscles. Then you will experience the flow of energy which creates the tension in those muscles. Finally you will become aware of how you can direct the flow of energy to them. As you practice you can mentally repeat: 'The greater the will, the greater the flow of energy.'

Learning to direct energy has a practical benefit because we can apply these principles on mental and spiritual levels as well. The more aware you are of the flow of energy, the more you can direct that energy by willpower or willingness, not only to the body, but to anything that you do – towards self-improvement, service to others, your work, creative inspiration, the Divinity within you in meditation. In fact, when you are attuned with this energy it can be harnessed and used in all aspects of your life to transform it.

Guidelines for practising the Energisation Exercises:

- **Practise the exercises with willingness, enthusiasm and joy.** When you have willingness, and are happy and positive, you will experience an increase in energy. The more you become aware of using your willingness to direct that energy, the more you will be able to increase the flow. Remember Yogananda's maxim: 'The greater the will, the greater the flow of energy.'

- **Contract and relax the muscle group gradually in a continuous wave from low, to medium, to high tension, vibrating with great willpower.** 'Tense with will, relax and feel.' Hold the tension for three or four seconds, but do not tense so hard that you cause physical discomfort, or soreness. After tensing, relax gradually, in a wave from high, to medium, to low, and completely relax and feel the flow of energy suffusing the area that has been energised. If you find it difficult to isolate a specific muscle or body part, concentrate and focus your mind there and the energy and *prāṇa* will automatically flow to that part – energy follows thought.
- **Many of the exercises are practised with a double breath**. Double breathing is a short, sharp inhalation through the nose followed directly by a longer, smoother inhalation, completely filling your lungs. Then, without pause, exhaling through the mouth and nose with the same double breath ('Ha-haaa').
- **Modify or leave out exercise if necessary.** There should be no pain or discomfort associated with them. If you have been ill or had neck, spinal, or any other physical disabilities, you can practise the exercises with low tension, or visualise the energy flowing in a current of light to the affected body part as you mentally do the exercise.
- **Feel that through the power of your will, you are consciously drawing and directing a limitless current of cosmic energy or light force into your body.** After tensing a body area with will, completely relax and feel the results. Conscious relaxation after each exercise is very important. Tensing and relaxing not only recharges the body cells with energy, but more importantly, trains you to bring the flow of *prāṇic* energy under control. As you practise the Energisation Exercises keep this affirmation in your mind: '*My will is attuned to Divine Will, the unlimited and Infinite Source of all power and accomplishment.*'
- **Practise the Energisation Exercises daily** in the morning and evening, preferably outdoors, or if indoors then with a window open so that you can oxygenate your lungs with fresh air and draw *prāṇa* into them. Each of the exercises is practised from three to five times. When you have learned all 39 exercises in the correct sequence by practising them it will take you no longer than 15 minutes to do them. Practise them before meditating to release mental and physical tensions. This will allow you to go deeper into the stillness of meditation. These exercises can be practised at any time, anywhere, and because they are all performed from a standing position you need very little space.

  If you have little time, then it is suggested that you just practise the 20-part recharging exercise (step 20 of the 39 Energisation Exercises).

After having learned and memorised the practice of the Energisation Exercises, you can practise them with your eyes closed or half closed, with your gaze directed to the midpoint between the eyebrows, the centre of spiritual perception and willpower. This will help you to interiorise your consciousness and keep your mind in superconsciousness.

Caution

If you suffer from high blood pressure, it is advised that you use medium rather than high tension during practice of the exercises. If you have an injured muscle, then apply only light tension when sending energy to that muscle or group of muscles. If you are unable to tense the muscle at all, then send energy to it only mentally. If you have a condition which prevents you from practising any of the Energisation Exercises through physical movement, then do them mentally, even if you have to sit on a chair or lie down. Remember, energy follows thought, so you can still direct energy to anywhere in your body through conscious will and awareness.

PRACTICE OF THE 39 ENERGISATION EXERCISES

Begin by standing upright with your hands folded in prayer at your chest and pray:

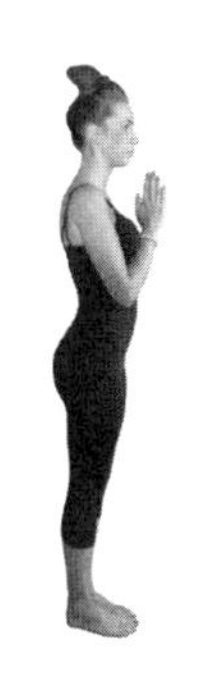

> O Infinite Spirit, recharge this body with Thy cosmic energy, this mind with Thy deep concentration, clarity and determination, and this soul with Thy ever-new joy. O eternal youth of body and mind, abide in me forever and ever. Aum, Amen.

1. Double breathing (with palms touching)

Begin the Energisation Exercises from the standing position, with your arms extended out to the side at shoulder level, and with a double breath exhalation, bringing your arms together in front of you, with your palms touching, and your knees bent. With a double inhalation, tense your entire body upwards in a wave, as you straighten your legs and pull your arms back outward against a resisting force.

Then, with a double exhalation relax downward in a wave through your body, bringing the arms together again and bend the knees. Repeat three to five times.

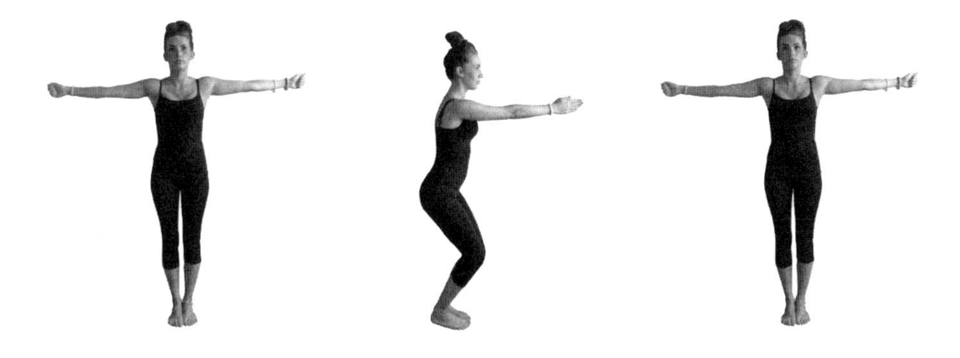

2 and 3. Calf recharging and ankle rotation

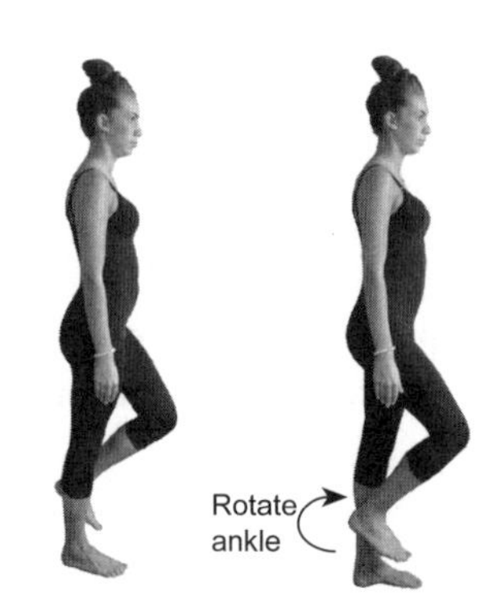

Balance on your right leg, with your left knee slightly bent. Then slowly pull your left leg upward, bending at the knee, while tensing your calf muscle, as if you are pulling your leg up against a resisting weight. Relax briefly, and then push the leg down against a resisting weight.

Practise three to five times and then, lifting your left foot a few inches from the floor, lightly tense your ankle and rotate it in small circles three to five times in each direction. Repeat with the other leg.

4. Calf and forearm; thigh and upper arm

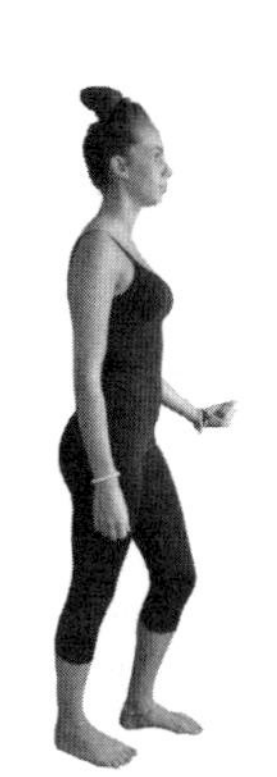

Stand with the weight on your right leg, place your left leg slightly in front, and simultaneously tense your left calf muscle and left forearm gradually from low, to medium, to high tension, and then vibrate them. Relax the muscles gradually in reverse order – from high, to medium, to low, then completely relax and feel the energy.

Repeat this with your thigh and upper arm muscles. Alternating between the upper and lower muscles, do this three times on the left side, then three times on the right.

Then with your weight equally balanced on both legs, tense both calves and both forearms simultaneously, and relax; and then both thighs and both upper arms, and relax. Repeat three to five times.

5. Chest and buttock recharging

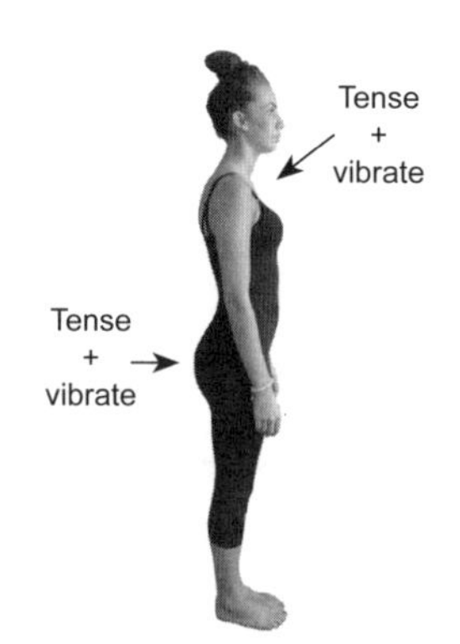

Simultaneously, gradually tense your left buttock and left chest from low, to medium, to high tension, and vibrate with energy. Then gradually relax them, and repeat on your right side. In this way, alternate from the left side to the right three to five times.

6. Back recharging

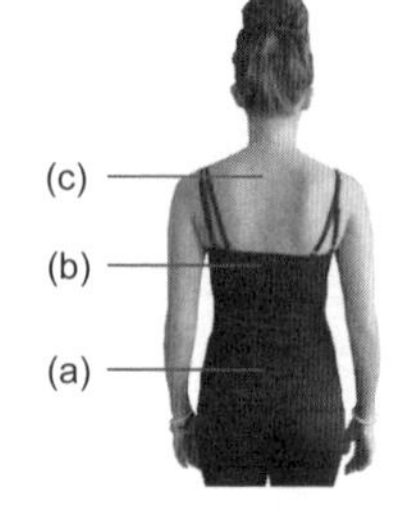

a) Tense and relax the lower back muscles, in the lumbar area, alternating left and right three to five times.
b) Then, tense and relax the middle back muscles, between the shoulder blades.
c) Finally, tense and relax the upper back muscles, above your shoulder blades.

7. Shoulder rotation

Rest your fingers on your shoulder blades, and rotate the shoulders with tension in large circles three to five times in each direction.

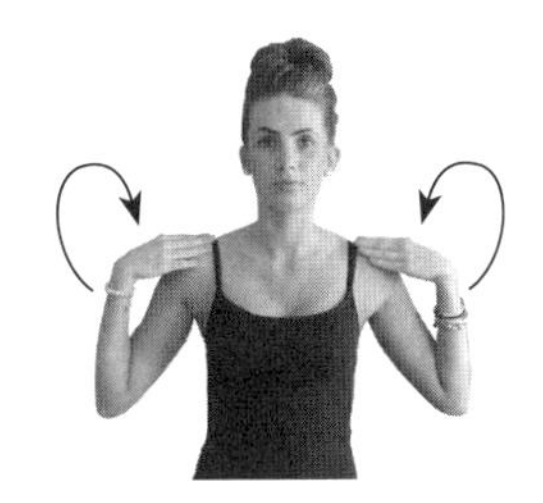

8. Throat recharging

Tense and relax your entire throat and neck muscles three to five times and then alternately tense and relax the left side of your neck, followed by your right side, three to five times.

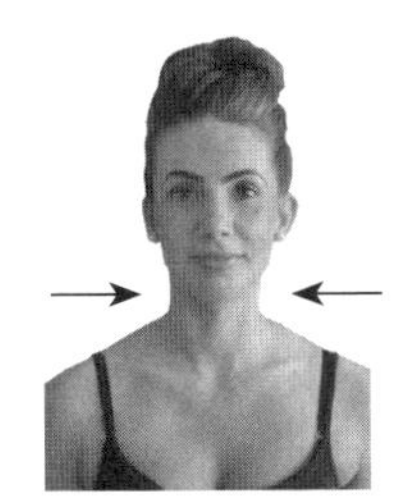

9. Neck recharging

With a double exhalation, slowly lower your head until your chin is close to your chest. Then, as if your chin were tied to the chest, and with a double inhalation, pull your head slowly up and back, vibrating the neck muscles. Relax slowly downwards with a double exhalation, and repeat three to five times.

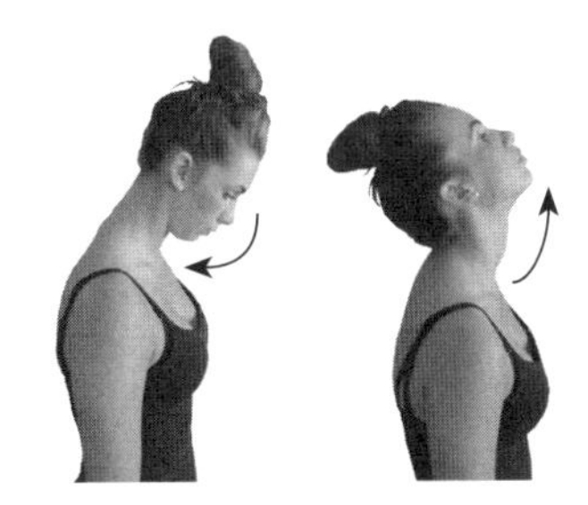

10. Neck rotation

Tensing the muscles on the inside and outside of your neck, rotate your head three times in one direction, and then in the other direction. Repeat the rotations, without tension, three to five times.

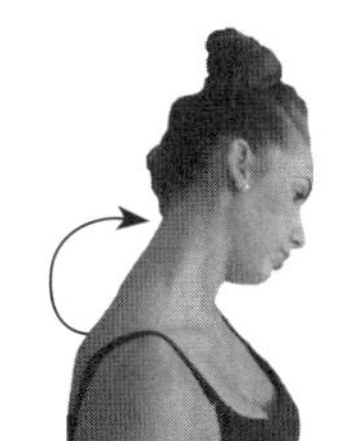

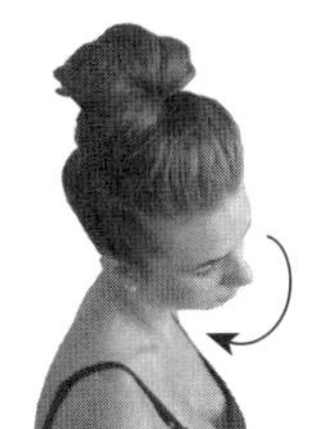

11. Spinal recharging (lower spinal adjustment)

Stand with your feet hip-width apart, with your arms bent at the elbow and placed at the level of your hips. Twist your hips and lower body to the right while simultaneously moving your shoulders to the left. Alternate the twisting to the left and right several times with brisk, defined movements. Repeat three to five times.

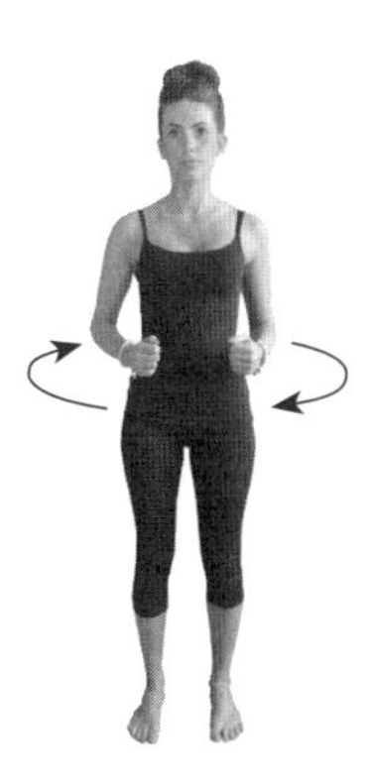

12. Spinal rotation

Stand with your feet hip-width apart with your hands on your waist. Then with your head aligned with the spine and looking straight ahead, bend slightly forward arching your spine. With tension in the arched spine, rotate your trunk three to five times in each direction, while keeping your hips and legs still.

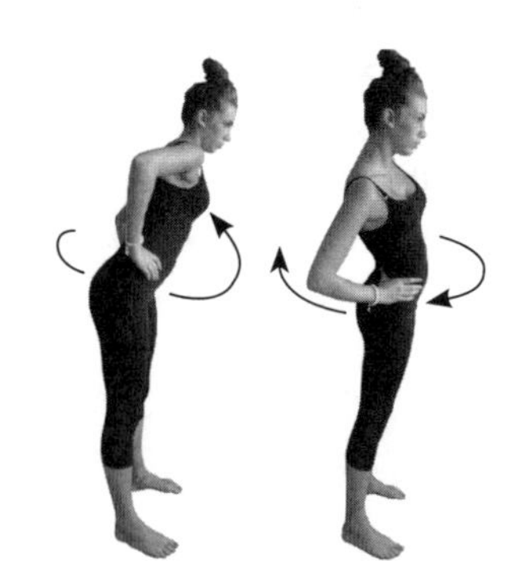

13. Lateral spinal stretching

Stand with your feet hip-width apart and your hands on your hips and, with tension in your spine, push against the tension to the left, and then to the right. Repeat three to five times.

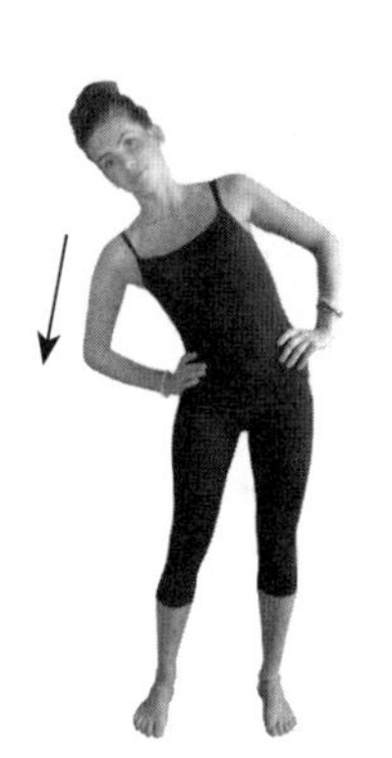

14. Vertebrae adjustment

Bend slightly forward with your fists pressing firmly on the muscles on each side of your spinal column. Starting at the base of the spine, and pressing inward and upward with your knuckles, arch your spine and thrust your upper body backward, while coming up onto your toes. Repeat this movement with the knuckles positioned one vertebra higher with each cycle.

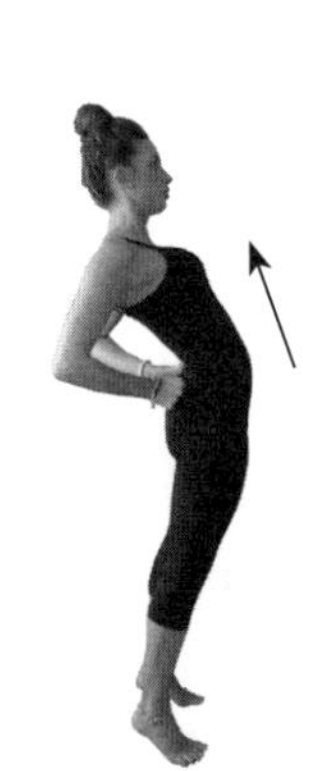

15. Upper spinal adjustment

Stand with your feet hip-width apart with your arms straight out in front of your body at the level of the shoulders. Keeping your hips and legs still, draw your arms back to the left with tension, bringing your right hand to the chest. The head and eyes simultaneously follow the motion of the outstretched arms. Relax back to the starting point, and repeat to the right side. Practise three to five times, alternating to the left and right sides.

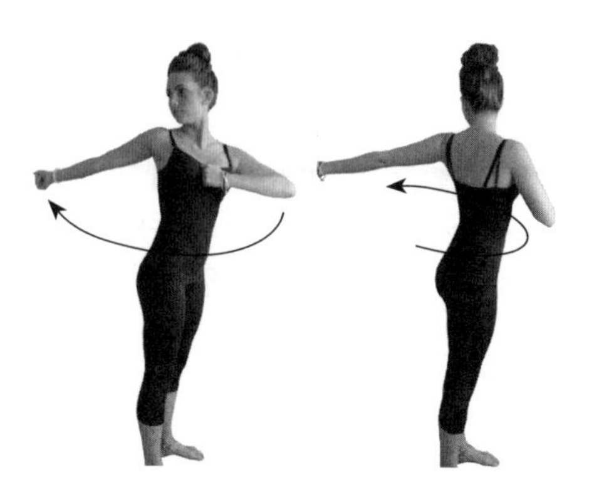

16. Brain cell recharging

Briskly and gently rap your entire skull and forehead with your knuckles to stimulate the energy in the brain cells. Visualise your brain cells being awakened with Cosmic Energy.

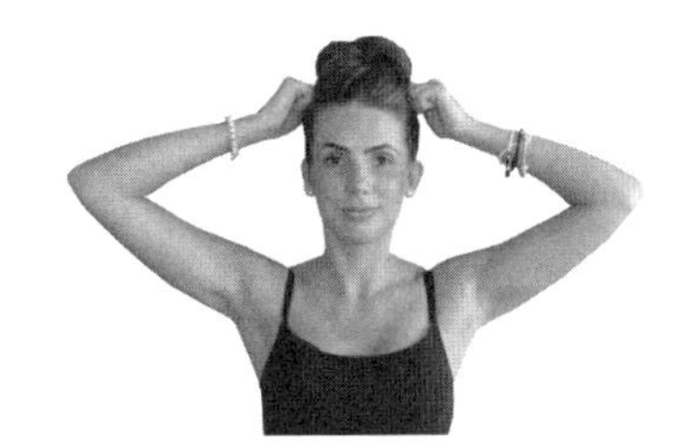

17. Scalp massage

Press your fingertips firmly on your scalp and move the scalp forwards and backwards, left and right, and then rotate in each direction. Then move your fingers to another position on the head and repeat until your entire scalp has been massaged.

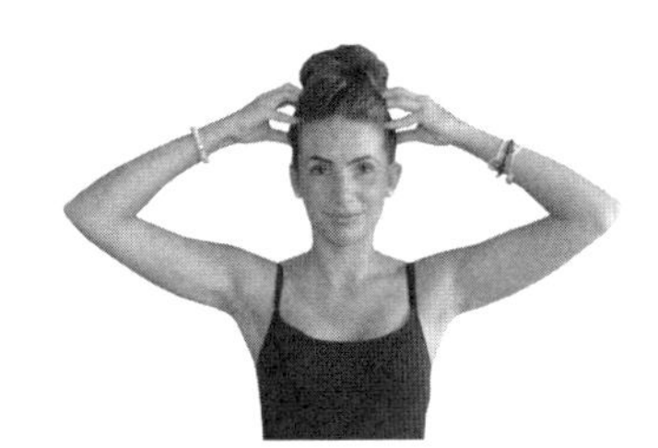

18. Medulla memory exercise

Joining together your forefinger, middle finger and ring finger of each hand, position them at the medulla oblongata (the hollow at the back of the neck where it meets the skull) and, applying pressure there, rotate them in small circles in each direction several times. Then bring your head slowly back against the pressure of your fingers as you take a double inhalation. Feel the energy entering through the medulla oblongata, then with a double exhalation, relax the tension and bring your chin down to the chest with a firm but not too strong movement. Repeat three to five times.

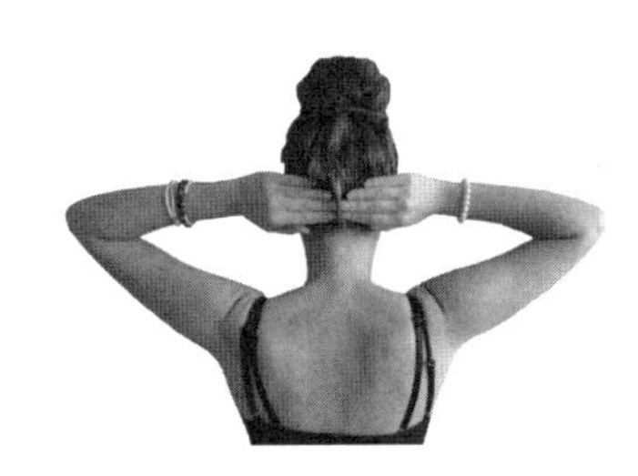

19. Biceps recharging

Clasp your hands above your head and gradually tense your bicep muscles (low–medium–high), vibrate and then relax. Alternate to the left and right several times.

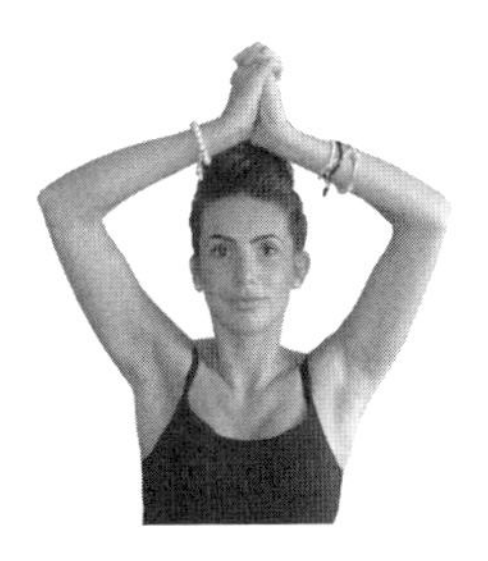

20. Twenty-part body recharging

Phase one: Stand with your feet hip-width apart with your arms down by your sides. With a double inhalation, simultaneously and gradually tense all your body muscles (low–medium–high), vibrate the whole body strongly, then relax gradually (high–medium–low) with a double exhalation.

Phase two: Gradually tense and relax each of the 20 body parts individually, alternating from left to right: starting with the feet, then calves, thighs, buttocks, lower and upper abdominal muscles, forearms, upper arms, chest muscles, neck (left side, right side, front and back).

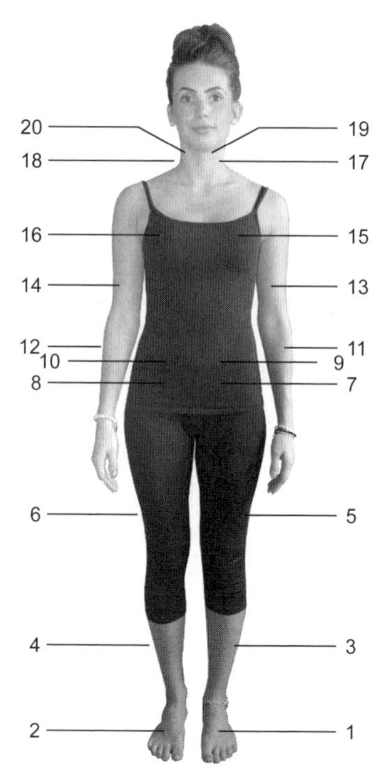

Phase three: Repeat the exercise, this time maintaining the tension at a medium level in each body part, as you slowly inhale, synchronising the inhalation to last until you have completely tensed all the body parts. When the entire body is tense, vibrate it briefly with high tension.

Phase four: Then, relax each muscle individually in the reverse order as you slowly exhale, again synchronising your exhalation to last until you have relaxed down through all the body parts. Begin the relaxation phase by bringing your chin to the chest, relaxing all the muscles in your neck, and continue down the body releasing first the right side and then the left, until you have completely relaxed your whole body. Relax and feel your body is a dynamo of energy.

Phase five: With your chin still on the chest, take a double inhalation and gradually tense, and vibrate your whole body with energy, and then gradually relax with a double exhalation.

21. Weight lifting in the front

Stand with your arms down at your sides with your fists facing each other, and tense your arms as if you are pulling up heavy weights. Vibrating the arms with energy, bring your fists to your chest, relax briefly, and push them down with the fists still facing each other. Repeat several times. *Optional:* double inhalation with the upward movement and exhalation with the downward movement.

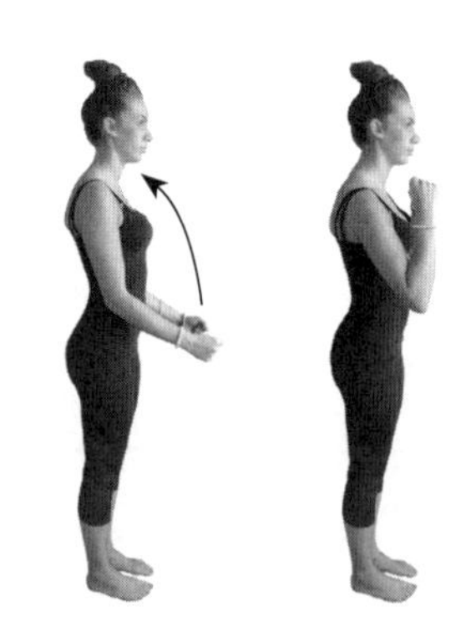

22. Double breathing with elbows touching

With your elbows bent at right angles, raise your arms to the sides of your head at shoulder level. With a double exhalation, bring your elbows together in front of your chest as you bend at the knees. With a double inhalation, vibrate with energy and pull your arms back to the starting position, as you tense the lower body in a wave upwards, similar to the first exercise. Repeat several times.

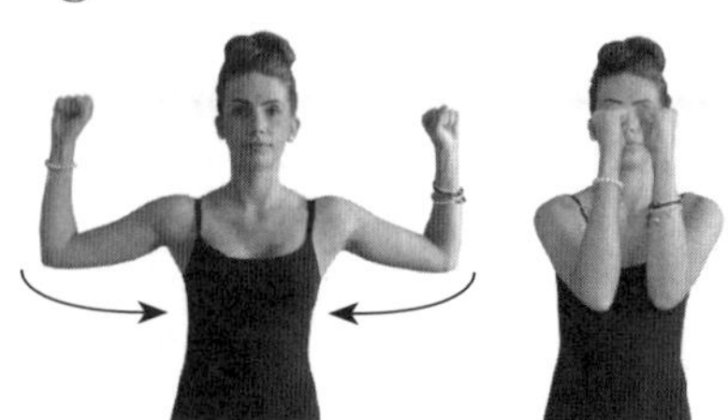

23. Weight pulling to the side

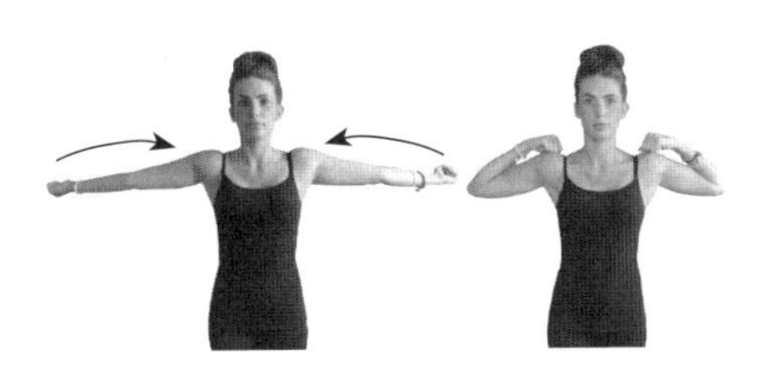

With your arms extended to the side at shoulder level, parallel to the floor, clench your fists in an upward position, and draw your arms towards the head, as though pulling heavy weights towards you. Relax briefly and push your arms out again, making them vibrate with energy. Repeat several times. *Optional:* double breathing.

24. Arm rotations in small circles

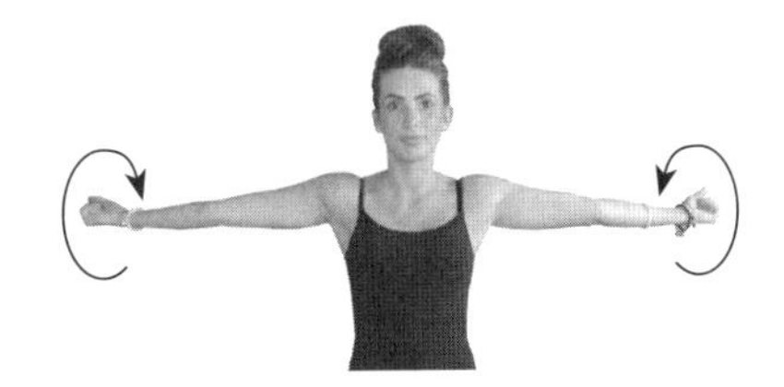

Stand with your arms extended to the side at shoulder level with your fists facing upwards, and rotate your arms in small circles, tensing strongly all the time. Then relax momentarily, and rotate in the opposite direction.

25. Weight pulling to the front

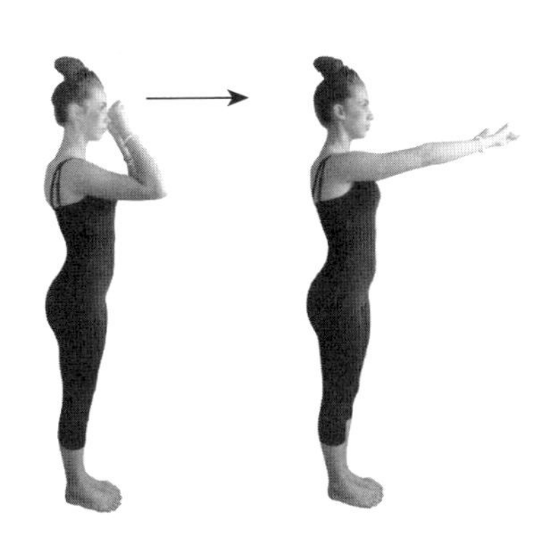

Position your arms bent at right angles in front of you, so that the backs of your fists are close to your forehead. Then extend your arms straight out in front, vibrating them with energy, as though pushing weights. Relax briefly, and pull the weights back in towards your head. *Optional:* double breathing.

26. Finger recharging

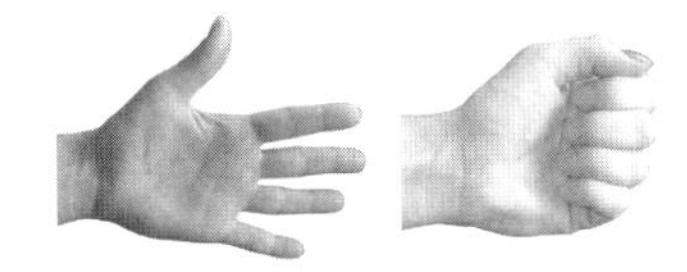

Stand with your arms relaxed down at your side, and open and close your hands vigorously several times with tension. Repeat the exercise with your arms extended laterally, then again with your arms extended at shoulder level in front of your body, and finally with your arms extended straight above your head.

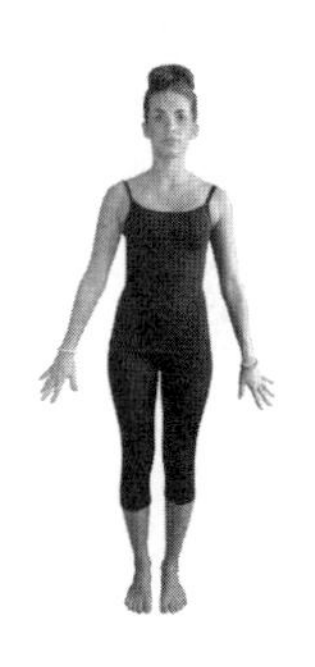
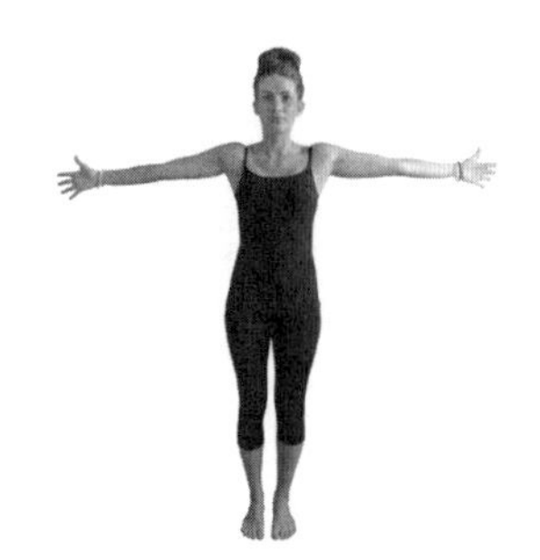
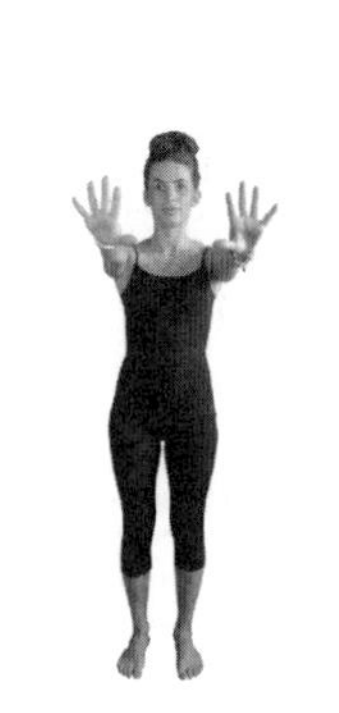
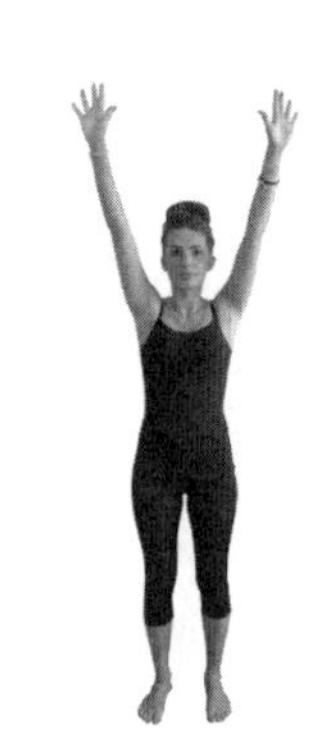

27. Arm recharging in four phases

In the starting position bring your fists up to your chest, and imagine you have weights in your hands, so you can feel the tension in your arms as you perform the following exercises.

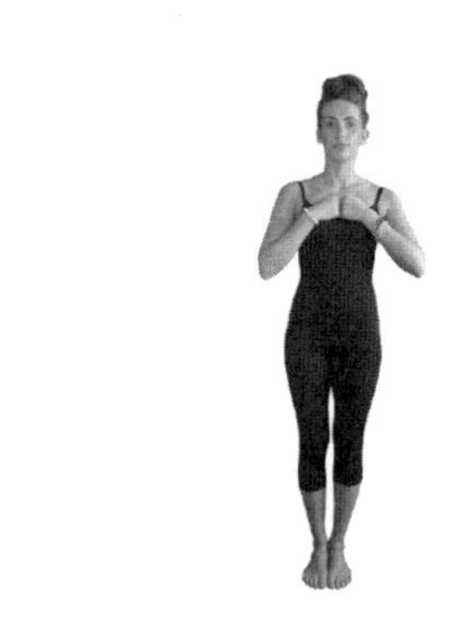

a) While inhaling with a single breath, push your arms out to your sides with tension in the arm muscles, relax briefly, and then pull them back with tension to the starting position, and relax briefly.

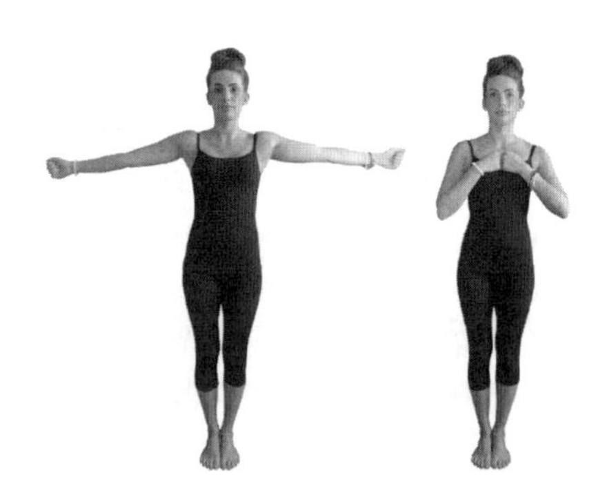

b) With tension again in the arms, and a single exhalation, push the arms out in front of you, relax briefly, and pull them back with tension to the starting position.

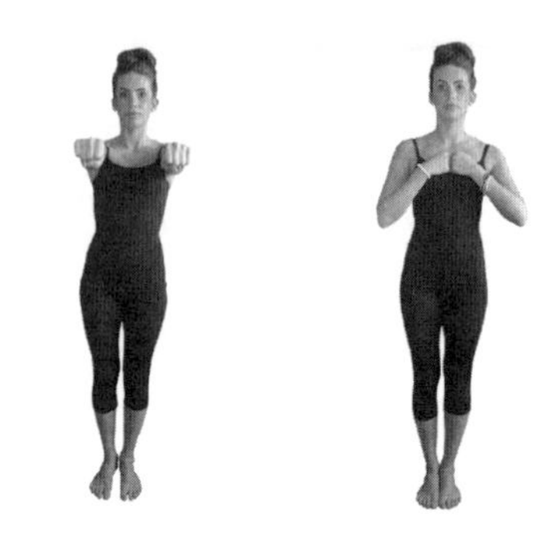

c) Now with tension and a double inhalation, lift them over your head, while rising up onto your toes.

d) With relaxed arms and a double exhalation, bring the imaginary weights down to your chest, and then down to your sides, as you come down off your toes.

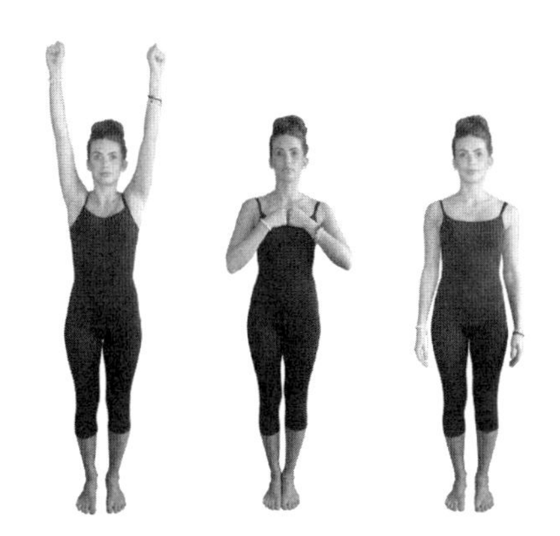

28. Overhead weight lifting (single arm raising)

Tense your left arm as though you are holding a weight in your hand, and inhale with a double breath as you lift it over your head, coming up onto your toes. Then with a double exhalation, relax your arm as you bring it back down. Repeat with alternate arms several times.

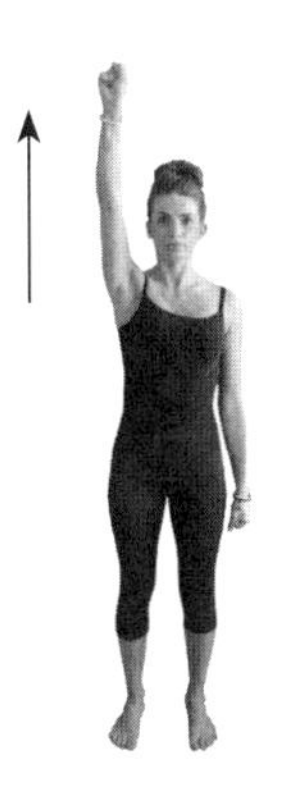

29. Lateral weight lifting

With your feet hip-width apart, tense your left arm as though holding a weight, and with a double inhalation bring your arm up laterally until the upper arm touches your head, bending very slightly to the right side. With a double exhalation relax your arm downwards, and repeat with alternate arms several times.

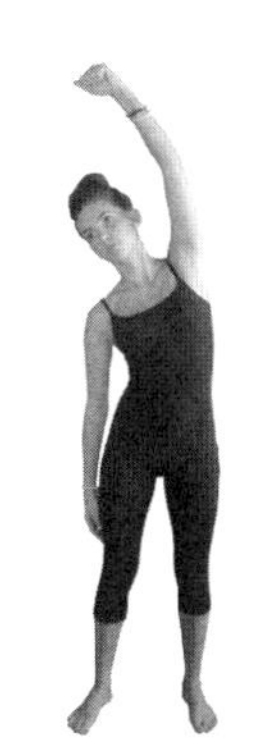

30. Walking in place

Walk in place with an exaggerated marching step, lifting your knees high and swinging the opposite arm to the opposite leg. Continue for 50 to 100 steps, remaining aware of the energy flowing to, and through, your body.

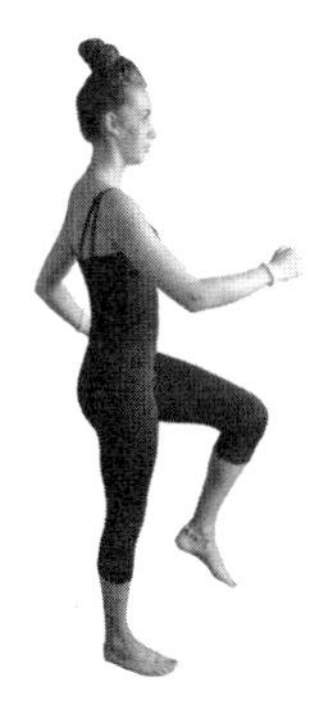

31. Running in place

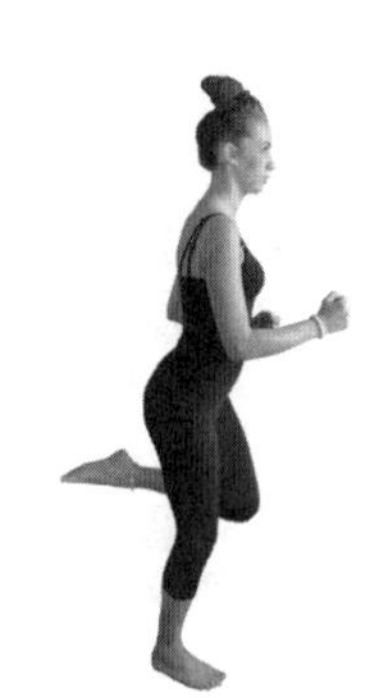

Run in place, lifting your knees as before, and at the same time bring your heels up to touch your buttocks if you can. The arms remain stationary, bent at the elbows. Practise 50 to 100 steps, being aware of the flow of energy to, and through, your body.

32. Fencing

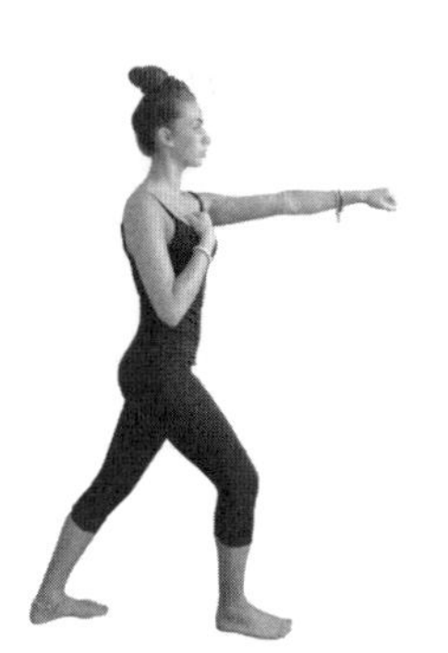

With both fists on your chest, step forward with your left leg and, with a double exhalation, thrust your right arm and fist to the front, as though you are pushing a very heavy door. Keep your spine straight and tense, with tension as well in the chest, the back leg and the extended arm, as you move from the standing to the thrusting position. Both feet are flat on the floor. With a double inhalation, relax and return to the standing position, and repeat the exercise with the other leg and arm, alternating several times.

33. Arm rotation in large circles

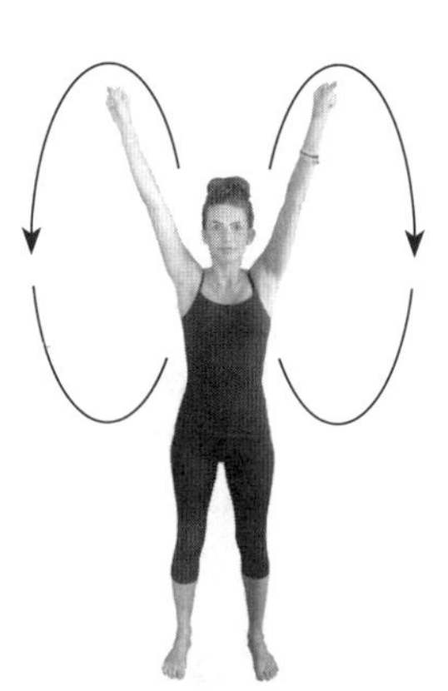

Inhaling, lift your tensed arms in a large arc over your head, and with an exhalation bring them down behind you, relaxing them. Repeat at least three times in each direction.

34. Abdomen recharging

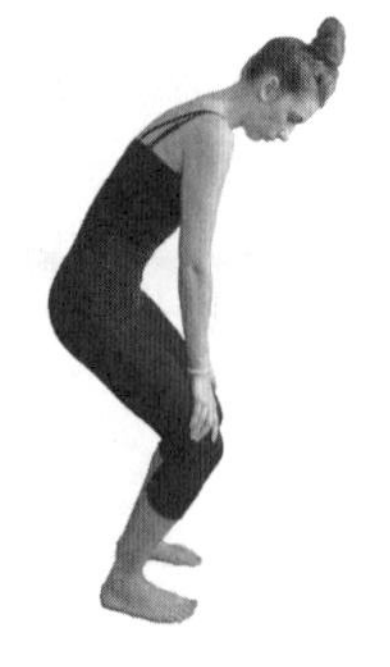

First phase: This phase is known as *udyana bandha*. Exhale completely as you bring your upper body forward, resting the heels of your hands on the thighs. With the breath still held out, contract the abdominal muscles as far as possible inward and upward towards the spine, and hold for as long as comfortable, without strain. Slowly relax the abdomen, then inhale, and return to the upright position.

Second phase: The second phase is known as *agnisar kriyā*. Exhale again and resume the forward position, resting the palms of your hands on the thighs. This time, contract and expand the abdominal muscles repeatedly, for as long as you are able to retain the breath externally. Relax, inhale, and return to the upright position. This is a very good exercise for awakening energy in the navel centre or *maṇipūra chakra*, as well as stimulating the digestion and toning the abdominal organs and glands.

Caution

People suffering from high blood pressure, heart disease or acute peptic or duodenal ulcers should not practise these stomach exercises, nor should pregnant women or persons who have undergone abdominal surgery in the last six to nine months.

35. Double breathing with palms touching

Stand with your arms straight out to your side at shoulder level, and exhale with a double breath. Bend your knees slightly and bring your arms to the front, so that your palms touch. With a double inhalation, tense the entire body upwards in a wave, as you straighten your legs and pull the arms back outward against a resisting force. With a double exhalation, relax the body downward in a wave. Repeat three to five times.

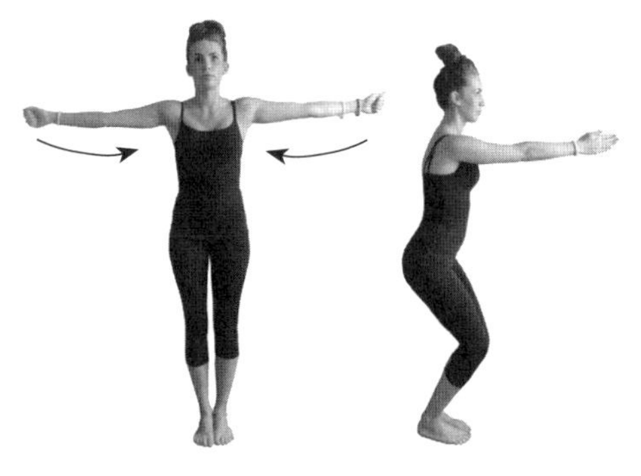

36 and 37. Calf recharging and ankle rotation

Repeat steps 2 and 3. Balance on your right leg, with your left knee slightly bent. Then slowly pull your left leg upward, bending at the knee, while tensing your calf muscle, as if you are pulling your leg up against a resisting weight. Relax briefly, and then push the leg down against a resisting weight.

Practise three to five times, and then lifting your left foot a few inches from the floor, lightly tense your ankle and rotate it in small circles three to five times in each direction. Repeat with the other leg.

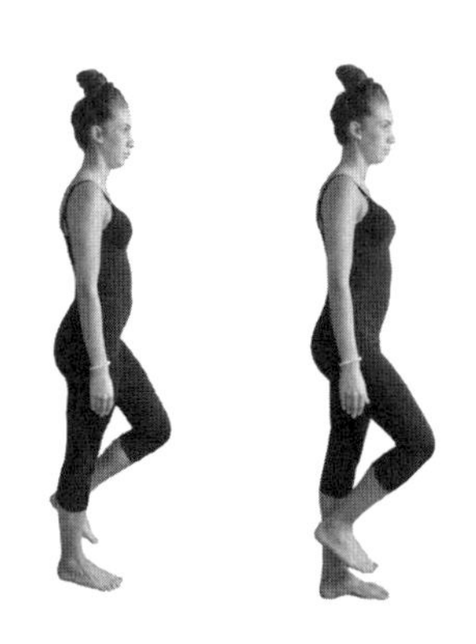

38. Hip recharging

Balance with your weight on your right leg, extend your left leg about a foot forward with the foot close to the floor, and rotate your foot three or more circles in each direction. Repeat on the right side.

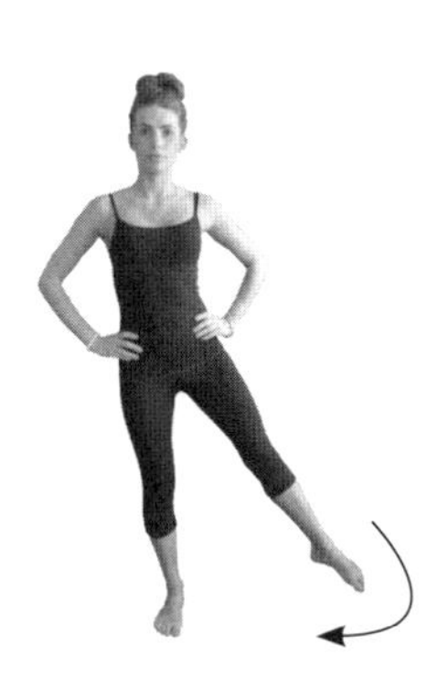

39. Double breathing without tension

With your mind calmly focused at the midpoint between the eyebrows and looking inwardly with closed eyes, bring your fists to your upper chest, holding them forward. With complete relaxation, and a double exhalation, extend your arms slowly in front of you. Pause and enjoy the flow of energy you feel throughout your body. With a double inhalation slowly draw the arms back to your chest, pausing again to feel the energy flow. Repeat six to ten times.

With your eyes closed, continue to focus your attention inwardly at the midpoint between the eyebrows. Feeling relaxed, peaceful and energised, enjoy the pauses between the breaths, and mentally affirm: '*I am eternal! I am blissful! I am free!*'

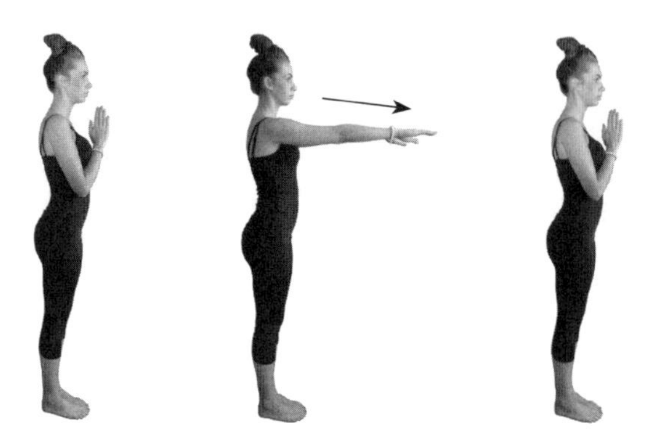

7.6.3 *AUM* TECHNIQUE – INNER SOUND MEDITATION

> 'Patañjali speaks of God (in the *Yoga Sūtras*) as the actual Cosmic Sound of *Aum* heard in meditation. *Aum* is the Creative Word, the sound of the Vibratory Motor. Even the yogi-beginner soon inwardly hears the wondrous sound of *Aum*. Receiving this blissful spiritual encouragement, the devotee becomes assured that he is in actual touch with divine realms.'
>
> *Yogananda 1946, p.233*

> *'Tasya vācakaḥ Praṇavaḥ.'*
> 'The manifest expression of Īsvara is the sacred sound Aum (Praṇavaḥ).'
>
> *Yoga Sūtras 1:27*

> 'That indwelling omnipresent sole reality is verbally alluded to as *Oṁ*, which is the ever-new and eternal Cosmic Sound that is heard in all natural phenomena (thunderclap, roaring of the ocean, wind rustling trees in the forest) and even in the reverberations of the musical instruments, the hum of engines, and the distant din of the carnival crowd.'
>
> *Venkatesananda 1998, pp.80–81*

Oṁ (pronounced *Aum*), also known as the *Praṇava*, is the Divine Cosmic Vibration that is God. In the Bible, the Word that St John refers to is the Creative Vibration: 'In the beginning was the Word, and the Word was with God and the Word was God'

(John 1:1). And similarly in the *Vedās* it is said: 'In the beginning Prajapati, or the Lord of Creation, alone existed; He alone was the universe; He had Vak as His own and as second to Him, and Vak, or the Word, was verily the Supreme *Brāhman*.'

From the centre of God's Consciousness of Absolute stillness and Oneness vibrated the omnipresent Cosmic Sound, *Aum*, into all Creation. This Divine Intelligence is in every atom and cell, vibrating with the Cosmic Sound of *Aum*. Paramhansa Yogananda referred to *Aum* as the Holy Spirit, the 'Comforter', that gives supreme comfort to the soul, inwardly attuned to it.

> '*Brāhman* is the indestructible and supreme Spirit. *Adhyatma* is *Brāhman's* manifestation as the essential soul of all beings. Cosmic *karma* is *Aum* (the Cosmic Vibration) which causes the birth, sustenance, and dissolution of all creatures, and also the diversity of their nature.'
>
> *Bhagavad Gītā 8.3*

There are numerous names, words and symbols used to symbolise God. But there is no other word that can convey the significance and direct experience of the Ultimate Reality so profoundly and accurately as the word-sound symbol, *Aum* (*Oṁ*). Even the word God in comparison to *Aum* is insufficient and limited in its function and significance. The word God has been widely used by adherents of monotheistic religious systems to indicate one Ultimate Reality or a concept of it. The word God has been thought to be related to an Anglo-Saxon word 'good', and as *gad*, pronounced 'gohdt', found in a Germanic manuscript from the sixth century. It could be from the Proto-Indo-European *ghau* meaning 'to invoke'. It is not in Hebrew, Aramaic, Greek or Latin Judeo-Christian scriptures or original major religious texts of India.

All the sacred scriptures born out of India, from the *Vedās* to the *Upaniṣads*, and from Yoga and *Vedānta,* maintain that the eternal Word *Aum* (the *Praṇava*) signifies the Supreme Reality. *Aum* is that which expresses the inexpressible. It is the true and highest symbol of *Brāhman* both as the Absolute (God), and as the personal God (*Iśvara*), that has been chanted, contemplated and meditated upon by rishis, sages and yogis down through the ages. According to the *Śiva Mahāpurāṇa* (an ancient Hindu religious text of 24,000 verses, devoted to Lord Śiva) a spiritual devotee who repeats *Aum* 1,080,000 times becomes pure, and a spiritual devotee who completes 90,000,000 repetitions of *Aum* attains enlightenment.

Aum transcends all the conceptions of symbols and anything that is signified by the symbols. *Aum* is a unique symbol; there is no other symbol that represents all the different aspects of the Ultimate Reality in one sound. It is all-inclusive; it includes all sounds, and all thoughts and concepts of God. The subtlest of all vibrations is *Aum*, the sound-form of the Ultimate Reality or God, that is omnipresent, omniscient and omnipotent, and has infinite energy and power.

It is out of this eternal primordial sound vibration *Aum* that the entire Cosmos has been created. It is the 'great seed' (*mahā bīja*), the source of all there is.

> '*Oṁ* has become the one symbol for the religious aspiration of the vast majority of human beings. Take, for instance, the English word God. It covers only a limited function, and if you go beyond it, you have to add adjectives, to make it

Personal, or Impersonal, or Absolute God. So with the words for God in every other language; their signification is very small. This word *Oṁ*, however, has around it all the various significances. As such it should be accepted by everyone.'

Vivekananda 2011, p.114

'Continue to listen to that *Omkar* sound and contemplate its meaning as God Itself.'

Niketan 2005, p.236

'One who has known *Aum*, which is soundless and of infinite sounds, and which is ever-peaceful on account of negation of duality, is the true sage and none other.'

Gaudapada Karika 1.12.29

HOW TO HEAR THE COSMIC SOUND VIBRATION

In this technique, the energy that normally flows out through the senses is redirected within. The outer senses of seeing and hearing are closed by using a hand *mudrā*, so that the awareness and attention can be attuned inwardly to perceive the subtle sounds of *Aum*. When your mind is interiorised with your awareness focused on the midpoint between the eyebrows at the Spiritual Eye, and concentrated there for some time, it awakens the subtle sounds of the *chakras*. The mind then becomes deeply absorbed in these inner subtle astral sounds, leading to the pure sound of *Aum*. At first you may only hear the sounds of your own physical body, such as your heart beating, blood pumping through your veins or the sound of your breathing, but as your consciousness is withdrawn deeper within you may hear the astral sounds emanating from your *chakras*, which can draw you still deeper into the all-compelling, all-captivating and all-absorbing cosmic sound of *Aum*. Deeply merged in the vibrationless calm of *Aum* one can enter into the blissful and expansive state of *samādhi* in oneness with the Ultimate Reality, God.

Your inner attunement to the Cosmic Sound of *Aum* can also attract the grace and presence of divine light. Also manifested in the Divine are the qualities of divine love, heavenly bliss, ineffable peace, perfect wisdom, perfect calmness and stillness.

'A yogi should sit in *Siddhāsana* ("Adept pose" meditation posture) and perform *vaiṣṇavī mudrā* (Seal of Vishnu is the same as *shambhavi mudrā*). Then he should listen through the right ear, to the subtle inner sounds.'

Nādabindūpanisad 31

This meditation of inner perception – listening with the ear of intuition – to the Cosmic Vibration of *Aum* is best practised when the mind is calm and focused in the stillness after practising *Hong Sau* meditation. For beginners, practise *Hong Sau* for at least three months to help you deepen your concentration and calm the restlessness of the mind, before you start to practise this *Aum* Inner Sound Meditation. Then you will be able to go deep in your meditation to feel a deep sense of inner calmness, and attunement in oneness with Ultimate Reality, God.

1. Before practising the *Aum* Inner Sound Meditation, begin with a few rounds of *prāṇāyama* (*kapālabhāti* and *nāḍī śodhana* – alternate nostril breathing). Then calm the mind by practising *Hong Sau* meditation for 10–15 minutes, or until you are calmly centred within in inner stillness.
2. Sit in a comfortable meditation posture with the head, neck and spine aligned. Place your upper arms on a wooden T-shaped arm rest ('*Aum* Board'), parallel to the floor with the elbows in line with your shoulders. Make sure the arms and shoulders are at a comfortable height. There should be no strain on your hands, arms, back or neck.
3. Raise your hands up to your head and position the fingers in the *Aum mudrā*: first close your ears by gently pressing the earflaps (*tragi*) inward with your thumbs. An alternative is to use earplugs to close the ears, which are available from a pharmacy. Rest the little fingers gently and lightly on the outer corners of each closed eyelid. Rest the other fingers on the forehead pointing inward towards the midpoint between the eyebrows to direct energy towards the Spiritual Eye.
4. While holding the *Aum mudrā*, breathe normally, and with your eyes closed, gaze with deep attentive awareness into the Spiritual Eye. Then in a natural rhythm, mentally chant *Aum, Aum, Aum, Aum*...continuously at the Spiritual Eye, so that it vibrates and resonates in that centre.
5. As you gaze inwardly into the Spiritual Eye mentally chanting *Aum*, listen in your right ear for the subtle inner sound-frequencies of the *chakras*. If you hear the sounds in the left ear, gradually bring them to your right ear. If you hear one distinct sound, focus your awareness totally on that one sound. As sensitivity develops, another fainter sound will be heard behind it. Leave the first sound and transfer your awareness to the fainter sound. Again, a third sound will begin to emerge behind the second sound. With awareness, continue discarding the grosser sounds for the more subtle sounds. Your aim is to reach the source of all sound – the Primordial Sound, *Aum*. As your listening to *Aum* deepens, your consciousness expands, and you begin to feel omnipresent, beyond the mind, body, ego and the senses. Your consciousness dissolves into that omnipresent *Aum* sound-current of the power of Consciousness, and you feel complete oneness with *Aum*, experiencing the reality of God.
6. After listening to the inner sound vibration of *Aum*, remain sitting calmly and joyfully in the stillness of your meditation and experience pure awareness of Being or a perception of oneness. Mentally affirm: '*The quiet stillness of the Infinite permeates my being. I melt into the ocean of Bliss.*'

THE INNER SOUNDS OF THE *CHAKRAS*

> 'In the beginning stage of the practice, one hears different types of strong or gross inner sounds. When the practice increases one hears subtle and subtler sounds.'
>
> *Nādabindūpaniṣad 33*

As a beginner, when you first practise the *Aum* Inner Sound Meditation you may only hear the inner sounds of the physical body: heartbeat, blood circulation and breathing. You may also hear a very high-pitched electrical sound from the electrical field of energy of the astral body. If you hear any of these distinct sounds, concentrate on them until they recede into the background, then transfer your awareness to the next fainter sound that you hear, and then to the more subtle astral sounds. If your mind is deeply interiorised and calm while listening to these inner sounds, you will eventually be able to tune into and hear the subtle sounds of the *chakras*. Listening to the inner *chakra* sounds will lead you to hear the Primordial Sound vibration, *Aum*.

In the *Hamsopaniṣad* (16), the classical ten different inner sounds are described as: sounds of the honeybee or bumblebee, crickets singing in the forest, sound of a temple bell, blowing of a conch shell, sound of stringed instruments (such as a lute, harp, vina, sitar or tamboura), cymbals, flute, double-ended drum like a *mridaṅga*, a low-pitched drum, and the roar of thunder.

THE *CHAKRA* SOUNDS AS HEARD IN MEDITATION

Mūladhāra chakra. The humming or drone of bees, a low vibratory sound. When heard less perfectly it may sound like a motor or a drum.

Svādhiṣṭhāna chakra. Like a flute. When heard less perfectly it may sound like crickets singing in the forest, or like running water of a mountain spring.

Maṇipūra chakra. Stringed instrument sound, like a sitar or harp.

Anāhata chakra. Like the flowing peal of deep bells, or a gong. Less perfectly it sounds like tinkling bells.

Viśuddha chakra. Thunder or the ocean's roar. When heard less perfectly it may sound like wind or a waterfall.

Ājñā chakra (Spiritual Eye/medulla). A symphony of sounds; *Aum*.

> '*Brāhman* is beyond the silence, the state is of the Supreme Self (*Paramātma*). While there is sound there is the mind, at the end of sounds the mind does not exist.'
>
> *Nādabindūpaniṣad 48*

When the mind concentrates on the subtle inner sounds, it recognises the different types of sounds, but still the mind has not been transcended. It is only when the mind completely merges with the subtle sounds that both the subtle sounds and the mind cease to exist. The ultimate goal is for the Self (*ātman*) to merge in the *Brāhman*

(God), the Universal Consciousness, That which is beyond all sounds, and which is to be known and realised.

All that we experience and perceive in this world is dependent upon there being both a subject and an object, or a seer and a seen. Nothing can be experienced or perceived without the subject, the seer. And vice versa, if there is only an object without a subject or seer to perceive it nothing is experienced. If a tree falls in the stillness of a forest, and no one hears it fall, was there really a sound?

7.6.4 *NĀBHI KRIYĀ* – AWAKENING *PRĀṆA* IN THE NAVEL CENTRE

Nābhi Kriyā is one of the original preparatory techniques of the *Kriyā Yoga* meditation that was taught by Yogiraj Sri Lahiri Mahasaya (1828–1895), who was taught the supreme science of *Kriyā Yoga* meditation by Mahavatar Babaji, the great immortal Himalayan yogi.

The purpose of this technique is to stimulate and awaken the *prāṇic* energy at *maṇipūra chakra*, in the navel centre, and then to draw the energy from *maṇipūra* up the spine to the Spiritual Eye of the *ājñā chakra*. While practising this technique, a calm energy is experienced in the lower part of the abdomen. The *prāṇic* current there is called *samāna vayu*, whose role is in guiding all the *prāṇa* present in the body into the subtle *suṣumnā* channel (the main *nāḍī* in the astral spine).

The *maṇipūra chakra* is the centre in which the *prāṇa* and *apāṇa* currents are united after they have been activated and balanced through *Kriyā prāṇāyāma*.

For directing *prāṇic* energy up the spine to the higher *chakras*, *Nābhi Kriyā* is a good preparation technique for *Kriyā* meditation, and particularly helpful during longer meditations.

PRACTISING *NĀBHI KRIYĀ*

Before beginning *Nābhi Kriyā* it can be beneficial to practise a few rounds of *kapālabhāti* (the skull or brain cleansing breath), while concentrating on the *maṇipūra chakra* at the navel. This purification breath technique has a stimulating effect on activating both the brain cells and the navel centre. It cleanses the frontal part of the brain, and purifies the five elements: earth, water, fire, air and ether in the body. Carbon dioxide is expelled from the blood and more oxygen is circulated throughout the body. The *ājñā* and *maṇipūra chakras* are particularly awakened with *prāṇic* energy by *kapālabhāti*.

After practising *kapālabhāti*, the breath becomes quiet, the mind calm, and due to concentration at the *maṇipūra*, the vibrations can be there (for *kapālabhāti* technique see 'The five purifications', in Chapter 6.5).

1. Sit in a comfortable meditation posture with your head, neck and spine aligned. Relax your whole body, close your eyes and bring your attention for a moment to the midpoint between the eyebrows, at your Spiritual Eye, the positive pole of *ājñā chakra*.

2. Then bring your awareness to *mūladhāra chakra*, at the base of your spine, and slowly inhale and mentally chant *Oṁ* as if you were sending the *mantra*'s energy into this *chakra*.
3. Repeat this internal chanting of the *mantra Oṁ* at each of your ascending *chakras* in succession, sending the energy there each time:

   svādhiṣṭhāna – at the genital area

   maṇipūra – at your navel

   anāhata – at your heart

   viśuddhi – at your throat

   the medulla oblongata – the negative pole of *ājñā chakra*, located in the brain stem at the back of your head, below the base of the brain.

   the Spiritual Eye – the positive pole of *ājñā chakra*, which is located at the midpoint between your eyebrows.
4. Slowly tilt your chin down towards your neck, forming a throat or chin lock (*jālandhara bandha*), and bring your awareness to the *maṇipūra chakra* at your navel.
5. As you continue to breathe normally (do not synchronise your breathing with the chanting of *Oṁ*), mentally chant *Oṁ* 100 times to activate this *chakra* and bring energy up from the lower two *chakras*: *mūladhāra* and *svādhiṣṭhāna*. A calm energy is usually perceived gathering around the navel; this is the *prāṇic* current called *samāna vayu* guiding your *prāṇa* into the subtle *suṣumnā* channel of the astral spine.
6. Maintaining your awareness at *maṇipūra chakra*, with your inner gaze at the midpoint between your eyebrows, release the throat lock, raise your chin to the normal upright position, and slowly tilt your head back as far as is comfortable without strain. See if you can feel your energy moving into the area at the base of your skull at the back of your head known as the medulla oblongata, and then back down through your spine to *maṇipūra chakra* at your navel centre.
7. Holding your head back in this tilted position, mentally chant *Oṁ* 25 times, directing the *mantra*'s energy into the counterpart of the navel on the back of your spine.
8. Now slowly raise your head to its normal position, and with concentration, once again mentally chant *Oṁ* successively at each of the six *chakras*, this time starting at the Spiritual Eye and medulla of *ājñā chakra* and moving downward to *viśuddhi*, *anāhata*, *maṇipūra*, *svādhiṣṭhāna* and *mūladhāra chakras*.

This completes one round of *Navi Kriyā*. Aim to practise six to 12 rounds, then sit quietly, go into stillness with your inward attention at your Spiritual Eye. When you return to your normal activities, carry this natural sense of inner stillness and energy with you to give you the inner strength to overcome life's trials and tribulations.

MEDITATION

After your practice of *Navi Kriyā*, focus your attention within, in the stillness of your inner Self. As you meditate, keep your inner vision at the Spiritual Eye, at the midpoint between the eyebrows. Feel the upward flow of energy in the *suṣumnā* in the subtle spine flowing to the medulla oblongata at the top of the spine. Concentrate there first for a short while, then feel that you are dissolving the ego-consciousness (seated at the medulla) into superconsciousness at the Spiritual Eye. With a steady inward gaze, concentrate your attention deeply at that midpoint between the eyebrows. Then feeling joy within, expand that blissful consciousness into the Infinite.

Mentally affirm: '*I am pure consciousness awakening in God.*'

7.6.5 *MAHĀ MUDRĀ* – AWAKENING ENERGY IN YOUR SPINE

> 'Out of the many *mudrās*, the following ten are the best: (1) *Mahā mudrā*, (2) *Mahābandha*, (3) *Mahāveda*, (4) *Khecarī*, (5) *Jālandhara*, (6) *Mūlabandha*, (7) *Viparītkaraṇī*, (8) *Uḍḍīyāna*, (9) *Vajroli*, (10) *Śakticālana*.'
>
> *Siva Saṃhitā 4.15*

Mahā mudrā and other classical Yoga *mudrās* are listed and explained in the ancient *Haṭha Yoga* treatises: *Śiva Saṃhitā*, *Gheraṇḍa Saṃhitā* and *Haṭha Yoga Pradīpikā*. The path of *Haṭha Yoga* was formulated and laid out by the great *siddha* yogis: Matsyendranath, his disciple Gorakshanath, and others – 14 altogether.

The Sanskrit word *mahā* means 'great' and *mudrā* means 'gesture' or 'attitude'. As a flow of energy *mudrā* is an 'attitude'. By practising *mudrā*, our intention is to align our own individual *prāṇic* flow of energy with the source of cosmic *prāṇa* that surrounds and suffuses us with life. Another meaning of the word *mudrā* is that it expresses the inner state of the practitioner performing the *mudrā*.

YOUR SPINE IS THE PATHWAY TO GOD

The practice of *mahā mudrā* awakens and enlivens the subtle energy in the seven-centred astral *suṣumnā* passage in the cerebrospinal axis (the Pathway to God), through which all aspirants seeking liberation must pass to reach God consciously. It is a specific process by means of which one is able to awaken dormant forces in the lower three *chakras* and cause them to flow upward to the *ājñā chakra* and the thousand-rayed lotus at *sahasrāra*, at the crown of the head.

Mahā mudrā also controls the vital airs in the body known as *vyāna* and *udāṇa*. *Vyāna* permeates throughout the entire body and is the aura of the body. It helps the other *vayus* (vital airs) to function properly. It controls both the physical nerves and the subtle or astral nerves (*nāḍīs*).

Udāṇa functions in the body above the throat and the crown of the head. It controls the automatic functions of the cephalic divisions of the autonomic nervous system. It controls speech, sense of balance, memory and intellect. *Udāṇa* has an upward movement – it carries *kuṇḍalinī* to the *sahasrāra* at the crown of the head, and separates the astral body from the physical body at the time of death.

The spinal cord can be likened to an electrical wire. In the astral wire are located seven subtle centres of light (*chakras*) which are the sub-centres for the conduction and distribution of *prāṇic* life currents throughout the body. From the medulla oblongata (the negative pole of the two-rayed lotus, *ājñā chakra*) energy flows into the cerebrospinal axis through the physical body. Just as electricity flows into a bulb through a wire passage, so the Cosmic Energy enters the medulla and flows through the brain (where it is stored) into the cerebrospinal axis and its seven subtle centres (*chakras*), it is distributed throughout a network of subtle wire passages called *nāḍīs* to the whole body.

MAHĀ MUDRĀ: PREPARATION FOR *KRIYĀ* MEDITATION

The *Haṭha Yoga* technique of *mahā mudrā* is a good preparation for the practice of meditation. It is a powerful practice, and when practised properly, provides not only various kinds of physical benefits, but it also balances and opens the *iḍā* and *piṅgala nāḍīs* (see Chapter 4.4). In the *Kriyā Yoga* tradition *mahā mudrā* is used to great effect in opening the spinal passage, allowing the life-force (*Prāṇa Shakti*) to flow upward in the central subtle channel of the *suṣumnā*. This magnetises the spine with energy, and helps you to gain control over the *prāṇic* energy currents in the spine, bringing a deeper awareness and concentration in your meditation.

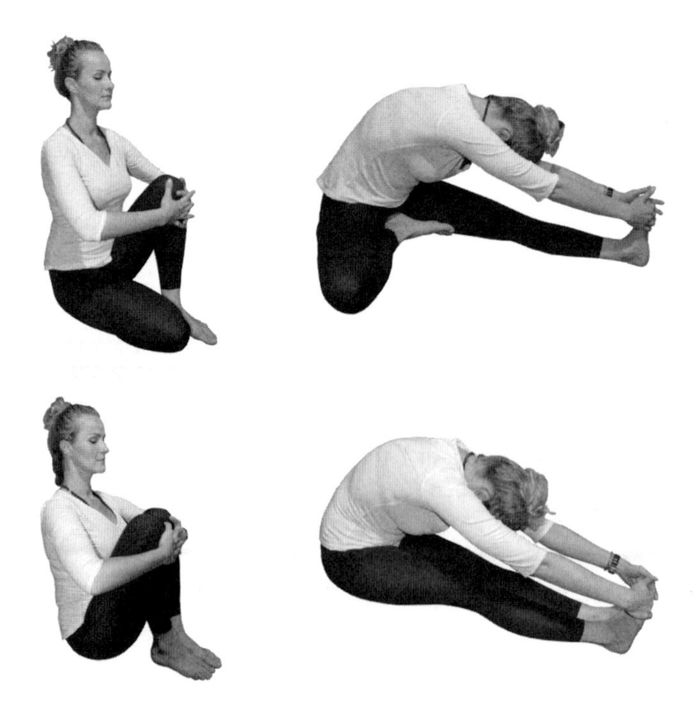

The *Kriyā Yoga* version of *mahā mudrā* that you will practise is modified with a different knee position. If you have problems with your knee, like a tear in the meniscus, or other knee injuries, then you may find this posture easier to practise, as it does not require a rotation or twist to the knee as in the *Haṭha Yoga* version.

The two *mudrās* – anal lock and chin lock – that are held in the *mahā mudrā* retain the magnetised energy in the spine, so it can be directed upward into the higher centres in the brain.

In *mahā mudrā*, stretching individually over the left leg and right leg while pulling on the big toe opens the left and right subtle *prāṇic* channels (*nāḍīs*), allowing the *prāṇic* energy to move more easily into the central channel (*suṣumnā nāḍī*). *Mahā mudrā* also releases the psychic knot (*granthi*) at the *mūladhāra chakra* at the base of the spine. When this is released, *prāṇa* is able to flow more easily into the *suṣumnā nāḍī* between the three lower *chakras*: *mūladhāra*, *svādhiṣṭhāna* and *maṇipūra*.

Note: The full *Kriyā Yoga* version of *mahā mudrā* is taught with the *Kriyā prāṇāyama*, a different breathing technique to the one described here. You would need to be initiated into the practice of *Kriyā prāṇāyama,* as taught by Paramhansa Yogananda on the spiritual *Kriyā Yoga* path, to be taught this technique.

THE IMPORTANCE OF *MAHĀ MUDRĀ*

Do not underestimate the power of this technique, or neglect its practice, for besides keeping the spine flexible, it can greatly increase the awareness of the *suṣumnā nāḍī* (central subtle channel) in the astral spine, and awaken the energy within it.

Three is the minimum number of *mahā mudrā* to be practised in one session. After that it is recommended that for every 12 *Kriyā prāṇāyamas* practised, one should perform one complete cycle of *mahā mudrā*. So if you are practising 60 *Kriyā prāṇāyamas* then you would practise *mahā mudrā* five times.

There are some advanced *Kriyāvāns* (initiated practitioners of *Kriyā*) who have been practising 48 complete cycles of *mahā mudrā* in two sessions daily. Practising one cycle of *mahā mudrā* takes approximately two minutes to complete, so to perform 48 would take approximately 96 minutes. One cycle of *mahā mudrā* is the equivalent to practising three *Kriyā prāṇāyamas*.

MAHĀ MUDRĀ PRACTICE

Stage one

1. Sit upright with the head, neck and spine aligned, on a firm carpeted surface or a Yoga mat to protect your ankles. Sit on your left foot, with the heel pressing against the anal region, or with the sole of your left foot resting under your left hip. Bend your right leg and place the foot flat on the floor. Then, interlocking the fingers of both hands together, clasp your hands around the right knee and draw the thigh in against your torso, or as close as possible. Keep your spine straight, and while pulling on the right knee, inhale (breathing in *ujjayi* breath) slowly to a count of ten. Keeping your concentration and awareness in the spine, feel that you are drawing a cool current of *prāṇic* energy up the spine.

2. Then hold the breath in, and stretch your right leg out in front of you. Bend forward, and with the fingers of each hand interlocked, grasp your big toe and pull, so that you extend your trunk forward with your forehead towards the knee as close as is comfortable. (If you are not supple enough, then bend the knee slightly. The most important thing is to feel the spine stretching and a sensation of energy rising through it.) As you hold the breath in, apply the chin lock (*jālandhara bandha*), and with your focused attention at the Spiritual Eye, mentally chant *Oṁ* six times. Feel a sensation of energy rising up through the spine and then pulsating at the Spiritual Eye, radiating waves of bliss throughout the brain.
3. Release the chin lock (*jālandhara bandha*), and with the clasped hands around the right knee draw the knee back up against your torso, while slowly exhaling to a slow count of ten. Keeping your concentration and awareness in the spine, feel a warm current of energy flowing down through the spine.

Stage two

Now change sides. Begin by tucking your right foot under, so it presses against the anus, and pull the left knee to the torso with your clasped hands. Repeat the previous instructions.

Stage three

1. Sit upright with your both knees bent, and with your clasped hands (fingers interlocked) around the knees, pull in your thighs against your torso. Inhale (breathing in *ujjayi* breath) for a slow count of ten. Feel that you are drawing a cool current of *prāṇic* energy up the spine.
2. Now stretch both legs out together in front of you, and grasping the big toes with the interlocked hands, pull on the big toes and stretch your torso forward, feeling the stretch in the spine. Apply the chin lock (*jālandhara bandha*) and bring your forehead towards the knees. Hold the breath in, and with your focused attention at the Spiritual Eye, mentally chant *Oṁ* six times. Feel a sensation of energy rising up through the spine and then pulsating at the Spiritual Eye, radiating waves of bliss throughout the brain.
3. Release the chin lock (*jālandhara bandha*), and slowly exhale to a count of ten. Keeping your concentration and awareness in the spine, feel a warm current of *prāṇic* energy flowing down the spine.
4. Then bring your knees and thighs back up against your torso, by pulling on the knees with clasped hands. Relax and return to normal breathing.

This completes one round of *mahā mudrā*. Practise three complete rounds. As you progress with this practice, you may increase the number of rounds to six to 12 complete rounds.

Caution

Due to the strong effects of contraction and relaxation of the abdomen, *mahā mudrā* is to be avoided by women during menstruation and pregnancy. Avoid strain and tension in the knees, spine and back, particularly if you have a knee or back problem.

Benefits

The entire abdominal cavity and its organs are massaged, and rejuvenated by more blood being supplied to them. The brain cells are stimulated, and the *tamasic* quality of inertia is removed from the body. The spine and the posterior back muscles are stretched, making them more flexible. Pressure placed at the perineum from sitting on the heel stimulates and encourages the vital energy (*prāṇa*) to flow upwards in the inner spine, energising the whole spine and brain.

MEDITATION

After your practice of *mahā mudrā*, focus your attention within, in the stillness of your inner Self. As you meditate, keep your inner vision at the Spiritual Eye, at the midpoint between the eyebrows. Continue to feel the energy vibrating in the spine. Feel and visualise it radiating out into every atom and cell in your body, until your body is permeated with divine Bliss. Then expand that blissful consciousness into the Infinite.

Mentally affirm: '*I am the ocean of Spirit that has become the wave of human life.*'

> 'To be Self-realised is to know your Self as the great ocean of Spirit by dissolving the delusion that you are a little ego, body, or personality.'
>
> *Paramhansa Yogananda*

7.6.6 *YONI MUDRĀ* – AWAKENING THE INNER LIGHT

> 'When the two eye currents are concentrated and thrown back in the medulla by focusing the eyes on the point between the eyebrows, they are perceived as one single Spiritual Eye of light.'
>
> *Yogananda 2003, p.14*

> 'The light of the body is the eye: if therefore thine eye be single, thy whole body shall be full of light.'
>
> *Gospel of Matthew 6:22*

Yoni mudrā, also known as *jyoti mudrā* ('Gesture of Light', 'Inner Light') is the gesture by which light is created. In sacred yogic texts this *mudrā* is referred to as *yoni mudrā*. The Sanskrit word *yoni* denotes the womb of creation, the source of origin, because like the baby in the womb, the yogi practising *Yoni mudrā* has no contact with the external world, and therefore no externalisation of consciousness. *Yoni* is also used to name the female sexual organs, and is regarded as the dispenser of *bhaga* (fortune, good luck, wealth, greatness), a word also used as a synonym for *yoni*. From the Sanskrit word *bhaga* comes the title *Bhāgavan*, 'God', 'Supreme Lord', and *bhagat*, 'devotee', from the root *bhaj*, 'to honour, adore'. The word *mudrā* in this case denotes a physical practice which has an effect on the mind.

In India there are specially carved stones in the form of a *yoni* in which the *Śiva lingam* rests, representing the source which supports and sustains spiritual consciousness. When *yoni* unites with *linga*, it becomes a symbol of divine procreative energy. *Linga* is the mind, *yoni* is the *kūtastha*, the midpoint between the eyebrows, where the spiritual light manifests. *Ājñā chakra* is the root of *kūtastha*. Everything evolves from *kūtastha-yoni*, and is traditionally referred to in the yogic scriptures as the 'seal of the creation'. When the *linga*-mind settles in *kūtastha-yoni* the yogi experiences a state of infinite Bliss; the meditator experiences the presence and oneness of the whole universe.

Yoni mudrā is also known as *shanmukhi mudrā*. *Shan* means 'seven' and *mukhi* means 'gates'. *Shanmukhi* means 'closing of the seven gates or doors of sense-perception (the two eyes, two ears, two nostrils and the mouth)'. *Jyoti mudrā* and *shanmukhi mudrā* are both *Haṭha Yoga* practices that are mentioned in the *Haṭha Yoga Pradīpikā* (Light on *Haṭha Yoga*) by Yogi Swatmarama. *Pradīpikā* actually means 'self-illuminating' or 'that which illumines'.

In the practice of *yoni mudrā* the mind is brought to a point of relaxed absorption within itself. By closing the outer doors or gates of the senses *yoni mudrā* redirects the energy of the senses inward, which induces *pratyāhāra* (sense-withdrawal).

During the practice of *yoni mudrā*, certain nerves in the body are affected and rejuvenated, similar to an acupressure rejuvenation treatment (though this is not the main purpose of *yoni mudrā*). Around the head and eyes are many acupuncture points which can be targeted to direct energy. The nerves that are affected when the fingers and thumbs are in position on the face in *yoni mudrā* are as follows:

The **thumbs** indirectly inhibit sensory stimulation of the eighth cranial nerve.

The **index fingers** touch over the infratrochlear branch of the opthalmic and the infraorbital branch of the maxillary.

The **middle fingers** depress the nasal rami (branches) of the infraorbital nerve.

The **little fingers** affect the inferior labial branch of the mandibular nerve (sensory branch).

> 'The yogi, sitting in *muktāsana*, concentrated in *śambavī mudrā*, should listen closely to the *nāda* heard within the right ear.
>
> Closing the ears, eyes, nose and mouth, a clear distinct sound is heard in the purified *suṣumnā* (astral spine).'
>
> *Haṭha Yoga Pradīpikā 4:67–68*

The Sanskrit word *śambavī* means an attitude or gesture of peace and concentration of mind in which one gazes at the midpoint between the eyebrows. *Shambhu* is Śiva sitting in *Pādmāsana* (Lotus pose), his eyes half-opened and raised upwards, fixed inwardly at the midpoint between the eyebrows. He is in the *khecāri* state. A yogi practising *Kriyā Yoga* assumes this posture and a coordination of the eye position *khecāri mudrā* (tongue lock) and *pādmāsana* is *śambavī mudrā*.

The purpose of *yoni mudrā* is to take the energy awakened by the *Kriyā prāṇāyama* (First *Kriyā*) in the spine, and draw it upward to focus it at the midpoint between the eyebrows at the Spiritual Eye. *Yoni mudrā* calms the breath in the region from the throat to the midpoint between the eyebrows, enabling you to see the radiant light of the Spiritual Eye within the radiance of stirring light in the form of absolute stillness and absolute peace.

YONI MUDRĀ TECHNIQUE

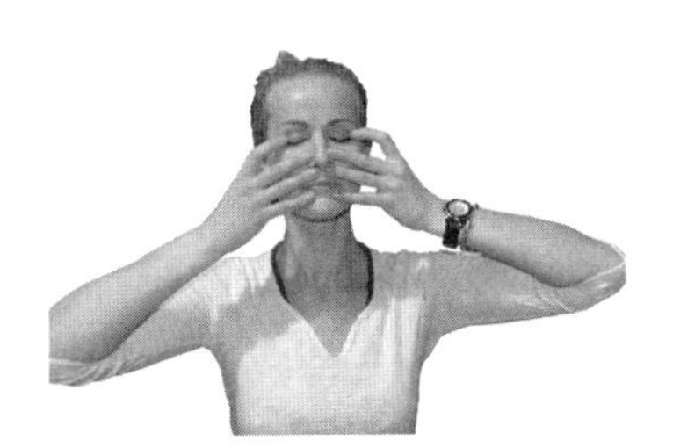

To practise *yoni mudrā*, sit upright with your head, neck and spine aligned in a comfortable and steady posture. Relax your whole body and, with your eyes closed, bring your focused attention to the midpoint between your eyebrows, at your Spiritual Eye. If you are able to perform *kecharī mudrā* (tongue lock) then do it, otherwise keep your tongue relaxed.

1. As you inhale slowly to a mental count of 10–12, drawing a current of *prāṇic* energy up the spine, raise your arms in front of your face with your elbows parallel to the floor and pointing sideways (if necessary prop your elbows up on a T-shaped elbow rest) so that you are ready to take up the finger positions of *yoni mudrā* at the end of the inhalation.
2. Hold the breath and the *prāṇic* energy you have drawn up your spine, focused at the midpoint between your eyebrows (Spiritual Eye). While holding your breath, close off all the sense openings in your head with the fingers and thumbs of both hands, so that all the energy lights up the region between your eyebrows. Close your ears by pressing the ear flaps (*tragi*) in with your **thumbs**. Place the **index fingers** on the corners of your eyelids, resting on the lower bony eye sockets, and lightly press the eyes shut (do *not* put pressure on the eyes as it could harm them). Use your **middle fingers** to close the two nostrils by pressing the soft nares of the nose just below the nasal bones. Place your **ring fingers** above the lips and the **little fingers** below the lips, squeezing your mouth shut, with the fingertips touching each other.
3. Now, while holding *yoni mudrā*, feel that your fingers are directing the *prāṇic* energy to your Spiritual Eye, and with deep focused awareness, turn your gaze inward towards the inner light of the Spiritual Eye. If you perceive light at the Spiritual Eye, experience it and merge into it, and feel that you are one with the light.

   Hold your breath in for as long as is comfortable without strain, and while gazing into the Spiritual Eye, mentally and continuously chant *Oṁ*, directing the energy of the *mantra* at the midpoint between your eyebrows. See if you can see the light of the Spiritual Eye that is gathering and intensifying at that point into a golden ring and expanding to surround a sphere of deep-blue light with a silvery-white five-pointed star at its centre.

4. Release *yoni mudrā* by removing your fingers from the sense openings. Keep your fingers and thumbs gently resting on your face, so that you are ready to practise another round of *yoni mudrā.*
5. Exhale slowly to a mental count of 10–12, feeling the current of *prāṇic* energy descend through the spine to the *mūladhāra chakra* at the base of your spine.

This completes one round of *yoni mudrā.* Practise three rounds, then sit in stillness in meditation. *Yoni mudrā* can be practised at any time, but the best time is in the deep calmness at night. After calming your mind and relaxing your body with deep breathing in *ujjayi prāṇāyāma* (see page 291), practise *mahā mudrā* to awaken the energy in your spine (see page 465), then a few rounds of *anuloma-viloma prāṇāyama*, followed by the *Hong Sau* technique to calm and concentrate the mind (see page 440), then *yoni mudrā.* Then remain concentrating for as long as possible at the midpoint between the eyebrows, to experience the inner light of the Spiritual Eye. To go deeper into meditation, the *Aum* technique can be practised after the *yoni mudrā.* Finally, sit in meditative stillness for as long as you comfortably can. Lahiri Mahasaya referred to it as enjoying the 'after-effect-poise'.

7.6.7 *KECHARĪ MUDRĀ*

> 'When the tongue is turned back into the hole in the skull and the eyes fixed firmly between the eyebrows, this is *kecharī mudrā.*'
>
> *Haṭha Yoga Pradīpikā 3:32*
>
> 'He who knows *kecharī mudrā* is not afflicted by disease, death, intellectual torpor, sleep, hunger, thirst or clouding of the intellect.'
>
> *Haṭha Yoga Pradīpikā 3:39*
>
> 'The body becomes beautiful; Samādhi is attained, and the tongue touching the holes obtains various juices (it drinks amrita nectar).'
>
> *Gheraṇḍa Saṃhitā 3:30*

In *Haṭha Yoga*, and in the *Kriyā Yoga* tradition of Lahiri Mahasaya, there is a mystical technique that he taught to his disciples called *kecharī mudrā.* It is a very difficult practice for most persons, and is not easily attained, which is probably why Paramhansa Yogananda did not teach it to his Western disciples. But for advanced yogis, *kecharī mudrā* can bring total absorption of mind, known as the state of *laya* (originating from the Sanskrit root *li*, meaning 'to become dissolved'). The yogi in this state of *laya* dissolves the mind, intellect and ego into the transcendental Being-Consciousness-Bliss (*Sat-chit-ānanda*). This revival of memory in the mind is itself the eternal life of a human being: pure Consciousness, pure Existence and pure Bliss – the state of the essential inner Being, the Divine Self.

In Sanskrit, *kecharī* consists of two words: *khe* ('sky') or *kha* (*ākāśha*, 'space') and *char* ('moving'). *Kecharī* therefore means 'one who flies or moves in the sky or space of Supreme Consciousness'. The symbolic meaning of this is that the upper part of the skull that corresponds with the brain is known as 'the sky of the yogi's body'. The practice of *kecharī mudrā* involves the tongue entering the 'sky' or 'space' of the yogi's body through a particular cavity in the skull. In *kecharī mudrā* the tongue is fastened securely within a hidden passage above the nasopharynx. Because the tongue is locked within this passage it is also sometimes referred simply as *jivabandha* (tongue lock). *Kecharī mudrā* has also been referred to as 'Inner-Outer-Space *Kriyā*', meaning that the very advanced *Kriyā* yogi is not bound or limited to the physical body. By changing the vibration of his physical body to a higher ethereal vibration, the yogi can travel both inside and outside of it.

Some advanced yogis who have experienced the effects of *kecharī mudrā* have expressed that the true *kecharī mudrā* is not actually accomplished through the manipulations of physical technique, but that it occurs spontaneously through a natural process which is activated by an automatic process of a powerful release of *prāṇa* (inner vital force). This natural and spontaneous process of *kecharī mudrā* is revealed only when the tongue is spontaneously activated through the force of *prāṇic* energy. A secret opening is uncovered, a hidden cavity in the skull located above the nasopharynx, which forms a part of the base of the skull where the brain sits. The tongue is inverted, drawn back, and enters this hidden internal passage; and when it is fully locked inside, and the internal gaze of the yogi is fixed between the eyebrows, the mind becomes absorbed there in the state known as *laya* (complete mental absorption).

> 'Turning the tongue upwards, it is inserted into the *triveṇī* (the junction of the three *nāḍīs*: *iḍā*, *piṅgala* and *suṣumnā*), which is known as the *vyoma chakra*. This is called *kecharī mudrā*.'
>
> *Haṭha Yoga Pradīpikā 3:37*

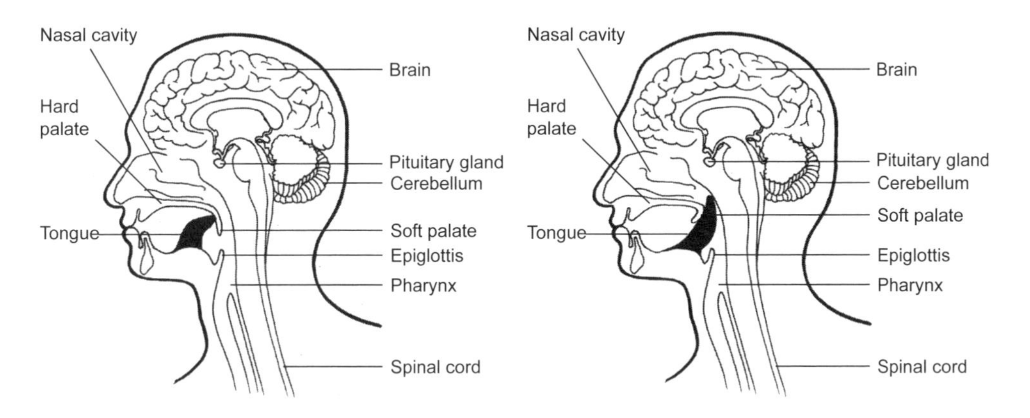

For the tongue to rise up beyond the air passage and into the region of the brain where the 'nectar of immortality' (*amrita*) flows from, the tongue would have to actually create an opening at the base of the skull and penetrate the sinus cavity. Because the passage does not exist, an opening can only be created by the automatic and spontaneous force of *prāṇa*, in which the tongue is forced through the rostrum bone at the base of the sphenoidal sinus and into its cavity. It is in this cavity, when the tongue is fully inserted, that it experiences the taste of nectar (*amrita*) exuding from the pituitary gland in the brain. This sweet tasting nectar generates strength and optimum health and longevity in the physical body, and causes inner tranquillity with spiritual realisation of the Divine Self, which is pure Consciousness.

> 'Upon the spontaneous emergence of wisdom, occurs *kecharī mudrā*, which is the state of *Śiva* (Supreme Consciousness).'
>
> *Śiva Sūtras 2:5 (Vasgupta, eighth century CE)*

The traditional practice of *kecharī mudrā* by very advanced yogis in India, under the strict direction and guidance of a guru, involves having the lower membrane of the tongue (*frenulum linguae*) gradually cut over a period of months, until the membrane that connects the tongue with the lower part of the mouth is severed. The reason for this is to make the tongue as long as necessary, so that when it is retroverted it can be made to enter the upper back cavity, above the palate. The tip of the tongue is pressed towards the eyebrow centre, where the three *nāḍīs* (*iḍā*, *piṅgala* and *suṣumnā*) meet.

Some very advanced yogis with the retroverted tongue in *kecharī mudrā* actually close the *rima glottidis* (the elongated opening between the true vocal cords and the arytenoid cartilages). This completely closes the air passage and controls the impulse to breathe in, so that the period of breath suspension can be lengthened.

Very advanced yogis of this technique with perfect control over their body, mind and *prāṇa* have been known to sit perfectly still in the Lotus pose (*Pādmāsana*) and suspend the breath for 40 days.

TECHNIQUE: THREE STAGES OF THE *KECHARĪ MUDRĀ*

In the *Haṭha Yoga Pradīpikā* three main stages are given for reconditioning and preparing the tongue for *kecharī mudrā*:

1. ***Chedan* (dissecting).** *Chedan* involves cutting the *frenulum linguae* (the mucosal fold running from the floor of the mouth to the underside of the tongue), which frees the tongue from the floor of the mouth. This is achieved by gradually and very carefully making a hair's-breadth cut to the *frenulum linguae* every seven days over a period of six months. The fine blade that is used must be sterilised, sharp and smooth. The cut is then cleaned by applying a mixture of rock salt and turmeric; amalaki powder (*Emblic myrobalan*) from the fruit of a tree grown in India can be substituted for turmeric.

The next two steps gradually lengthen the tongue and make it supple, until it is long enough to enter inside the skull to the level of the eyebrow centre.

2. ***Chalan* (loosening).** The tongue is loosened by grasping it with the thumb and fingers, and pulling it on all sides until it becomes supple.
3. ***Dohan* (milking).** The tongue can be lengthened by applying butter or sesame oil to it, and kneading and drawing it out with the hands as if milking a cow's udder.

***Warning:* Under no circumstances cut the membrane (frenulum linguae) of your tongue as outlined above.** It is definitely not recommended in the *Kriyā Yoga* tradition. Lahiri Mahasaya was extremely against it and Swāmi Kriyananda related a true story of how our guru, Paramhansa Yogananda, once spoke out severely against this practice when one of his young enthusiastic students began to cut the membrane of the tongue to lengthen it.

Within the tongue there are five main nerves, blood vessels and arteries, mucous glands and lymphatic vessels. To cut the *frenulum linguae* of the tongue could sever nerves, resulting in the tongue becoming numb, and it could also leave it without a proper blood supply.

Safe exercises for stretching your tongue

Exercise one

1. First, turn your tongue back and touch your uvula (the fleshy grape-like structure that hangs down from the back of your soft palate). Look in a mirror as you practise, to see what is happening.
2. Turn your tongue backwards and reach the uvula with the underside. With your mouth closed, push the base of your tongue up towards the roof of your mouth until you feel a stretch underneath your *frenulum linguae*. Gently but firmly practise without straining. Practise as often as you want to.

Exercise two: Tālavya Kriyā

This is pronounced 'Talabya Kriyā'.

1. Begin with your mouth closed and your tongue relaxed, with the tip of the tongue gently touching the back of the upper teeth.
2. Press the upper side of your tongue up against the roof of your mouth. Then create a suction by sucking your tongue hard to the roof of your mouth. Then gently open your mouth, still with your tongue sucked up against the roof of the mouth, until you feel the *frenulum linguae* being stretched.
3. The final position of this exercise involves opening your mouth wider, so that the suction is released, making a 'plucking' sound, and the tongue is pushed forward and downward towards your chin.

In order to avoid straining the *frenulum linguae*, in the beginning only practise ten repetitions a day. Later, you can aim to practise 25 to 50 times a day.

With daily practice of the tongue stretching exercises it can take three to six months or longer for the tongue to lengthen.

Keeping the tongue raised

Lahiri Mahasaya recommended practising *Kriyā* meditation with the mouth closed and with the tongue in the *kecharī mudrā* position so that the energy is directed up towards the eyebrow centre (*ājñā chakra*). Although Yogananda taught beginners after taking their first *Kriyā* initiation to breathe through the mouth when practising *Kriyā*, it was not his intention for the student to continue in this way indefinitely. In *Kriyā* meditation, the superior way to breathe is with the mouth closed and the tongue in the *kecharī mudrā* position. Most persons will not achieve the complete *kecharī mudrā*, but it is still beneficial to roll the tongue back, and keep the tip of the tongue touching the roof of the mouth at the point close to the uvula. This has a subtle and magnetic effect of drawing the energy towards the eyebrow centre (*kūtastha*).

1. Sit in a comfortable meditative posture, relax your body and close your eyes. Direct your inner gaze to the midpoint between the eyebrows.
2. With your mouth closed, roll your tongue back, so that part of the lower surface of the tongue and its tip touches the upper palate of your mouth. Without straining, draw the tip of your tongue as far back as possible, and press it upward against the back part of your mouth close to the uvula.

Retain this position while practising *ujjayi prāṇāyāma*. Practise for as long as comfortable, then relax your tongue.

> 'The positive and negative energies in the tongue and nasal passages, when joined together, create a cycle of energy in the head, which instead of allowing the energy to flow outward to the body, generates a magnetic field that draws energy from the body and from the base of the spine to the brain.'
>
> *Swāmi Kriyananda (a direct disciple of Paramhansa Yogananda)*

KECHARĪ MUDRĀ: THE FULL PRACTICE

This is the complicated practice that involves the artificial elongation of the tongue.

The tongue goes behind the uvula of the soft palate, and is inserted up into the nasal cavity. The tip of the tongue presses upward and forward, stimulating certain nerves in that area. Breathing is performed through the nose, because the mouth is blocked by the tongue.

The tongue in this position actually creates a short-circuit of energy in the medulla oblongata (base of brain in brain stem) and directs it to the eyebrow centre (*ājñā chakra*). Normally, the energy enters through the medulla oblongata, then comes down and goes out through the body.

This helps to awaken the *kuṇḍalinī* and higher states of consciousness. It purifies the body, subdues the senses and brings calmness to the mind.

7.6.8 *NABHO MUDRĀ*

> 'The yogi who knows *mahā mudrā*, *nabho mudrā*, *uddīyāna bandha*, *jalandhāra bandha*, and *mūlabandha* attains liberation.'
>
> *Goraksha Paddhati 1:57*

Another *mudrā* that is similar to *kecharī mudrā,* in which the tongue is turned upward, is the advanced practice called *nabho mudrā*. The Sanskrit word *nabh* means 'sky' or 'space'. It refers to the space in the region of the brain known as 'the sky of the head'.

The difference between *kecharī mudrā* and *nabho mudrā* is that *nabho mudrā* includes the very advanced practice of *kevala kumbhaka* (continuous retention or suspension of the breath, that occurs automatically), whereas *kecharī mudrā* does not.

The advanced yogi who practises *nabho mudrā* is able to maintain concentration (*dhāraṇā*) on the elements (*mahābhūtas*): ether, air, fire, water and earth. When the yogi achieves success in *nabho mudrā* all the seeds of past *karmas* (actions) are burnt.

7.6.9 *AUM JAPA* IN THE *CHAKRAS*

Your aim in practising *Aum japa* in the *chakras* is to interiorise your concentration and intuitively or mentally touch (by mentally chanting *Aum*) the centre of each *chakra* and perceive its subtle rays. For beginners, it is suggested that you chant *Aum* aloud (in this technique pronounce *Aum* as 'ong', as in 'song'). Then chant it silently when you are able to concentrate and locate the *chakras*.

BEGIN WITH A PRAYER

> Heavenly Father, transfer my consciousness from the physical body to the astral spine and from it through the seven chakras to Cosmic Consciousness, where Thy glory and Light reign in the fullness of Thy manifestation; where the Life Force reigns in all Thy power. Aum, Peace, Amen.

Aum japa can be practised before *Kriyā prāṇāyāma* to stimulate or activate the *chakras*. Practise with deep concentration, intuitively feeling the inner energy of each *chakra* as you briefly pause to mentally chant *Aum* at each one.

PREPARATORY PRACTICE

Before you begin *Aum japa* in the *chakras*, it is helpful to practise a few rounds of *nāḍī shodhana prāṇāyāma* (alternate nostril breathing) to purify and balance the subtle astral channels. This practice will help you to become aware of the subtle currents flowing up and down your spine, and it will also calm your mind, in preparation for both *Aum japa* and *Kriyā prāṇāyāma*. Practise three to 12 rounds.

AUM JAPA PRACTICE

Sit comfortably and deeply relax in a meditative posture with the head, neck and spine aligned. Close your eyes, and bring your awareness to your breath, as you breathe in feel the spaciousness expanding in the spine. Sense the presence of a subtle channel of energy in your spine. Change the centre of your consciousness from the body and senses to the spine… Feel the subtle astral spine by slightly and gently swaying the upper body from left to right… Then, feel your consciousness with the breath move slowly up and down the spine several times, from the *mūladhāra chakra* at the base of the spine to the midpoint between the eyebrows at the Spiritual Eye… Your attention should be internalised on the *chakras* and the breath… Now exhale and take your awareness to the root of the spine in *mūladhāra chakra*, and mentally chant *Aum* (pronounced *Oṁ*) there.

Now as you inhale, moving your breath and awareness up through your spine, mentally chant *Aum* in each *chakra – mūladhāra, svādhiṣṭhāna, maṇipūra, anāhata, viśuddha*. Pause, and hold your breath as you mentally chant *Aum* at the sixth *chakra*: *ājñā* (first at the medulla oblongata, then at the midpoint between the eyebrows, then again at the medulla).

Reverse the process, with the exhalation, descend through the spinal passage and *chakras* mentally chanting *Aum* at each *chakra*, returning back down to *mūladhāra*. As you do so, try to perceive the subtle radiation of each *chakra*.

Practise six to 12 rounds or continue the practice until you feel that your consciousness is transferred from the body into the astral spine.

Then meditate in the stillness, feeling your consciousness expanding into the Infinite. Feel the *Aum* vibration expanding up to the crown *chakra* (*sahasrāra*) into silence, stillness and spaciousness.

7.6.10 *KRIYĀ PRĀṆĀYĀMA*

> 'In the same way that a human draws water through a stem of a lotus, the yogi established in Yoga draws the air (up through the inner spine: *suṣumnā*).
>
> Making the sound like that of *ardhamātrā* through the stem of a lotus, the breath is to be sucked up through the inner canal (inner spine: *suṣumnā*) and merged at the midpoint between the two eyebrows.'
>
> *Dhyānabindhūpaniṣad 38–39*

The Primordial Vibratory Sound *Aum* is composed of four sounds: *a*, *u*, *m* and *ardhamātrā*. The sound vibration *ardhamātrā* cannot be pronounced properly; however, it can be compared with the lengthening sibilant sound of a breath practice such as *ujjayi prāṇāyāma*, in which the breath is drawn slowly, constricting the breath passage in the throat.

Prāṇa is not breath in its gross form. *Prāṇa* is the omnipresent vital force or life energy that has a subtle form, that is the link between the gross and the subtle world. The body, mind and *prāṇa* are internally linked and related – they affect each other. It is the movement of *prāṇa* that energises and activates the mind, body and senses. So to control your mind you need to control or regulate your breath, through *prāṇāyāma*. When the breath is still, the mind also becomes still. The mind is like a candle flame, and *prāṇa* is like the wind. When the wind blows, the candle flame restlessly flickers; similarly, the movement of *prāṇa* makes the mind restless.

If your mind is continually restless, scattered and dispersed, then nothing within yourself is seen, or realised. But if your mind becomes quiet, still, and unified in its subtle state, then you will begin to discover your own spiritual essence – the Self.

For *Kriyā* meditation, calming the mind is of primary importance, because the mind is the internal mechanism behind the movement of the breath. This is why the *Hong Sau* technique is practised first before the *Kriyā* breath meditation, to concentrate the mind and bring it to a state of inner calmness. Then when the mind is steadied, the *prāṇa* settles down of its own accord. If the mind is unsteady, disturbed, and upset by emotions and desires, then it is very difficult to practise meditation. The senses first have to be restrained through *pratyāhāra* (withdrawal of the senses from their respective objects) and *prāṇāyāma* (regulation of the vital energy through the breath). When breathing is regulated, the *prāṇa* is also regulated, which gives support to concentration. Then the breath, through deep concentration, becomes extended and subtle. The calm mind can then become one-pointed in its concentration on the Infinite.

The senses are the instruments by which the *prāṇa* operates, which is a means of satisfaction for the mind. The mind acts as the dynamo which generates the energy passing through the *prāṇa,* which moves through the pathways of the senses towards particular objects of sense.

> '*Kriyā*, controlling the mind directly through the life force, is the easiest, most effective, and most scientific avenue of approach to the Infinite.'
>
> *Yogananda 1946, p.236*

Kriyā prāṇāyāma (also known as *Kriyā* Breath, First *Kriyā*, *Kriyā* Proper, Spinal Breathing, *suṣumnā* breathing), the most superior of all *prāṇāyāmas*, is the most important technique of *Kriyā Yoga,* acting on the life energy (*prāṇa*) in the body, the breath, and *prāṇa* mastery. In *Kriyā Yoga prāṇāyāma*, the concentration is focused directly on the *suṣumnā* (central channel) in the subtle or inner astral spine, rather than the *iḍā* and *piṅgala*, the subtle lunar and solar *prāṇic* channels. When these two channels, *iḍā* and *piṅgala*, are balanced, the breathing becomes long and deep in *suṣumnā*, the subtle spine.

If the *prāṇic* life force flows uninterrupted continuously through the *suṣumnā*, then the path to spiritual progress opens up. In the *Kriyā* breath, the mind's attention is withdrawn from the sense-objects and focused with attentive awareness at the midpoint between the two eyebrows. Simultaneously, the concentration is on the breath within the spine. The breath ascends and descends in the deep inner spine or astral spine (the pathway to Supreme Consciousness) from the *mūladhāra chakra* at the base of the spine to the Spiritual Eye located between the eyebrows, directly opposite the *ājñā chakra*. The controlled breath is subtle, smooth and long. It is extended in both the inhalation and the exhalation as it moves slowly up and down the spine through the *chakras*, with a very short breath retention at the end of the inhalation, held at the Spiritual Eye or *ājñā chakra*. This rotation of the *Kriyā* breath up and down the spine magnetises it with *prāṇic* energy, and redirects the *saṁskāras* (latent seed-impressions of past actions) towards the brain to be burnt at the Spiritual Eye. The inner heat (*tapas*) created by *Kriyā prāṇāyāma* burns and purifies all impurities of the body and mind.

The *prāṇa* then withdraws from the spine and merges at the Spiritual Eye of divine perception (*ājñā chakra*), bringing a deep inner calmness and tranquillity.

In the very advanced state of breath mastery in *Kriyā prāṇāyāma* there is an automatic suspension of the movements of the inhalation and exhalation. With the breath suspended, the mind is also suspended in deep tranquillity. In *Kriyā Yoga* this is the state known as *kevala kumbhaka*. This 'breathless and thoughtless state' is described in the *Bhāgavad Gītā*:

'One practice of Yoga offers the upward force of breath (*prāṇa*) into the downward force of breath (*apāṇa*), and the *apāṇa* into the *prāṇa*, thereby, through *prāṇāyāma*, rendering the breath unnecessary.'

Bhāgavad Gītā 4.29

The regular practice of *Kriyā Yoga prāṇāyāma* (First *Kriyā* in the tradition of Paramhansa Yogananda) with devotion – offering the breath and energy upward in the *suṣumnā* to the higher centres in the brain – brings subtlety to the *Kriyā* breath, that is further increased by the deepening of concentration. As the mind becomes more perfectly stilled, the breath calms even further, moving into the spontaneous 'breathless' meditative state, in which the breath goes into temporary suspension. The *vṛttis* of the mind and life airs (*prāṇa-vayus*) in the body become perfectly tranquil.

MENTAL *PRĀṆĀYĀMA*

Although this technique is similar to *Aum japa* in the *chakras*, it is not the same. The subtle difference between these two techniques is that in *Aum japa* the *chakras* are stimulated during a short pause by the *Aum mantra*, whereas in mental *prāṇāyāma* the *chakras* are not stimulated by *Aum*, and the pauses at the *chakras* are much longer to allow for one's awareness to perceive their inner sounds and inner light. For best results practise mental *prāṇāyāma* after doing *Kriyā prāṇāyāma*.

Mental prāṇāyāma practice

After your *Kriyā prāṇāyāma* (First *Kriyā*) practice, continue to sit comfortably and deeply relax in a meditative posture with the head, neck and spine aligned. Close your eyes, and bring your awareness to your breath, as you breathe in feel the spaciousness expanding in the spine. Sense the presence of a subtle channel of energy in your spine. Change the centre of your consciousness from the body and senses to the spine… Feel the subtle astral spine by slightly and gently swaying the upper body from left to right… Then, feel your consciousness with the breath move slowly up and down the spine several times, from the *mūladhāra chakra* at the base of the spine to the midpoint between the eyebrows at the Spiritual Eye… Your attention should be internalised on the *chakras* and the breath… Now exhale and take your awareness to the root of the spine in *mūladhāra*.

Breathing normally, with your attention and awareness in *mūladhāra chakra*, pause for ten to 20 seconds. Be aware of the sensation you feel there and the perception of the subtle radiation of this *chakra*. Then, move your awareness up to *svādhiṣṭhāna*, the second *chakra*, and again pause at this *chakra* and become aware of the subtle perceptions you experience there. Continue in this way as you gradually ascend through the other *chakras*: *maṇipūra*, *anāhata*, *viśuddha*, *ājñā* – pause first at the medulla oblongata (located in the brain stem at the rear of the brain), then pause at the midpoint between the eyebrows, then return to the medulla to begin the descent. As you descend your spine, maintain your awareness in each of the *chakras*, pausing in each one – *viśuddha*, *anāhata*, *maṇipūra*, *svādhiṣṭhāna*, and finally to *mūladhāra chakra* at the base of the spine.

Practise rotating your awareness up and down the *chakras* for as long as it is comfortable for you, or until your consciousness rests in calm tranquility.

KRIYĀ: THE SUPREME *PRĀṆĀYĀMA*

> '*Kriyā Yoga*, the scientific technique of God-realisation will ultimately spread in all lands, and aid in harmonising the nations through man's personal, transcendental perception of the Infinite Father.'
>
> *Mahavatar Babaji, in Yogananda 1946, p.337*

The *Kriyā Yoga prāṇāyāma* is superior to the *prāṇāyāma* practised by *Haṭha* yogis because it does not require the discomfort of mechanically holding the breath for a long duration. The suspension of the breath in the *Kriyā* breath of *Rāja Yoga* (the supreme path of meditation) occurs naturally as a result of being absorbed in the Infinite. The more the *Kriyā* meditator's mind is focused on the Infinite Consciousness or Supreme Self, the more calm and still it becomes. When there is suspension of the breath with the mind completely absorbed in the Divine or Infinite, the mind and body are transcended. Patañjali in his *Yoga Sūtras* (2:51), refers to this as the fourth (*chaturthaḥ*) *prāṇāyāma*: 'The fourth *prāṇāyāma* transcends the external and the internal.' This is when the breath naturally and automatically stops by itself. Both the internal and the external operations of the respiration are suspended when the breath becomes subtle. The external operation of the breath (*bāhya vṛtti*) refers to the natural extension of the breath after a complete exhalation. The internal operation of the breath (*antar vṛtti*) is when the breath is inhaled completely and then there is a natural suspension of the breath. When the breath can be naturally and effortlessly suspended for long periods of time it becomes very supportive for deep meditation (*dhyāna*) and *samādhi*.

The benefits of the Kriyā breath

> '*Kriyā Yoga* is a simple, psychological method by which the human blood is decarbonised and recharged with oxygen. The atoms of this extra oxygen are transmuted into life current to rejuvenate the brain and spinal centres.'
>
> *Yogananda 1946, p.231*

The average person breathes 15 to 18 breaths per minute, but one who practises *Kriyā prāṇāyāma*, which is long, smooth and deep, breathes only 3 breaths per minute. It does not take long to work out the arithmetic – a *Kriyā* meditator practising one hour of continuous *Kriyā* breathing (60 min x 3 *Kriyā* breaths) uses 180 breaths, whereas the average person breathing (60 min x 15 normal breaths) uses 900 breaths! Therefore, the *Kriyā* meditator is saving 720 breaths.

In ancient times when yogis in India lived a renunciant life in the forest, they made detailed observations of the animals living there – their lifespan, the way they moved, and their breathing. They discovered that the lifespan of every living creature is determined according to their respiration. It was found that elephants, tortoises and snakes have a slow rate of breathing, giving them a long lifespan. For example, the giant tortoise native to the Galapagos islands breathes four times per minute and can live up to 200 years. Whales breathe 6 times per minute and the oldest known whale – an Arctic Bowhead Whale – was at least 211 years old. A snake breathes seven to eight times per minute and can live to 150 years. In comparison, dogs, rabbits and birds, which have a faster breathing rate, are considerably short-lived. A dog, for example, breathes 28 to 30 times per minute and only has an average lifespan of ten to 20 years, although in some cases dogs of a certain breed have lived to 29 years. Cats can live from 12 to 18 years old, and the average lifespan of a horse is 25 to 30 years.

With this awareness and observation the yogis came to the conclusion that those who breathe shallow and quick have a shorter lifespan than those who breathe long and deep. They realised that the human being normally breathes 15 to 18 times per minute (21,600 breaths in 24 hours), and that by slowing down the respiration one could not only increase health and longevity, but also a yogi could gain greater control over his own mind and *prāṇic* energy. By taking long, deep breaths as in the practice of *Kriyā prāṇāyāma* the alveolar air in the cardiovascular system becomes more oxygenated. The reduction in carbon dioxide in turn affects oxygen and carbon dioxide concentration in the blood leaving the pulmonary capillaries. The removal of carbon dioxide and more oxygenated blood makes the body fluids alkaline, around the level of pH of 7.2.

One thousand Kriyās

> 'Meditate unceasingly, that you may quickly behold yourself as the Infinite Essence, free from every form of misery. Cease being a prisoner of the body; using the secret key of *Kriyā*, learn to escape into Spirit.'
>
> *Lahiri Mahasaya, in Yogananda 1946, p.315*

In reference to *Kriyā prāṇāyāma*, Paramhansa Yogananda states in his *Autobiography of a Yogi*:

> 'One thousand *Kriyā* practised in eight hours gives the yogi in one day, the equivalent of one thousand years of natural evolution: 365,000 years of evolution in one year. In three years, a *Kriyā* yogi can thus accomplish by intelligent self-effort the same result which nature brings to pass in a million years. The *Kriyā* short-cut, of course, can be taken only by deeply developed yogis. With the guidance of a guru, such yogis have carefully prepared their bodies and brains to receive the power created by intensive practice.
>
> The *Kriyā* beginner employs his yogic exercise only fourteen to twenty-eight times, twice daily. A number of yogis achieve emancipation in six or twelve or twenty-four or forty-eight years. A yogi who dies before achieving full realisation carries with him the good *karma* of his past *Kriyā* effort; in his new life he is harmoniously propelled towards his Infinite Goal.'
>
> *Yogananda 1946, p.234*

7.7

INITIATION INTO KRIYĀ

'Because so many people thirst after higher knowledge and only a few find entry into its realm, to be initiated is surely obvious evidence of God's redemptive grace.'

Roy Eugene Davis (a direct disciple of Paramhansa Yogananda)

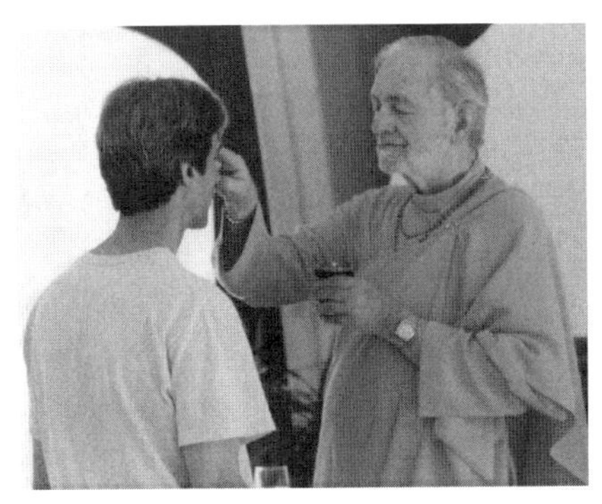

Stephen Sturgess receiving blessings from Swāmi Kriyananda

The original method of *Kriyā* was given by Sri Yogiraj Shyama Charan Lahiri Mahasaya (1828–1895), the disciple to whom Babaji revealed the almost lost science of *Kriyā Yoga*. But the *Kriyā* techniques have been altered and adapted to some extent by both Swāmi Sri Yukteswar (a direct disciple of Lahiri Mahasaya) and Paramhansa Yogananda (a direct disciple of Swāmi Sri Yukteswar). So these three main branches of *Kriyā Yoga* will be found to have some differences in the way the *Kriyā* techniques have been taught.

This can be confusing for those spiritual seekers who are new to the path, especially if they start mixing techniques from the different ways they are taught by Lahiri Mahasaya, Sri Yukteswar and Yogananda. Think of it like a family tree: each of these three great *Kriyā* Masters had direct disciples, who then passed the *Kriyā Yoga* teachings down to further disciples. The teachings are not necessarily diluted but each guru naturally had their own illumined insights, and divine creative inspirations and innovations, and so made additions, modifications, alterations and variations.

For instance, Paramhansa Yogananda has added the Energisation Exercises to his *Kriyā Yoga* techniques, an innovation of his own making, not taught by Babaji, Lahiri Mahasaya or Sri Yukteswar. He is certainly welcomed for these exercises as they give a whole new way of understanding energy and how to experience and direct that energy in one's own body for meditation and healing.

> 'A significant feature of Lahiri Mahasaya's life was his gift of *Kriyā* initiation to those of every faith. Not Hindus only, but Moslems and Christians were among his foremost disciples. Monists and dualists, those of all faiths or of no established faith, were impartially received and instructed by the universal guru.'
>
> *Yogananda 1946, p.314*

Lahiri Mahasaya at times would modify his *Kriyā* techniques to suit the personal needs of each one of his disciples. Sri Yukteswar also made slight modifications and variations to *Kriyā Yoga* techniques. This is perfectly natural if the modification, variation or addition facilitates progress towards the ultimate spiritual goal, especially so if it is coming from a spiritual master such as these great *Kriyā* Masters.

These kinds of changes are natural. There would be stagnation and crystallisation of our thinking if there was no change in some way. We have progressed from the industrial age of the nineteenth century, and are now in a technological age (ascending *Dwapara Yuga*) that is far more advanced. Medicine, science, technology and communication have progressed in tremendous leaps. Ideas are communicated and expressed in new and innovative ways, and information is now shared world-wide as it has never been before.

Teaching methods, including the teachings of *Kriyā Yoga*, have been improved in the way they are communicated to us, and they can be more refined and perfected without diluting the original message they were intended to impart. The problems of dilution only arise when the *Kriyā* techniques are modified to such an extent that they become unrecognisable from the original, and so they no longer have the power to spiritually transform an individual.

It can be confusing and overwhelming if you start curiously trying to follow two or three different gurus and ways of practising *Kriyā* techniques at the same time, because there are many techniques, and finding the many hours you would need to practise them all would not be possible for the majority of persons. It would be like digging many shallow holes trying to find water, rather than digging one deep well.

It is suggested that once you have found your genuine *Kriyā Yoga* guru and his particular way of teaching the *Kriyā* methods and techniques, then follow your heart, allow your soul-intuition and inner wisdom to guide you. Do not just passively accept blindly, but sincerely question, to know and to understand the teaching and techniques you are following. If you are sincere and discriminate wisely you will be guided to Truth. Once you have found your true guru and spiritual path, be loyal to them. Stay with it and persevere until you succeed. You will not be successful if you keep chopping and changing spiritual path, guru and *Kriyā* techniques.

WHO IS QUALIFIED TO INITIATE OTHERS INTO *KRIYĀ*?

To be a *Kriyā* disciple is to have three main qualities:

1. **Loyalty.** Yogananda said that loyalty is the first law of God: loyalty and dedication to your spiritual path, guru and God.
2. **Attunement.** Inner attunement to the guru's consciousness and teaching.

3. **Commitment.** Commitment to the *Kriyā* practices, steadfast in daily meditation and in becoming a channel of service to others

A disciple becomes a qualified representative to initiate others as a result of inner realisation. The disciple has to be a *Kriyāvan* (one who has been initiated by his or her authentic guru or guru's authorised representative into the *Kriyā Yoga* tradition), and be experienced in practising the teachings and techniques of *Kriyā Yoga*. Such a disciple will also be steadfast in Self-realisation, spiritually aware, sincere, honest, showing loyalty and respect towards the guru and his teachings, and with right attitude and willingness following the *yamas* and *niyamas*. The disciple will also be steadfast in practising *Kriyā Yoga* with attention and devotion, regularly meditating every day. Without these qualifications the spiritual vibrations and forces and flow of grace through the line of *Kriyā* gurus cannot be effectively transmitted.

The guru will acknowledge the disciple's qualifications, and if the necessary requirements are fulfilled the guru will give permission to that disciple to initiate others.

One who has departed from the guru line because of inability to adhere to the *Kriyā* teaching tradition cannot successfully transmit the teaching. If you are invited to be initiated by a person who does not honour the *Kriyā* guru line, or who is being promoted as a special teacher without legitimacy, avoid that relationship. You will only waste your time and the results will be unsatisfactory. No one should follow blindly. Trust your direct soul intuitive higher experience, and discriminate wisely in making your decisions and choices in spiritual matters, whether it is with an individual or an organisation.

WHO CAN SERVE YOGANANDA AND HIS TEACHINGS?

My spiritual teacher, Swāmi Kriyananda, who first gave me discipleship and initiated me into *Kriyā* in 1983, and gave me the approval to serve Yogananda by guiding others in *Kriyā Yoga*, made some very interesting points about *Kriyā* disciples serving and continuing Paramhansa Yogananda's work of disseminating *Kriyā Yoga*.

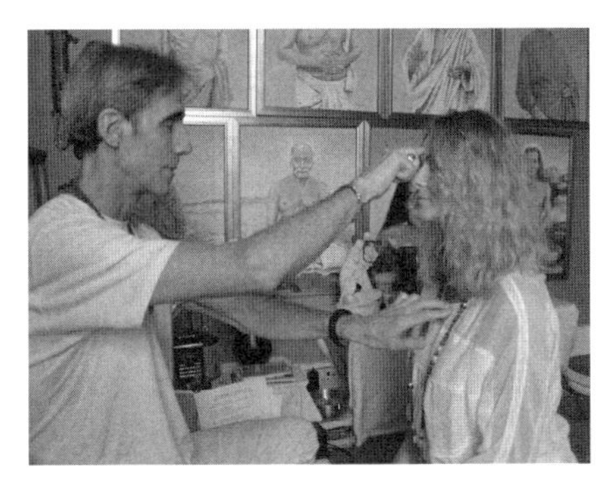

STEPHEN STURGESS GIVING A *KRIYĀ* BLESSING DURING *KRIYĀ* INITIATION

'Give *Kriyā* freely to all who humbly ask for help.'

Mahavatar Babaji, in Yogananda 1946, p.307

Yogananda had stated that he was the last in the line of his *Kriyā* gurus, but Kriyananda said that if Yogananda was the last one who could guide or inspire anyone spiritually, it would mean that no one on this path could or should ever take special pains to offer spiritual help to others, and that such a prohibition would raise doubts as to the very authenticity of these teachings. Kriyananda explained that Yogananda's statement that he was 'the last of our line of gurus' meant in a more personal sense that he would continue to work through all those who dedicate themselves to deepening their attunement with him. Kriyananda said that teachers in Yogananda's work who sincerely try to develop spiritually, whether or not they have achieved Self-realisation, *can* be channels for our line of Masters.

Kriyananda went on further to say that the requirement is that the disciples follow Yogananda and his teachings humbly and sincerely, giving service to others, and remaining attuned to him. Yogananda can and does work through his loyal disciples – those who have received the 'touch' from some other true disciple, and who deeply accept Yogananda in their hearts as their guru. Anyone who, now and in the future, teaches in Yogananda's name will certainly be helped and guided in his or her sincere, humble and loving efforts to be of service to others.

LAHIRI MAHASAYA'S *KRIYĀ* INITIATION

When a student was initiated into the First *Kriyā*, Lahiri Mahasaya gave five techniques to practise in order to bring under control the five main vital airs (*vayus*) in the body – *prāṇa*, *apāṇa*, *samāna*, *vyāna* and *udāṇa*. This was important because when these five airs had been steadied, all other minor airs in the body were effortlessly controlled.

The five main *Kriyā* practices that Lahiri Mahasaya gave were:

1. *Tālavya* (*Talabya*) with *kecharī mudrā*
2. *Kriyā prāṇāyāma* (controls *prāṇa* and *apāṇa*)
3. *Nabhi* (*Navi*) *Kriyā* (controls the *samāna vayu*)
4. *Yoni mudrā* (for experiencing the inner Light)
5. *Māha mudrā* (controls *Vyāna* and *Udāṇa vayus*).

The *Kriyā prāṇāyāma* (First *Kriyā*) technique is traditionally given to the disciple on *Kriyā* initiation. Practising the technique alone will not have any spiritual benefit without the personal guidance of an experienced *Kriyā* teacher or guru and the spiritual vibration and transmission of the guru's blessings. So it is advised that you find an experienced *Kriyā* teacher or guru to impart the teaching to you.

This is the way I was first initiated into *Kriyā Yoga* by Swāmi Kriyananda, in London, 1983. There was just a small group of us, and *swāmiji* held this initiation informally in my house.

Swāmi Kriyananda never charged any money for teaching us *Kriyā Yoga,* nor for giving *Kriyā* Initiation. He was not interested in material gain for himself, but was dedicated in joyfully serving and blessing others by sharing with them the *Kriyā Yoga* teachings of Paramhansa Yogananda.

I was blessed with *swāmiji*'s presence twice more over the years, when he came to give *Kriyā* initiations at my house. I remember him sitting in the full lotus pose (*pādmāsana*) in my meditation room, playing the harmonium and singing with joy Yogananda's beautiful devotional chant, 'Door of My Heart', and then guiding us into a deep meditation. *Swāmiji* was in his sixties during that time. He was healthy, energetic and enthusiastic, and had tremendous inspiration to give us. Unfortunately, his physical health deteriorated in his later years, but his mind was alert, and he still had that tremendous inspiration and warmth of heart that he gave freely to all those who came in contact with him.

It should be clearly understood that to take up the study and practice of *Kriyā Yoga* is to make a genuine and sincere commitment and spiritual effort towards Self- and God-realisation. It is not for the undisciplined casual seeker who like a butterfly flits from one flower to another, nor for those who are superficially interested, constantly restless, and lack definite purpose. For success and spiritual awakening in *Kriyā Yoga* one needs to be disciplined with unswerving purpose and unfailing effort, to have an inner, intuitive attunement with the consciousness of the guru. The divine qualities of sincerity, loyalty, love, devotion, dedication and service to others need to be cultivated.

> 'Truth is for earnest seekers, not for those of idle curiosity.'
>
> *Lahiri Mahasaya, in Yogananda 1946, p.308*

One must practise meditation regularly every day. Once you have decided to take up *Kriyā Yoga*, knowing and understanding intuitively in your heart and soul that this is your spiritual path to follow, then resolve to follow it with all your mind, heart and soul and, to be successful in your spiritual aim, make everything serve that purpose.

> 'I am ever with those who practise Kriyā. I will guide you to the Cosmic Home through your everyday perceptions.'
>
> *Lahiri Mahasaya, in Yogananda 1946, p.317*

> 'To those who think me near I will be near.'
>
> *Paramhansa Yogananda*

For *Kriyā* to be completely effective, and successful, it needs to be received with the spiritual vibrations and blessings of the original *Kriyā Yoga* Masters – Mahavatar Babaji, Lahiri Mahasaya, Swāmi Sri Yukteswar and Paramhansa Yogananda. The spiritual contact of these great *Kriyā Yoga* gurus can be transmitted to a new disciple through those who are sincere disciples themselves, who have made a lifetime commitment to the spiritual path of *Kriyā Yoga*, and who have been ordained as a *Kriyācarya* (*Kriyā* teacher and initiator).

After serving Yogananda through Kriyananda's Ananda organisation for 27 years, and being initiated into *Kriyā* also by Roy Eugene Davis (a direct disciple of Paramhansa Yogananda), I was ordained as a *Kriyā* minister by Roy Eugene Davis in 2011 to teach and initiate others into *Kriyā*.

As my First *Kriyā* teacher and initiator, Swāmi Kriyananda (a direct disciple of Yogananda) said, 'A magnet is created either by electrical realignment of the molecules, or by close proximity to another magnet. Attunement with a God-awakened guru influences the *saṁskāras* (comparable to the material molecules) to flow upward to the brain.'

'A worthy leader has the desire to serve and not to dominate.'

Swāmi Sri Yukteswar, in Yogananda 1946, p.126

For the teacher–student (guru–disciple) relationship to be worthy of the teacher's time and attention and of benefit to the student, one who wants personal spiritual instruction and guidance on the path of *Kriyā Yoga* should have the right attitude and following qualifications:

Sincerity.

Loyalty.

Commitment.

Respect for the *Kriyā Yoga* tradition, its line of gurus, and the teacher.

Willingness to learn and to practise what is learned.

A holistic, balanced, positive and constructive lifestyle that supports your physical, mental and spiritual wellbeing.

'The guru–discipleship relationship is destined. A seeker of Truth is led to the contact which is most suitable for the unfoldment of his or her highest good. In this matter, Higher Intelligence does not make a mistake. Once the relationship is established, it remains until the disciple awakens completely in God, whether in a few years or a few incarnations.'

Roy Eugene Davis

At this moment in time there are very few direct disciples of Paramhansa Yogananda still living, and those few who are still with us are in their eighties. But the transmission of *Kriyā Yoga* has to continue. The direct disciples of Yogananda, like my teachers Swāmi Kriyananda and Roy Eugene Davis, have initiated their own direct disciples, like myself, who in turn can initiate others. Such *Kriyācaryas* or *Kriyā* teachers serve as representatives of the *Kriyā* tradition. They are not impelled by self-centred compulsions to be of service, and they are not interested in personal fame or material gain.

NO FEE FOR *KRIYĀ* INITIATION

'A true spiritual teacher must never charge money for giving spiritual instruction. Hindu, Buddhist and Jain traditions strongly forbid it. But the teacher may accept gifts given by students out of gratitude.'

Bhaskarananda 2002, p.16

It has been the *Kriyā* tradition to not charge money for teaching and initiating *Kriyā*. It was never intended to be made into a profitable business. Some persons claiming to be authoritative *Kriyā* gurus are trying to get as many people as they can for a one-day or weekend session to give a *Kriyā* initiation – people who perhaps have never even meditated or practised Yoga before. The so-called guru charges each of them £100 or more, and if he has even 50 people he can make a nice profit of £5000. Obviously, their interest lies in making money and probably egotistic fame, too, not sincerely serving others in God. If such a person's consciousness is thinking about money and business all the time how can it be focused on spiritual consciousness, or how can it be aware of the Presence of God?

Beware of non-genuine, self-appointed gurus of today, who bestow the title of *Paramhansa* on themselves and profess that in a dream Babaji gave them the title, and that they were authorised by Babaji to initiate others into *Kriyā*, especially if they try to coax or coerce money from you for it.

Roy Eugene Davis told us that in the early 1950s, at the Self-Realization Fellowship headquarters in Los Angeles, California, he was with some brother disciples gathered near Paramhansa Yogananda's car, who was preparing to be driven to an appointment somewhere. As Yogananda settled in the back seat of the car, he left the door open and talked with his disciples for a few minutes. During that conversation he said, 'After I am gone, several people in India will claim to be our Babaji and some mediums in America will say that I talk through them. Don't believe such stories. They will not be true!'

And starting in 1970, a young Indian man in the Hariakhan region in Northern India was falsely promoted by his followers as the Babaji in the *Kriyā* lineage of Lahiri Mahasaya. Several Europeans and Americans who had visited his ashram told Roy Eugene Davis that, when they were there, use of marijuana and other mind-altering substances was permitted. After some illnesses, he died in 1984.

Both Lahiri Mahasaya and Swāmi Sri Yukteswar told disciples not to seek Babaji in the Himalayas; that it would be more beneficial for them to attend to their secular duties and improve their spiritual practices.

> '*Kriyā Yoga* teachers do not attempt to convert or persuade, nor do they accept money for personal spiritual instruction or initiation. Donations for charitable purposes may be accepted.'
>
> *Roy Eugene Davis*

Lahiri Mahasaya, the great *Kriyā* yogi, whom Mahavatar Babaji first imparted these teachings to, did not initiate anyone on a casual basis. He only initiated one, two or three persons at a time. He never built an organisation around himself, and advised against the establishment of institutions in the name of *Kriyā Yoga*. Although it is said that he charged a set fee of five rupees to each person he initiated into *Kriyā Yoga*, he did not keep the money for himself but gave it to his own guru, Mahavatar Babaji, who used it to feed the poor and provide other charitable services for village people in the foothills of the Himalayas. Babaji did not come himself to collect it, instead he sent a devotee to collect it. The fee of five rupees for the *Kriyā* initiation was more a symbol representing a disciple's inner spiritual yearning and commitment to a new beginning on the spiritual path of *Kriyā Yoga*. It is understood that a monetary offering at the time of initiation is not payment for services rendered, for the *Kriyā* teachings are freely given. It should be understood that resources, including money, are not to become objects to which we become attached, but are to be used for constructive purposes.

Lahiri Mahasaya was a householder yogi, with a family to support, but he had sufficient income to keep both himself and his family.

> 'Never did I hear him (Swāmi Sri Yukteswar) ask or even hint for money for any purpose. His hermitage training was given free to all disciples.'
>
> *Yogananda 1946, p.133*

Swāmi Sri Yukteswar, Paramhansa Yogananda's guru, did not charge a fee for teaching *Kriyā Yoga* or giving *Kriyā* initiation.

Roy Eugene Davis told me that when he was living with Yogananda at the Self-Realization Fellowship (SRF) in the early 1950s and was present at *Kriyā* initiations, he did not see money being donated. The disciples just offered a fruit and a flower and Yogananda put a few rose petals in their hands to take with them.

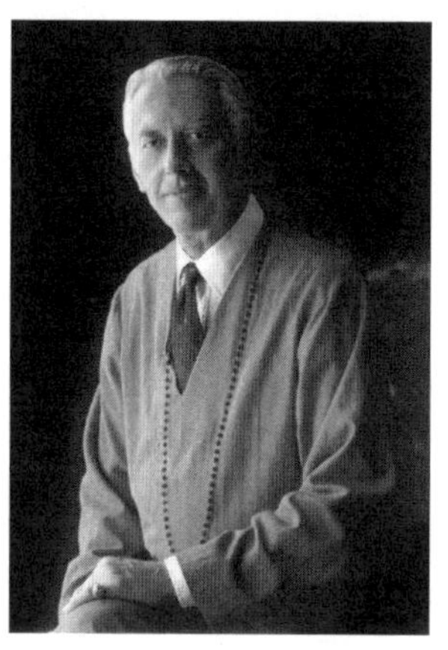

Roy Eugene Davis

When I was initiated by direct disciples of Paramhansa Yogananda into *Kriyā* by Swāmi Kriyananda, Roy Eugene Davis and monks of the Self-Realization Fellowship, none of them charged money for *Kriyā* initiation. There was only the offering of a flower, a fruit, and a spiritual offering of a small donation in an envelope. Swāmi Kriyananda came to my house in London a few times in the 1980s and 1990s and taught my meditation group the *Kriyā* techniques and gave *Kriyā* initiation completely free of charge. Roy Eugene Davis was also very generous, coming to London a few times to teach *Kriyā Yoga* and gave *Kriyā* initiations free of charge. His generosity went further by giving everybody free copies of his books.

7.8

WHY THE SECRECY IN KRIYĀ?

'Let the fragrance of the *Kriyā* flower be wafted naturally, without any display; its seeds will take root in the soil of spiritually fertile hearts.'

Lahiri Mahasaya, in Yogananda 1946

For many years *Kriyā* had been cloaked in a veil of secrecy and mystery and was not available as easily as it is today. But now we are in a completely new and revolutionary age (ascending *Dwapara Yuga*) in which the development of science, medicine and new technologies have rapidly advanced. Information on every conceivable subject is now easily and quickly obtainable. More and more hidden secrets and mysteries from the past are being revealed and explained as never before. With the internet widely disseminating every possible kind of knowledge and information one can think of, it is not surprising that it is no longer possible to keep secret information hidden.

The more that teachings and techniques are kept secret, the more people seeking those truths become curious and inquisitive to know them. Whether out of curiosity, frustration, or the zeal to want to know the Truth, they eventually find ways to reveal them.

The turning point was in 2013 when two complete books on the details of the *Kriyā* techniques were published, one by the author J.C. Stevens, who has written in detail the complete *Kriyā* techniques as taught by Lahiri Mahasaya, in his book *Kriyā Secrets Revealed*; and the other authored by Swāmi Nityananda Giri, who has given in detail the *Kriyā* techniques as taught by Swāmi Sri Yukteswar in his book *Kriyā Yoga: The Science of Life-force*. Both authors are practising *Kriyā* yogis. Even before they had published their books a vast amount of material on *Kriyā* had been put up on websites by many different people who wanted to share the knowledge and secrets of *Kriyā*. Now there are many of the original writings of the *Kriyā* Masters available that have been translated into English through the Yoga Niketan, thanks to Sri Sailendra Bejoy Dasgupta (1910–1984), a direct disciple of Swāmi Sri Yukteswar Giri. Yoga Niketan was created in order to present, protect and preserve the *Kriyā* writings within Acharya Dasgupta's guru lineage.

If you want to take up the practice of *Kriyā Yoga* seriously, then I strongly advise you to learn it properly from an experienced *Kriyā Yoga* teacher, and remember that the real spiritual connection to *Kriyā*, the *Kriyā* Masters and God is through the spiritual vibration and blessings that one receives from the *Kriyā* initiation and not the technique alone. *Kriyā* has to be practised with a spirit of devotional self-offering, cooperation and loyalty to the guru, and with the awareness of God's presence. This is essential to progress spiritually. Practising *Kriyā* mechanically with the wrong attitudes is detrimental to spiritual progress.

In this book I have not given the *Kriyā* technique or the higher *Kriyās* (the more advanced techniques that need to be received from a *Kriyā* guru or an experienced *Kriyā* teacher who is practising them). In my guru's tradition the *Kriyā* technique is only learned when taking *Kriyā* initiation, when one becomes a *Kriyāvan* (male *Kriyā* yogi) or a *Kriyāvati* (female *Kriyā* yogini). Paramhansa Yogananda states in his *Autobiography of a Yogi*, in Chapter 26, 'The Science of *Kriyā Yoga*': 'Because of certain ancient yogic injunctions. I cannot give a full explanation of *Kriyā Yoga* in the pages of a book intended for the general public. The actual (*Kriyā*) technique must be learned from a *Kriyāvan* or *Kriyā* yogi; here a broad reference must suffice.'

A prerequisite to practising the higher *Kriyās* would be to have the physical ability to practise *kecharī mudrā* (see section 7.6.7). Lahiri Mahasaya called the second *Kriyā*, *Thokar Kriyā*; and the third *Kriyā*, *Omkar Kriyā*. The fourth *Kriyā* is difficult to perform unless the third has been mastered. Sri Sailendra Bejoy Dasgupta said that Swāmi Sri Yukteswar had given the fourth *Kriyā* to only one disciple, and that disciple had taught only one or two more.

No one person has exclusive ownership or possession of *Kriyā*, and no organisation can monopolise *Kriyā Yoga* as their own. To do so would be in opposition to Truth itself, for Truth is everyone's birthright. To hide and conceal the Truth from others (especially from sincere seekers), whether it takes the form of a spiritual teaching or a technique, is a contraction of energy. It goes against the true nature of the Self or Spirit, which is ever-expanding. Divine Spirit holds no secrets, it is transparent, allowing Light to pass through so that truth can be distinctly seen. There are no boundaries, it is omnipresent, it is freely available to all. All life is an expression of Divine Consciousness. Spiritual truths are to be freely shared, not secretly hidden away; nor used for gaining power or fame or controlling others, or sold for financial gain.

It is the ego that obscures Reality; Consciousness reveals it. Control is always the defensive position of the ego. Attachment is also involved – unwillingness to let go or to share with others. Attachment is also about need, and the fear of losing control. Attachment itself constrains and limits not only ourselves but others around us too. There is no freedom in attachment, whether that object of attachment is a technique, a perspective or a person.

> '"The *Kriyā Yoga* which I am giving to the world through you in this nineteenth century," Babaji told Lahiri Mahasaya, "is a revival of the same science which Krishna gave, millenniums ago, to Arjuna, and which was later known to Patañjali, and to Christ, St John, St Paul, and other disciples."'
>
> *Yogananda 1946, p.232*

From another perspective it can be said in regard to the *Kriyā* techniques that they have always been freely available to those who might look into the scriptures and the *Haṭha Yoga* and Tantric texts of India, that date back to antiquity. One has only to seek them out. These ancient texts were recorded long before Lahiri Mahasaya was given the *Kriyā* techniques by Mahavatar Babaji in the nineteenth century. For example, the *Haṭha Yoga Pradīpikā*, a treatise on the practices and techniques of *Haṭha Yoga* by the yogi Svatmarama, dates back to the fifteenth century. The several hundred works of the *Upaniṣads* that were transmitted by great sages at the end of the Vedic period include, in some of the later texts, practices of Yoga and Tantra. The great Adi Saṅkara (Shankaracharya) wrote commentaries on 11 of the principal *Upaniṣads* between the eighth and ninth centuries of the Common Era, and the *Bhāgavad Gītā* itself is a devotional *Upaniṣad*, which includes *Kriyā Yoga* teachings. So the question arises, if these scriptures do not hide the teachings and techniques then why should books written on *Kriyā Yoga* not also describe them?

Scriptures, texts and books are necessary to clarify teachings and for reference, and also so that the teachings and techniques are not modified or lost and are kept pure over the duration of time. In the 1970s, one well-respected and long established school of the ancient Tantric Yoga tradition, the Bihar School of Yoga in India, that was started by Swāmi Satyananda Saraswati (a direct disciple of Swāmi Sivananda Saraswati of Rishikesh), openly made available all of its Yoga and *Kriyā* techniques in a number of practice manuals for study and for reference. The Bihar School of Yoga has a world-wide and successful following of devotees practising Yoga and *Kriyā* techniques.

Of course, readers are always advised to learn not just from books, but from an expert, an experienced teacher or master of the subject. The subtle details cannot always be communicated through a book. And so with *Kriyā Yoga* it is always good to have both – personal instruction from a *Kriyā* teacher, and reference books or manuals on *Kriyā Yoga* including guidance on methods and techniques for reference and support. It should not be secret. Even scientists and physicists share their information on the internet now with those who are interested to know.

When I studied at university for my Bachelor of Arts in *Āyurveda* (*Āyurveda* is a sister science to Yoga, dating back 5000 years; it is the 'Science of Life', healing and health from India), all the knowledge was available in Āyurvedic text books and manuals on the subject – the knowledge was not secret or hidden. If I could not understand what I had read in the book I would ask my experienced tutors to explain and clarify a technique or the meaning. I could not learn through books alone.

So, as with all learning, adequate preparation is essential for positive results and success. If you want to learn and perfect a skill, whether it be *yogāsana*, *prāṇāyāma*, *Kriyā* techniques, or anything else, you will need to start from the basic principles, methods and techniques. An experienced teacher is essential but it is also normal to have learning resources at hand, such as books, manuals and the internet for study and research.

Of course, for *Kriyā Yoga* to work successfully and effectively in the individual practising it, it needs to be received not only intellectually but through the spiritual vibration and transmission of a *Kriyā* initiation, in which the disciple becomes intuitively and devotionally attuned to the God-realised guru's spiritual guidance. Being merely casual and lackadaisical about *Kriyā Yoga* while practising *Kriyā* techniques mechanically without inner attunement and devotion to God and guru will not bring one to spiritual realisation. To be a disciple on the *Kriyā Yoga* path one needs to be sincere and steadfast in meditation with devotion and loyalty to God and guru. One also has to have the attitudes of the *yamas* and *niyamas* (as outlined by Patañjali in his *Yoga Sūtras*), as well as humility, willingness, even-mindedness, openness, understanding and compassion towards others.

Even if someone discovers the secrets of practising the *Kriyā* techniques, or reads it in a book, unless they are spiritually aware and awakened they will not have the motivation and sustained discipline to establish the constant routine of practising it. Those who are just casually looking for instant enlightenment, collecting gurus and techniques, will not succeed either. *Kriyā Yoga* is a gradual process of spiritual unfoldment; a disciple on this path has to gain spiritual understanding and attunement with gurus who are the channels through which it is transmitted.

KNOWLEDGE IS POWER

Knowledge is not merely abstract information. Knowledge is power. There is a danger that religions, spiritual organisations, individual teachers and gurus can use that power to control and condition their followers to think in a certain way. This is how unnecessary myths and simplifications are created, and that is why there needs to be transparency, truthfulness, sincerity, honesty and openness. Knowledge can be withheld and made secret, even altered and modified to change the original meaning, by those who possess the secret knowledge, which can take the form of a spiritual teaching, its methods and techniques.

Knowledge that should be available and open becomes secret, obscure and divisive in the hands of those controlling it. Why should spiritual truths be kept from those who are sincerely seeking it? Why should those in control of knowledge obscure the path to Reality for others? For those sincerely seeking the truth, this creates a barrier of separation. True spiritual masters or gurus of pure heart and understanding do not experience any separation – they encourage unity. Their spirit is unfettered and boundless and their knowledge is available to all who sincerely seek it.

IS *KRIYĀ* YOGA DANGEROUS?

> 'Master (Yogananda) said to all of us at Mt Washington (SRF Headquarters, Los Angeles), "Do 108 *kriyās*, twice a day." I was quite surprised when he said that and I asked, "Is it safe?" He replied, "Yes, it is safe. Get that thought out of your mind that it is not!"'
>
> *Swāmi Kriyananda*

Life can be dangerous. Wherever you go in the world and whatever you do, there can be potential dangers – crossing the road and the possibility of being hit by a car; flying in an aeroplane that might crash; slipping on ice; falling from a ladder; being bitten by a poisonous snake or even a dog; taking *Ayahuasca*, a hallucinogenic drug from the Amazon jungle – the list is endless.

Awareness, common sense, discrimination, respect, understanding, knowing when to be careful, and anticipating the danger ahead and taking necessary precautions are all needed in order to avoid danger. I think the majority of us choose to embrace the adventure of life, rather than be in fear and paranoia and playing it safe by staying at home all the time.

Kriyā practised under the guidance of an experienced *Kriyā* teacher is completely safe. I have been practising *Kriyā* for 31 years and I have known many people practising *Kriyā*, but I have never known anyone (including myself) who has been practising *Kriyā* to have been hurt by it or to have had a bad experience with it. As long as you are mentally and physically healthy, practising within your limits, and under the guidance of an experienced teacher, there should be no problem.

Before I was initiated into *Kriyā Yoga* in 1983 by Swāmi Kriyananda, I had been practising *Haṭha Yoga* for ten years, and never once witnessed any harmful effects from practising Yoga. But there is some danger and risk in performing the Lotus posture (*Pādmāsana*) in which tendons can be torn if not performed correctly, and in practising excessive *prāṇāyāma* in which the breath is held for long duration. Holding the breath for more than a minute without expert guidance present and without using *bandhas* (locks for controlling the *prāṇic* energy) could be damaging to the brain, nervous system, heart and *prāṇic* circuits.

To minimise any harm or danger to yourself in practising any form of Yoga, ensure that you are not going further than your body is ready for, whether you are doing *yogāsanas*, *prāṇāyāma* or *Kriyā Yoga* techniques. Forceful effort should not be used. You should not force or push excessively or too quickly beyond your safe limit, but develop your capacity gradually and systematically and aim for steady progress. If you have any disabilities or injuries then use modifications whenever necessary. If unsure, then always be guided by an experienced teacher.

> 'All the methods of *Haṭha Yoga* are meant for gaining success in *Rāja Yoga*.'
>
> *Haṭha Yoga Pradīpikā 102*

> '*Haṭha Yoga* cannot be obtained without *Rāja Yoga*, nor can *Rāja Yoga* be attained without *Haṭha Yoga*. Therefore, let the yogi first learn *Haṭha Yoga* from the instructions of the wise guru.'
>
> *Śiva Samhitā 5.181*

There are numerous practical manuals published on *Haṭha Yoga* that give detailed instructions and precautions. These are not secret and are widely available. As in *Kriyā Yoga*, they responsibly recommend that you find an experienced teacher to guide you in practising the techniques.

Practising *Haṭha Yoga* is a very useful step towards *Rāja Yoga/Kriyā Yoga*, while also leading a balanced and healthy diet and lifestyle following Āyurvedic regimens. These will not only help you to achieve optimum physical health, but will also help you to be emotionally and mentally balanced. The powerful practices of *Haṭha Yoga,* which include purification *kriyās* and *prāṇāyāma*, strengthen the physical body and the nervous system, and balance the *chakras and nāḍīs* (subtle *prāṇic* channels), preparing you for *Kriyā* meditation practices. This is why a person who has had a *Haṭha Yoga* training is prepared for *Kriyā Yoga*. I remember when I first came on to the *Kriyā Yoga* path that the *Kriyā* techniques were familiar to me. This was because I had been practising *Haṭha Yoga* and Tantric Yoga for ten years, from which these *Kriyā* techniques have originated.

7.9

SPIRITUAL GUIDELINES FOR PRACTISING KRIYĀ YOGA

It is not enough to be just practising *Kriyā Yoga* techniques – you also need to have a wholesome lifestyle that nurtures and supports your total being in body, mind and spirit, and to develop your spiritual qualities of love, compassion, understanding, forgiveness, peace, harmony, friendship and goodwill towards all. You need to remember that there is no separation between spiritual and material realities. Reality is omnipresent; wherever you are, it is around and within you, *as* you – the inner, unchanging, eternal Self – and can be easily discovered at any moment. Anything that changes cannot be your true Self.

While engaging in your daily duties be established in Self-awareness and wisely use your knowledge of how your consciousness, mental states, desires, intentions, attitudes and behaviours influence your life, other people and the environment. Be constantly aware of your true nature and relationship with the Infinite, and choose to live wisely in ways that support, nourish and are beneficial and harmonious to the wellbeing of yourself and others. Live always with positive and conscious intention to improve your spiritual awareness and to remain spiritually awake. Conserve your energy so that you can channel it into useful creativity that can inspire others to awaken spiritually. Be regular in your meditation – every day, meditate deeply into calm superconsciousness to clarify your awareness, refine your brain cells, and experience direct inner realisation of the Divine. Meditate to go more deeply into your essence of being to know your true nature and your oneness with the infinite Divine Reality. Aspire to know the higher purpose of your being and fulfil your spiritual destiny.

May you be blessed and guided to that inner freedom, eternal peace and limitless joy which is your birthright!

Oṁ Tat Sat

Appendix 1

AN INTRODUCTION TO SANSKRIT

> 'The Sanskrit language, whatever be its antiquity, is of wonderful structure, more perfect than the Greek, more copious than the Latin and more exquisitely refined than either.'
>
> *Sir William Jones (British Orientalist, 1746–1794)*

The word Sanskrit is a Western name that originates from *saṃskṛta* ('perfectly composed', 'refined'). In the Western world, Sanskrit, like Latin, is usually considered to be an unspoken language. However, Sanskrit is very much a spoken language today. In India there are nine Sanskrit universities with about 600 branches where all subjects are taught in the Sanskrit medium, and India publishes many magazines in the Sanskrit language, which address contemporary issues. The news service offered by the Government of India through television and radio continues to feature daily Sanskrit programmes covering local as well as international news. The grammar of Sanskrit has attracted scholars worldwide. It is very precise, up-to-date and remains well defined even today.

Sanskrit is a language for humanity and not merely a means for communication within a society. There is sufficient evidence available today that shows that Sanskrit is the oldest language in the world. In fact, Sanskrit is known as the 'Mother of all European Languages'. Among the current languages which possess an antiquity, such as Latin or ancient Greek, Sanskrit is the only language which has retained its pristine purity. It has maintained its structure and vocabulary even today as it did in the ancient past. Sanskrit distinguishes itself from other languages in that it is the only known language which has a built-in scheme for pronunciation, word formation and grammar.

The oldest surviving literature of the world – the *Vedās* – encompasses knowledge in virtually every sphere of human activity. The early Brāhmanical texts of the *Rigveda* written in the pre-Classical form of Vedic Sanskrit are the oldest, dating back to as early as 1500–1200 BCE. The oldest surviving Sanskrit grammar that evolved from the earlier Vedic form is Pānini's *Eight-Chapter Grammar* (*Astādhyāyī*), consisting of 3990 *sūtra*s (aphorisms), which define correct Sanskrit. About a century after Pānini (around 400 BCE), Kātyāyana composed *Vārtikas* on Pānini's *sūtra*s. Around the middle of the second century BCE the great sage Patañjali, who formulated the *Yoga Sūtras*, also wrote the *Mahābhashya* (the 'Great Commentary'), a commentary on the earliest extant Sanskrit grammar (the *Astādhyāyī* and *Vārtikas*) of Pānini. Patañjali, who lived three centuries after Pānini, formulated certain new grammatical rules (*ishtis*) to supplement the earlier ones; this would mean that Sanskrit had by now undergone changes.

Around the mid-first millennium BCE, Vedic Sanskrit began the transition from a first language to a second language of religion and learning.

Sanskrit abounds in philosophy-related and theology-related issues. There are so many words one encounters within Sanskrit that convey subtly differing meanings of a concept that admits of only one interpretation when studied with other languages. The Sanskrit language thus has the ability to offer links between concepts using just the words. For every sound there is only one letter and for every letter there is only one sound. This principle is hardly seen in any other language. Also, in the Sanskrit alphabet, all the vowels are listed first and then all the consonants. This is different from the alphabets used for Western languages, which are mostly based on Egyptian hieroglyphics and the old Phoenician alphabet. The order a, b, c, d…mixes vowels and consonants indiscriminately and is generally unsystematic.

Sanskrit is a spiritual language full of spiritual significance. Like most things in Sanskrit, the grammar has roots tracing back to a divine origin. The mythological story of the seven great Seers, the *Saptarsi*, describes how they went to Lord Śiva seeking the essence of language. Lord Śiva played his tiny two-ended drum (*damaru*), and from it came sounds that are known as the *mahesvārasūtrani*. These sounds were 14 *sūtra*s (aphorisms) that became the basis of Sanskrit grammar as recorded by Pānini.

For those who are sincerely practising Yoga, meditation, and chanting *mantras*, Sanskrit words give meaning and clearer explanation on a spiritual level. It is useful to understand the exact connotations of Sanskrit terms, as it can be difficult to equate certain Sanskrit terms with English words. For example, 'mind' and 'consciousness' are two words that get confused in translation. Usually in Sanskrit *manas* is translated as 'mind', but the connotations are certainly different. *Manas* is subtle material and objective, it is not the brain. The brain is gross matter and is an instrument of *manas*. The physical brain dies when the physical body dies, but *manas,* which is made of subtle matter, leaves the body at the time of death.

It is also worth taking some time to learn correct pronunciation of Sanskrit. Correct pronunciation helps to bring out the subtle effects in chanting *mantras*, adding a beneficial effect through their vibrations.

Devanāgari script of Sanskrit is a phonetic alphabet that consists of 13 vowels (*svāra*) and 34 consonants (*vyanjana*). It is known as a syllabic script. Every letter has a unique sound and is a single syllable of each word. Each letter in the *Devanāgari* script of Sanskrit has a mystic value.

According to the *Bīja-Code* each letter of the Sanskrit *varnamāla* (alphabet) represents certain instincts. Since each letter has a different acoustic root, each one of them creates a different vibration which often corresponds to the psyche of the persons being addressed. For the students of the science of *mantra* it is important to know the acoustic root and the power of all letters used in Sanskrit.

The seed syllable has a magical aura around it. According to the Tantric tradition, every seed syllable must have a nasal sound which results in a divine union. Since *Śiva* and *Śakti* are considered to be two lips, their union leads to the birth of seed, that is, *bīja*.

The nasal sound (*anusvāra*) as in ṁ, is supposed to have the germ of a complete doctrine. Through *bīja-akshar* (seed syllable) a huge treatise can be compressed in a few lines. A seed syllable, by virtue of being short, is good for the repetitions of a *mantra* as it creates cerebral vibrations which keep reverberating. With the help of the nasal sound, one can transfer the seed syllable to the back of the head or between the eyebrows. At a later stage the accumulated energy of a *mantra* can be projected anywhere in order to achieve the desired result. *Mantras* chanted in Sanskrit reveal the mystery of sound. The result can be multi-dimensional – some *mantras* can bring enlightenment, while other *mantras* bring disenchantment.

The aim of *mantra* is to experience the non-dualistic experience. The great yogis have stated that a *mantra* (in Sanskrit) does not give any results if it is not chanted properly, as it represents *Śabda-Brāhman*, which stands for 'Cosmic sound waves'.

Sanskrit is the eternal spiritual language. The eternal syllable *Oṁ* is the Primordial Transcendental Sound, the divine sound vibration from which all other sounds originate. *Oṁ,* the *Praṇava*, is the root of all the *mantras*. From *Aum* (*Oṁ*) emanated all the other sounds of the alphabet, including the seven primary notes of music: *ṣaḍja*, *ṛṣabha*, *gāndhāra*, *madhyama*, *pañcama*, *dhaivata* and *niṣāda* (known as *Sa*, *Re*, *Ga*, *Ma*, *Pa*, *Da*, *Ni*).

> 'The word *Oṁ* should be used in the beginning. It is the Supreme Reality. It is used as a synonym for *Brāhman*.'
>
> *Atharvaśikhopaniṣad*

GUIDE TO SANSKRIT PRONUNCIATION

Too often, in Western books on Yoga, there is an over-simplification of translation of a Sanskrit word into English, where the original meaning tends to get diluted, mistranslated or lost. In this book I have tried to keep as many Sanskrit words as possible in their original meaning.

Since the late eighteenth century, Sanskrit has been transliterated using the Latin alphabet. The system most commonly used today is the IAST (International Alphabet of Sanskrit Transliteration), which has been the academic standard since 1888/1912.

The following guide to pronunciation gives approximate equivalents in English to the Sanskrit sounds.

Diacritical marks used in this translation

ā ī ū ṛ ḷ ḥ ṁ ṅ ñ ṇ ṭ ḍ ś ṣ

Vowels

a ā i ī u ū r ṛ ṝ l ḷ e ai o au

These vowels are further divided into simple vowels (*a*, *ā*, and so on) and combined vowels (*e*, *ai*, *o*, *au*). The simple vowels are listed in pairs (*a-ā*, *i-ī*…). In each pair the first vowel is short and the second is exactly twice as long. In the English transliteration the long vowels are marked with a bar (-). The diphthongs are also pronounced twice as long as the short vowels. Thus in the words *nī-la* 'blue' or *go-pa* cowherd', the first syllable is held twice as long as the second.

Simple

a short *a* as in '**a**bout'

ā long *a* as in 'f**a**ther'

i short *i* as **e** in '**e**ngland'

ī long *i* as in **ee** in 'f**ee**t'

u short *u* as in **oo** in 'f**oo**t'

ū long *u* as in 'r**u**le'

ṛ as in 'w**r**itten'(but held twice as long)

ḷ **le** as in 'turt**le**'

ḹ longer '**le**'

Diphthongs

e as in 'they'

ai as in '**ai**sle' '**i**ce' 'k**i**te'

o as in 'go'

au as in '**ow**l'

Aspiration

ḥ (*visarga*) a final 'h' sound that echoes the preceding vowel slightly; as in 'aha' for ***aḥ***; ***iḥ*** as ihi; ***uḥ*** as uhu.

Nasalised vowel

ṁ (*anusvāra* – marked with a dot) a nasal sound pronounced like *mm*, but influenced according to whatever consonant follows, as in 'bingo'. The nasal is modified by the following consonant: *Sāṃkhya* as 'saankhya'.

Consonants

Consonants are generally pronounced as in English, but there are some differences. Sanskrit has many 'aspirated' consonants; these are pronounced with a slight 'h' sound. For example, the consonant *ph* is pronounced as English *p* followed by an *h* as in ha*ph*azard. The *bh* is as in a*bh*or.

k as in 's**k**ip'

kh as in 'E**ckh**art'

g as in '**g**ame'

gh as in 'do**gh**ouse'

ṅ as in 'si**ng**'

c as in 'ex**ch**ange'

ch as in '**ch**urch'

j as in ‘**j**am’

jh as in ‘he**dg**ehog’

ñ as in ‘ca**n**yon’

ṭ as in ‘**t**ub’; the tongue curls back and hits the upper palate

ṭh as in ‘ligh**t-h**eart’; the tongue curls back and hits the upper palate

ḍ as in ‘**d**ove’; the tongue curls back and hits the palate

ḍh as in ‘a**dh**ere’; the tongue curls back and hits the palate

ṇ as in ‘ti**n**t’; tip of tongue touches the back of the upper teeth

t as in ‘**t**ub’; tip of tongue touches the back of the upper teeth

th as in ‘**th**ick’; tip of tongue touches the back of the upper teeth

d as in ‘**d**ove’; tip of tongue touches the back of the upper teeth

dh as in ‘re**d-h**ot’; tip of tongue touches the back of the upper teeth

n as in ‘**n**ame’; tip of tongue touches the back of the upper teeth

p as in ‘**p**a**p**a’

ph as in ‘ha**ph**azard’

b as in ‘**b**alloon’

bh as in ‘a**bh**or’

m as in ‘**m**um’

y as in ‘**y**ellow’

r as in ‘**r**un’

l as in ‘**l**ove’

v as in ‘**v**ine’

ś as in ‘**sh**ell’

ṣ as in ‘**s**ilk’

h as in ‘**h**ill’

Double consonants

In double consonants, both letters are pronounced distinctly separately.

śraddhā (faith) is pronounced *śrad-dhā*

icchā (desire) is pronounced *ic-chā*

jagannātha (Lord of the Universe) is pronounced *jagan-nātha*

jña (to know) as in *Jñana Yoga* (the path of wisdom or higher knowledge) is widely pronounced ‘gya’. More accurate is ‘gnya’, and best is to combine a correct *ja* with a correct *ña*.

Appendix 2

PROPERTIES OF THE CHAKRAS

The table on the following pages details the properties of the *chakras*.

Subject	Mūlādhāra	Svādhiṣṭhāna	Manipūra	Anāhata	Viśuddhi	Ājñā	Sahasrāra
Location	Perineum/ cervix	Sacral centre/ sex organs	Lumbar centre/ navel	Dorsal centre/ heart	Cervical centre/ throat	At the centre of the brain	At the crown of the head
No. of lotus petals	4	6	10	12	16	2	1000 or infinite
Element	Earth	Water	Fire	Air	Ether	Mahat, i.e. mind, ego and intellect	Beyond all elements
Bija mantra	Laṁ	Vaṁ	Raṁ	Yaṁ	Haṁ	Kṣam or Oṁ	Visarga or Oṁ
Colour of petals	Deep red	Orange-red	Yellow	Blue	Purple	White	Multi-coloured
Physiological relationship	Sacro-coccygeal plexus	Pelvic plexus	Solar plexus	Cardiac plexus	Pharyngeal and laryngeal plexus	Cavernous plexus	Hypothalamic pituitary axis
Endocrine relationship	Perineal body	Testes, ovaries	Adrenal glands	Thymus gland	Thyroid gland	Pineal gland	Pituitary gland
Vedic astrological sign and ruling planet	Aquarius Capricorn Saturn	Sagittarius Pisces Jupiter	Aries Scorpio Mars	Libra Taurus Venus	Gemini Virgo	Leo – Sun Cancer – Moon	
Inner sounds	Bumble bee, rumbling motor	Flute, Crickets, trickling water	Stringed instrument, sitar, harp	Deep bell or gong	Wind in the trees, rushing water	*Aum* (*Oṁ*), like the roar of the sea	
Positive qualities	Courage, loyalty, steadfastness, perseverance	Open, willingness, intuitive, creative	Enthusiasm, self-control, loving leadership	Devotion, unconditional love, compassion	Expansive, deeply calm, silence	Selfless service, attunement, strong willpower, Divine surrender	Beyond all duality, omnipresent, omniscient, samadhi bliss

cont.

Subject	Mūlādhāra	Svādhiṣṭhāna	Manipūra	Anāhata	Viśuddhi	Ājñā	Sahasrāra
Negative qualities	Stubborn, prejudice, intolerant	Indecisive, vague	Misuse of power and ruthless	Attachment, harmful emotions: anger, rage, hatred	Restless, boredom, worldly desires	Egotistic, proud, too intellectual, strong sense of 'I, me, mine'	
Prāna vāyu (vital force)	*Apāṇa*	*Vyāṇa*	*Samāna*	*Prāṇa*	*Udāṇa*	All five *prāṇa vāyus*	Beyond
Ḳośa (sheath)	*Annamāyā* (physical body)	*Prāṇamāyā* (subtle vital body)	*Prāṇamāyā* (subtle vital body)	*Manomāyā* (mental body)	*Vijñānamāyā* (intellectual body)	*Vijñānamāyā* (intellectual body)	*Ānandamāyā* (blissful causal)
Tattva (elements)	*Pṛithvī* (earth)	*Apās* (water)	*Agni* (fire)	*Vāyu* (air)	*Akaśa* (ether)	*Manas* (mind)	Beyond
Yantra (symbolic form)	Yellow square	Silver or white crescent moon	Red inverted triangle	Smoky six-pointed star	White circle	Clear or grey circle	Beyond
Tanmātrā	Smell	Taste	Sight	Touch	Hearing	Mind	Beyond
Jñānedriya	Nose	Tongue	Eyes	Skin	Ears	Mind	Beyond
Kārmendriya	Anus	Sex organs, kidneys, urinary system	Feet	Hands	Vocal cords	Mind	Beyond
Loka (spiritual world)	*Bhūr*	*Bhuvaḥ*	*Svaḥ*	*Manaḥ*	*janaḥ*	*tapaḥ*	*Satyam*
Devi (goddess)	*Savitri* or *Dākinī*	*Saraswati* or *Rākinī*	*Lakshmi* or *Lakini*	*Kali* or *Kākinī*	*Sākinī*	*Hākinī*	*Śakti*
Deva (god)	*Gaṇeśa*	*Viṣṇu*	*Rudra*	*Isha*	*Sadaśiva*	*Paramśiva*	*Śiva*
Animal	Elephant (*airavata*)	Crocodile (*makara*)	Ram	Antelope	White elephant		

Yoni	*Tripura*			Triangle		Triangle	
Lingam	*Swayambhu*	*Dhumra*		*Bana*		*Itarakhya*	
Granthi	*Brahma*			*Viṣṇu*		*Rudra*	*Jyotirmāyā*
Alphabet sounds related to the petals	*Vaṁ* *Saṁ* *Saṁ* *Saṁ*	*Baṁ* *Bhaṁ* *Maṁ* *Yaṁ* *Raṁ* *Laṁ*	*Ḍaṁ* *Ḍham* *Ṇam* *Taṁ* *Thaṁ* *Daṁ* *Dhaṁ* *Naṁ* *Paṁ* *Phaṁ*	*Kaṁ* *Khaṁ* *Gaṁ* *Ghaṁ* *Ṇaṁ* *Caṁ* *Chaṁ* *Jaṁ* *Jhaṁ* *Naṁ* *Taṁ* *Ṭhaṁ*	*Aṁ* *Aṁ* *Iṁ* *Iṁ* *Uṁ* *Uṁ* *Rṁ* *Rṁ* *Lrṁ* *Lrṁ* *Aiṁ* *Aiṁ* *Oṁ* *Auṁ* *Aṅ* *Aḥ*	*Ham* *Kṣam*	All the alphabet sounds

Appendix 3

THE FIVE GREAT ELEMENTS

	Ether *Akaśa*	**Air** *Vāyu*	**Fire** *Tejas*	**Water** *Apās*	**Earth** *Pṛithvī*
Principle	All-pervasive	Motion	Illumination	Cohesion	Stability
Qualities	Expansive, light, clear, subtle, cold, infinite, all-pervasive	Light, like the wind, mobile, clear, rough, dry, erratic	Hot, sharp, penetrating, fluid, luminous, light, ascending, dispersing	Wet, fluid, heavy, cool, lubricating, cohesive, soft, stable	Dense, solid, thick, heavy, stable
Sense	Sound	Touch	Sight	Taste	Smell
Organ	Ear	Skin	Eyes	Tongue	Nose
Action	Speech	Holding	Walking	Procreation	Excretion
Organ of action	Mouth	Hand	Feet	Genitals	Anus

Appendix 4

THE SEVEN CHAKRAS CENTRES OF CONSCIOUSNESS

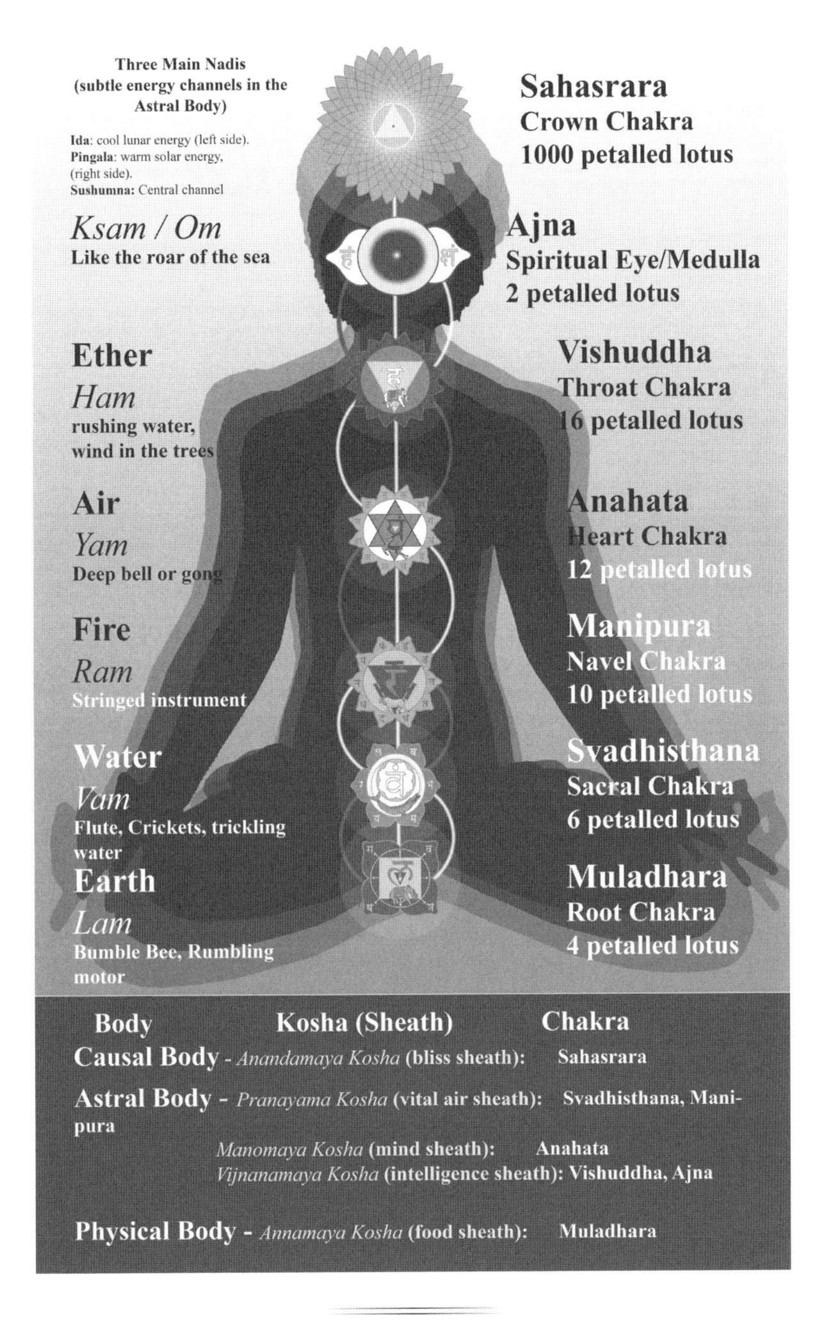
Three Main Nadis
(subtle energy channels in the
Astral Body)
Ida: cool lunar energy (left side).
Pingala: warm solar energy,
(right side).
Sushumna: Central channel
Ksam / Om
Like the roar of the sea
Ether
Ham
rushing water,
wind in the trees
Air
Yam
Deep bell or gong
Fire
Ram
Stringed instrument
Water
Vam
Flute, Crickets, trickling
water
Earth
Lam
Bumble Bee, Rumbling
motor
Sahasrara
Crown Chakra
1000 petalled lotus
Ajna
Spiritual Eye/Medulla
2 petalled lotus
Vishuddha
Throat Chakra
16 petalled lotus
Anahata
Heart Chakra
12 petalled lotus
Manipura
Navel Chakra
10 petalled lotus
Svadhisthana
Sacral Chakra
6 petalled lotus
Muladhara
Root Chakra
4 petalled lotus
Body
Kosha (Sheath)
Chakra
Causal Body - Anandamaya Kosha (bliss sheath): Sahasrara
Astral Body - Pranayama Kosha (vital air sheath): Svadhisthana, Manipura
Manomaya Kosha (mind sheath): Anahata
Vijnanamaya Kosha (intelligence sheath): Vishuddha, Ajna
Physical Body - Annamaya Kosha (food sheath): Muladhara

GLOSSARY

A

Abhyāsa: Persistent repeated practice.

Adhyatmika: Pain within oneself (physical, mental and emotional).

Adhbhautika: Pain caused by other beings (including wild animals and insects).

Adhidaivika: Pain caused by natural forces (sound, air, fire, water, earth, heat, cold, and planetary forces).

Adiśvara: The first Lord, Śiva.

Āgamas: Literally, 'that which is received or acquired; acquisition of knowledge'. This is usually applied to non-Vedic texts that are regarded as revelation.

Āgāmi karmas: The actions which are being done in this present life and will bear fruits in a future life. It is this karma which preserves our free-will with certain limitations and ensures our future success.

Agni: Digestive fire. In *Āyurveda*, *agni* is the internal digestive fire responsible for nutrient transformation and tissue and cellular assimilation.

Ahaṁkāra: Ego.

Ajapā japa: Repetition of a *mantra* is called *japa*. The *japa* becomes *ajapā* when the *mantra* gets repeated in the mind on its own. *Ajapā japa* is continuous repetition of a *mantra* on the subconscious level of the mind.

Ājñā: The sixth *chakra*, located at the eyebrow centre. It has two poles: the negative pole is at the medulla oblongata; the positive pole is at the midpoint between the eyebrows, the Spiritual Eye, the seat of concentration.

Ajñanā: The word *'jña'* means 'knowing' or 'conscious'. *'Ajña'* (as in *ajñanā*) describes the condition of the individual soul (*jiva*) as limited in the capacity to know. The *jiva* or soul is not devoid of consciousness but only unaware of its own original nature. This ignorance or not knowing is *ajñanā*.

Ākāśha: Space, ether element, infinite void.

Alasya: Laziness.

Anavasthitatvā: Instability.

Anāhata: Heart *chakra*, the fourth centre in the *suṣumnā*, the subtle spine.

Ānanda: Bliss, infinite joy.

Ānandamaya-kośa: The bliss sheath, corresponding to the causal body.

Antar: Inner, internal.

Antar vṛitti: The internal operation of the breath.

Antaḥkaraṇa: Internal instrument of cognition; consisting of consciousness, intellect, ego and mind.

Antahphala: The female gonads, the ovaries.

Anusvāra: Nasalised vowel 'marked with a dot' (*ṁ*) used in Sanskrit pronunciation (a nasal sound pronounced like 'mm'), but influenced according to whatever consonant follows.

Apāṇa: Downward moving aspect of *prāṇa*; one of the five major *vayus*; functions in the region of the navel to the feet.

Āsana: Seat, posture; pose for meditation, the third of eight limbs of *Aṣṭāṅga Yoga*.

Asmitā kleśa: Affliction of ego.

Astādhyāyī: Pānini's 'Eight-Chapter Sanskrit Grammar'.

Aṣṭāṅga: Eight limbs (*Aṣṭāṅga Yoga* – Eight Limbs of Yoga).

Aśvinī: Horse (*aśvinī mudrā* – Horse Gesture). The practice is so-called because the anal contraction resembles the movement a horse makes with its sphincter immediately after evacuation of its bowels.

Ātma; ātman: The innermost Self, or soul.

Ātmavidyā: Self-knowledge.

Aum: The primordial *mantra* sound vibration of creation.

Avidyā: *Avidyā* means the false identification of purusha with buddhi, ignorance, nescience (first of five kleshas, afflictions).

Avirati: Attachment to sense-pleasure.

Āyurveda: 'Science of Life'. *Ayus* means 'life' or 'lifespan'; *veda* means 'science' or 'knowledge'. *Āyurveda* deals with the fundamental principles in nature that underlie the creation, preservation, and restoration of health and the promotion of longevity.

B

Bahir: External (*bahir kumbhaka* – external breath retention).

Bāhya vṛitti: The external operation of the breath.

Bandha: Literally translates as 'lock'. *Bandhas* are inner actions that direct the subtle power of the breath or *prāṇa*, locking it into a particular part of the body.

Bhūr: Represents earth.

Bhuvaḥ: Represents the subtle worlds with their demigods.

Bhrāmarī: Humming bee (as in *bhrāmarī prāṇāyama*).

Bīja: Seed, source (*bīja mantra* – seed-syllable *mantra*).

Bījarakta: Ovum, human female egg.

Brāhmarandhra: 'The Door of God'.

Brāhman: From the Sanskrit verb root *brha*, meaning 'expansion, knowledge, all-pervasiveness'. It indicates the Absolute Supreme Consciousness, Absolute Reality.

Brāhmacharya: Literally 'walking the path of God'; control of vital energy; control of sexual passion (one of the five *yamas*).

Brahmā muhūrta: 'Time of God'. (*Brāhma* – God, *muhurta* – time). The auspicious time, one and a half hours before sunrise.

Brāhmavidyā: The Absolute Truth.

Bhuta shuddhi: *Bhuta* means 'elements', *shuddhi* means 'purification'; *bhuta shuddhi* is purification of the five subtle elements: earth, water, fire, air and space (ether).

C

Chakra: Wheel, vortex of energy, energy centre within the body, of which there are seven main centres. The *chakras* are transformers for the *prāṇic* life-energy and consciousness flowing through them. They store energy and distribute it throughout the body.

Chyavanaprash: The famous general Āyurvedic tonic in the form of a jam-like paste, containing a formula of herbs, minerals, honey and ghee, but chiefly composed of the *amla* fruit (*Phyllanthus emblica*).

Cin: Consciousness (*cin mudrā* – gesture of consciousness); *cit* – consciousness.

Citriṇī: Pale like the moon. *Citriṇī* is one of the *nāḍīs* within the *suṣumnā* (the central subtle channel in the spine).

Citta: Mind-field; mind, field of consciousness.

D

Damaru: A tiny two-ended drum that Lord Śiva played.

Dandāsana: 'Stick'. This is the basic sitting position with the spine straight and the legs straight out in front of the body. It is from this position that the forward bending positions are performed.

Daurmanasya: Despair, frustration.

Devanāgari: Sanskrit script.

Dhātus: 'Supports' from *dhā* 'to give','to give support'. The three forces, *vāta, pitta* and *kapha*, that govern the biological processes of the body/mind in the normal state of equilibrium that constitutes health. The word *dhātus* is also used to denote the seven tissues of the body.

Dhyāna: Meditation.

Doṣas: 'Faults', from *duṣ* 'to soil, 'to spoil', 'to impair'. When the *dhātus* are in disequilibrium the three forces *vāta, pitta* and *kapha* are called *doṣas*.

Draṣṭuḥ: The Seer.

Duḥkha: Pain, suffering and sorrow.

Dveṣa: Repulsion, aversion (fourth of five *kleṣas*).

G

Gāndhāra: One of the seven primary notes (Ga) of Hindu music.

Gāyatrī: The most sacred prayer of the *Ṛigveda*, that is known to all Hindus concerns *Savitṛ*. It is the great *Gāyatrī mantra*.

Gheraṇḍa Saṃhitā: The Tantrik Sanskrit text on *Haṭha Yoga*, which is in the form of a dialogue between the sage Gheraṇḍa and an inquirer Chaṇḍa Kāpāli.

Guṇas: 'Strands' or 'ropes' that bind the soul to material existence. The three energy-forces (*guṇas*) that materiality operate through are *sattva* (subtle matter of pure thought), *rajas* (energy) and *tamas* (inertia).

H

Haṁsa: A *mantra* meaning, 'I am He'. When repeated continuously it becomes *so'ham*, which means 'He (the Absolute) am I'. Either way it means the same. *Haṁsa* is also the word for 'swan', the migratory white bird that can fly to places unknown to ordinary people. *Haṁsa* is the ever-perfect Self. One who dwells in this consciousness is called a *Parāmhaṁsa*.

Haṭha Yoga: A system of purifying techniques and Yoga postures to control the body and mind, through control of *prāṇa. Haṭha Yoga* is a preparation for *Rāja Yoga*, the path of meditation.

Haṭha Yoga Pradīpikā: A classic guide to the practice of *Haṭha Yoga* from the seventeenth century by Yogi Swatmarama.

Hiranyagarbha: Golden Womb; Universal mind.

Hong Sau: *Kriyā* meditation *mantra*, that means 'I am He'. It deepens the concentration and brings inner calmness.

I

Icchā: Desire, pronounced *ic-chā*.

Iḍā: One of the three major *nāḍīs* (subtle channels) that runs on the left side of the spine, from the *mūladhāra chakra* to the *ājñā chakra*. It is associated with lunar energy.

J

Jāgrat: Waking state; conscious mind.

Jala neti: Nasal cleaning.

Jālandhara bandha: Chin lock.

Jīvātma: Individual self; *puruṣa*.

Jña: 'To know', as in *Jñana Yoga* (the path of wisdom or higher knowledge). Widely pronounced 'gya', though more accurate is 'gnya', it is best to combine a correct *ja* with a correct *ña*.

Jñanā mudrā: Gesture of intuitive knowledge.

Jñānendriyas: Organs of perception: the ears, eyes, skin, tongue, nose.

Jñānī: The one endowed with self-Knowledge.

K

Kaivalya: Liberation. It expresses the *Sāṃkhya* view that liberation is the isolation of *puruṣa* from *prakṛiti*. In *Advaita Vedānta*, *kaivalya* means 'absolute nonduality', for the liberated Self *is* the one reality.

Kanda: Located between the anus and the root of the reproductive organs, just above *mulādhāra chakra*. From this source 72,000 *nādīs*, invisible vital *prāṇic* current channels, flow out to the entire subtle circuitry of the astral body.

Kāraṇa-śarīra: Causal body.

Kapālabhāti: *Kapāla* means 'skull' and *bhāti* means 'shine'. A *Haṭha Yoga* frontal brain purification technique using invigorating breathing.

Karma: Actions that have a binding effect; the law of cause and effect.

Karmendriyas: Organs of action: the vocal cords, hands, legs, reproductive organs and anus.

Kokanada rakta-kāmāla: Reddish lotus.

Koṣas: The five sheaths: *annamaya* (food), *prāṇayamas* (vital), *manomaya* (mind), *vijñānamaya* (intellect) and *ānandamaya* (bliss).

Kriyā Yoga: *Kri* from the Sanskrit root *Kriyā* means 'to do, to act'. *Kriyā Yoga* is 'union with the Infinite through the action of *Kriyā'*. An ancient sacred Yoga science that includes advanced techniques of meditation leading to Self and God realisation, *Kriyā Yoga* was revived in this age by Mahavatar Babaji and passed down through a succession of Masters to Paramhansa Yogananda.

Kriyāvān: An initiated practitioner of *Kriyā*. Usually pronounced 'kriyaban'.

Kuṇḍalinī śakti: *Kundala* means 'coiled'. Ś*akti* means primordial cosmic energy. The coiled-up, dormant, primordial cosmic energy that gives power and energy to all the *chakras*; lies dormant at the *mūladhāra chakra*, at the base of the spine.

Kūtastha: 'That which remains unchanged.' *Kūtastha Caitanya* means 'Christ Consciousness' (the cosmic intelligence of Spirit that is omnipresent in creation). The *kūtastha* is also used as another name for the Spiritual Eye, located at the midpoint between the eyebrows.

L

Lam: Seed-syllable (*bīja*) *mantra* representing the energy of earth element at the *mūladhāra chakra*.

Lahiri Mahasaya: A *Kriyā* yogi, known as one of the greatest yogis of nineteenth century India, written about extensively in Yogananda's *Autobiography of a Yogi*.

Laya: Dissolution; merging (the word *laya* originates from the Sanskrit root *li*, meaning 'to become dissolved'). The yogi in this state of *laya* dissolves the mind, intellect and ego into the transcendental Being-Consciousness-Bliss (*Sat-chit-ānanda*).

Linga: Mark; characteristic; gender; sign; symbol; distinctive sign through which it is possible to recognise the nature of something. Usually a reference to a column-like egg-shaped symbol of Śiva.

Linga sharīra: Subtle body; astral body (also called *sukshma sharīra*).

M

Mahābīja: *Oṁ* is the 'great seed'.

Mahā mudrā: 'Great Gesture'.

Mahā Śakti: Cosmic Energy, the great infinite Cosmic Force that enlivens and sustains this universe.

Māhat: Cosmic consciousness; cosmic mind.

Mahesvārasūtrani: Sounds that are known as the *Mahesvārasūtrani* came from Lord Śiva's tiny two-ended drum (*damaru*) that he played.

Malas: Three excretory waste products of the body – faeces, urine and sweat; impurities.

Mālā beads: 108 beads strung together like a rosary. Used for *mantra japā*, counting repetitions of *mantras* in meditation.

Maṇipūra chakra: *Maṇipūra* means 'Jewelled City'. The third *chakra* located at the navel centre in the astral spine.

Manas: Recording mind, seat of thinking, mind as receiver of sensation.

Mantra: From *manas,* meaning 'mind', and *tri,* meaning 'to cross over'. A subtle transcendental sound that liberates the consciousness.

Mitrāya: Friend.

Mokṣa: Liberation

Mudrā: 'Gesture.' A *mudrā* is an energy seal that helps in controlling the *prāṇic* energy in the body.

Mukti: Liberation.

Mūlabandha: Anal lock. *Mūla* means 'root', and refers to the region between the anus and the perineum. *Bandha* means 'lock'.

Mūladhāra chakra: The first *chakra*, at the base of the spine.

N

Nāda: Inner sound, subtle sound vibration. Eternal pure cosmic sound reverberating throughout endless space.

Nāḍī: 'Flow.' Subtle channel in the astral body, through which *prāṇic* energy flows.

Nāḍī śodhana: Purifying subtle channel breath. A *prāṇāyama* breath that uses alternate nostril breathing to purify the *nāḍīs* (subtle *prāṇic* channels).

Nāsikāgra mudrā: An alternative and comfortable hand position to use when practicing *nāḍī śodhana*. With the index and second finger positioned at the eyebrow centre, use the thumb to open and close the right nostril and the third finger to open and close the left nostril.

Neti: Nasal cleaning.

Niralambapuri: 'Dwelling place without support.'

Nyāya: Valid knowledge through logical criticism. The *Nyāya* system of Indian philosophy was founded by a great sage named Gautama (Gotama), who is also known as Akṣopāda, and Dīrghatapas.

O

Oṁ: The *Praṇava*, the primordial sound vibration, a *mantra* that symbolises God. It is the supreme verbal symbol of *Brāhman* both as the Absolute and as the personal God (*Īśvara*). It is written as *Aum*, and repeated or chanted as *Oṁ*.

P

Pādma: Lotus.

Pañchamahābhūta: Five Great Elements: ether, air, fire, water and earth; the fundamental material building blocks of the body and all material substances.

Panchikarana: A process of quintuplication that takes place between the five elements (*mahābhūtas*).

Patañjali: A great sage who around the third century of the common era formulated the *Yoga Sūtras* (also known as *Yoga Darśana*), and includes *Aṣṭāṅga Yoga* (Eight Limbs of Yoga).

Paramātma: Supreme Self.

Parāmhaṁsa: 'Supreme Swan.' A title bestowed on Self-realised gurus or yogis, signifying a spiritual master. 'Swan' (*haṇsa*) symbolises spiritual discrimination.

Piṅgala: One of the three major *nāḍīs* (subtle channels) that runs on the right side of the spine, emerging opposite *iḍā*, from the right side of the *mūladhāra chakra* and intersecting each *chakra* until it reaches the right side of the *ājñā chakra*. It is associated with solar energy. The 'tha' of *Haṭha Yoga* indicates the sun or solar energy.

Prakruti: The individual body type or constitution of a person; the structural and functional expression of the individual's genetic code.

Prājñā: 'Knower', undivided consciousness.

Prārabdha karmas: Results of past actions which are producing fruit in the present. This is also called ripe karma, because it is a debt which is overdue and it is time that it should be paid in the form of sorrow and suffering, gain and loss, whether we like it or not.

Prakṛiti: The eternal material principle.

Prakruti: 'The first action.' *Prakruti* in *Āyurveda* refers to an individual's inherent 'nature', the inborn tendencies which influence consciousness and activity. It is one's basic constitution that remains unchanged throughout their lifetime.

Pramāṇa: The sources of knowledge.

Prameya: The object of knowledge.

Prāṇa: The cosmic vibratory life force that is omnipresent and sustains the universe. *Prāṇa* is also the specific vital energy, the vital air within our bodies. There are five main *prāṇa* currents in the body (*prāṇa*, *vyāna*, *samāna*, *udāṇa*, *apāṇa*).

Praṇava: 'Sounding' or 'reverberating'; refers to the vibration of consciousness itself. *Aum*, the primordial sound vibration.

Prāṇāyama: *R*egulating and harmonising the energy or subtle life force within the body. The Sanskrit word *prāṇāyāma* is formed by two words: *prāṇa* means energy or subtle life force; *ayāma* has two meanings: to regulate, and to extend, lengthen or expand.

Pratyāhāra: Withdrawal of the senses from their respective objects.

Pundarika: White lotus.

Pūraka: Inhalation.

Purānas: Sacred texts that contain many of the ancient legends of Hinduism. There are 18 major *Purānas* or *Mahāpuranas*, as they are also known.

Puruṣa: The Supreme Self, the eternal principle of consciousness.

Puruṣārthas: The four principles of life: *dharma* (righteousness), *artha* (material wellbeing), *kāma* (enjoyment) and *mokṣa* (liberation).

R

Rāga: Attraction, attachment (third of five *kleṣas*).

Rāja Yoga: *Rāja* means 'royal' or 'king'. The Royal path of Yoga. The highest path of meditation for realising God.

Ram: Seed-syllable (*bīja*) *mantra* representing the energy of fire element at the *maṇipūra chakra.*

Rasa: Plasma, one of the seven body tissues. *Rasa* also means 'taste' of a substance (the six tastes – sweet, sour, salty, pungent, bitter, astringent – used in *Āyurveda* to classify the quality of foods and herbs). *Rasa* can mean the 'essence' of something, and 'spiritual enjoyment'. Food after being chewed is converted into chyle that is termed as *ama rasa* in *Āyurvedic* texts.

Rasāyana: Rejuvenation therapy.

Ravaya: 'Shining One.'

Recaka: Exhalation.

Ṛṣis: Seers who produced the divinely intuited *Vedās*. Pronounced 'rishis'.

S

Sādhana: From the root verb *sadh*, 'to accomplish one's goal', or 'to hit the target'. Spiritual practice that is practised regularly for attainment of realisation of the Self and cosmic consciousness.

Sahasrāra: Crown *chakra* at the top of the head, which contains all the six main *chakras*; thousand-petalled rayed lotus.

Śakti: The vital power and energy of consciousness. The active creative female principle of the universe.

Samādhi: *Sam*, 'with'; *ādhi*, 'Lord': 'union with the Lord'. Or *sam-ā-dhā,* 'to hold together', 'to concentrate upon'. The state of superconscious absorption that is attained when the meditator, the process of meditation, and the object of meditation (God) become One.

Samāna vayu: One of the five major *vayus*; the *prāṇic* air current functions between the heart and navel in the body; facilitates assimilation.

Śambavī mudrā: A *Haṭha Yoga* practice of concentration by gazing at the midpoint between the eyebrows. The practice activates the third eye or *ājñā chakra*.

Saṁsāra: Cycle of suffering, wheel of birth and death, worldly existence, flow of the mind to the world.

Saṁskāras: Latent impressions stored in the subtle body and subconscious mind; deep mental impressions produced by past experiences; dormant impressions of our past lives; innate tendency.

Saṁskṛta: Sanskrit. Sanskrit is a refined and literary language; it is also capable of communicating in a direct, practical manner the important facts of the spiritual life. Sanskrit possesses many precise terms for spiritual concepts and disciplines.

Samśaya: Doubt, or the state of uncertainty.

Sanatana Dharma: 'The Eternal Natural Law or Way'. The Sanskrit word *Sanatana* denotes that which is *anadi* (beginningless) and *anantha* (endless) and does not cease to be, that which is eternal. *Sanatana Dharma* represents a code of conduct and a value system that has spiritual freedom as its centre.

Sañchita karmas: Those actions that have accumulated in several previous lifetimes.

Sapta dhātus: The seven tissues of the body according to *Āyurveda*: *rasa* (chyle), *rakta* (blood), *māmsa* (muscle), *meda* (fat), *asthi* (bone), *majjā* (marrow) and *sukra* (reproductive tissue, semen ovum).

Saptarsi: Seven great Seers that appeared in a mythological story.

Sarāsvāti: The goddess of the creative arts, science and knowledge, and speech; bestower of wisdom. Consort of *Brāhma*. She is the creative power and the knowledge behind the power of *Brāhma*.

Śarīra: Body.

Sat-chit-ānanda: Ever-Existing, Ever-Conscious, Ever-New Bliss. This is the best definition describing the nature of the Self, God, or the Absolute.

Satsanga: Fellowship with those who embody spiritual values and truth; or association with spiritually oriented people.

Śāstra: Indian scripture.

Savitṛ: 'Vivifier' or 'one who brings forth or inspires'; connotes *Sūrya*'s power. *Savitṛ* is the guiding principle in the heart that leads one to higher states of consciousness. *Savitṛ* is known to us through the *Gāyatrī Mantra Prayer*.

Siddhārtha: The name given to the Gautama Buddha ('Enlightened One') at birth. *Siddhārtha* means 'he who attained his goals' or 'every wish fulfilled'.

Śiva: 'In whom all things lie'; 'The Auspicious One'; 'Great Lord'. Pure Consciousness. Name of the deity representing the cosmic state of consciousness.

Śiva lingam: A symbol of *ātma*, the soul or inner spirit; consciousness. *Linga* or *lingam* is a natural oval-shaped stone representing the subtle bodies.

Śiva Mahāpurāṇa: Also known as the *Śiva Purāṇa*, an ancient Hindu religious text devoted to Lord Śiva. The original *Purāṇa* was thought to have consisted of 12 *Saṁhitās* and 100,000 verses. However, the existing text, after abridgement from the great Sage Vedavyasa, consists of 24,000 verses only. It is said that Vedavyasa taught the verses to his disciple Lomaharshana, who later recited it to sages who wanted to expand their knowledge of Lord Śiva.

Śivasvarodāya: A scripture in the form of a dialogue between Śiva and Shakti which begins with the nature of the universe and the essential knowledge on living a happy, healthy and inspired life.

Śiva-Śakti: In Tantra, *Śiva* is *Param Puruṣa*, the Male Principle, and *Śakti* is the Female Principle, and the Cosmos has evolved from their union. *Śiva* and *Śakti* are inseparable. God is inseparable from His energy or power. There are images and statue deities known as *Ardhanarisvara* or *Hara Gauri*, the one half of which is *Śiva* and the other half is *Śakti* or *Gauri*; that is, the one is inseparable from the other.

Śiva Saṃhitā: A Sanskrit text on Yoga. The five chapters discuss and elaborate on the essentials necessary for the practice of Yoga, the importance of Yoga, principles of *prāṇāyama*, *āsanas*, *kuṇḍalinī* and its awakening, and the various forms of Yoga.

Savikalpa samādhi: In the state of *Savikalpa samādhi* the mind is conscious only of the Blissful Spirit within, it is not conscious of the exterior world.

Śodhana: Purification.

Sparśa: Touch.

Śraddhā: Faith.

Sthiti: Stability.

Styāna: Dullness.

Śukra: Semen, male sperm.

Sūkshma Prāṇa: Subtle vital air.

Sūrya namaskāra: Salutations to the Sun. A sequence of 12 Yoga poses.

Suṣumnā: The main subtle channel running through the spine, along which the six *chakras* are located. When awakened, the *kuṇḍalinī śakti* rises upward through the *suṣumnā*.

Suṣhupti: Deep sleep state – unconscious mind.

Svādhyāya: Self-study, study of the scriptures (one of the five *niyamas*).

Svapna: Dream state – subconscious mind.

Svāra: Vowels of Sanskrit, of which there are 13.

Svāra Yoga: A precise science, it has an emphasis on the analysis of the breath and the significance of *prāṇic* rhythms

Svādhiṣṭhāna chakra: 'One's own abode.' The second *chakra* located in the sacral region.

Svaḥ: Represents the third dimension or celestial region, known as *svarga loka* and all the luminous *lokas* (spheres) above.

Svāsthya: Self-abiding. A *svāstha* in *Āyurveda* is one who enjoys normal health. *Svā* means position 'one's own'; 'self' (being present or centred in one's own self), which in *Āyurveda* is *ayus*, 'life'. *Sthā* means stability of maintenance, 'one who stands.' He is stable, who, in preference to other attractions, attends to the requirements of the body.

Svāsthvṛtta: Healthy regimen.

T

Tāḍāsana: Mountain pose, a standing Yoga posture. In this pose you stand straight like a mountain, firm and strong at the base and ascending upwards. The standing ā*sanas* all start from this position.

Taijasa: 'Luminous one.' The manifestation of the individual in the subtle body that develops a false identification of the self with ego.

Tapasya, tapas, tapaḥ: Literally 'to burn'. Discipline, austerity (one of the five *niyamas*).

Turīya: Transcendent; the fourth state of consciousness in *Vedānta* philosophy. *Turīya* is distinguished from the three states (waking, dream, dreamless sleep).

U

Upaniṣads: The *Upaniṣads* form part of the tradition of the Vedic literature, and they form the completion or end (*anta*) of the *Veda* and are called the *Vedānta*. The *Upaniṣads* contain the teachings of the ancient seers on the identity of the Self (*ātman*), and the ultimate reality (*Brāhman*) and the means to liberation (*mokṣa*) through knowledge. They were composed from about 700 BCE.

V

Vairagya: Derived from *viraga*. The prefix *vi* means 'devoid of; free from; very special and unique'; *raga* means 'colouring; influencing; attachment'. *Vairagya* refers to the state in which the mind is stable and is not coloured or affected by thoughts, speech or deeds. *Vairagya* is a state of awareness free from all attachment, and freedom from worldly desires.

Vaiśeṣika: Analysis of the aspects of reality. Originates from the Sanskrit word *Viśeṣa* meaning 'uniqueness'. *Vaiśeṣika* philosophy was founded by the sage Kaṇāda, who wrote the *Vaiśeṣika Sūtra* (third century BCE).

Vajrāsana: Thunderbolt pose. A kneeling posture.

Vajriṇī: 'Sunlike.' One of the inner *nāḍīs* within the *suṣumnā*, the subtle spine.

Vam: Seed-syllable (*bīja*) *mantra* of *svādhiṣṭhāna chakra*.

Varnamāla: Sanskrit alphabet.

Vāsanā: Means 'colouring', and is a more active and stronger form of *samskara*, a subtle karmic impression.

Vayus: The five main vital airs in the body – *prāṇa*, *apāṇa*, *samāna*, *vyāna* and *udāṇa*.

Vedānta: Literally means 'the end (*anta*) of knowledge or wisdom (*veda*)'.

Vichāra: Reflection, enquiry, analytical thought process.

Virat: Cosmic manifestation.

Viśuddha chakra: The fifth *chakra*, which corresponds to the cervical plexus at the level of the throat.

Viṣṇu: 'The all-pervading one'; name of one of the gods of the Hindu Trinity. He is the Preserver and descends to Earth in the form of a divine incarnation when the world especially needs His grace. *Viṣṇu* is mainly worshipped in the form of his incarnations *Kṛṣṇā* (Krishna) and *Rāma*.

Viṣṇu mudrā: A hand position that becomes a *mudrā* or 'seal' for directing and regulating the breath in each nostril, as in alternate nostril breathing.

Viśva: The individual self, the experiencer of the waking state bound and conditioned by matter, and associated with the phenomenal world and the gross body.

Viveka: Discrimination.

Vṛttis: Subtle vortices of energy created by *samskāras* (karmic actions), and waves of like and dislike that create our mental tendencies desires and habits, enter the subconscious mind and then get submerged in the lower *chakras*.

Vitaṇḍā: Irrational reasoning.

Vyāhṛtis: Rhythms.

Vyanjana: Consonants of Sanskrit, of which there are 34.

Y

Yantra: Diagrammatic symbol used as a focal point for concentration and meditation.

BIBLIOGRAPHY

Aïvanhov, O.M. (1984) *What is a Spiritual Master?* Fréjus, France: Éditions Prosveta.
Ashley-Farrand, T. (2000) *Healing Mantras.* Dublin: Gateway (an imprint of Gill & Macmillan).
Atmananda (1982) *Words of Anandamayi Ma.* Calcutta: Sri Sri Anandamayi Charitable Society.
Avalon, A. (1974) *The Serpent Power: The Secrets of Tantric and Shaktic Yoga.* New York: Dover Publications.
Bhaskarananda, S. (2002) *Meditation, Mind and Patañjali's Yoga: A Practical Guide to Spiritual Growth for Everyone.* Chennai: Sri Ramakrishna Math.
Bryant, E.F. (2009) *The Yoga Sūtras of Patañjali.* New York: North Point Press.
Chopra, D. (2006) *Power, Freedom, and Grace: Living from the Source of Lasting Happiness.* San Rafael, CA: Amber-Allen.
Clarissa (2009) *Drg Drsya Viveka: The Yoga of Seer and Seen.* Chup-Sadhana. Available at www.lulu.com/shop/clarissa/drg-drsya-viveka/paperback/product-6553964.html, accessed on 10 December 2014.
Dasgupta S. (2006) *A History of Indian Philosophy, Volume One.* Cambridge: Cambridge University Press
Dasgupta S.B. (2006) *Kriyā Yoga.* Michigan: Yoga Niketan.
Feuerstein G. (2008) *The Yoga Tradition.* Arizona: Hohm Press.
Feuerstein, G., and Feuerstein, B. (2011) *The Bhāgavad-Gītā: A New Translation.* Boston, MA: Shambhala.
Feuerstein G., Kak, S., and Frawley, D. (2008) *In Search of The Cradle of Civilisation: New Light on Ancient India.* Delhi: Motilal Banarsidass.
Ganguli, A. (1995) *Anandamayi Ma: The Mother, Bliss-Incarnate.* Calcutta: Sri Sri Anandamayi Charitable Society Publications Division.
Giri Swāmi Nityananda (2013) *Kriyā Yoga: The Science of Life-force.* Delhi: Munshiram Manoharlal.
Keshavadas, S.S. (1997) *Gāyatrī: The Highest Meditation.* Delhi: Motilal Barnarsidass.
Kriyananda, S. (1990) *The Essence of Self-Realization: The Wisdom of Paramhansa Yogananda.* Nevada, CA: Crystal Clarity.
Kriyananda, S. (2003a) *The Art and Science of Rāja Yoga: 14 Steps to Higher Awareness.* Delhi: Motilal Barnarsidass.
Kriyananda, S. (2003b) *God is for Everyone.* Nevada City, CA: Crystal Clarity.
Kriyananda S. (2009) *Religion in the New Age and Other Essays for the Spiritual Seeker.* Nevada City, CA: Crystal Clarity.
Laird, M. (2006) *Into the Silent Land.* London: Darton, Longman and Todd.
Lipski, A. (1988) *Life and Teaching of Sri Anandamayi Ma.* Delhi: Motilal Banarsidass.
Madhavananda, S. (2003) *Vivekacudamani of Sri Sankaracarya (Translation).* Calcutta: Advaita Ashrama.

Maharshi, Sri R. (1972) *The Spiritual Teaching of Ramana Maharshi.* Boston, MA: Shambhala.

Maharshi, Sri R. (2014) *How to Practice Self Inquiry.* The Freedom Religion Press.

Maharshi, Sri R., and Shankara (2002) *Ramana, Shankara and the Forty Verses: The Essential Teachings of Advaita.* London: Watkins.

Mother Theresa (1998) *Everything Starts from Prayer: Mother Teresa's Meditations on Spiritual Life for People of All Faiths.* Ashland, OR: White Cloud Press.

Niketan, Y. (2004) *A Collection of Biographies of Four Kriyā Yoga Gurus by Swāmi Satyananda Giri.* New York: iUniverse.

Niketan, Y. (2005) *The Scriptual Commentaries of Yogiraj Sri Sri Shyama Charan Lahiri Mahasaya: Volume 1.* New York: iUniverse.

Nikhilananda, S. (1949) *The Upaniṣads: Volume I.* New York: Ramakrishna-Vivekananda Center.

Nityaswarupananda, S. (1996) *Ashtavakra Samhita.* Calcutta: Advaita Asrama.

Prakash, P. (1998) *The Yoga of Spiritual Devotion: A Modern Translation of the Narada Bhakti Sūtras.* Rochester, VT: Inner Traditions.

Sankaracarya, S. (1978) *Vivekacudamani.* Calcutta: N.K. Mitter at the Indian Press.

Scofield, C.I., Schuyler English, E., Mason, C.E., Sherrill Babb, W., and Karleen, P.S. (1984) *Oxford NIV Scofield Study Bible: New International Version.* New York: Oxford University Press.

Shastri, H.P. (2012) *Understanding 'That Thou Art': Shankara's Vakya Vrihi.* London: Shanti Sadan.

Shearer, A., and Russell, P. (1989) *The Upaniṣads.* London: Unwin Paperbacks.

Sinh, P. (2001) *Haṭha Yoga Pradīpikā.* Delhi: Munshiram Manoharlal.

Stevens, J.C.(2013) *Kriyā Secrets Revealed.* North Charleston, SC: Golden Swan Publishing & CreateSpace Independent Publishing Platform.

Sturgess, S.R. (2002) *The Yoga Book.* London: Watkins.

Sturgess, S.R. (2014) *The Book of Chakras and the Subtle Bodies.* London: Watkins.

Sturgess, S.R. (2014) *Yoga Meditation.* London: Watkins.

Swatmarama, Y., and Vishnu-Devananda, S. (1999) *Haṭha Yoga Pradīpikā: The Classic Guide for the Advanced Practice of Haṭha Yoga.* New York: Oṁ Lotus Publishing.

Thapan, A.R. (Ed.) (2005) *The Penguin Swāmi Chinmayananda Reader.* Delhi: Penguin Books India.

Vasu, Rai Bahadur Srisa Chandra (1996) *The Siva Samhita.* Delhi: Munshiram Manoharlal.

Vasu, Rai Bahadur Srisa Chandra (1996) *The Gheranda Samhita.* Delhi: Munshiram Manoharlal.

Venkatesananda, S. (1998) *The Yoga Sūtras of Patanjali.* Rishikesh, India: The Divine Life Society.

Vishnudevananda, S. (1987) *Haṭha Yoga Pradīpikā.* New York: Oṁ Lotus Publishing.

Vishnudevananda, S. (1995) *Meditation and Mantras.* New York: Oṁ Lotus Publishing.

Vivekananda, S. (2011) *Conquering the Internal Nature: Rāja Yoga.* Calcutta: Advaita Asrama.

Walters, J.D. (1996) *Superconsciousness: A Guide to Meditation.* New York: Warner.

Yogananda, P. (1946) *Autobiography of a Yogi.* New York: The Philosophical Library.

Yogananda, P. (2003) *Super Advanced Course Number 1, Lessons 1 to 12.* Whitefish, MT: Kessinger.

Yogananda, P. (2006) *How to be Happy All the Time: The Wisdom of Yogananda, Volume 1.* Nevada City, CA: Crystal Clarity.

Yogananda, P. (2007a) *Spiritual Relationships: The Wisdom of Yogananda, Volume 3.* Nevada City, CA: Crystal Clarity.

Yogananda, P. (2007b) *Karma and Reincarnation: The Wisdom of Yogananda, Volume 2.* Nevada City, CA: Crystal Clarity.

Yogananda, P. (2008a) *The Essence of Bhāgavad Gītā.* Nevada City, CA: Crystal Clarity.

Yogananda, P. (2008b) *How to Be a Success: The Wisdom of Yogananda, Volume 4.* Nevada City, CA: Crystal Clarity.

Yogananda, P. (2010) *How to Have Courage, Calmness and Confidence: The Wisdom of Yogananda, Volume 5.* Nevada City, CA: Crystal Clarity.

Yogananda, P. (2011) *How to Achieve Glowing Health and Vitality: The Wisdom of Yogananda Volume 6.* Nevada City, CA: Crystal Clarity.

Yukteswar, S.S. (1990) *The Holy Science.* Los Angeles, CA: Self-Realization Fellowship.

Yukteswar, S.S. (2013) *Kriyā Yoga: The Science of Life-force.* Delhi: Munshiram Manoharlal.

KRIYĀ YOGA RESOURCES

KRIYĀ YOGA MEDITATION TEACHERS, ORGANISATIONS AND CENTRES FOLLOWING THE TEACHINGS OF PARAMHANSA YOGANANDA

Stephen Sturgess (UK)

Stephen Sturgess, Kriyācarya, is a disciple of Paramhansa Yogananda and a direct disciple of Swami Kriyānanda for 30 years, from whom he first received Kriyā Initiation in 1983. He was ordained in 2011 as a Kriyācarya by Roy Eugene-Davis (another direct disciple of Yogananda) to teach and initiate sincere Truth seekers into Kriyā Yoga meditation. Stephen feels blessed to be of spiritual service to others in teaching Rāja and Kriyā Yoga. He teaches the preparation Kriyā meditation techniques in London, and gives Kriyā Initiation only to those who are sincerely interested in Yogananda's teachings and spiritual awakening and have done the necessary spiritual training. Awakening to Self-knowing and Self-realisation is a gradual process and requires self-discipline and diligent practice with love, devotion, willingness, right attitude and perseverance.

email: stephensturgess@hotmail.com
website: www.yogananda-Kriyāyoga.org.uk

Roy Eugene Davis (USA)

Roy Eugene Davis is a direct disciple of Paramhansa Yogananda. He offers spiritual support and resources, seminars and Kriyā meditation retreats based on the teachings of Paramhansa Yogananda.

Center for Spiritual Awareness, PO Box 7, Lakemont, Georgia, GA
tel: 30552-0001
email: info@csa-davis.org
website: www.csa-davis.org

Self-Realization Fellowship (USA)

Paramhansa Yogananda founded the Self-Realization Fellowship (SRF) in America in 1920, to make available the teachings of Kriyā Yoga universal. The Self-Realization fellowship (SRF) has its headquarters in Los Angeles, California. SRF has more than 500 temples and centres around the world and has members in 175 countries. In India and surrounding countries, Paramhansa Yogananda's work is known as Yogada Satsanga Society of India (YSS; www.yssofindia.org), which he founded in 1917. The SRF Lessons, an in-depth home study course which provide Paramhansa Yogananda's step-by-step instructions in his Yoga methods, including the Kriyā Yoga science of meditation and his 'How-to-live' teachings, are available from the Self-Realization Fellowship (SRF). The SRF have many books available for sale written by Paramhansa Yogananda, a selection of DVD and CD talks and devotional music.

Self-Realization Fellowship, International Headquarters, 3880 San Rafael Avenue, Los Angeles, CA 90065-3219, SA.
tel: (323) 225-2471; (818) 549-5151 (telephone orders)
website: www.yogananda-srf.org

London Centre of Self-Realization Fellowship (UK)

London Centre of Self-Realization, 82a Chiltern Street, London, W1U 5AQ
website: www.srf-london.org.uk

ANANDA COMMUNITIES

Ananda communities have a selection of instructional DVDs and CDs that cover preparation techniques for practising *Kriyā Yoga*, including Yogananda's 'Energisation Exercises'. Both Ananda and the Self-Realization Fellowship sell the 'Arm-rests' or 'Aum-boards' for practising the *Aum* Technique.

Ananda Sangha (USA)

Ananda Sangha is a worldwide organisation founded by Swāmi Kriyānanda, a direct disciple of Paramhansa Yogananda, which offers spiritual support and resources based on the teachings of Paramhansa Yogananda. There are Ananda spiritual communities in Nevada City, Sacramento, Palo Alto and Los Angeles, California; Seattle, Washington; and Portland and Laurelwood, Oregon.

website: www.ananda.org; www.expandinglight.org

Ananda Assisi (Italy)

Ananda Assisi is a spiritual community and Kriyā Yoga retreat.

Ananda Assisi, Via Montecchio, 61, 06025 Nocera Umbra (PG), Italy
website: www.ananda.it

Ananda India (India)

Ananda India has spiritual communities at Gurgaon near New Delhi and Pune in North India.

email: ananda@anandaindia.org
website: www.anandaindia.org

MĀLĀ BEADS FOR MEDITATION AND JAPA (REPETITION OF A MANTRA)

Maha Mala (India)

Maha Mala is a small company based in New Delhi, India, which specialises in making beautifully made health and wellness and meditation jewellry in the form of 108 bead necklaces, these necklaces can be used for japa (chanting with a mantra) or as jewellry. The term Maha Mala stems from two Sanskrit words; maha meaning 'the great' and mālā meaning 'garland'.

Maha Mala started out as an idea to create sacred healing objects for use in personal rituals, this manifested into the stringing and restringing of mālās back in 2009. The mālās are designed by Nora Wendel and Piya Jain, the beautiful semi-precious stones and silver are hand sourced from Jaipur, Northern India for their quality and lustre. Each mālā is hand strung using extra grade wire for durability and suppleness. Rudraksha, Tulsi and Sandalwood beads are also used in the making of their mālā necklaces and bracelets.

Matrika Creations Pvt. Ltd., 34 Aurobindo Place Market, New Delhi 110016
tel: +91 98100 81415
email: info@mahamala.com
website: www.mahamala.com

ABOUT THE AUTHOR

Stephen Sturgess was born in London. His first experience of practising Yoga and meditation was when he was 19. In 1970, he met for the first time a Yoga teacher in south west London, named Laya Garady (now known as Swāmi Pragyamurti Saraswati), one of Britain's first and dedicated disciples of Swāmi Satyananda Saraswati (1926–2009) of the Bihar School of Yoga, India. This beginning in authentic Yoga gave Stephen a thorough grounding in the *Haṭha Yoga* practices of the *Shat kriyās*, *Yoga āsanas*, *prāṇāyāma*, *Yoga Nidra*, *mantra japa*, *kirtan* (devotional chanting) and meditation.

The 1970s was a particularly inspiring time in London, as authentic and spiritually inspiring gurus and swamis visited from India. Stephen was blessed to meet and study under many of them at their Yoga workshops and retreats, including: Swami Dr Gitananda (1906–1993), an expert on *prāṇāyama*, who founded the Ananda ashram in Pondicherry, Tamil Nadu, India; and Swami Satyananda Saraswati (1923–2009), Swami Vishnudevananda (1927–1993), Swami Ventakesananda (1921–1982), and Swami Satchidananda (1914–2002), who were four enlightened direct disciples of Swami Sivananda of Rishikesh (1883–1963). These disciples have now passed on leaving their inspiring and practical spiritual legacies to their followers.

In 1974 Stephen had his first experience of Yoga discipline and austerity living in a Yoga ashram by going on a Satyananda Ashram one-month course in Belfast, Ireland, under the teaching of Swāmi Atmananda Saraswati (1939–2003).

Then a few years later in 1979 at the Dublin Yoga Convention, Stephen was given *Guru Diksha* (Initiation), with the spiritual name *Shankara* and a personal *mantra,* by Swāmi Satyananda Saraswati.

During the years 1973 to 1976 Stephen followed the teachings of Krishna Consciousness founded by the guru, Swāmi Bhaktivedanta Prabhupada, and travelled with the Hare Krishna devotees in 1976 as a full devotee with them on their Lord Caitanya Pilgrimage to Brindāvāna and Māyāpur (West Bengal) in India for one month. There he lived a very disciplined and austere life in their ashrams, going to bed at 9 pm and rising at 3 am every day to practise *Bhakti* and *Karma Yoga.*

During this time Stephen read Paramhansa Yogananda's classic Yoga book *Autobiography of a Yogi*, which inspired him immensely. It had sown a spiritual seed in his heart, but it was not the right time to meet his true guru until later in the 1980s. For 12 years Stephen studied and practised different Yogas: *Haṭha*, *Karma*, *Jñanā*, *Bhakti*, *Rāja* (Patañjali's Eight Limbs of Yoga), *Tantric* and *Kuṇḍalinī*, under various teachers. This was to give him a good understanding of authentic Yoga and he achieved purification of his body and mind through the yoga practices.

It was during the eighties, in 1981 at Brockwood, Hampshire, in England, that Stephen met another enlightened and well-known spiritual teacher named Jiddu Krishnamurti (1895–1986), who was born in India. During his youth Krishnamurti met the well-known Theosophists Annie Besant and C.W. Leadbeater, who believed him to be the new spiritual World Teacher whose coming the Theosophists had predicted. They tried to groom him as a Messiah, but Krishnamurti renounced the role he was expected to play, and for the rest of his life travelled the world giving talks on the nature of mind, with meditation and self-inquiry. In private conversation with Krishnamurti at Brockwood, Stephen personally experienced this great soul's deep spiritual awareness, spiritual insights, and aura of love and compassion.

In the summer of June 1982, for the first time Stephen had the fortunate blessing of meeting Swāmi Kriyananda (1926–2013; a direct disciple of Paramhansa Yogananda and founder of the spiritual community Ananda Village in Nevada, California) at the Mind-Body-Spirit Festival at Olympia in London. Kriyananda was on a lecture tour of Europe, and London was one of the places where he gave a *Kriyā Yoga* lecture titled 'Divine Life'. In his own words of this experience, Stephen says:

> 'After meeting Swāmi Kriyananda, I went home with great feelings of joy and happiness in my heart. My inspired thoughts were continually revolving around what *swāmi* had sung, said and shown to us. Throughout my life, I had been searching for something of great value, some intangible, ultimate blessing. I had been given many wonderful gifts – in the beauty of nature, in family and friends, and other spiritual teachers and their paths, yet these blessings were but a glimpse of the wonder and goodness of God. They were like the many layers that form a pearl and contribute to the depth of its beauty. My search for Truth had led me to this discovery: The precious pearl I was seeking was the Kingdom of God, and it was within me. All I ever need or want is part of that kingdom, the kingdom that holds the riches of life itself. Through Paramhansa Yogananda, and his direct disciple, Swāmi Kriyananda, I was introduced to and made aware of that inner Kingdom of God.
>
> 'That night, after seeing Swāmi Kriyananda, I had an extraordinary dream experience. A superconscious dream, that to this day is very vivid in my memory. A dream that was important in giving me faith, purpose, and direction in life. I awoke the next morning with a great feeling of joy and exuberance! It was an overwhelming feeling and blessing that filled my heart – a life-changing realisation. In my superconscious dream both Paramhansa Yogananda and Swāmi Kriyananda had appeared to me. They came to affirm to me that *Kriyā Yoga* was my spiritual path. I could see Yogananda's radiant form very clearly as he stood in front of me and said, "Fear not, for I am Paramhansa Yogananda, your true guru. This is your spiritual path, come follow me!"
>
> 'Inspired by Yogananda's words, that incredible feeling of joy and inspiration I experienced in his presence gave me great inner fulfilment, in knowing that at last I had found my true guru. I knew without doubt that Yogananda was my true guru. It was strange, but over the next two nights Yogananda and Kriyananda continued to appear to me in my dreams. I knew intuitively that this was a confirmation of what Yogananda had said to me. That he was my guru and I was to follow the path of *Kriyā Yoga*, guided by the wisdom of my spiritual teacher, Swāmi Kriyananda.
>
> 'I met many spiritual teachers, *swāmis* and gurus on my spiritual journey through life, to whom I'm also grateful for sharing with me their teachings. But Paramhansa

stands clearly above the others as a perfected Spiritual Master. He is a true authentic Guru, like a faultless diamond, without any imperfections. His inspiring teachings are perfect.

I was first initiated into *Kriyā* at my house in London in May 1984 by Swāmi Kriyananda, and later also by the monks of the Self-Realization Fellowship and by Roy Eugene Davis, who was initiated into *Kriyā* with blessings by Yogananda himself in August 1951.

In 2011 I was ordained as a *Kriyācarya* (*Kriyā* teacher) by Roy Eugene Davis to teach and initiate others into *Kriyā Yoga*.'

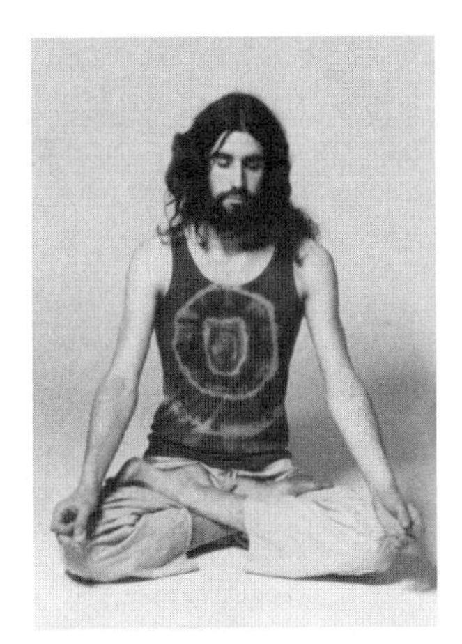

Stephen Sturgess, 1972

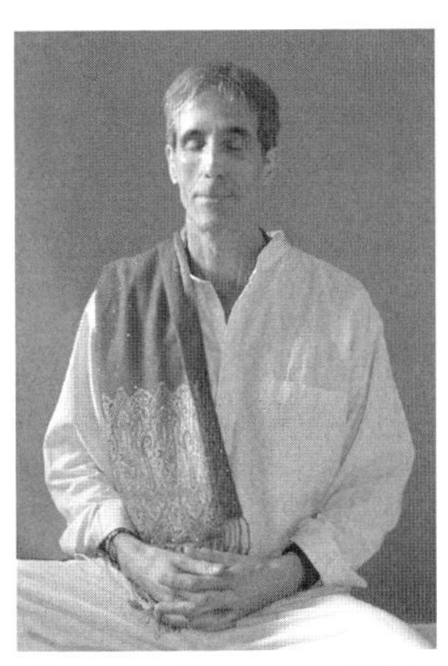

Stephen Sturgess, 2014

INDEX